Enhancing Human Capacities

Enhancing Human Capacities

Edited by
Julian Savulescu, Ruud ter Meulen,
and Guy Kahane

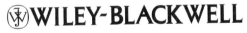

WILEY-BLACKWELL

A John Wiley & Sons, Ltd., Publication

This edition first published 2011
© 2011 Blackwell Publishing Ltd.

Blackwell Publishing was acquired by John Wiley & Sons in February 2007. Blackwell's publishing program has been merged with Wiley's global Scientific, Technical, and Medical business to form Wiley-Blackwell.

Registered Office
John Wiley & Sons Ltd, The Atrium, Southern Gate, Chichester, West Sussex, PO19 8SQ, United Kingdom

Editorial Offices
350 Main Street, Malden, MA 02148-5020, USA
9600 Garsington Road, Oxford, OX4 2DQ, UK
The Atrium, Southern Gate, Chichester, West Sussex, PO19 8SQ, UK

For details of our global editorial offices, for customer services, and for information about how to apply for permission to reuse the copyright material in this book please see our website at www.wiley.com/wiley-blackwell.

The right of Julian Savulescu, Ruud ter Meulen and Guy Kahane as editors of this editorial material in this work has been asserted in accordance with the UK Copyright, Designs and Patents Act 1988.

Library of Congress Cataloging-in-Publication Data
Enhancing human capacities / edited by Julian Savulescu, Ruud ter Meulen, and Guy Kahane.
    p. ; cm.
  Includes bibliographical references and index.
  ISBN 978-1-4051-9581-2 (hardcover : alk. paper) 1. Medical innovations–Moral and ethical aspects.
2. Medical innovations–Government policy. 3. Medical innovations–Social aspects. I. Savulescu, Julian.
II. Meulen, R. H. J. ter (Ruud H. J.), 1952- III. Kahane, Guy, 1971-
  [DNLM: 1. Biomedical Enhancement–ethics. 2. Genetic Engineering–ethics. 3. Health Policy. W 82]
  RA418.5.M4E536 2011
  610.28–dc22
                                                                          2010034211

A catalogue record for this book is available from the British Library.

This book is published in the following electronic formats: eBook [ISBN]; Wiley Online Library [ISBN]; ePub [ISBN]

Set in Galliard 10/12.5 pt by Thomson Digital, Noida, India
Printed in Malaysia by Ho Printing (M) Sdn Bhd

01   2011

Contents

Part III   Mood Enhancement

Part IV   Physical Enhancement

Part V Lifespan Extension

Part VI Moral Enhancement

Part VII General Policy

Notes on Contributors

Gustaf Arrhenius is Torgny Segerstedt Pro Futura Fellow and Docent (Reader) in Practical Philosophy at Stockholm University and the Swedish Collegium for Advanced Study since 2006. He is also an Affiliated Researcher at the Oxford Uehiro Centre for Practical Ethics, University of Oxford, and at the Centre de Recherche Sens, Ethique, Société, CNRS, Paris.

Gaia Barazzetti is a Teaching Fellow in Ethics at the College of Humanities of the Ecole Polytechnique Fédérale de Lausanne (EPFL) and at the Faculty of Philosophy of San Raffaele University in Milan.

Ron Berghmans is an Assistant Professor at the Department of Health, Ethics and Society, Maastricht University.

Ineke Bolt is Senior Lecturer at the Ethics Institute of Utrecht University and at the Department of Medical Ethics and Philosophy of Medicine of Erasmus Medical Centre, Rotterdam.

John Bond is Professor of Social Gerontology and Health Services Research, Ageing, Health and Society Research Group, Institute of Health and Society, Newcastle University.

Nick Bostrom is Professor and Director of the Future of Humanity Institute, Faculty of Philosophy and James Martin 21st Century School, University of Oxford.

Bengt Brülde is Associate Professor of Practical Philosophy at the Department of Philosophy, Linguistics, and Theory of Science, University of Gothenburg, and Senior Lecturer in Ethics at the Department of Nursing, Health, and Culture, University West, Sweden.

Allen Buchanan is James B. Duke Professor of Philosophy and Investigator, Institute for Genome Sciences and Policy, Duke University. He is also a Distinguished Research Associate of the Oxford Uehiro Centre for Practical Ethics, University of Oxford.

Steve Clarke is a Research Fellow, Program on the Ethics of the New Biosciences, James Martin 21st Century School and Faculty of Philosophy, University of Oxford.

Christopher Coenen is a Senior Researcher at the Institute for Technology Assessment and Systems Analysis (ITAS), Karlsruhe Institute of Technology (KIT).

Thomas Douglas is a D.Phil. student in the Faculty of Philosophy, University of Oxford, and a Research Associate at the Oxford Uehiro Centre for Practical Ethics.

Bennett Foddy is Deputy Director of the Program on the Ethics of the New Biosciences, James Martin 21st Century School and Faculty of Philosophy, University of Oxford.

Henry T. Greely is Deane F. and Kate Edelman Johnson Professor of Law, Stanford law School, Stanford.

Hidde J. Haisma is Professor of Therapeutic Gene Modulation and Chair of the Department of pharmaceutical Gene Modulation, Groningen Research Institute of Pharmacy, University of Groningen.

Søren Holm is Professor of Bioethics, Centre for Social Ethics and Policy, Institute of Science, Ethics and Innovation, University of Manchester, and Section for Medical Ethics, University of Oslo.

Tony Hope is Professor of Medical Ethics at The Ethox Centre; Honorary Consultant Psychiatrist; and Fellow of St Cross College, University of Oxford.

Steven Horrobin is a Researcher at the College of Medicine, University of Edinburgh.

Charlotte R. Housden is a Ph.D. student at the Department of Psychiatry, University of Cambridge.

Kenneth Howse is a Senior Research Fellow at the Oxford Institute of Ageing, University of Oxford.

Niklas Juth is a Senior Lecturer at the Stockholm Centre for Healthcare Ethics, Department of Learning, Informatics, Management, and Ethics, Karolinska Institutet, Stockholm University.

Guy Kahane is Deputy Director of the Oxford Uehiro Centre for Practical Ethics Faculty of Philosophy, University of Oxford.

Laurens Landeweerd is Researcher at the Department of Health Ethics and Society, Maastricht University.

S. Matthew Liao is Associate Professor in the Center for Bioethics with an affiliation in the Department of Philosophy, New York University.

Sigmund Loland is Professor of Sport Philosophy in the Department of Social and Cultural Studies, The Norwegian School of Sport Sciences, Oslo.

Mike McNamee is Professor of Applied Ethics at the Department of Philosophy, History and Law in Healthcare, School of Health and Human Sciences, Swansea University.

Andrea Malizia is a Consultant Senior Lecturer in the Psychopharmacology Unit, University of Bristol.

Ruud ter Meulen is Professor and Director of the Centre for Ethics in Medicine, University of Bristol.

Andy Miah is Chair of Ethics and Emerging Technologies in the Faculty of Business & Creative Industries, University of the West of Scotland, Fellow of the Institute for Ethics and Emerging Technologies, USA, and Fellow of the Foundation for Art and Creative Technology, UK.

Roberto Mordacci is Professor of Moral Philosophy and Coordinator of the Centre for the Study of Public Ethics (CeSEP), Faculty of Philosophy, Università Vita-Salute San Raffaele, Milan.

Sharon Morein-Zamir is a Research Associate at the Department of Psychiatry, University of Cambridge.

Lisbeth Witthøfft Nielsen is a Research Fellow at the Centre for Biomedical Ethics (CBmE), Yong Loo Lin School of Medicine, National University of Singapore.

Christine Overall is Professor of Philosophy and Queen's University Research Chair, Department of Philosophy, Queen's University, Kingston, Ontario.

Ingmar Persson is Professor of Practical Philosophy, University of Gothenburg and Distinguished Research Fellow, Oxford Uehiro Centre for Practical Ethics.

Russell Powell is a Research Fellow at the Oxford Uehiro Centre for Practical Ethics, Faculty of Philosophy, University of Oxford.

Massimo Reichlin is Professor of Moral Philosophy and Bioethics at the Faculty of Philosophy, and member of the Centre for Research in Public Ethics, Università San Raffaele, Milan.

Rebecca Roache is a Research Fellow at the Future of Humanity Institute, Faculty of Philosophy and James Martin 21st Century School, University of Oxford.

Barbara J. Sahakian is Professor of Clinical Neuropsychology at the Department of Psychiatry, School of Clinical Medicine, University of Cambridge.

Anders Sandberg is a Research Fellow at the Future of Humanity Institute, Faculty of Philosophy and James Martin 21st Century School, University of Oxford.

Julian Savulescu is Uehiro Chair in Practical Ethics, University of Oxford and Director of the Oxford Uehiro Centre for Practical Ethics, the Program on the Ethics of the New Biosciences, and the Wellcome Centre for Neuroethics.

Maartje Schermer is Associate Professor of Medical Ethics and Philosophy of Medicine, Erasmus Medical Centre, Rotterdam.

Mirjam Schuijff is a Researcher in Technology Assessment at the Rathenau Institute, The Hague.

Martijntje Smits is a Researcher in Technology Assessment at the Rathenau Institute, The Hague.

Torbjörn Tännsjö is Professor of Practical Philosophy at the Department of Philosophy, Stockholm University, and Co-director of the Stockholm Centre for

Health Care Ethics at Karolinska Institutet, Stockholm University, and The Royal Institute of Technology, Stockholm.

Claudio Tamburrini is a researcher at the University of Göteborg, and an associated researcher at the Stockholm Bioethics Centre, Stockholm University.

Larry Temkin is Professor of Philosophy at Rutgers, The State University of New Jersey.

Rein Vos is Professor at the Department of Health, Ethics and Society, Maastricht University.

Acknowledgments

The majority of the chapters in this volume are based on presentations at workshops organized by the ENHANCE project which was funded under the Science and Society Program within the Sixth Framework Program of the European Commission. (Project full title: Enhancing Human Capacities: Ethics, Regulation and European Policy, Contract no.: SAS-CT-2005-017455.) Chapters 26, 27, 34, and 35 have previously been published in the *Journal of Applied Philosophy*: Temkin, L. (2008), Is living longer living better? **25**(3), 193–210; Arrhenius, G. (2008), Life extension versus replacement, **25**(3), 211–27; Douglas, T. (2008), Moral enhancement, **25**(3), 228–45; Persson, I. and Savulescu, J. (2008), The perils of cognitive enhancement and the urgent imperative to enhance the moral character of humanity, **25**(3), 162–77. We are grateful to the editors for permitting us to republish them. We are also most grateful to Wiley-Blackwell for their support. Finally, we would like to thank Lisbeth Witthøfft Nielsen, Miriam Wood and Nicholas Iles for their help in preparing this volume.

Preface

Guy Kahane, Julian Savulescu, and Ruud ter Meulen

The rise of modern science and technology has radically transformed the relation *[immutable - unchanging over time, or unable to be changed.]* between human beings and nature. Nature, which for millennia had seemed all powerful and <u>immutable,</u> has suddenly become an object for control and manipulation, something that can be systematically shaped to human ends. Yet throughout the dramatic upheavals of the modern era the fundamental constants of human nature – human mortality, a shared repertoire of emotions and moods, a range of basic perceptual and intellectual capacities – remained a relatively fixed reference point that could bridge cultural and ideological differences. But in recent decades, radical advances in genetics and the neurosciences, and in computing and other forms of technology, raise the possibility that we are on the brink of a further revolution, this time not in our relation to the natural world, but in our relation to ourselves. Our bodies, even our feelings, thoughts, and intellectual capacities, are also gradually entering the sphere of scientific control and manipulation. And as the scientific understanding of the biology of aging increases, some even begin to envisage technologies that would dramatically slow down, even stop, the aging process. It appears that soon we will be able to radically enhance human capacities well beyond the normal range. In some circles, there is even talk about an approaching post-human era, a prospect that is horrifying to many, but enticing to others.

Some aspects of this silent revolution are already around us, in the form of antidepressants and other drugs that control mood and attention, performance-enhancing drugs illicitly used by athletes, or cosmetic surgery to correct the results of the genetic lottery or to conceal the effects of aging. Others are only in early stages of speculative research: mind–machine interfaces, or neuropharmaceuticals that reduce aggression and increase cooperation. The use of pills to "brighten" mood, and the widespread diagnosis of controversial and pharmacologically treatable new psychiatric conditions such as attention deficit disorder, are putting in question the traditional conception of medicine as concerned only with the treatment and cure of disease. Traditional notions of human nature, normality and flourishing seem increasingly inadequate. Proponents of enhancement see these as positive developments. They argue that it is high time that we used biomedical science, not only to fight disease, but also to positively enhance human capacities and well-being. But opponents of enhancement see these developments as a grave threat to what is most dear in human life. These contrasting hopes and fears have already generated intense controversy.

A look back at similar disputes about past scientific and technological advances reveals that many past fears and hopes were deeply misguided or exaggerated. The real dangers were often overlooked, and the real benefits often misunderstood. If we are not to repeat this error, it is important that we set the debate on the right track. We will not find sound answers through armchair prophecy. Instead, the debate needs to be informed by detailed and accurate knowledge of the relevant science and its limits – an understanding of what is feasible and practicable, and what really is just science fiction – as well as by a clear view of the relevant concepts and values. It cannot, for example, be simply assumed that ethical conceptions and principles that have served us well in the past will be useful guides in this uncharted territory.

This volume, we hope, will contribute to setting the debate about human enhancement on the right path. It aims to offer a comprehensive view of the latest scientific developments in human enhancement, and a wide range of perspectives on its ethical significance. The chapters in this volume represent a diverse range of perspectives from several disciplines. Some focus on philosophical discussion of fundamental concepts, others engage in ethical analysis and argument. Others review the very latest empirical research in biology, neuroscience, and the social sciences, and attempt to predict future developments. Then others try to offer concrete policy prescriptions.

The first part of this volume discusses key concepts and issues about enhancement, and is followed by parts focusing on the main categories of enhancement: cognitive, mood, and physical enhancement, lifespan extension, and, finally, moral enhancement. Except for the short section on moral enhancement, each of these sections begins with an introductory chapter that surveys the current state of the science and introduces some of the main conceptual and ethical issues, and ends with a chapter on the policy implications of that form of enhancement. The book ends with two chapters examining the general policy issues raised by human enhancement in the United States and European Union contexts.

Part I: Key Concepts and Questions

The chapters in this section attempt to clarify general issues in the debate about enhancement. What is meant by "enhancement"? Is it a descriptive or normative concept? What is its relation to human flourishing and well-being? The chapters also clarify the role of the concepts of nature and autonomy in current thinking on enhancement, and examine the ways our understanding of evolution might affect our attitude to human nature and its modification.

Part II: Cognitive Enhancement

Cognitive enhancement involves increasing human cognitive capacities: intelligence, memory, and attention. Such "upgrading" of our brains can be achieved using neuropharmacology or genetic intervention, but also through participation large-scale networking, not to mention "traditional" education. The chapters in this section review the latest scientific advances in cognitive enhancement, and examine its possible benefits and risks, both in terms of individual well-being and the broader social impact.

Part III: Mood Enhancement

The widespread use of Prozac and other antidepressants, not to mention various forms of recreational drugs, is by now a familiar aspect of contemporary life. Do such drugs rob people of authenticity or do they rather enable their true selves to shine through? Might they corrupt our ability to properly appreciate the darker aspects of life? Chapters in this section also highlight the way mood enhancement raises questions about the proper goals of medicine, and about the viability of the treatment/enhancement distinction.

Part IV: Physical Enhancement

Radical forms of physical enhancement allowing humans to radically augment their physical abilities are already available – and extremely controversial. In certain forms they have been banned in sport, but it's assumed they are nevertheless being used by some athletes. The chapters in this section ask whether this ban on "doping" in sports is justified. Is there a useful line to draw between permissible forms of physical enhancement and forms of it that amount to cheating? Does physical enhancement really contravene the "ethos" of sport?

Part V: Lifespan Extension

Reflection on mortality has been central to philosophy since its inception. Some philosophers have taken the limit imposed by death to be a fundamental source of meaning. But, at least in Western societies, the human lifespan is already far longer than that of our distant ancestors, and as science advances, it is no longer unthinkable that we might be able to radically slow, or even stop, the aging process. But if we could live for hundreds of years, would our present identity survive – and if not, how could this be a benefit to us, as we are now? And even if our selves could survive into the far future, wouldn't this eventually lead to unbearable boredom? The possibility of radical lifespan extension thus raises profound questions about the value and meaning of life itself.

Part VI: Moral Enhancement

An area of enhancement that is vital but so far largely neglected in the current debate is the prospect of moral enhancement: using scientific means to increase the precious but frail human capacity to engage in moral behavior. Is this aim even coherent? Would, for example, pharmacologically induced altruism amount to genuine moral behavior or only to artificial mimicry of true morality? Indeed, given the urgent global crises facing humanity, and the biologically limited human capacity for altruism and empathy, might moral enhancement be our most urgent task?

Part VII: General Policy

The volume ends with general discussions of legal and policy issues in the U.S. and European context. How should one deal with enhancements in a European context, with different cultures and diverse legislations in the various European Member States? Does the European Union have any role in the regulation of enhancement, or should it be left to the Member States? Do we need new regulations or new policy bodies to develop public policies on enhancement? What kind of normative framework should guide such public policies? Who should be involved in the development of such a framework and what could be the role of public deliberation in policy development?

Part I
Key Concepts and Questions

1

Well-Being and Enhancement

Julian Savulescu, Anders Sandberg, and Guy Kahane

Many chapters in this volume review current and future possibilities for enhancing human physical ability, cognition, mood, and lifespan. These possibilities raise the ethical question of whether we *should* enhance normal human capacities in these ways. We are not likely to agree on answers to this question without a clear and shared understanding of the concept of enhancement. The aim of this chapter is to offer such an account of enhancement. We begin by reviewing a number of suggested accounts of enhancement, and point to their shortcomings. We identify two key senses of "enhancement": *functional* enhancement, the enhancement of some capacity or power (e.g. vision, intelligence, health) and *human* enhancement, the enhancement of a human being's life. The latter notion, we suggest, is the notion of enhancement most relevant to ethical debate. We argue that it is best understood in welfarist terms. We will then illustrate this welfarist approach to enhancement by applying it to the case of cognitive enhancement.

Definitions of Enhancement

Although there is much debate about the ethical implications of new technologies, only a few authors have attempted to provide an explicit definition of enhancement. Often discussion focuses on a particular application such as muscle strength, memory or lifespan, or a definition of enhancement is implicitly assumed. However, without an adequate shared understanding of what is meant by "enhancement," we are not likely to resolve these debates and reach sound ethical conclusions.

The sociological pragmatic approach

In the literature there is a great deal of uncertainty and confusion about the term "enhancement." Erik Parens (1998) states that:

> ... some participants think the term *enhancement* is so freighted with erroneous assumptions and so ripe for abuse that we ought not even to use it. My sense is that if we didn't use enhancement, we would end up with another term with similar problems.

Enhancing Human Capacities, edited by Julian Savulescu, Ruud ter Meulen and Guy Kahane.
© 2011 Blackwell Publishing Ltd

He then continues by using the term as a focus for a discussion of the goals of medicine and society. A similar pragmatic approach is taken by Paul Root Wolpe (2002) who also states that enhancement is a slippery socially constructed concept: "Yet, ultimately, any exclusive enhancement definition must fail, in part because concepts such as disease, normalcy, and health are significantly culturally and historically bound, and thus the result of negotiated values." Likewise, he then turns to discuss issues of reimbursement, public policy, and normative behavior. James Canton (2002) stresses the relativism inherent in such an approach:

> The future may hold different definitions of human enhancement that affect culture, intelligence, memory, physical performance, even longevity. Different cultures will define human performance based on their social and political values. It is for our nation to define these values and chart the future of human performance.

This approach is broadly social and pragmatic: Enhancement captures a certain historically and culturally specific value-laden domain of discourse related to human performance rather than having a substantive transcultural independent meaning. The sociological pragmatic approach describes how particular social groups delineate and value (or disvalue) various technological advances. It is less helpful when we want to ask whether these valuations are valid. This account merely tells us that, for example, some cultures or groups value intelligence more than others.

The ideological approach

Another superficially similar approach is to avoid defining the term at all. This move is made both by proponents and opponents of enhancement. Typically a list of technologies or enhancement goals are stated and the field is defined or marked by them (Kass, 2003; Naam 2005). For example, the President's Council on Bioethics delineates the domain of discourse, after stating the problems of definition and the smooth blending between therapy and enhancement, as one related to human desires and goals. As stated by Kass: "The human meaning and moral assessment must be tackled directly; they are unlikely to be settled by the term 'enhancement,' any more than they are by the nature of the technological intervention itself."

This approach differs from the sociological pragmatic approach by aiming directly at deep values, invoking concepts of metaphysics or spirituality. It is an ideological approach: A set of often controversial values are applied to a range of possible technological advances, and these are directly classified as morally wholesome or problematic. Thus the ideological approach offers a range of specific and contentious value claims but no general conceptual framework for thinking about enhancement.

The "not-medicine" approach: treatment vs. enhancement

Another influential approach has been to define enhancement in terms of going beyond health-restoring treatment or health. Eric T. Juengst (1998) defines it as: "The term *enhancement* is usually used in bioethics to characterize interventions designed to improve human form or functioning beyond what is necessary to sustain or restore good health."

(Handwritten margin notes:)

Pragmatic: dealing with things sensibly & realistically in a way that is based on practical rather than theoretical considerations.

Discourse: written or spoken communication or debate.

Delineate: describe or portray (something) precisely.

Edmund D. Pellegrino (2004) uses a similar definition just for the purpose of arguing against enhancement on the grounds that it goes beyond medicine as a healing enterprise:

> ... my operating definition of enhancement will be grounded in its general etymological meaning, i.e., to increase, intensify, raise up, exalt, heighten, or magnify. Each of these terms carries the connotation of going "beyond" what exists at some moment, whether it is a certain state of affairs, a bodily function or trait, or a general limitation built into human nature ... For this discussion, enhancement will signify an intervention that goes beyond the ends of medicine as they traditionally have been held.

One problem with this approach is that the definition of medicine and treatment itself is contested. Even a maximally inclusive definition such as medicine being the "science and art of diagnosing, treating, curing, and preventing disease, relieving pain, and improving and preserving health" (McKechnie, 1961) still leaves us to define disease and health, equally complex terms (Smith, 2002). For example, Robert Freitas Jr. (1999) reviews nine disease concepts (disease relativism, statistical disease, disease idealism, functional failure, and so forth), and if enhancement is defined as going beyond preventing disease/improving health, this will give us nine different enhancement concepts. The not-medicine approach is thus indeterminate. Indeed, there is some doubt whether it is even possible to draw a consistent and useful distinction between treatment and enhancement.

It is worth mentioning, however, one influential view of disease – Christopher Boorse's (1975) "species-typical functioning" account. By determining the natural functional organization of members of a species it is possible to create a normal function model, which should be, according to Daniels (2000), the standard of functioning a society has an obligation to help reach. This model has been employed influentially by Norman Daniels in addressing enhancement (Sabin & Daniels, 1994). On this view, disease is defined as:

> **Normal species-functioning conception of disease**: Any state of a person's biology or psychology which reduces species-typical normal functioning below some statistically defined level.

And enhancement can be thus defined as improvement in human functioning that goes beyond what is needed for medical treatment:

> **Normal species-functioning definition of enhancement**: Any change in the biology or psychology of a person which increases species-typical normal functioning above some statistically defined level.

For example, low intelligence is defined as intellectual disability and treated as a disease when Intelligence Quotient (IQ) falls below 70. On this species-functioning or naturalistic conception of disease and enhancement, raising someone's IQ from 60 to 70 is treating a disease and raising someone's IQ from 70 to 80 is enhancement.

On a normal distribution of function, about 2.5% of the population will have a disease. Improvements in function of the other 97.5% counts as enhancement. For example, the bottom 2.5% of hearing counts as deafness. The other 97.5% of people are counted as having "normal hearing" even though those at the bottom of that distribution will have impairments in hearing almost identical to those classified as "deaf." But they fell on the wrong side of the statistical line to be eligible for "medical treatment." Improving their hearing, even if they hear very little at all, would, on this view, be an enhancement.

The functional approach

A related fourth approach is the functional approach. Rather than avoiding defining enhancement or mainly seeing it as not-medicine, it is defined in terms of enhanced functions of various kinds (whether cognitive function generally or vision or hearing more narrowly).

The archetypal example of this approach is Douglas C. Engelbart's (1962) *Augmenting Human Intellect*: "By 'augmenting human intellect' we mean increasing the capability of a man to approach a complex problem situation, to gain comprehension to suit his particular needs, and to derive solutions to problems."

Here, cognitive enhancement is defined simply in terms of improved general information-processing abilities. The difference from the Daniels' approach is that no weight need be given to some level of normal, species-typical functioning which would determine whether some manipulation is to count as treatment or enhancement. On this view, any increase in IQ or hearing could count as an enhancement.

The Welfarist Account of Human Enhancement

Enhancement of what?

Enhancement is, indeed, a wide concept. In the broadest sense, it means "increase" or "improvement." For example, a doctor may *enhance* his patient's chance of survival by giving the patient a drug. Or a doctor may enhance the functioning of a person's immune system or memory – enhancement in the functional sense. These are no doubt enhancements of a sort – enhancements in an attributive sense. But enhancing a permanently unconscious person's chance of surviving might not be good for the person. It might not constitute *human* enhancement. It might not enhance intrinsic good – or good in a predicative sense.

As the example of life extension shows, these two senses of enhancement can come apart. Consider memory. Genetic memory enhancement has been demonstrated in rats and mice. In normal animals during maturation expression of the NR2B subunit of the NMDA receptor is gradually replaced with expression of the NR2A subunit, something that may be linked to less brain plasticity in adult animals. Tang *et al.* (1999) modified mice to overexpress NR2B. The NR2B mice (commonly known as the "Doogie" mouse) demonstrated improved memory performance, both in terms of acquisition and retention. This included unlearning of fear conditioning, which is believed to be due to learning a secondary memory (Falls, Miserendino, & Davis 1992). The modification also made them more sensitive to certain forms of pain, showing a potentially nontrivial trade-off (Wei *et al.*, 2002). It is possible that even though memory is improved, their lives are worse.

The term human enhancement is itself ambiguous. It might mean enhancement of functioning as a member of the species *homo sapiens*. This would be a functional definition. But when we are considering human enhancement, we are considering improvement of the person's life. The improvement is some change in state of the person – biological or psychological – which is good. Which changes are good depends on the value we are seeking to promote or maximize. In the context of human enhancement, the value immediately in question is the goodness of a person's life, that is, his or her well-being.

The welfarist definition

These reflections suggest a fifth possible definition of human enhancement:

> **Welfarist definition of human enhancement**: Any change in the biology or psychology of a person which increases the chances of leading a good life in the relevant set of circumstances.

In line with the welfarist definition of enhancement, we can classify states of a person as *enhancing* or *advantageous states* or *abilities*:

> Any state of a person's biology or psychology which increases the chance of leading a good life in the relevant set of circumstances.

And similarly define contrary *disadvantageous states* or *disabilities*:

> Any state of a person's biology or psychology which decreases the chance of leading a good life in the relevant set of circumstances (Kahane & Savulescu, 2009).

This account of enhancement makes no use of the distinction between medical treatment and enhancement. On this view, any increase in IQ could count as enhancement – so long as it tends to increase a person's well-being. But, contrary both to the species-functioning and functional approaches, in contexts where increase in IQ is not beneficial to some person, such increase would not count as an enhancement, even if it raises the person to (or well beyond) the level of normal functioning, that is, even if it were a functional enhancement.

Unlike the sociological pragmatic and functional approaches, the welfarist account is inherently normative. It ties enhancement to the value of well-being. Unlike the ideological approach, however, it offers a general framework for thinking about enhancement. It offers more than a mere list of value claims. It singles out well-being as one dimension of value that is constitutive of genuine human enhancement. But it leaves open substantive and contentious questions about the nature of well-being, and important empirical questions about the impact of some treatment on well-being. Moreover, whereas the ideological approach only offers us all-things-considered value judgments about various treatments, the welfarist approach distinguishes ways in which some treatment might benefit a person from other relevant values, such as justice. It thus allows us to say that although some treatment is an enhancement (i.e. contributes to individuals' well-being), it might nevertheless be bad overall, because its employment in the current social context will lead to far greater injustice.

On the welfarist account, common medical treatments are enhancements, or more precisely, a subclass of enhancements, and diseases are best seen as a subclass of disabilities or disadvantageous states.

Folk usage of the term enhancement supports this account (Pellegrino in fact gestures towards this definition in his account). According to the *Oxford English Dictionary*:

Enhancement
The action or process of enhancement: the fact of being enhanced

Enhance
to raise in degree, heighten, intensify (qualities, states, powers, etc.)
to raise (prices, value)
to raise or increase in price, value, importance, attractiveness, etc.
(Formerly used *simply,* = "to increase in price or value"; *esp.* to raise the intrinsic value of (coin). Also *(rarely)* = "to increase in attractiveness", to beautify, improve.)

The spirit of all these definitions is that to enhance is *to increase value*. In the context of human enhancement, to enhance is to increase the value of a person's life. This notion is best captured by the welfarist account. Henceforth, we will refer to human enhancement simply as enhancement for brevity's sake.

Subclasses of enhancements

Enhancements include different kinds of improvements:

1. Medical treatment of disease.
2. Increasing natural human potential – Increasing a person's own natural endowments of capabilities within the range typical of the species *homo sapiens*, e.g. raising a person's IQ from 100 to 140.
3. Superhuman enhancements (sometimes called posthuman or transhuman) – Increasing a person's capabilities beyond the range typical for the species *homo sapiens*, e.g. giving humans bat sonar or the capacity to read minds.

By accepting the welfarist definition of enhancement, the question of when should we enhance becomes: when should we increase human well-being?

One of the advantages of a welfarist account of enhancement is that it reframes existing debates in a more productive manner. The ideological approach is really a debate about what constitutes a good life and resistance to enhancement is often not really resistance to enhancement *per se*, but resistance to accepting an overly narrow or mistaken conception of human well-being.

Applying the Welfarist Account:
The Case of Cognitive Ability

Expected value

An intervention constitutes an enhancement when it is expected to increase the chances of a person leading a good life. It is important to recognize that something expected to increase the chances of leading a good life may, in a probabilistic world, not result in a good life. Those born with the greatest gifts and talents may squander them while those born to great biological and social hardship may overcome enormous obstacles to lead the best of lives.

The term "expected" thus does not mean "will." It is a technical term taken from decision theory. The expected value of an outcome is the value of that outcome multiplied by the probability of it occurring. In the debate around enhancement, the outcome of value is a person's life and how well it goes.

This approach derives from decision theory. The standard way of making decisions under uncertainty is to choose that option which maximizes expected value. While this may not be the way we make decisions all the time in ordinary life, it is one standard norm of rationality for how an ideal agent who has no computational limitations should make decisions. In general terms, the expected value of adopting any course of action can be given by:

Pr(good outcome given that course taken) $\times$ V(good outcome) $+ Pr$(other outcomes given that course taken) $\times$ V(other outcomes).

We often use this approach in a rough and ready way in everyday decisions. Consider a person trying to decide whether to buy a house or rent. The decision will usually be made by weighing the pros and cons, how bad these are and how likely they are. She needs to know how far each residence is likely to be from work, schools, friends and amenities. She needs to know how big the house and land of each are likely to be, and the quality of each. And of course she needs to know the cost of each both in the short term and long term, and how this will affect her financial position overall.

This approach can be formalized. The golfer Tiger Woods is reputed to have had laser surgery to give him better than 20/20 vision. Imagine someone like Woods, a professional golfer wanting to win the British Open, but who is also knowledgeable about decision theory. He is trying to decide whether to have laser surgery to give 20/20 vision. The following figures are purely hypothetical.

Assume that without surgery, his life will go very well and he will win many golf tournaments. If 1 is the perfect life, his life overall will be of value 0.96. If he has laser surgery, he will win slightly more tournaments. His life will be slightly better (0.97). However, there is a risk (1/1000) that the surgery will damage his eyesight and he will win slightly fewer tournaments and his life will go slightly less well (0.95):

The expected value of life without surgery is 0.96
The expected value of life with surgery $= V$(life, given successful surgery)
$\times Pr$(surgery successful) $+ V$(life, given unsuccessful surgery)
$\times Pr$(surgery unsuccessful)
$= 0.97 \times 999/1000 + 0.95 \times 1/1000$
$= 0.96998$

Even though the benefits of surgery are small, it is rational to have the surgery given its risks are also very small. As the probability of harm rises, or it becomes more serious, there is less reason to opt for surgery.

Dimensions of well-being

Whether, on the welfarist account, something counts as a human enhancement depends on how we understand the notion of well-being. There are various theories of well-being: hedonistic, desire-fulfillment, objective list theories (Griffin, 1986; Parfit, 1984). According to hedonistic theories, what matters is the quality of our experiences, for example, that we experience pleasure. According to desire-fulfillment theories, what matters is the degree to which our desires are satisfied. According to objective list theories, certain activities are good for people, such as achieving worthwhile things, possessing dignity, having children and raising them, gaining knowledge of the world, developing talents, appreciating beautiful things, and so on.

As an example, consider cognitive enhancement, such as improvement of memory. Improving memory is, by definition, a form of functional enhancement. But is cognitive enhancement also a human enhancement? The answer to the question lies in the answer to the question: Is cognitive enhancement likely to lead to a better life, to a life with more well-being?

It is clear enough how enhancing human cognition is likely to increase human well-being. First, cognitive capacities are the required for deployment of any kind of instrumental rationality – the capacity to reliably identify means to one's ends and projects. Better cognition means better access to information about one's surroundings and about one's own biology and psychology, as well as better abilities to use this information in rational planning. Persons need to exercise instrumental rationality in order to obtain pleasure and avoid pain, in order to fulfill their desires, and in order to realize objective goods. So cognitive enhancement should promote well-being on all major theories of well-being.

Second, on some views of well-being certain cognitive capacities are necessary conditions for a good life. For example, on a Millian view of pleasure, forms of pleasure that do not involve the exercise of sophisticated cognitive abilities have less value. Persons with greater cognitive capacities will have access to higher hence more valuable pleasures. Human beings with cognitive capacities far beyond those available to existing people may thus have access to far higher pleasures than those accessible to existing humans. Similarly, Mill placed great value on the power of "vivid imagination" to decide which of two pleasures is more valuable, when we are unable to experience both. Such imaginative powers require complex cognition involving memory, logical inference, and other higher order faculties.

Similar remarks apply to objective theories that emphasize the value of knowledge and achievement. Persons with low cognitive capacities will, on objective views, be able to achieve only moderate levels of well-being even if they lead healthy and happy lives. Only cognitive enhancement will offer them access to the greater objective goods which require sophisticated cognition. The same will be true to a lesser extent of most human beings with normal cognitive capacities. Most people cannot fully grasp the intricacies of quantum mechanics or enjoy complete appreciation of the highest aesthetic achievements of human culture. Some great objective goods are now accessible only to a few.

Although improvement of cognitive ability is a major form of enhancement in all of these ways, it is partly an empirical question whether human beings with great cognitive capacities actually successfully use them to promote their well-being. It is a common view that great intelligence, for example, can be an obstacle to happiness. The empirical data currently available to test this claim is limited, and is typically limited to the relation between intelligence and subjective well-being. But although intelligence is a central cognitive capacity, it does not exhaust cognition. And subjective well-being is the whole of well-being only on hedonistic theories, although it is a significant component of well-being on all plausible views. Furthermore, the existing empirical evidence may tell us only about the subjective well-being of highly intelligent people in a world populated and controlled by people with lesser intelligence. Nevertheless, this evidence is of some interest. It suggests that while general intelligence does not directly predict happiness, it is nevertheless a protective factor against mental and health problems. Thus even if higher intelligence does not directly make a person happier, it does contribute to her having a longer and healthier life. As such it is a significant contribution to a person's overall well-being even on the narrowest hedonistic theory.

All-purpose goods

General intelligence is only one aspect of cognition. Many other biological and psychological characteristics can also profoundly affect how well our lives go. In the 1960s Walter Mischel conducted impulse control experiments where four-year-old children were left in a room with one marshmallow, after being told that if they did not eat the marshmallow, they could later have two. Some children would eat it as soon as the researcher left, others would use a variety of strategies to help control their behavior and ignore the temptation of the single marshmallow. A decade later, the children were re-interviewed and found that those who were better at delaying gratification had more friends, better academic performance, and more motivation to succeed. Whether the child had grabbed for the marshmallow had a much stronger bearing on their SAT scores than did their IQ (Mischel, Shoda & Peake, 1988). Impulse control has also been linked to socioeconomic control and avoiding conflict with the law.

Shyness too can greatly restrict a life. A newspaper story described a woman who blushed violet every time she went into a social situation. This led her to a hermitic, miserable existence. She eventually had the autonomic nerves to her face surgically cut. This revolutionized her life and had a greater effect on her well-being than the treatment of many diseases (Drott, Claes, & Rex, 2002).

Following Rawls, Buchanan and colleagues have discussed the value of "all-purpose goods" (Buchanan *et al.*, 2002). These are traits that are valuable regardless of which kind of life a person chooses to live – valuable on all plausible conceptions of well-being. They give us greater all-round capacities to experience a vast array of lives. Examples include memory, self-discipline, patience, empathy, a sense of humor, optimism, and just having a sunny temperament. All of these characteristics – and perhaps many of the moral virtues – may have some biological and psychological basis capable of manipulation with technology. Intelligence is a clear example of an all-purpose good.

Cognitive disability

Many cognitive deficits are obstacles to a good life. They are disabilities in our stipulated welfarist sense. Correcting such disabilities is one central aim of cognitive enhancement. Indeed we argue that even normal human cognition can constitute a disability – an obstacle to well-being – in the current social context.

In the case of low intelligence, what ultimately matters is not whether low normal intelligence is called a disability but whether it is bad and should be avoided if possible. The answer to this question turns, in significant part, on the expected value of a life with low intelligence compared to life with high intelligence. One way to answer this question is to ask: Should a person with low intelligence attempt to have his or her intelligence increased? Or, should a person with high intelligence attempt to have intelligence reduced? This is like the question: Should a normally sighted person attempt to achieve better than 20/20 vision?

Some disability advocates deny that the profound cognitive impairment that characterizes Down syndrome is a genuine disability – that it is any kind of misfortune or makes life worse. Such a view is implied by remarks like the following (Hogan, 2006):

> People with Down's syndrome are entirely capable of having what we would understand to be a good quality of life, defined by achieving satisfactory personal goals, making a wide range of friends, holding down a job, contributing to the well-being of others and by and large making some sense of the environment that surrounds them.

Parents of children with Down syndrome often deny that their lives are in any interesting way worse than those of people with normal cognitive capacities or that it makes good sense to compare their respective well-being.

Whether Down syndrome is a disability depends on many variables including the value of more intelligent life, the chance of the intervention working, its risks, the value of a less intelligent life and the risks and benefits of any other courses of action. The value of a more intelligent life (like a life with better than 20/20 vision) depends on how that intelligence enables one to realize various possible good lives, and the probabilities of achieving these.

Elsewhere, two of us have developed a welfarist definition of disability (Kahane & Savulescu, 2009; Savulescu & Kahane 2009):

> **Disability**: Any state of a person's biology or psychology which decreases the chance of leading a good life in the relevant set of circumstances.

Is low intelligence a disability in this sense? As we have argued earlier, low intelligence is likely to mean that one is less effective at achieving one's ends (instrumental rationality) and less likely to achieve various objective goods. It is also likely to compromise health and happiness in various ways. It is likely to a form of disability in this broad welfarist sense, even if not a disease.

Is it possible that there is something unique, and valuable, in a life that realizes less good? Even if intellectual disability affords a unique perspective on the world, it seems false that this perspective is equally desirable. This perspective entails numerous difficulties and hurdles to attaining many of the goods which uncontroversially are a part of the good life: to gain knowledge and understanding of the world and others, be capable of forming a wide variety of friendships and relationships, having, raising and caring for a family, achieving independence, etc.

A "normal intelligence" is defined as IQ which is within two standard deviations of the mean of 100. The standard deviation is 15 points—that is, an IQ between 70 and 130, which accounts for 95% of all people. Intellectual disability is defined statistically as that IQ which is below two standard deviations from the mean, which accounts for 2.5% of the population. It is subdivided into:

Mild   50 – 70
Moderate   35 – 49
Severe   Below 34

However, this definition of when low intelligence constitutes a disease or disability is entirely arbitrary. One needs an IQ of about 90 to complete a tax return in the United States, which means that more than 15% of normal people in the United States will not be able to complete a tax return, severely hampering their employment opportunities. With an IQ of 120, you have enough cognitive ability to enter university and to have virtually any job you choose. In a technologically advanced society, those with low but normal IQ may be severely disadvantaged and have a restricted range of options. We could redefine significant intellectual disability as any IQ below 120. If we were concerned to give everyone a substantial chance of the best life, we could say that those with an IQ of less than 120 have a significant intellectual disability because their IQ holds them back from full participation in a technologically advanced society with complex social institutions and global conflicts.

These claims are controversial and contestable. But consider this hypothetical example. Imagine that you have a child with normal intelligence, say an IQ of 110. A man knocks at your door one day. He says he is the health inspector. He suspects you have old lead water pipes. You ask what the consequences are: "It's not life-threatening. But it may reduce your child's IQ by a few points. I would recommend that you change them."

Should you be concerned if your child's IQ were to drop from 110 to 105? Perhaps such a small change would have minimal affect on the child's well-being. But if it were likely to have some effect, you should be concerned. You should remove the lead pipes.

Disability is ubiquitous and even those with normal IQ are disabled

One might argue that there is no such thing as a better or best life. This, as we have argued, is false. All of us will have some cognitive strengths and weakness. Those with great mathematical intelligence may have lower emotional intelligence. And our cognitive abilities deteriorate normally over time. Memory deteriorates after the age of 40. In this way all of us will have some cognitive disabilities in our lives, though these will vary in degree from one individual to another, and from time to time. In this way, *all of us are disabled in some ways* which make it more difficult to lead a very good life. *Enhancement is an issue of vital concern to all of us.*

Another objection is that it is impossible to achieve the best life. This is virtually always the case because, among other things, we lack complete information and the ability to process such information. But it is a feature of all decision making in a less than ideal world. We are never sure that we have performed the act which has the best consequences, or bought the best house or the best TV or helped our friends as much as we could, even if we wanted to. This is an objection to any theory which aims to bring about a certain state of affairs in a probabilistic world. It applies whenever we try to do our best or merely even try to affect the world. Though we can rarely if ever do our best, we can try. We cannot be certain of the effects of our actions – we can only rationally estimate them.

It is important to recall that on our definition of disability, we all suffer from disabilities which are conditions inherent to our nature (biological, psychological or other) which either reduce the value of our lives or which make it more difficult to realize (in the sense that that they reduce the chances that we will achieve) a good life. Poor concentration, poor memory, poor visuospatial skills, poor emotional intelligence are just like asthma, a lame foot, pigheadedness and weakness of will. They are all disabilities on this definition.

Such an approach allows us to explain why we treat disease and classify those with an IQ as suffering from a disease, and the extent to which we believe a diseased person should be treated. The extent of the claim that a diseased person has to be treated depends on the extent to which that disease is a disability. Some diseases have so little impact on a person's life that such diseased people have very little claim to treatment. A symptomless disease which had no impact on the length or quality of a person's life would be irrelevant. The IQ is set at 70 for disability simply because this picks out the 2.5% of the population who are worst off.

Thus on our view medical treatment is a subclass of enhancement or improvement. In general, disease has significant impact on our well-being. Medical treatment makes a greater improvement in well-being than most other enhancements. For this reason medical treatment should generally have greater priority than other enhancements. But it leaves open whether there might be nonmedical enhancements that have a much greater influence on well-being than medical treatment and so have greater priority. Imagine we could raise the IQ of everyone who had an IQ of between 70–80 by 10 points. This would not count as medical treatment. However, this might (depending on which theory of justice you accepted) have greater priority than raising the IQ of a few people with an IQ of 60 by 10 points, even though the latter is medical treatment.

Biopsychosocial correction of disability

Our biology evolves slowly, over thousands if not millions of years. Our social life has radically changed over the last 100 years. Doctors are keen to tell us that our biology is not suited to our current high fat, low fiber diet and sedentary lifestyle. But our biology and psychology are probably more globally out of synchrony with our way of life. It is not merely that we are prone to "lifestyle disease," it is that we are prone, to some degree, to lifestyle unhappiness. And our cognitive abilities are hardly adapted to the massive technological and social changes which have happened in a blink of human history.

Whenever there is a mismatch between biology, psychology, and social/natural environment resulting in a bad life, we have a choice. We can alter our biology, our psychology, or our environment. This is occurring in medical practice when doctors advise diets which are low in fat, high in fiber, high in antioxidants, lower our cholesterol, and which basically mimic the diet to which our bodies are basically designed to tolerate. The most extreme example of this is the Stone Age diet which attempts to replicate the diet of primitive man. But another approach is not to change our environment (in this case diet) but to change our biology through drugs. The polypill is designed to allow the body to tolerate a modern diet by lowering chemically for example our cholesterol and/or blood pressure.

When it comes to questions of enhancement, we can enhance our biological and psychological capacities to suit our natural and social environment, or we can attempt to alter our environment to suit our unenhanced selves. Our own view is that all routes must be considered. In some cases, it is reasonable and practicable to alter the environment. So giving people with current intellectual disabilities a fair and equal opportunity might be preferable to cognitive enhancement, if it were cheaper, more effective, or had beneficial externalities. But in at least some cases, it is going to be difficult to change the modern environment to allow all possible people to flourish. For example, it may be most effective to choose children with more melanin pigment in their skin to protect them from the sun in areas of high ozone layer damage, rather than attempting to close the hole in the ozone layer in that area or enforcing sunscreen, coverage of the skin, and fear of the sun.

The consequences of low intelligence can be lethal. Low intelligence is correlated with the development of disease and with lethal accidents. Improving cognition, in the way the world is likely to be, may be a matter of life and death.

Summary: The Case in Favor of Enhancement

How do we decide?

There are four possible ways in which our psychology and biology will be decided (Savulescu, 2009).

1. Nature or God
2. "Experts" – philosophers, bioethicists, psychologists, scientists
3. "Authorities" – government, doctors
4. By people themselves – liberty and autonomy

It is a basic principle of liberal states the state should be "neutral" between different conceptions of the good life. This means that we allow individuals to lead the life that they believe is best for themselves – respect for their personal autonomy or capacity for self-rule. The sole ground for interference is when that individual choice may harm others. Advice, persuasion, information, and dialogue are permissible. But coercion and infringement of liberty are impermissible.

There are limits to what a liberal state should provide:

1. Harm to others – The intervention (like some manipulation that increases uncontrollable aggressiveness) should not result in significant harm, whether direct or indirect, for example, by causing some unfair competitive advantage.

2. Distributive justice – The interventions should be distributed according to principles of justice.

John Stuart Mill argued that when our actions only affect ourselves, we should be free to construct and act on our own conception of what is the best life for us. Mill was not a libertarian. He did not believe that such freedom was solely valuable for its own sake. He believed freedom was important for people to discover for themselves what kind of life is best for themselves. It is only through "experiments in living" that people discover what works for them, and others can see the richness and variety of lives that can be good. Mill strongly praised "originality" and variety in choice as being essential to discovering which lives are best for human beings (Savulescu, 2002). Such experiments and originality require cognitive skills and creativity, insight, and many other skills.

Conclusion

What is enhancement? According to a

> **Welfarist definition of human enhancement**: Any change in the biology or psychology of a person which increases the chances of leading a good life in the relevant set of circumstances.

When should we bring about some modification of biological or psychological alteration of a person which is a putative enhancement? On a welfarist account, whether we should intervene depends on:

1. The account of well-being we employ.
2. Whether the modification is expected to increase the chances of the person in question leading a good life in the circumstances likely to be obtained.
3. Whether there are reasons to prefer modifications of the natural or social environment.
4. Whether the modification will harm others or create or exacerbate injustice.

Questions about enhancement are questions in value theory about the account of well-being we should employ. They are questions in science about what brings about well-being. And they are questions about the limits of the pursuit of self-interest or beneficence.

In this chapter, we applied the welfarist approach to the example of cognitive ability. We argued that cognitive enhancement is likely to be a form of human enhancement. Cognition plays a central role in our well-being as members of the species *homo sapiens*. In addition, it may provide significant social and economic benefits. These are all strong reasons to support cognitive enhancement. In many cases, cognitive enhancement will have to be done early in life to have maximum benefit. Parents will have to make choices for their children. Thus, as technology advances, parents will have a duty to enhance their children.

While we have focused on cognitive enhancement, our arguments, and the welfarist account of enhancement, can also be easily applied to potential examples of mood or physical enhancements. What aspects of our biology and psychology we should alter will depend, in major part, on their contribution to a good life.

References

Boorse, C. (1975). On the distinction between disease and illness. *Philosophy and Public Affairs*, **5**, 49–68.

Buchanan, A., Brock, D., Daniels, N. & Wikler, D. (2002). *From Chance to Choice*. Cambridge: Cambridge University Press.

Canton, J. (2002). The impact of convergent technologies and the future of business and the economy. In M.C. Roco & W.S. Bainbridge (eds.), *Converging Technologies for Improving Human Performance: Nanotechnology, Biotechnology, Information Technology and Cognitive Science*. New York: Springer.

Daniels, N. (2000). Normal functioning and the treatment-enhancement distinction. *Cambridge Quarterly of Healthcare Ethics*, **9**(3), 309–22.

Drott, C., Claes, G. & Rex, L. (2002). Facial blushing treated by sympathetic denervation – long-lasting benefits in 831 patients. *Journal of Cosmetic Dermatology*, **1**, 115–19.

Engelbart, D.C. (1962). *Augmenting Human Intellect: A Conceptual Framework*. Summary Report AFOSR-3223 under Contract AF 49(638)-1024, SRI Project 3578 for Air Force Office of Scientific Research, Stanford Research Institute, Menlo Park, CA, October. www.bootstrap.org/augdocs/friedewald030402/augmentinghumanintellect/1introduction.html

Falls, W.A., Miserendino, M.J.D. & Davis, M. (1992). Extinction of fear-potentiated startle: Blockade by infusion of an NMDA antagonist into the amygdale. *Journal of Neuroscience*, **12**, 854–63.

Freitas Jr., R.A. (1999). *Nanomedicine, Volume I: Basic Capabilities*. Georgetown, TX: Landes Bioscience. www.nanomedicine.com/NMI.htm

Griffin, J. (1986). *Well-Being*. Oxford: Clarendon Press.

Hogan, J. (2006). Abortion decisions and people with Down's syndrome. *The Independent* (London), May 30.

Juengst, E.T. (1998). What does *enhancement* mean? In E. Parens (ed.), *Enhancing Human Traits: Ethical and Social Implications*. Georgetown, TX: Georgetown University Press.

Kahane, G. & Savulescu, J. (2009). The welfarist account of disability. In K. Brownlee & A. Cureton (eds.), *Disability and Disadvantage*. Oxford: Oxford University Press.

Kass, L. (ed.) (2003). *Beyond Therapy: Biotechnology and the Pursuit of Happiness*. The President's Council on Bioethics, Washington, DC, October, Chapter 1.

McKechnie, J.L. (ed.) (1961). *Webster's New Twentieth Century Dictionary of the English Language*, unabridged, 2nd edition. New York: The World Publishing Co.

Mischel, W., Shoda, Y. & Peake, P.K. (1988). The nature of adolescent competencies predicted by preschool delay of gratification. *Journal of Personality and Social Psychology*, **54**(4), 687–96.

Naam, R. (2005). *More Than Human: Embracing the Promise of Biological Enhancement*. Portland, OR: Broadway Books.

Parens, E. (1998). Is better always good? The Enhancement Project. In E. Parens (ed.), *Enhancing Human Traits: Ethical and Social Implications*. Georgetown, TX: Georgetown University Press.

Parfit, D. (1984). *Reasons and Persons*. Oxford: Oxford University Press.

Pellegrino, E.D. (2004). *Biotechnology, Human Enhancement, and the Ends of Medicine*. The Center for Bioethics and Human Dignity, November 30. www.cbhd.org/resources/biotech/pellegrino_2004-11-30.htm

Sabin, J.E. & Daniels, N. (1994). Determining medical necessity in mental health practice. *Hastings Center Report*, **24**(6), 5–13.

Savulescu, J. (2002). Deaf lesbians, "designer disability," and the future of medicine. *British Medical Journal*, **325**(7367), 771–3.

Savulescu, J. (2009). Genetic interventions and the ethics of enhancement of human beings. In B. Steinbock (ed.), *The Oxford Handbook of Bioethics*. Oxford: Oxford University Press.

Savulescu, J. & Kahane, G. (2009). The moral obligation to create children with the best chance of the best life. *Bioethics*, **23**(5), 274–90.

Smith, R. (2002). In search of "non-disease". *British Medical Journal*, **324**, 883–5.

Tang, Y.P., Shimizu, E., Dube, G.R., Rampon, C., Kerchner, G.A., Zhuo, M. *et al.* (1999). Genetic enhancement of learning and memory in mice. *Nature*, **401**, 63–9.

Wei, F., Wang, G.D., Kerchner, G.A., Kim, S.J., Xu, H.-M., Chen, Z.-F. & Zhuo, M. (2001). Genetic enhancement of inflammatory pain by forebrain NR2B overexpression. *Nature Neuroscience*, **4**, 164–9.

Wolpe, P.R. (2002). Treatment, enhancement, and the ethics of neurotherapeutics. *Brain and Cognition*, **50**, 387–95.

2

The Concept of Nature and the Enhancement Technologies Debate

Lisbeth Witthøfft Nielsen

It is often said that biotechnology is a challenge to our notion of nature and that introducing technologies for the main purpose of enhancing human capacities may change our views on both human nature and the nature that surrounds us. While a lot of attention is being paid to the "nature" of the technologies in this context (i.e. what do the technologies actually do, what are their target areas etc.), little attention is being paid to the complexity of the concept of nature, and the influence this complexity has on debates on emerging biotechnologies. Many bioethicists will dismiss naturalness arguments as obfuscatory arguments, because of the lack of a uniform definition of concepts such as "nature" and "human nature." However, to claim that the concept of nature has no moral relevance in the debate is a different matter. No matter whether we are arguing for or against the use of biotechnologies for the purpose of enhancing both nonhuman and human capacities, we assume the concept of nature as a frame of reference, because "nature" is the common reference to the world that *is*. Nevertheless, there is no such thing as a universal definition of what "nature" is. Therefore, as Collingwood (1965, p. 176) has expressed it: "if nature is a thing that depends for its existence on something else, this dependence is a thing that must be taken into account when we try to understand what nature is."

But how does the concept of nature contribute to the ethical and philosophical debate arising from the introduction of biotechnologies that can be used for the purpose of enhancing human capacities, such as physical or mental capacities?

In this chapter I will analyze the concept of nature and naturalness and its contribution to the debate on biotechnology as enhancement, and in particular enhancement of human capacities. I am not attempting to give an exhaustive analysis of the concept of nature's appearance and of the ethical issues exposed by the debate on biotechnology applied for enhancement of human capacities. The purpose of the chapter is first and foremost to throw light on the complexity with which the concept of nature appears and the challenges this complexity pose to the ethical debate when "nature" or the

Enhancing Human Capacities, edited by Julian Savulescu, Ruud ter Meulen and Guy Kahane.
© 2011 Blackwell Publishing Ltd

"natural" is used as a normative argument, either explicitly or as an underlying presumption of a defined "(human)nature" used as a reference state.

In the first part of the chapter, I outline how biotechnology can be seen as a challenge to our notion of nature, and how the complexity of the concept of nature in itself is a challenge in the debate on enhancement of capacities in humans, animals and plants by means of biotechnology. In the second part, I explore how the same concept contributes to the ethical arguments both for and against enhancement of human capacities. In this part I focus on two central aspects of the enhancement debate namely: (i) the debate that focuses on enhancement as an overreaching form of therapy and: (ii) the debate that focus on enhancement as the goal in itself.

Finally I will summarize the contribution of the concept of nature in terms of the challenges that its inherent complexity poses to the ethical and philosophical debate on enhancement technologies. I will briefly go on to discuss how "nature" and "naturalness" can be said to have moral relevance in the enhancement debate.

Enhancement by Means of Biotechnology and the Challenge to the Notion of Nature

Modern biotechnology, such as gene technology, raise ethical concerns that relate to humans, animals, and plants.[1] The possibility to transfer genes from one species to another means that scientists are able to engineer changes in living organisms that are far more radical and far more targeted than has previously been considered technologically feasible. For some, the possibility of *changing* capacities in animals and humans by using gene technology is a significant ethical concern. They claim that it potentially changes the position of human beings in the natural order of things: Human beings are part of "nature," but they have also become creators of new species and/or even new life forms. It is as if humans were "playing God" instead of recognizing the interdependency between humans and the "nature" that is altered. Others would argue that the development of new technologies is a way of expressing a fundamental creativity, that is seen as something constitutive and unique to human nature.

In the first position, "nature" (and "human nature") has inherent value in its existence *without technological interference*. In the second it is the fundamental element of creativity within human nature, that is accredited a value.

Two frameworks and the challenge of biotechnology

Erik Parens describes the debate on the enhancement of human capacities as circling around two different ethical frameworks. He describes these frameworks as "built of answers to questions that do not have only one good answer." Parens (2005, p.38) mentions the question on whether one can meaningfully distinguish between "natural" and "artificial human interventions into nature", as an example of a question that can be answered from two different frameworks. He describes how these frameworks form the arguments for and against the technological enhancement of human capacities:

When we observe scholars and others debate about "enhancement technologies," I believe that we often see people who have at least for the moment adopted either the gratitude or creativity framework, as I am calling them. As one side emphasizes our obligation to remember that life is a gift and that we need to learn to let things be, the other emphasizes our obligation to transform that gift and to exhibit our creativity. As one framework emphasizes the danger of allowing ourselves to become, in Heidegger's famous formulation, "standing reserve," the other emphasizes the danger of failing to summon the courage to, as Nietzsche put it, "create" ourselves, to "become who we are."

The gratitude framework tends to be critical of enhancement technologies, whereas the creative framework is mainly pro-enhancement of human capacities. Parens (2005, p.37–8) emphasizes that the gratitude framework and the creative framework are used depending on how intrusive people find the particular technology in question. The particular debater may consider some technologies as acceptable and others as intrusive, and may therefore argue from both frameworks, although not concurrently.

When considering the ethical aspects of biotechnologies as applied to either humans or to animals and plants, it is not enough to focus on the aspect of improvement introduced by a new technology in comparison with previously used techniques. It must also take into consideration whether a society is prepared for the potential risks that such a technique involve, and more importantly, whether a society and people in general are ready for the changes the technology in question may bring. It is in this particular context that biotechnology can be said to be a challenge to our notion of nature. The general ethical concerns that are emerging from the introduction of new biotechnologies are twofold: On the one hand, there are the risk factors to be considered, such as the long-term impacts if we modify the human genome or fuse human and animal tissue or genes, or alter plants and animals: Will modifying the human genome make people stronger and better able to survive? Will fusion of human and animal genomes to form chimeras make people more vulnerable to new disease patterns? How will it change the diversity of species if genetically modified plants and animals are released into the environment? These are only some of the practical risk factors to be considered when dealing with new biotechnologies, whether it is for improvement of "human or nonhuman nature."

On the other hand, there are also the more fundamental philosophical/ethical concerns about the intrusiveness of such technologies to "nature" (and "human nature"), such as: Is there a limit to the changes that can be made to the human body and mind, in animals and in the environment, before it is no longer possible to consider humans as such, or the specific animal as belonging to the same species as before? Do such changes, even if they are not causing harm, violate some fundamental values that are embedded in nature (human nature and nonhuman nature) in its current state?

To summarize one can say that biotechnology – whether it is developed or applied for medical or enhancement purposes – forces us to consider what kind of society we want to live in the future, and what values we want to protect and pursue in relation to being human and part of "nature".[2] Having this in mind, I will now turn the focus to the analysis of the complexity of the concept of nature and its contribution to the ethical debate on enhancement by way of (bio) technologies.

The complex nature of "nature"

The concept of nature plays a central role in this debate on enhancement, as the concept is often used as a reference state for the purpose of describing what *is*, and to justify moral arguments. The problem, however, is that "nature" and/or "human nature" is referred to as if it were a clearly defined concept, and not a nebulous concept that embraces a host of meanings. The complexity is embedded in the concept, in the sense that the word "nature" in itself refers to different things. "Nature" or the "natural" is used as a reference to something substantive (some sort of phenomenon) and in a normative context, where "nature" or the "natural" express a reference state that plays a central role in order to justify different moral viewpoints.

In the debate on biotechnology and enhancement, "nature" is represented in at least three different meanings:

- "Nature" understood substantively where it represents the world as a whole in the sense of everything that exists and/or the order or system with which everything that exists, *is* or interacts.
- "Nature" understood as the *essence* of living beings or a biological process/system, i.e. animals and humans are referred to as having a nature which implies their species specificity or in some cases a specific personality.
- "Nature represents that which is in and of itself, and untouched by man. Hence what is "natural" is by itself as opposed to what is artificial.

The three meanings are interpreted in many different ways, yet are sometimes used concurrently in debate, despite the fact that they function differently in different contexts. The distinction between the substantive reference and the normative is rarely clear cut, in the sense that only some of the three meanings are used in a normative context. The reason is that "nature" in all three meanings represents something undefined. In short it can be agreed that "nature" exists, but *what* "nature" *is* and *what* is "natural" depends on the interpretation of the world. "Nature" and "natural" are notions that appear when one tries to either distance oneself from the world around or places oneself in it. We do this when we try to grasp the world through science (natural and social), and through philosophy and religion. But by doing so, it is also revealed what "nature" *does* to us. In light of this an analysis of the concept of nature and what this concept does is an important instrument in the attempt to understand the fundamental disagreements in the ethical debate on enhancement of human capacities.

The different employment of "nature" in debates on biotechnology as an enhancement

When analyzing what "nature" or the "natural" *do*, and the challenge to ethical debate, it is necessary to distinguish between the contexts which concern nonhuman nature and human nature.

In the nonhuman nature debates, "nature" is the common term that embraces animals, plants, ecosystems, and the like. The concept is a descriptive term that seems to refer to something substantive. What is "natural" is what is by "nature," i.e. what is according to its nature in the natural world. Depending on whether the focus is on environmental ethics, food ethics, or animal ethics, "nature" is used as a frame of reference to life processes, the diversity between ecosystems, or living organisms such as animals and plants. But "nature" and the "natural" also represent a normative value, and this value depends on how "nature" as a whole is perceived. A central dispute in this type of debate is whether the ethical value of "nature" is intrinsic or whether the ethical value is assigned by humans, as an aesthetic value or a value that is perceived through the experience of the interdependency between man and "nature".[3]

Some would claim that the diversity entails an intrinsic value, others that the life processes or reproduction processes have a value that requires ethical attention. A strong interpretation of the intrinsic value is to claim that nature has a value that is independent of whether anyone values it. Such a value can be explained as a value embedded in the species specificity, i.e. what makes a cat a cat; or it can be a value intrinsic in the "order of nature" or in the "interaction" between species and biological systems (Kaebnick, 2008, p. 29).

In the ethical debate on biotechnology and enhancement that concerns "human nature" and the "natural," "nature" tends to be understood as the essence of what it means to be *human*.[4] The interpretation of ethical principles such as human dignity and integrity depends on the initial perception of human nature that is used as frame of reference for the argument. This interpretation, however, also depends on how human nature is perceived in the context of "nature" as a whole. One of the most well-known examples of using "nature" as an argument in the debate on enhancement of humans by means of biotechnology, is presented by the German philosopher Jürgen Habermas in his book *The Future of Human Nature*. Habermas (2003) argues against the use of genetic techniques for the purpose of enhancement of human life, because he sees such technologies as a potential threat to human nature, or rather a potential threat to what he considers as constitutive for human nature, namely the ability of self-reflection and with that, freedom and autonomy to choose one's own life path:

> May we consider the genetic self-transformation and self-optimization of the species as a way of increasing the autonomy of the individual? Or will it undermine our normative self-understanding as persons leading their own lives and showing one another equal respect. If the second alternative is true, we surely don't immediately have a conclusive moral argument, but we do have an orientation relying on an ethics of the species, which urges us to proceed with caution and moderation (Habermas, 2003, p. 29).

Habermas refers to the ability of self-reflection as something species specific for "human nature." For Habermas "human nature" represents an intrinsic good. The problem is, however, that in his moralizing of "human nature," he indirectly presupposes that it is universally definable and that it in itself is morally relevant as a legitimate normative argument against enhancement of human beings by means of biotechnology.[5] However, Habermas' definition of "human nature" is but one interpretation of many and all emphasize different elements of "human nature." Hence, when using "nature" as normative argument, we may refer to the same concept, but the value we attribute to this concept may be very different from the value attributed by other people to the same concept.

To Habermas, and many others (among some of the better known in the enhancement debate are Francis Fukuyama (2002) and Leon Kass (President's Council on Bioethics, 2003),[6] nature seems to represent something *sacred*, that potentially can be violated by technology and Habermas uses this "sanctity" to argue against the use of certain biotechnologies (Fenton, 2006, p.36).

In his article "On the Sanctity of Nature" Gregory E. Kaebnick emphasizes that sanctity does not necessarily lead to an absolute dismissal of biotechnologies, but can be seen as an attempt to adopt a precautionary approach. In relation to this, Kaebnick (2000, pp.22–3) argues:

> Similarly, what kinds of requirements the sacred generates depend on what can be said in each of these various cases. This is only to be expected: if to regard something as sacred is to find some value in its being the way it is, then we would not expect to make any general claims about what the sacred enjoins. It will depend on the nature of the thing we are talking about, and so should vary from case to case.

There is, however, no consensus with regard to the constitution of such sanctity (which is a point that Kaebnick also recognizes), and hence, using "nature," "human nature," or "the natural" as a reference state to something assumed "sacred" is highly problematic.

The way "nature" and "human nature" is interpreted in relation to the emerging new technologies is highly dependent on tradition – the ways nature has been interpreted in culture, history, and religion. The idea of an intrinsic good in "nature" and the "natural" might, of course, be based on specific religious grounds, but it is also embedded in other ideas. For example in the ancient Greek tradition, "nature" represented a single, complex living organism and each part of "nature" has its role and place in this organism. Likewise, one might not feel quite as offended by evolutionary reinterpretations of "transhumanism" when considering the Darwinian interpretation of nature as a historical process, and where human nature (and "dolphin nature" and "snail nature" could be argued as equally relevant here) and "nature" are in constant change over time. Similarly, one could consider nature as a "machine," which can not only be tamed but also mastered.[7] As Philip Hefner (2003, p.190) expressed it in his analysis "Nature Good and Evil":

> There is a consensus that our experience of nature is inseparable from our ideas of nature. Obviously, there are important reasons for saying that nature is prior to and independent from humans. Nevertheless, it also seems to be true that we have no conscious experience of nature that is not significantly under the impact of our human ideas.

So far I have tried to outline how the concept of nature, by virtue of its complexity becomes a challenge when employed in the ethical debate, and particularly the debate surrounding biotechnological enhancement of nonhuman and human capacities. In the following parts of the chapter, I will explore how the concept of nature contributes to two of the most central areas of the enhancement debate: enhancement as something distinct from therapy, and the contentious idea that enhancement represents a moral good.

The Contribution of "Nature" and the "Natural" in the Debate on Enhancement of Human Capacities

In the following section I will take a closer look at the contribution of "nature" and the "natural" in the debate that deals with enhancement of human capacities. In this context, I will refer to enhancement technologies in general; and not only enhancement by means of biotechnology as I outlined in the previous part of the chapter. I will explore the concept of nature and its complexity as reference state in two aspects of the enhancement debate: (i) the perception of nature and the natural and the problem of distinguishing enhancement from therapy; and (ii) the perception of nature and the natural and the idea of enhancement as a moral value.

"Nature" and "naturalness" and the distinction between "therapy" and "enhancement"

Despite the positive value embedded in the word "enhancement,"[8] the ethical status of enhancing human capacities by means of biotechnology lacks consensus. The arguments, both for and against enhancement of specific human capacities which include mood, intelligence, physical capacities, or significant extension of human lifespan, are many, and deal with issues such as autonomy, dignity, integrity, distributive justice, intergenerational justice, to mention just a few. I shall not address these issues as such here, but shall instead focus on the fundamental discussion in which these issues appear, namely the discussion on whether there is a distinction to be made between therapy and enhancement in terms of the nature debate. The main issue in this debate is whether "going beyond therapy" by using technology for the purpose of enhancing human capacities equals "going beyond what is naturally human," and to an extent that can be said to violate values embedded in our perceptions of nature and human nature.

One can describe the distinction between therapy and enhancement as a way to voice a concern that a "technology creep" is taking place. Most technologies that are referred to as enhancement technologies were originally developed for therapeutic purposes. But as they emerge from the context of medicine, they also have prospects for being used for other specifically nonmedical purposes, i.e. their mood, cognitive, or physical enhancing effect if used on "healthy" people. It is the prospect of using such technology on "normal" or "healthy" persons that assigns the name "enhancement" to such technologies. The problem of using "nature" and the "natural" to distinguish between therapy and enhancement is that the argument reveals a paradox: The diseases that cause the need for therapy are also "natural," i.e. part of "nature" understood as what *is in and of itself.* Likewise, one can claim that biotechnologies have an aspect of "naturalness" in their "artificiality," in the sense that they copy and/or make use of biological processes.

An additional aspect to this paradox is the aspect of medicalization. As knowledge about the human genome and different biological processes is expanded, new technologies are being developed in parallel. This development can in itself be said to contribute to a gradual medicalization process. What was previously considered to be "normal"/"natural" human behavior or "natural" conditions of human life may gradually be perceived as a disease or a condition one can choose not to have to live with. The reason is that technologies become available for use, in order to prevent or overcome some existing or gradually occurring behavioral or physical traits that may not previously have been considered as conditions that needed treatment. From this perspective, even aging can be seen as a disease or an imperfect aspect of being human that can be, if not cured, then at least treated for the purpose of living longer.

In this context "nature" and the "natural" play a central role as the *norm* for what is considered as "healthy" or "naturally human" behavior. However, norms tend to change over time: What is "naturally human" in the context of medicine and therapy today, may not be "naturally human" a few years from now. More importantly, what is considered "naturally human" in the context of therapy today is also very different from society's perception of it only 100 years ago. In other words the technology developed for medical purposes may also be said to change our perception of what is "naturally human." The normative employment of "nature" and the "natural" to distinguish between ethical uses of enhancement technologies is therefore rather dubious.

Whereas most people do not consider a technology to be problematic if used for therapeutic purposes, the prospect of using the techniques outside a therapeutic context in order to enhance "normal" functions in humans raises concerns. Therapy is seen as a way of *restoring* or *assisting* the "natural" healing process back to a "naturally human state." This is to be compared with "(technological) enhancement," which, in this context, is defined as an *"improvement," "increase,"* or *"expansion"* beyond the "normal."[9] It is important to emphasize that this distinction between therapy and enhancement must not be mistaken for an attempt to make a moral distinction between the "natural" and the "artificial." It is not the technologies as such, but the *intentions* behind these technologies that are ethically questionable. Hence, it is not a question of whether the method we use is "natural" or "artificial," but rather whether we intend to employ this method for the purpose of *restoring* or *enhancing* what is considered "naturally human."

Arguments that refer to therapy and enhancement as a dichotomy in order to justify use of different technologies for certain purposes but not for others, tend to indirectly presume that there is a certain state of "naturalness," or a "human nature" essence, which can be applied as a reference state in the assessment of the use of a particular technology.[10]

In this particular context, "nature" and the "natural" play an important normative role, which makes it possible to describe "therapy" and "enhancement" as a dichotomy in order to defend technology for therapeutic purposes and reject enhancement of human capacities. An example of such a way of using "nature" and the "natural" as a state of reference is presented in the President's Council on Bioethics" report, *Beyond Therapy* (2003, pp.287–8):

> When a physician intervenes therapeutically to correct some deficiency or deviation from a patient's natural wholeness, he acts as a servant to the goal of health and as an assistant to nature's own powers of self-healing, themselves wondrous products of evolutionary selection. But when a bioengineer intervenes for nontherapeutic ends, he stands not as nature's servant but as her aspiring master, guided by nothing but his own will and serving ends of his own devising.

According to the report there is a moral difference between therapy and enhancement (i.e. in the purpose for which humans use the technology). This moral difference is defined in the relation between human beings and "nature," the latter of which is understood as the world as a whole. Such arguments presuppose that "nature," and therefore everything that can be said to be natural, has a positive value *per se*. The report defends an idea of the "natural" as *that which is given by nature*. In this particular context the value is embedded in "nature's ability to restore itself and in the process of evolution that 'nature' reflects" (Parens, 2005, p.37; President's Council on Bioethics, 2003, p.289). However, as the President's Council on Bioethics also recognizes:

> Respect for the 'giftedness' of things cannot tell us which gifts are to be accepted as is, which are to be improved through use of training, which are to be housebroken through self-command or medication, and which opposed like the plague (President's Council on Bioethics, 2003, p.289).

It is important to emphasize here, that the debate is not about whether technology is "good" or "bad" in itself, and that it should not be mistaken for discussion on whether the "natural" is to be valued against the "artificial." Technology is in this particular debate context, mainly referring to neutral terminology. After all, the ability to develop new technologies is what makes it possible for human beings to overcome some of the ontological challenges that "nature" poses.

Most debaters cherish the aspect of creativity in humans, which is expressed in the ability to develop technologies for the purpose of dealing with challenges encountered in "nature." Nevertheless, it is this very element of human nature that is central to the enhancement debate. The way "nature" and the "natural" are referred to in the enhancement debate, depends on how this "creativity" is perceived and how it is held against other elements of human nature. Kaebnick (2007, p.578) has described the role of "nature" and the "natural" as follows:

> Within the debate about human nature, for example, we might find that considerations about enhancement differ depending on context. We may find that what counts as "natural" is unproblematic in some cases, contestable in others, and too indeterminate to be of any use in others. If there are domains and cases in which the application of the term natural seems appropriate, we will have to think further about the questions of whether and how what is natural is valued.

Arguing for a precautionary approach by using "nature" and the "natural" as a reference state can be a way of expressing a fear of the unknown: it implies recognition of the limits of human nature and of interdependency between human beings and the surrounding world. Furthermore, it suggests the conception of "nature" as an organism; an order of things; or a historical process in which human beings are intrinsically involved. This perception of the relation between humans and "nature" opposes the traditional anthropocentric worldview, where nature is considered as a mere resource available to human beings for our own improvement, exploration, and protection.

Using "nature" or the "natural" as an argument against enhancement can, however, also be a way to express our immediate dislike of something new, that clearly challenges our social norms and our perception of what is "normal". In other words, it may be a way of expressing what some bioethicists have described as the "yuck" factor or "wisdom of repugnance."[11]

Bearing in mind these different representations of "nature" and the "natural" and the complexity with which these appear in the enhancement debate, it is highly problematic to use "nature" and the "natural" as a reference state and as a moral justification of technology applied for therapy but not for enhancement of human capacities.

"Nature" and the "natural" and the idea of enhancement as a moral good

So far I have noted the creative element of human nature as used by skeptics of technology as a means to enhance human capacities beyond the sphere of therapy. In these arguments, human creativity is potentially threatening to other central elements of "human nature" (i.e. dignity in the ability to self-reflect, authenticity, freedom to chose ones own life history etc.). In this last section of the chapter I shall turn to the idea of transhumanism and the claims of enhancement as a moral good. Specifically, I will look at how the concept of nature is applied in pro-(bio) technology positions.

Often, pro-enhancement proponents do not try to make (and normally oppose) any distinction between therapy and enhancement. In this way, it is possible to focus on enhancement as an *a priori* good. Such arguments are often representative of libertarianism ethics, where autonomy, in terms of individual freedom to decide and pursue what is good for "me," is the core value of "human nature," and as such is to be protected above all else.[12] Thus, preventing people from using technology to enhance their physical and mental capacities can be seen as an unacceptable restriction of their autonomy. Such a view dismisses any egalitarian systems of positive or negative rights, in the objective assessment of the benefits of enhancement technologies. Furthermore, although a certain perception of "human nature" (i.e. the element of autonomy) is necessary (i.e. what is a rational agent?), deliberate reference to "nature" or the "natural" is normally to be avoided.

A counter argument in this context is that "what is an enhancement for you, may not be an enhancement for me." Hence, in order to protect people's freedom to act in general, we may choose to reject some enhancement technologies and accept others (Capps, 2010).

However, the transhumanist, for whom enhancement by means of technology is seen as a way of overcoming the limits of "human nature," is apt to employ the concept of nature in a more central role when discussing enhancement.[13] Thus, while libertarian approaches to enhancement in line with views represented in the enhancement debate by John Harris, try to avoid defining what enhancement is,[14] the transhuman approach requires that we return to such questions as the involvement of creativity in the positive enhancement enterprise. For example Nick Bostrom (2008, p.6) emphasizes that when we say "enhancement," we do not express any very precise thought, unless we make clear what it is we understand by "enhancement." Bostrom (2008, p.6) defines enhancement as

> an intervention that improves the functioning of some subsystem of an organism beyond its reference state: or that creates an entirely new functioning or subsystem that the organisms previously lacked.

The definition illustrates the underlying perception of nature as an evolutionary process. "Human nature," and "nature" as a whole, is seen in terms of the (un-)natural selection and modification of beneficial traits and capacities. However, this "natural" evolutionary process is not considered to be unambiguously good in itself and therefore it will not do to merely defend enhancement as an unequivocal good (Harris, 2005, p.16). This is the reason why Bostrom needs to specify what is to be understood from the idea of enhancement. There is, however, as Bostrom (2008, p.6) also recognizes, a problem in defining enhancement, by using "nature" or the "natural" as a reference state:

> There is some indeterminacy in this definition of the reference state. It could refer to the state that is normal for some particular individual when she is not subject to any specific disease or injury. This could either be age-relative or indexed to the prime of life. Alternatively, the reference state could be defined as the "species-typical" level of functioning.

If the definition refers to an individual, it follows that the answer to the question "what is an enhancement?" is subjective and that "enhancement" is a relative term. If instead, the definition is to referring to some species-typical level of functioning, it implies that there is an agreed perception of what it means to be human, from which the enhanced person (transhuman or not) can be distinguished. The problem is, however, as is also the case in the arguments against enhancement technologies, that such a universal definition of "nature" and "human nature" is not available.

The debate on enhancement as it unfolds itself both within and without the context of therapy is an example of how the complexity embedded in the normative references to "nature" and the "natural" becomes a challenge to the debate on enhancement of human capacities. The challenge lies within the complexity of the concept itself, and in the fact that we refer to different aspects at different times and attribute different elements of what we call "nature" or "natural." However, the challenge also lies within the way we use the concept as a normative argument, where it reflects different worldviews, which may be fundamentally irreconcilable.

Conclusion

In this chapter I have outlined the central meanings of "nature" and the "natural" which applies to the debate on enhancement by way of biotechnology. I have shown how these meanings contribute differently depending on whether we are discussing enhancement by means of biotechnology in a food–, environmental– or animal–ethical context, or if we are focusing on enhancement of human capacities. I have focused on the role of "nature" and the "natural" in the more fundamental disagreement on the intrusiveness of biotechnologies as enhancement. In this context, I have outlined the contribution of the concept of nature in what corresponds to the two frameworks introduced by Parens: the "gratitude framework" and the "creativity framework." Furthermore, I have shown how "nature" or "human nature" contributes to the debate in terms of representing or capturing some sort of sacredness towards change. In particular, I have described how the complexity of the concept itself, when applied in its different meanings in the defense of different ethical viewpoints, poses a challenge to the ethical debate. This challenge is twofold: First, the complexity represented by the concept makes it difficult to ensure that we debate on the same grounds. We may think we know what we mean by "nature" and the "natural" but in fact we may refer to different meanings, and use these different meanings in various ways, depending on our more general perception of the world. Second, the analysis of the concept and its role in arguments both for and against enhancement technologies, reveals the problem of finding a common ground on which we can discuss how best to proceed in terms of developing ethical guidelines for future use of enhancement technologies. Bearing this in mind, would it then be plausible to claim that "nature" and the "natural" has a moral relevance in the enhancement debate? Considering the complexity of the concept, it is important that we do not attempt to turn to terms like "human nature," "nature," and the "natural" when looking for a reference state for a common ethical framework for enhancement technologies. Nevertheless, the first step towards reaching some sort of consensus around these technologies is through an understanding of the fundamental disagreements in such debates. An analysis of the contribution of "nature" and the "natural" is crucial in this particular context in order to help us understand why some technologies seem to challenge us more than others. It is in this sense, and only this, that nature can be said to have a moral relevance in the enhancement debate.

Acknowledgments

I am deeply grateful to Benjamin J. Capps and Jonathan Mackenney for their insightful comments and constructive corrections. Needless to say, any errors are those of the author.

Notes

1. I use a broad reference to biotechnology as technology that aims at altering biological processes through utilizing biological systems, living organisms, or derivations of living organisms (see definition of biotechnology in Oxford Online Dictionary: www.askoxford. com). Biotechnology must not be confused with enhancement technology. The term "enhancement technology" embraces many different types of technology, not only biotechnology, and refers to technologies that are mostly developed for the purpose of treatment of illness or a disability, but which also has potential to improve human capacities, when applied in healthy people. Furthermore it must be stressed that not all types of biotechnology are considered as controversial.

2. The enhancement debate is generally associated with debate about enhancement of human capacities. However, we also use biotechnology for the purpose of enhancing food products, and we do this by enhancing the capacities of animals and plants in various ways. It is important to keep in mind that enhancement in this context sometimes raises the same issues as the ones we see in the debate about humans. For example, a Danish survey on the public's attitude to animal cloning showed that most of the respondents could accept biotechnology applied to animals if the purpose was to find ways to improve health and cure existing diseases in humans and animals. However, the majority was against use of cloning and genetic engineering of animals if the purpose was to enhance food quality or productivity in animal farming (see Pedersen, Vincentsen & Andersen (2004). *Borgernes*

holdning til dyrekloning, report by Teknologiraadet for BioTIK-secretariatet, Copenhagen 2004 (this report about the citizens' opinions on animals cloning is only published in Danish). The report is available online: www.tekno.dk/pdf/projekter/p04_BioTik_bor-geres-holdning-til-dyrekloning.pdf. pp. 21–31 and pp.72–5). The idea of enhancement for the purpose of enhancing in itself, seems to cause concern, no matter whether it relates to humans or nonhuman living organisms.

3. Ethical debate on environmental issues that focuses on the value of nature has very often been outlined as a dispute between different worldviews, such as anthropocentrism, deep ecology, biocentrism etc. However, when looking at the debate on biotechnology applied to animals and plants, it is far more nuanced than what can be described in a basic outline of three different worldviews. The complexity with which the concept of nature appears in various contexts such as debates on environment, biotechnology applied in food production, cloning or genetic modification of animals for research purposes seems to suggest that we refer to "nature" or the "natural" as a value in cases where we find the technology particularly intrusive, but this may not mean that we reject the particular technology as unnatural or against "nature" in other cases.

4. "Nature" in the meaning of the essence of a being can refer to something species specific, but it can also refer to the individual human being's character. Whether "nature" refers to one or the other must be seen from the context. Nevertheless this aspect of the complexity with which nature is used complicates the debate even further.

5. Another critique one can draw from Habermas' moralization of human nature, is that Habermas seem to only assume that humans have the capacity for self-reflection. Nevertheless, it is difficult to prove presence or absence of this in animal behavior.

6. Leon Kass was chair of the President's Council of Bioethics in 2002–5.

7. Collingwood (1965) has traced the history of Western interpretation of nature through three normative ideas: the idea of nature as a living organism (ancient Greek); the perception of nature as a machine, which is dominant throughout medieval times to Enlightenment; and "nature" as a historical process, e.g. Darwin's view of nature as evolution.

8. The *Penguin Concise English Dictionary* (2002) defines enhancement as something that has been improved in terms of value desirability or attractiveness.

9. For transhumanists this literally refers to "progress" and the "upgrading" of human capacities.

10. An example of human nature, used as reference state can be found in the President's Council on Bioethics report *Beyond Therapy*: "If there are essential reasons to be concerned about these activities and where they may lead us, we sense that it may have something to do with challenges to what is naturally human, what is humanly dignified, or to attitudes that show proper respect for what is naturally dignifiedly human" (President's Council on Bioethics, 2003, pp. 286–7).

11. The "yuck" factor is usually associated with the notorious rejection of certain technologies based on an emotion-based argument, which claims that the technologies are intrinsically bad, without being able to offer rational objections. Mary Midgley has argued against the total rejection of "yuck" factor arguments in the debate on biotechnology, because, as she says: "debate, however, is hardly ever really between these two (rational arguments versus emotion based arguments)." She says: "On both sides we need to look for the hidden partners. We have to articulate the thoughts that underlie emotional objections and also note the emotional element in contentions that may claim to be purely rational" (Midgley, 2000, p.8). The "wisdom of repugnance" (WoR) is a reference used by Leon Kass that corresponds to the "yuck" factor in terms of the emotion-based element of the

argument. WoR does, however, differ slightly form the first, because it indicates that the repugnance reflects a wisdom, that to some extent call for ethical justification to reject a certain use of a technology: For an outline of the impact of WoR in the enhancement debate, see Kaebnick, 2008, pp. 36–7.

12. The *Stanford Encyclopedia of Philosophy* defines libertarianism as a political philosophy that "holds that agents initially fully own themselves and have moral powers to acquire property rights in external things under certain conditions." In the libertarian view, respect for the individual choice and individual freedom are the core values in the ideal society. The state must above all else be neutral in the ethical question about what can be considered as a good life.

13. McNamee and Edwards (2006, pp. 513–14) distinguish between radical and moderate transhumanism. The first refers to defenders of enhancement as part of a greater project towards improving humanity and overcoming the limits of human nature. The second is characterized by being in favor of enhancement of human capacities based on a libertarian approach to technology, where the individual's freedom to choose and decide whether he/she wants to enhance him/herself.

14. It is unclear on which basis Harris justifies a technology as an enhancement and whether he considers all technology as enhancement, or whether he believes that it is self-apparent what an enhancement is. However, he seems to suggest that the "definition" of what is an enhancement relies on an assessment of the risks and benefits of a specific technology in terms of evaluating the utility in the employment of that technology (Harris, 2005, p.17).

References

Capps, B. (2010): Libertarianism, legitimation, and the problem of regulating cognition-enhancing drugs. NeuroEthics, Online First: DOI 10.1007/s. 12152-010-9059-3, February 24, 2010.

Collingwood, R.G. (1965). *The Idea of Nature* (first published 1945). Oxford: Oxford Paperbacks.

Bostrom, N. (2008). Dignity and enhancement. In *Human Dignity and Bioethics* (chapter 8). Washington, DC: President's Council on Bioethics.

Fenton, E. (2006). Liberal eugenics and human nature – Against Habermas. *The Hastings Center Report*, 36(6), 35–42.

Fukuyama, F. (2002). *Our Posthuman Future: Consequences of the Biotechnology Revolution*. London: Picador.

Habermas, J. (2003). *The Future of Human Nature*. Cambridge: Polity Press (English translation from original German version: *Die Zukunft der Menschlichen Natur. Auf dem Weg zu einer liberalen Eugenik?*, Surhkamp Verlag, Frankfurt Am main, 2001).

Harris, J. (2005). Enhancements are a moral obligation. *Second Thoughts*, Wellcome Science, October.

Hefner, P. (2002). Nature good and evil: a theological palette. In W.B. Drees (ed.), *Is Nature Ever Evil? – Religion, Science and Value* (pp. 189–202). London: Routledge.

Kaebnick, G.E. (2000). On the sanctity of nature. *The Hastings Center Report*, 30(5), 16–23.

Kaebnick, G.E. (2007). Putting concerns about nature in context – The case of agricultural biotechnology. *The Hastings Center Report*, 50(4), 572–84.

Kaebnick, G.E. (2008). Reasons of the heart – Emotions, rationality, and the "wisdom of repugnance". *The Hastings Center Report*, 38(4), 36–45.

McNamee, M.J.& Edwards, S.D. (2006). Transhumanism, medical technology and slippery slopes. *Journal of Medical Ethics*, 32, 513–18.

Midgley, M. (2000). Biotechnology and monstrosity: Why we should pay attention to the "yuck factor". *The Hastings Center Report*, **30**(5), 7–15.

Parens, E. (2005). Authenticity and ambivalence – Toward understanding the enhancement debate. *The Hastings Center Report*, **35**(3), 35–41.

President's Council on Bioethics (2003). *Beyond Therapy. Biotechnology and the Pursuit of Happiness*. New York: Regan Books.

3

Enhancement, Autonomy, and Authenticity

Niklas Juth

Introduction

Some regard enhancement technologies as a threat to autonomy, while others regard enhancement technologies as a way to enhance autonomy. In the following, I will discuss some concerns regarding the effects of enhancement technologies on autonomy and authenticity, insofar as authenticity relates to autonomy. As a preliminary, I note how enhancement and autonomy should be understood in this context along with some examples of enhancement. I go on to explain why enhancement can promote autonomy. Three types of concerns regarding the effect of enhancement technologies on autonomy will be raised: (i) that medical technologies should not be used to enhance autonomy, since this is not the proper use of such technologies; (ii) that some enhancement technologies are inimical to our authenticity; and (iii) that the widespread use of some enhancement technologies have negative overall consequences on people's autonomy.[1]

In general, to enhance something is to raise that thing in degree, intensity, magnitude, or in some sense improve upon it.[2] In this context, we are concerned with enhancements, i.e. amplifications or extensions, of human capabilities, functions, or forms. Two more qualifications need to be made. First, in the spirit of how enhancement is usually discussed, I will confine myself to interventions that go beyond treatment defined (i) as interventions to prevent, cure, or ameliorate disease, illness, or, in general, maladies; or (ii) as interventions aimed at restoring normal (e.g. in the sense of typical species) functioning (DeGrazia, 2005, p.206; Juengst, 2003, pp.753–5).[3] Although the difference between enhancement and treatment is unclear and vague on both these definitions, I will stick with examples that are commonly considered to clearly be at the enhancement side of the distinction. Since I am interested in the common concerns regarding autonomy in the existing debate on

Enhancing Human Capacities,   edited by Julian Savulescu, Ruud ter Meulen and Guy Kahane.
© 2011 Blackwell Publishing Ltd

enhancement, it should be clear enough what I am aiming for: cases which are relatively uncontroversial cases of enhancement and therefore seen as ethically controversial. However, I will return to the enhancement/treatment distinction in the discussion.

Second, I will focus on medical technologies used for enhancement purposes, again in the spirit of how enhancement is usually discussed. Accordingly, conventional and largely uncontroversial measures of enhancement, such as training, education, or diet, will be disregarded unless for purposes of comparison and discussion. Instead, I will concentrate on more controversial measures, which consist of procedures normally used in medicine for treatment purposes, often of a high-technological kind, such as pharmacologic or genetic interventions.

Different kinds of enhancements typically arouse different kinds of concerns as regards autonomy. Four kinds of enhancement are relevant for the following discussion: cognitive, mood, physical, and aesthetic enhancement.

There are various methods to improve basic cognitive capacities, some more or less tested and others speculative.[4] Drugs that stimulate the cholinergic system by increasing acetylcholine levels are already used for the treatment of Alzheimer's disease (e.g. Cognex), but can most likely be developed to improve long-term memory and attention in healthy individuals. More speculative measures to the same effect include somatic genetic intervention, e.g. increasing the number of NMDA receptors. The drug Modafinil has been found to improve working memory, e.g. visual pattern recognition memory, as well as reducing the need for sleep.

Various selective serotonin reuptake inhibitors (SSRIs) constitute the already classic example of mood enhancers.[5] The first generations of these were developed for the treatment of major depressions, but in the same way that cholinergic stimulating drugs can probably be used for cognitive enhancement purposes, SSRIs can probably be more or less effective at improving mood for persons without any clinical symptoms. Due to development in brain imaging and biochips, more specific neuromodulators that target specific neurological receptors can be expected, leading to drugs that can improve cognitive capacities as well as mood with negligible side effects.

Examples of physical enhancement technologies are Erythropoietin (EPO), which can increase endurance through regulating the level of red blood cells; insulin-like growth factor-1 (IGF-1), which can increase muscular strength through anabolic effects; and endorphins, which can increase both endurance and explosiveness through preventing hyperacidity and pain.[6]

What is to be counted as aesthetic enhancement is not as obvious as the above-mentioned examples of physical, cognitive, and mood enhancement, since opinions on what is aesthetically appealing differ to a great extent. However, there are measures that are taken with the obvious purpose of becoming more beautiful and attractive in the eyes of at least some others, which are more invasive and involve medical technologies to a larger extent than everyday measures, such as exercise and sunbathing. An example here is cosmetic surgery, which includes facelifts, nasal reconstruction, and breast augmentation, not done in order to remedy some malformation or accident.[7] To be more speculative, there may be genetic interventions that increase propensity for height (Buchanan *et al.*, 2002, p.3).

Autonomy

As generally defined, to be autonomous is to govern oneself; and to live autonomously is to live in accordance with one's basic desires or values.[8] Accordingly, autonomy is a matter of degrees: A person can more or less lead the life she has chosen, more or less choose how to live, and her desires can be more or less her own. One can discern three components from this general characterization: will (or desire, or value, i.e. pro-attitude); decision; and action. How autonomous a person is in various parts of her life is determined by all these components and all can vary in degree. First, the pro-attitude a person acts from can be more or less authentic, that is, self-determined or truly the person's own. Second, one can be more or less decision competent, that is more or less capable of successfully performing the task of deliberation. Third, one can be more or less efficient, that is capable through action to carry out what one has decided.

This general characterization of autonomy says nothing in itself about how autonomy matters morally. Traditionally, in biomedical ethics, autonomy has primarily been considered as giving rise to negative rights or side-restrictions on how we are allowed to treat each other (Beauchamp & Childress, 2001): If an individual is adult and competent enough to make decisions, other individuals should not prevent that individual from making decisions and acting upon them, at least if he does not violate the rights of others (as Locke thought) or inflict damage on someone else (as Mill thought). According to this line of reasoning, we thus have a duty (at least of a *prima facie* kind) not to restrict the autonomy of others. In biomedical ethics, this line of reasoning has been taken as the ground for not being manipulated or coerced into accepting a medical treatment.

However, in the enhancement discussion, the considerations of autonomy have seldom been in terms of autonomy as a right. Rather, as we will see, it has been claimed that enhancement can decrease or increase individuals' autonomy: Enhancement can make us lead more autonomous lives or become more autonomous persons; or it could threaten our autonomy in various ways. In these claims, autonomy is presupposed to be a value that can be promoted or threatened. Therefore, it becomes important to try to evaluate in what way and to what extent enhancement could promote or threaten our autonomy.

Enhancement Promotes Autonomy?

Can enhancement technologies promote individuals' autonomy? The answer is *yes*. In general, plans require capacities in order for them to be put in effect and enhancement technologies can increase our capacities to do the things we need to do in order to effectuate our plans. For scholars, or indeed anyone for whom intellectual endeavors are part of important plans and projects, increasing long-term memory and attention can make people more efficient in realizing their self-determined plans. As mentioned, it is not impossible that drugs targeting specific cognitive capacities will be developed, e.g. visual pattern recognition memory, which may aid for instance graphic designers and architects in becoming better at fulfilling their most cherished projects.

More generally, enhancement technologies could target mental process capacities that are used in deliberation, e.g. information processing, that in principle could further anyone's capacity to make difficult decisions involving a great deal of relevant information (Juth, 2005, pp.152–5).

The border between cognitive and emotional capacities is far from clear cut, and autonomous decision making and action is also affected by mood. First, a better mood can help a person uphold the "mental energy" required to see an arduous plan through. Second, many consider the ability to scrutinize one's values, desires, and plans to be an essential component of autonomy (DeGrazia, 2005, pp.101–6; Juth, 2005, pp.142–6; Lindley, 1986, p.56). But such scrutiny can be a tough exploration into one's own psyche, facing up to parts of oneself that are difficult to accept and handle. A not-to-gloomy general outlook can make this scrutiny easier, facilitating avoidance of self-deception or depression.

Of course, for an athlete, or indeed anyone who tries to accomplish beyond the ordinary in athletic endeavors, the above-mentioned physical enhancements can be an aid. And if one has a well-considered desire to become more physically attractive in one's own eyes or in the eyes of someone else, then aesthetic enhancement can improve one's chances of fulfilling this goal.

At the same time, it is important to note that enhancement technologies do not in themselves *necessarily* promote any individual's autonomy. This depends on a lot of facts, e.g. what the actual and autonomous values, plans, and desires of a particular person are, to what extent using enhancement technologies is an efficient method to accomplish these plans as compared to other methods, to what extent enhancement methods compromise other important goals one has as compared to other methods etc. Nonetheless, it is not difficult to see how the use of enhancement technologies can make many of us more autonomous persons and increase our chances of living more autonomous lives, i.e. the lives that we would want to live according to our own standards.

Promoting Autonomy is Irrelevant?

The ability of at least some enhancement technologies to promote autonomy, at least sometimes, can be employed as an argument in favor of using such autonomy-promoting enhancement. However, some would regard this argument as irrelevant, although perhaps true, since they would say that medical measures should be used to prevent, cure, or ameliorate disease or improve health and not to enhance capacities or performance beyond this. This line of reasoning refers to the well-known distinction between treatment and enhancement in order to delimit the boundaries of legitimate health care.[9]

As already mentioned, the distinction between treatment and enhancement can be explicated in different ways. However, the familiar problem of explaining in a way that is clear and unambiguous enough to handle difficult cases in the gray zone remains, whichever way one chooses to make the distinction. What counts as disease or not varies over time and seems to be susceptible to changes in common opinions on what is normal, valued, and problematic. Familiar examples are today's discussions of the extent to which problems with reproduction, potency, fatness, and general mood should be regarded as proper medical problems (Brülde & Tengland, 2003). However, some of the examples mentioned at the beginning of the chapter clearly fall outside the scope, such as increasing the number of NMDA receptors or using the drug Modafinil in order to improve working memory for a person already working at a high level of memory functioning, or using IGF-1 in order increase muscular strength through anabolic effects. To say a distinction is vague or in some respects unclear is not to say that there is no distinction at all.

Even so, something has to be said in order to support why this distinction is relevant: Why is it that medical measures in general and medical technologies in particular are legitimate only when employed to preventing, treating, or ameliorating disease or restoring health? One line of reasoning of a communitarian kind is to claim that medicine has certain internal values or goals that determine whether a certain medical measure is justified or not.[10] How are we to determine these values and goals? By investigating the actual doings and sayings of those engaged in the practice in question, i.e. by looking into which medical interventions that physicians and patients in general agree are useful and proper and which are not (Engelhardt, 1990; Good, 1994). Most would agree that to prescribe Ritalin for ADHD is within a physician's professional purview, while to prescribe EPO to further enhance endurance for an elite cyclist is not.

This line of reasoning could be employed to argue against any kind of enhancement, but is particularly common within the debate on physical enhancement, especially the one related to doping in sports. In this debate, it has even been claimed that to use e.g. genetic technologies of the kinds mentioned at the outset in order to improve skills or performance is to use a medical means for a nonmedical end (or goal), which amounts to medical malpractice (Ljungqvist 2005).[11] Even though the communitarian thought that the internal goal of medicine to combat disease and restore health sets the limits for what is proper medicine is seldom explicitly mentioned in these discussions, something of the kind has to be presupposed in order for the argument to get off the ground.

However, this communitarian line of reasoning is problematic, for several reasons. For one thing, there are the general problems with this kind of view on morality: It makes it hard to see how one can question the values and goals of a practice, since it is the values and goals of the practice that determines what is right and wrong within the practice to start with. Perhaps this kind of morality stems from skepticism regarding the possibility of justifying external moral criticism at all; one may, like Walzer (1983), believe that there are no universal moral standards beyond those internal to different practices. Although this meta-ethical position cannot be properly evaluated here, it is highly debatable and, to my mind, not very plausible at all (Dworkin, 1985).[12]

However, even if one accepts this communitarian view on morality, it is increasingly difficult to say that enhancement for autonomy-promoting purposes cannot be within the proper bounds of medicine. This is so, since it is obvious that there are other goals than that of combating disease and improving health that are increasingly recognized by standard medical ethics as important goals for health care. The most conspicuous one in recent decades is none other than autonomy: It has become more common to defend various medical practices with reference to their ability to promote patients' autonomy.

The fact that autonomy is increasingly becoming an independent goal in health care is most salient in areas of medicine where there have been extraordinary recent developments, such as genetics, assisted reproduction, and prenatal diagnosis. Genetic counselors have considered the promotion of autonomy as the primary rationale for their work for quite some time now (Wertz & Fletcher, 1988). One of the most interesting features from "the point of view of autonomy" is the content of the rationale, in genetics especially regarding presymptomatic testing for diseases that cannot be treated or ameliorated in any way (and accordingly hard to justify with reference to the traditional goals of preventing or treating disease), e.g. Huntington's disease: If a patient possesses knowledge regarding her future health, she is in a better position to plan her life in accordance with her own basic wishes.[13] This line of reasoning has also been used to justify offering assisted reproductive technologies and prenatal diagnosis: these procedures should be allowed since they can help couples to realize their plans for a family, i.e. the technologies promote reproductive autonomy (Chadwick *et al.*, 1999).

In this line of reasoning, it is obvious that autonomy is not conceived only as a right that ought to be respected, as is the traditional way of conceiving autonomy in biomedical ethics. Instead, autonomy is conceived as a goal to be achieved or as a value to be promoted, which is used to justify *introducing* a medical practice. However, the exact same line of reasoning that is used by esteemed representatives of the medical profession to justify presymptomatic genetic testing, assisted reproduction, prenatal diagnosis, and other medical practices, can be used to justify genetic enhancement. For as we have seen, just as the increased information from a genetic test can help a person to better realize her own plans, the increased capacity to perform due to some enhancement procedure can also help a person to better realize her plans, i.e., live an autonomous life.

By now, it becomes clear that those who claim that genetic enhancement for other purposes than to prevent, cure, or ameliorate disease or improve health cannot be a part of legitimate health care are in a tight spot. They could say that autonomy should not be a goal of health care. If they say so and are from the medical profession, they will probably upset some of their colleagues, not least those from clinical genetics. These colleagues would probably be even more upset if they still hold that, for instance, assisted reproduction, prenatal diagnosis, or presymptomatic genetic testing for autonomy-promoting purposes amounts to medical malpractice. Or they could grant that promotion of patients' autonomy can be a legitimate goal for health care. However, in such case, procedures that enhance the capacities of persons so that they become more autonomous could be a legitimate part of medicine.

The general point is the following: Even if we grant that some genetic procedures should be allowed with reference to the internal goals, ends, or values of medicine, there are other such values than preventing, curing, or ameliorating disease or improving health. What is regarded as crucial goals for health care changes over time and autonomy is increasingly emphasized as a goal in its own right. So even if one tries to settle the issue of the limits of legitimate medical measures with reference to the internal values of medicine, it is far from obvious that these values do not already harbor the possibility of justifying the use of at least some enhancement technologies, since they promote the values many medical practitioners and much medical ethics actually regard as vital. For instance, the dramatic increase in the prescription of Ritalin in the United States for other purposes than treating ADHD can be interpreted as an expression of this (DeGrazia, 2005, p.210).

Authenticity and Enhancement –Physical and Aesthetic

A different kind of concern about enhancement technologies from the point of view of autonomy agrees that these technologies can give people what they want at a superficial level, but denies that they could or would promote individuals' autonomy in a deeper sense. These concerns typically involve considerations of authenticity. In general, being authentic is being true to oneself or being who one really is (Taylor, 1992). In the context of autonomy, authenticity is about the extent to which one's will really is one's own and, in effect, the extent to which one can succeed in really "being oneself" or "becoming oneself," since autonomy is about living in accordance with one's *own* will.[14] This kind of concern can be spelled out in different ways and typically looks differently depending on what kind of enhancement technology is being debated.

Regarding aesthetic and physical enhancement, the argument is often that using such enhancement is an expression of societal norms that are morally problematic or oppressive and reinforces such norms. Take for instance female breast augmentation; some would say that the desire to have larger breasts is really the result of specific patriarchal norms regarding how women should look in order to be attractive in the eyes of men, as well the general patriarchal norm that women should mold themselves into fitting these norms. To satisfy these kinds of desires is far from enabling the women in question to live more autonomous lives. Rather, it is to reinforce the oppression that impedes the living of an autonomous life for women.

A similar line of reasoning has been employed in the debate of the use of genetic technologies in order to increase physical performance in sports (Miah & Rich, 2006): If such technologies were available, this would reinforce exceedingly performance-oriented norms, our tendency to label people after inherited talent (at least regarding germ-line genetic modification and genetic testing performed to spot genetic susceptibilities of various sorts) and other kinds of questionable societal beliefs and norms. Would satisfying these requests really assist those who use the technologies to help them realize their own self-determined plans of life?

This kind of argument represents no novelty in the bioethical debate on new technologies. For instance, some opposing assisted reproduction claim that the desire of women to have biological children of their own at least to some extent is *the result* of technologies for assisted reproduction, for instance IVF, being offered, since they reinforce societal norms that a "real" woman should have biological children of her own.[15] So the desire is the result of a cultural indoctrination of a gender oppressive kind, by being part of common beliefs and norms that contribute to the subordination of women.

In fact, there are two distinct arguments at work in the line of reasoning just presented. One argument says that it is wrong, or at least morally questionable, to act on these oppressive or otherwise morally problematic norms since they will then be *reinforced*, i.e. one contributes to the problematic norm by acting on it. I will return to this kind of argument later. The other argument is that satisfying desires will not promote the autonomy of a person if the desire in question is the result of cultural indoctrination, at least if the indoctrination is of an oppressive kind.

This last idea is clearly about the authenticity of individuals and their values, desires, and plans. The idea seems to be that if one has a desire which is the result of an oppressive culture, this desire is not self-governed and if it is not self-governed then it cannot be authentic. This idea is in line with our general picture of autonomy: To be autonomous is to govern oneself or to determine one's own way. If the desires one acts on are not self-governed, then the person acting is not self-determined, since she is not effectu-ating her *own* plans (even if she is unimpeded to effectuate the inauthentic plans she has).[16]

However, what does it mean for a desire to be self-governed? It cannot be the self-governed *forming* of or *creation* of all one's desires from the start. Since all desires entertained by a person have a causal history that is (at least partly) uncontrolled by the person herself, the self-governance of the creation of the desire cannot very well be the mark of authenticity (unless we would like a theory of authenticity implying that no actual person can have authentic desires).[17] On the contrary, any conception of authenticity must be compatible with the obvious fact that we are all formed in a society with certain values, norms, and rules that take part in the shaping of persons.

However, one could claim that desires that are the result of *oppressive* indoctrination are inauthentic, even if other origins of desires are irrelevant for their authenticity. This would amount to a "moral" or "substantial" ideal of authenticity, since it refers to the inherently normative conception of oppression. However, there is a huge difference between what desires, values, and plans we ought to have and which are autonomously had. Perhaps we should try to avoid having or acting on desires that express or are the result of oppressive norms, but that is not to say that these desires cannot be authentic from the point of view of autonomy.

In general, it does not seem true of *any type of origin* that it makes a desire inauthentic from the point of view of autonomy. The problem with such a suggestion is that it disregards the person's own judgment of her situation and desires and thus the *self* of the idea of self-determination. Rather, it is the person's own attitude towards the origin that matters to authenticity.[18] In order to make this last point more credible, consider the example of hypnosis, which seems to present an intuitively strong image of inauthenticity. If hypnosis may cause someone to hold a desire, then, generally speaking, the forming of the desire is in a sense not self-governed. But there is a huge difference between, for instance, the hypnosis of an unsuspecting victim in order to use her for some end she would not approve of herself and the voluntary subjection to a hypnotist in order to quit smoking. Presumably, in the first case, the person would not approve of the desire she has come to hold in the face of knowledge about why she has come to hold it. This is probably not true of the last case. However, even if the person unsuspectingly and against her expressed desire were made to desire to quit smoking, she might not be inclined to give that desire up when she found out why she has this desire. And why should the desire then be considered to be inauthentic from the point of view of autonomy?

Similarly, if one learned that one's desire to have biological children or to undergo some performance enhancing technology, was the result of a norm, the general acceptance of which contributes to or is a part of one's subordination in some regard and one with full awareness of this still is no way inclined to revise this desire, why should it be considered as being not one's own in any autonomy-reducing way? To hold this would require some reference to a notion of a "true self" or impartial reasons that have little to do with authenticity in the sense relevant for autonomy (*self*-determination) and more to do with objective or impartial ideals of human welfare and flourishing. To govern oneself is not necessarily to do good. It is to voluntarily act on self-determined decisions and desires. And a desire is self-determined if the person having it would approve of it in the light of information of why she has it, not if she ought to approve of it in the name of social justice or the like.

If we accept this line of reasoning we see that there is no way in which desiring genetic enhancement *must* be inauthentic, *even if* such desires in general are the result of oppressive or in some other way morally problematic norms.

Authenticity and Enhancement – Cognitive and Mood

A partly different set of worries relating to authenticity has been raised with regard to cognitive and mood enhancement. It is less about compliance with problematic norms,[19] as in the case of physical and aesthetic enhancement, and more related to changing one's person or personality, which is probably taken to be closer related to cognitive and affective functions than physical appearance and performance.

A representative sample of this type of worries is voiced by Elliott (1999, pp.28–9):

> What is worrying about so-called "enhancement technologies" may not be the prospect of improvement but the more basic fact of altering oneself, of changing capacities and characteristics fundamental to one's identity... Making him smarter, giving him a different personality... mean, in some sense, transforming him into a new person.

The worry can be interpreted in at least three ways. First, the worry may be that enhancement can make someone cease to exist by changing her in a very fundamental manner, i.e. affecting the numerical identity of someone. This opinion has been successfully rebutted elsewhere and I will not repeat the arguments here (DeGrazia, 2005). Anyway, even if one holds that numerical identity in principle can be ended by qualitative changes in mental capacities, as the psychological view would have it, none of the enhancement technologies mentioned in this text could produce such a dramatic change.

Second, the worry may be regarding using medical enhancement technologies *as a means* for changing personality. This worry is clearly expressed in the following passage from Kass (2003, p.22):

> ...biomedical interventions act directly on the human body and mind to bring about their effects on a subject who is not merely passive but who plays no role at all. He can at best feel their effects without understanding their meaning in human terms... Thus, a drug that brightened our mood would alter us without our understanding how and why it did so —whereas a mood brightened as a fitting response to the arrival of a loved one or an achievement in one's work is perfectly, because humanly, intelligible.

From the point of view of autonomy, this argument cannot have much force. If one has a self-determined plan and using some enhancement technology, probably in combination with other measures, is the most efficient way to realize this plan, it is hard to see what the problem is from the point of view of autonomy. In terms of this not being understandable "in human terms" is difficult to see, both from the point of view of autonomy and in general: Why is it not even *possible* to understand why one becomes happier from using SSRI or more able to perform complicated graphic tasks from using Modafinil? And what does it mean to understand something "in human terms"? Is it not *typical* of humans to be able to understand how bodily changes can give rise to different mental states and events, unlike most other animals?

However, a third interpretation of both the worry of Elliott and Kass is that the use of some enhancement technologies not only effectuate the realization of the plans, values, and desires of a person, but may also change that person so much that it changes her very plans, values, and desires into others than those she had before using the enhancement technology in question, even to such an extent that the person before and after the changes deems these pro-attitudes differently.

This is probably not true of most enhancement technologies, for instance, the scenario in which reducing the need to sleep and gaining in some respects a better working memory by using Modafinil, changes one's deeply held convictions and plans of life is hard to imagine. However, it is not inconceivable that such a change could be the result of using more powerful cognition and mood enhancement drugs. Imagine a neuromodulator that could drastically change one's general mood in a (much) more cheerful direction. After using such an enhancement, someone might find her old interests in gothic subculture an expression of attitudinizing gloominess, while the person before the enhancement kicked in would find the enhanced person an intolerably dashing cheerful fellow. The problem here is that the attitudes of the person have changed to the extent that the "new me" disapproves of the "old me" and vice versa or, in other words, her very outlook on her life has changed.

However, radically changing one's outlook on one's life cannot in itself make the resulting outlook inauthentic. Otherwise the development of new outlooks would automatically make us inauthentic. Is the problem then that the change is allegedly faster than normal when using enhancement? It is hard to see why the speed of the process would matter in itself and, moreover, sometimes we drastically change rather quickly as a result of some unexpected experience.[20] Is it the lack of pain and effort? It seems to have little to do with autonomy and more to do with some kind of chauvinist work ethics to claim that changes of personality have to be arduous in order to be authentic.

Enhancement and Autonomy on a Larger Scale

Some concerns regarding enhancement technologies and autonomy primarily regards the effects of these technologies at the collective level. If we presuppose that we can to various degrees increase and decrease each other's autonomy depending on what we do, such concerns are not farfetched: Questions of autonomy are (sometimes) questions of distributive justice, given that autonomy is not conceived of only as a negative right to be respected. So even if someone can promote her autonomy by using a certain enhancement technology, it is conceivable that the more general use of such a technology decreases the total level of autonomy as compared to the situation where this technology is not used at all (or to a very limited extent). Of course, any such claim must be highly speculative, e.g. due to the difficulty of comparing levels of autonomy.[21]

Nonetheless, there are situations where such claims seem to have some credibility. For example, if the establishment and use of a certain enhancement technology creates a strong social pressure for others to use it as well.[22] For instance, if it becomes commonplace enough to use long-term memory enhancement, even those who have no initial plans to use such technology may feel compelled to so anyway, in order not to decrease their social opportunities. The same sort of claim can also be made about doping in sports (see Tamburrini and Tännsjö, chapter 20, this volume).

However, not all kinds of social pressure are bad even from the point of view of autonomy. A trivial example is the social pressure not to resort to violence when disagreeing or being upset with someone, a norm which likely has positive overall consequences in terms of our possibilities to fulfill our self-determined plans. With regard to the overall effects on autonomy, there seems to be an important distinction between two types of enhancement: those which primarily give competitive advantages and those which give advantages besides possible competitive ones, where the former are more likely to reduce overall autonomy if there is a strong social pressure to use them. An example of an enhancement technology in which the advantages are almost exclusively competitive is the use of IGF-1 in sports: It would primarily be used in order to gain a competitive edge where explosive strength matters, e.g. weightlifting. Of course, if such use became widespread among weightlifters, the pressure to use it would increase at the same time as the competitive advantage of using it decreases, with remaining risks to health related to anabolic measures that threaten most individuals' plans in general. On the other hand, cognitive and mood enhancements mentioned earlier have the potential to improve autonomy for individuals regardless of possible further competitive advantages, or so it was argued.

As previously mentioned, a related kind of concern regards reinforcing oppressive or morally problematic norms by using a certain enhancement. However, for most enhancement technologies mentioned in this chapter, it is unclear what norm that would be, if any.[23] Nonetheless, there are cases when this risk seems likelier than other cases. For instance, it is not farfetched to claim that the increasing use of cosmetic surgery, e.g. breast augmentation among women, reinforces sexist norms, e.g. that women transform themselves to become attractive in the eyes of men.

However, it is highly doubtful whether any single individual acting on the norm (e.g. by performing breast augmentation) thereby reinforces it. If anything, it is the widespread practice that reinforces the norm, not individual expressions of it. Moreover, the cost for the individual in terms of fulfilling her plans, dreams, and ambitions may be quite high if she abstains from using the technology in question. So we may have a prisoner's dilemma kind of situation: anyone using the technology may be better off in terms of autonomy, but everyone who does so may be worse off in terms of autonomy than if no one used the technology to start with. However, even in such an obvious example as breast augmentation, the problem is not this procedure as such, but the norm that is reinforced by using the technology.

Concluding Remarks

The use of various kinds of medical enhancement technologies can promote individuals' autonomy. However, there are autonomy-related concerns as regards such use. I have raised three such concerns. First, there is the claim that medical technology should be used to prevent, cure, or ameliorate disease or improve health and not to promote autonomy, since only combating disease is within the proper bounds of medicine, determined by its internal values and norms. However, even if one agrees that the internal goals of medicine determine what are the proper boundaries of medicine and which medical measures should be used, it is increasingly difficult to say that enhancement for autonomy-promoting purposes cannot be within the proper bounds of medicine, since autonomy is increasingly emphasized as a goal in its own right within health care in general.

Second, there are concerns regarding whether the use of medical enhancement technologies is compatible with individuals' authenticity. Several such concerns are related to autonomy. One is that the desires or values that one acts from using some medical enhancement technologies, especially as regards aesthetic and physical enhancement technologies, are the result of oppressive or otherwise morally problematic societal norms and thus cannot be autonomous desires or values. I have tried to indicate why such desires and values are not necessarily problematic for autonomy-related reasons, although they certainly can be so. As regards cognitive and mood enhancement, it has been claimed that such enhancement technologies are problematic due to the potentially personality changing effects such enhancement can have. I have argued that such effects do not have to be problematic from the point of view of autonomy, if the changes are rationally approved of by the resulting personality.

Third, there may be large-scale effects on individuals' autonomy from more widespread use of enhancement technologies. Although speculative, these are the most troubling concerns, especially with regard to enhancement technologies that have only competitive advantages or reinforce socially problematic norms. Regarding the last kind of enhancements, we may very well end up in prisoner's dilemma situation: Anyone using the technology in question may be better off in terms of autonomy, but everyone who does so may be worse off in terms of autonomy than if no one used the technology to start with. However, it is far from obvious how we should face up to these kinds of possibilities. Should we ban such enhancements, tackle the problematic norms in some other ways, or something else? To answer this crucial question is beyond the scope of this chapter but certainly a question that needs to be tackled.

Notes

1. In this chapter, no definite stand is taken on what should be done if these concerns are well founded, e.g. whether this means that the use of the enhancement technologies should be outlawed, that it should not be provided by public health care, that individual physicians ought not to offer them or individual patients ought not to use them, or something else.
2. According to the *Oxford English Dictionary*, quoted from the President's Council on Bioethics, 2003, p.17.

3. A third type of way to make the distinction between treatment and enhancement is in terms of what is generally considered to be within the domain of physician's professional purview. I will return to this kind of distinction later.

4. For more on present and future methods of cognition enhancement, see Sandberg, chapter 5, this volume.

5. For more on present and future methods of mood enhancement, see Berghmans *et al.*, chapter 10, this volume.

6. For more on present and future methods of physical enhancement, see Tamburrini and Tännsjö, chapter 20, this volume.

7. For more on cosmetic surgery, see Benatar, 2006.

8. For more on autonomy in general, see Juth, 2005, chapter III.

9. Or in order to determine which health care that should be publicly funded and which should not (see e.g. Daniels, 2008).

10. See Daniels (2008) for another way of drawing and justifying the distinction with reference to preserving "normal opportunity range" for patients through maintaining their functional capacities typical for humans within the reference group in question. This approach has been extensively debated elsewhere and I will therefore not try to evaluate it here. For a criticism of this way of making the distinction between treatment and enhancement, see Juengst, 1997.

11. Perhaps it is not a coincidence that this way of thinking is predominant in the area of sports, as it clearly connects with how many anti-doping proponents think about sports in general: What is to be allowed and not within sports should be determined with reference to the internal values and norms of the sport in question (Loland, 2002).

12. To mention only one problem with this kind of morality concerning the ought/is-distinction: How does one get from facts regarding the actual values and norms of practice to the claim that the practice ought to abide to these norms and values?

13. For numerous references to geneticists and ethicists presenting this line of reasoning, see Juth, 2005, especially chapter II.

14. According to some influential contributors to the autonomy debate, authenticity is the most fundamental or philosophically most interesting component of autonomy (see e.g. Christman, 1988).

15. This type of argument is most common among representatives from FINRRAGE (Feminist International Network of Resistance to Reproductive and Genetic Engineering), perhaps most famously by Corea, 1985. However, see Sherwin (1992) for a similar line of reasoning. Later feminist bioethicists tend to be skeptical against this type of argument (see e.g. Purdy, 1996 and Donchin, 1996). However, the argument still crops up now and then (see e.g. Sparrow, 2006, p.312).

16. This relates to the often-invoked idea from e.g. Marxism, existentialism, and feminism that real power and oppression is not to prevent people from doing what they want, but to make them want what you want them to want. To act from such wants is *mauvais foi*.

17. For much the same reasons, one should reject conditions that say that a desire that is the result of someone else's deliberate attempt to install that desire is inauthentic, since this would mean that all desires that are the result of ordinary parental efforts of raising are inauthentic. Not many basic desires may remain given such a strict condition.

18. This claim is of course controversial and has to be substantiated much more thoroughly than can be done in this context. For such an argument, see e.g. Juth, 2005, pp.129–51, and DeGrazia, 2005, pp.95–106.

19. Even if such worries could be raised, e.g. regarding hyper-competitiveness (DeGrazia, 2005, p.219).

20. This at least Kass must consider to be okay, given what he says in the quote above.
21. For more on comparisons and measurements of autonomy, see Juth, 2005, pp.187–97.
22. Another such situation may be if access to some enhancement is very unequally distributed and leads to a very strong competitive advantage for those with access to it: In such a situation those without access may have autonomy more circumscribed than those with access gain in terms of autonomy.
23. Take for instance the cognitive- and mood-enhancing technologies mentioned above: What problematic norms would be reinforced if people improved upon their memories or mood to a larger extent using these technologies? Even though there are conceivable answers, such as "social conformism" or "competitiveness" these are highly speculative (for instance, why should tolerance for unusual behaviour in general decrease if people in general are in a better mood?) and one might as well point to positive norms that could be reinforced, such as "critical attitude" (if people in general are more energetic and intellectually able they might become more eager to question persisting conditions). Nothing says that the last speculation is more incredible than the former.

References

Beauchamp, T.L. & Childress, J.F. (2001). *Principles of Biomedical Ethics*, 5th edition. New York: Oxford University Press.

Benatar, D. (ed.)(2006). *Cutting to the Core: Exploring the Ethics of Contested Surgeries*. Lanham, MD: Rowman & Littlefield.

Brülde, B. & Tengland, P.A. (2003). *Hälsa och sjukdom – en begreppslig utredning (Health and malady – a conceptual inquiry)* Lund: Studentlitteratur.

Buchanan, A., Brock, D., Daniels, N. & Wikler, D. (2002). *From Chance to Choice*. Cambridge: Cambridge University Press.

Corea, G. (1985). *The Mother Machine: Reproductive Technologies from Artificial Insemination to Artificial Wombs*. New York: Harper & Row.

Chadwick, R. *et al..* (eds.) (1999). *The Ethics of Genetic Screening*. Dordrecht: Kluwer.

Christman, J. (1988). Constructing the inner citadel: Recent work on the concept of autonomy. *Ethics*, 99(1), 109–24.

Daniels, N. (2008). *Just Health – Meeting Health Needs Fairly*. New York: Cambridge University Press.

DeGrazia, D. (2005). *Human Identity and Bioethics*. New York: Cambridge University Press.

Donchin, A. (1996). Feminist critiques of new fertility technologies. *Journal of Medicine and Philosophy*, 21(5), 475–98.

Dworkin, R. (1985). *A Matter of Principle*. Cambridge, MA: Harvard University Press.

Elliott, C. (1999). *A Philosophical Disease: Bioethics, Culture and Identity*. New York: Routledge.

Engelhardt, H.T. (1990). Human nature technologically revisited. *Social Policy and Philosophy*, 8(1), 180–91.

Good, B. (1994). *Medicine, Rationality, and Experience: An Anthropological Perspective*. New York: Cambridge University Press.

Juengst, E.T. (1997). Can enhancement be distinguished from prevention in genetic medicine. *Journal of Medicine and Philosophy*, 22(2), 125–42.

Juengst, E.T. (2003). Enhancement uses of medical technology. In S.G. Post (ed.), *Encyclopedia of Bioethics, 3rd edition*. New York: Macmillan.

Juth, N. (2005). *Genetic Information – Values and Rights: The Morality of Presymptomatic Genetic Testing*. Göteborg: Acta Universitatis Gothoburgensis.

Kass, L. (2003). Ageless bodies, happy souls. biotechnology and the pursuit of perfection. *The New Atlantis*, **1**, 9–28.

Lindley, R. (1986). *Autonomy*. London: Macmillan.

Ljungqvist, A. (2005). The international anti-doping policy and its implementation. In C. Tamburrini & T. Tännsjö (eds.), *Genetic Technology and Sport – Ethical Questions* (pp. 13–18) London: Routledge.

Loland, S. (2002). Sport technologies – A moral view. *Research in Philosophy and Technology*, **2**, 157–76.

Miah, A. & Rich, E. (2006). Genetic tests for ability? Talent identification and the value of an open future. *Sport, Education and Society*, **11**(3), 259–73.

President's Council on Bioethics (2003). *Beyond Therapy. Biotechnology and the Pursuit of Happiness*. New York: Regan Books.

Purdy, L.M. (1996). *Reproducing Persons. Issues in Feminist Bioethics*. New York: Cornell University Press.

Sherwin, S. (1992). *No Longer Patient*. Temple, PA: Temple University Press.

Sparrow, R. (2006). Cloning, parenthood, and genetic relatedness. *Bioethics*, **20**, 308–18.

Taylor, C. (1992). *The Ethics of Authenticity*. Cambridge, MA: Harvard University Press.

Walzer, M. (1983). *Spheres of Justice: A Defence of Pluralism and Equality*. Oxford: Blackwell.

Wertz, D.C. & Fletcher J.C. (1988). Attitudes of genetic counsellors: A multinational survey. *American Journal of Human Genetics*, **42**(4), 592–600.

4

Breaking Evolution's Chains: The Promise of Enhancement by Design

Russell Powell and Allen Buchanan

Only quite recently in the history of life has nature produced a species whose understanding of evolution makes possible the intentional modification of its own genome. There is mounting evidence, including successful genetic modifications of laboratory animals (Tang *et al.*, 1999), that human beings will eventually be able to change their physical, cognitive, and emotional capacities by modifying their genes.[1] To an extent that it is now impossible to gauge, human beings will be able to take charge of their own biological development and evolution. Evolutionary theory is becoming self-reflexive: Understanding how evolution works is enabling us to modify the course of our own evolution – if we choose to do so.

Some find the prospect of "intentional genetic modification" (henceforth IGM) repugnant or at least dangerously hubristic. The most vocal critics of IGM declare that it is foolish to disregard the wisdom of nature. Some who make this charge explicitly appeal to science rather than religion: They explicate the idea of the wisdom of nature by recourse to what we will call the master engineer analogy (MEA). They believe that from an evolutionary perspective, the human organism is like the product of an engineering genius – a "delicately balanced," completed, well-functioning masterwork. On this view, IGM is likely to be disastrously counterproductive, like the blundering efforts of a child to improve on the intricate, well-thought out work of an engineering genius. Consider, for example, the following assertions of the (U.S.) President's Council on Bioethics (2003, pp.287–88):

> The human body and mind, highly complex and delicately balanced as the result of eons of gradual and exacting evolution, are almost certainly at risk from any ill-considered attempt at "improvement"..... It is far from clear that our delicately integrated natural bodily powers will take kindly to such impositions, however desirable the sought-for change may seem to the intervener.

Enhancing Human Capacities, edited by Julian Savulescu, Ruud ter Meulen and Guy Kahane.
© 2011 Blackwell Publishing Ltd

Let us call the claim that *because evolution is like a master engineer, there should be at least a very strong presumption against IGM* the "MEA argument." Although those who employ the MEA argument sometimes condemn all efforts to use biomedical technologies to improve human life, they tend to be especially averse to IGM. Whether the MEA argument is sound depends upon how apt the MEA is.

In this chapter, we critically examine the evolutionary assumptions that underlie the notion that nature is like a master engineer. Our strategy is to compare and contrast IGM with unintentional genetic modification (UGM), or the ordinary descent with modification that occurs when human beings lack or refrain from using IGM technologies. More precisely, we compare UGM and IGM as to their potential for improving human life.

We use the label "*unintentional* genetic modification" rather than "*natural* genetic modification" for two reasons. First, because human beings are part of nature, the modification of genes that they intentionally undertake is no less natural than that produced by the so-called "blind watchmaker" of classical Darwinian theory. Second, in some contexts, including some of the literature that rejects IGM, the term "natural" is covertly used in a positive evaluative sense, the assumption being that the natural is good or at least preferable.[2] Steering clear of the term "natural" helps avoid prejudicing the comparative evaluation of IGM and UGM.

In the first section of this chapter, we argue for two main theses. (i) UGM operates under constraints that severely limit its ability to realize what human beings rightly value, including their own survival and improvement. Because IGM can remove these constraints, it is *more versatile* than UGM and hence potentially more effective in promoting human well-being. (ii) IGM is also potentially *morally preferable* to UGM, since the latter is wantonly destructive of life, often involves suffering on a massive scale, and is utterly insensitive to the requirement that the costs of improvement ought to be fairly distributed. In the second section, we articulate the kernel of truth in appeals to the wisdom of nature, arguing for the need to develop appropriate cautionary heuristics for IGM. We show that the set of cautionary heuristics offered in a recent article by Bostrom and Sandberg on the ethics of IGM betrays a Strong Adaptationist bias in its understanding and interpretation of evolution, and should be rejected in favor of criteria that are grounded not in adaptive etiology but causal ontogenetic relationships. We conclude that evolutionary theory, far from grounding a prohibition or even a strong presumption against IGM, instead supports a presumption *in favor of* developing technologies for IGM, so long as appropriate causality-based precautionary heuristics are adhered to. Not only should nature not get a free pass, but it should not even be afforded the benefit of the doubt.

Unintended versus Intended Genetic Modification as a Means of Improving Human Welfare

The master engineer of evolution

Biological function evaded naturalistic explanation for thousands of years. The puzzle was finally solved in 1859, when Charles Darwin introduced the theory of natural selection, which provided a non-teleological (mechanistic) account of the origin and evolution of biological design. If Darwinian theory effectively banished intelligent design from evolutionary explanation,[3] what could philosophers mean when they attribute "wisdom" to nature and then appeal to it as a reason against IGM? Their idea is that over eons of evolutionary trial and error, the Darwinian crucible has produced 'ingenious solutions' to challenging 'design problems', achieving a degree of perfection that humans are overwhelmingly unlikely to improve upon. According to this view, organisms (including human beings) are like the finished products of a master engineer.

Even scientifically sophisticated bioethicists with a generally positive view of IGM have a tendency to rely on the MEA. For instance, Bostrom and Sandberg (2008) caution that when "an over-ambitious tinkerer with merely superficial understanding of what he is doing [makes] changes to the design of a master engineer, the potential for damage is considerable and the chances of producing an all-things-considered improvement are small."

But organisms are remarkably *unlike* the work of a master engineer in two fundamental respects. First, unlike a master engineer, evolution never gets the job done: Organisms are not the endpoints of an evolutionary process that gradually but steadily climbs the ladder of perfection. Hence they are not delicately balanced finished products in danger of being upset or destroyed by human intervention. Second, evolution does not "design" what it produces according to a plan that exists (even if only in rough outline) at the beginning of production. Each of these points and their significance for the MEA argument will become clear as we carefully consider the constraints under which UGM operates. Once the severity of these constraints is appreciated, the force of the MEA evaporates, and the analogy becomes so attenuated as to be quite incapable of supporting a prohibition on or even a strong presumption against IGM. On the contrary, the fact that IGM has the potential to overcome these powerful constraints on UGM provides a strong justification of the former.

The notion of constraint is empty unless a context is supplied; more specifically, it is necessary to specify what is being constrained. Broadly speaking, constraint in evolutionary biology relates to circumstances limiting the nature of design problems and their set of possible solutions. Here we use the term very differently. The evolutionary features that we catalog in the remainder of this section are constraints on the effectiveness of UGM as a process by which to promote (or even preserve) human well-being.

(1) The ubiquity of suboptimal design It is ironic that proponents of the MEA argument regard the theory of natural selection as support for the analogy, since it is the *imperfection* of biological design that is among the strongest evidence for evolution by natural selection. Darwin himself frequently pointed to the faulty, irrational construction of organisms in the service of rebuking arguments for intentional (and intelligent) design. In a letter to his friend and mentor Joseph Hooker, Darwin (Dawkins 2003) exclaimed: "What a book a Devil's Chaplain might write on the clumsy, wasteful, blundering low & horridly cruel works of nature!" Examples of poor biological design abound: the urinary tract in male mammals, which passes through (rather than being routed around) the prostate gland, and which consequently can swell and block urinary function, leading to infection; the primate sinus which has a feeble

drainage system; the inability of humans to synthesize vitamin C due to a mutation that most mammals do not have, a physiological disability which over the course of history has led to disease and countless deaths; the "blind spot" in the vertebrate eye (resulting from quirks of embryological development) forcing vertebrates to develop elaborate and costly perception-correcting mechanisms; the human pharynx whose dual function of both ingestion and respiration significantly increases the possibility of choking to death; the birth canal passing through the female pelvis, dramatically increasing the dangers of childbirth, thanks to selection's hasty re-arrangement of hominid posture. The list goes on and on.

Let us now turn to the *mechanisms* that originate and maintain suboptimal design in nature. Once these mechanisms are understood, it will become clear that suboptimal design is not the exception but rather the rule; it is a pervasive, systematic feature of UGM.

(2) Insensitivity to the post-reproductive quality of life Beyond a certain age, humans (like many organisms) will contribute little to the gene pool of the next generation, and thus with some rare and controversial exceptions, natural selection tends not to act on the post-reproductive period of life. This simple truth has enormous implications for the MEA, for if natural selection is the sole driver of optimality, then the vast majority of post-reproductive traits do not benefit from evolution's putative engineering genius. Therefore, the notion that all or even most biological traits are the result or the necessary side effect of natural selection is patently false. Once its reproductive years are spent, the organism is allowed to "drift" (ontogenetically speaking), accumulating mutations in cell lines leading to cancer, cardiovascular deterioration, and neural degeneration. Natural selection puts little value on the physiological repair of post-reproductive traits, an evolutionary neglect which leads to debilitating disease and ultimately death. For these reasons, nearly all post-reproductive traits and ailments fall outside the sphere of the master engineer's activity. This state of affairs is particularly relevant to long-lived organisms like ourselves, for whom a large proportion of life is post-reproductive. That alone should give pause to those who invoke the MEA.

One of the chief advantages of IGM is that it can avoid or ameliorate the harms that humans suffer as a result of UGM's insensitivity to their post-reproductive quality of life. For example, modifications of oncogenes or tumor-suppressing genes could reduce the incidence of cancer in later life (Weinstein, 2002),[4] and changes in the genetic networks that regulate hormones could prevent or retard muscle loss and frailty in the elderly (Schroeder *et al.*, 2007).

(3) Selection does not imply optimality, and optimality does not correlate with survival The MEA argument hinges on two chief assumptions: (i) natural selection is the predominant cause of biological traits; and (ii) natural selection tends to produce traits that are optimal. We have good reason to question assumption (i), since there is a major controversy as to whether natural selection is the default or even the predominant force in evolution (Brandon & Rausher, 1991), especially when it comes to larger patterns in the history of life where stochastic processes may play a more significant causal role (Raup, 1991). Population bottlenecks, mass extinctions, and founder effects can impose a highly circumscribed set of initial conditions that severely constrain the

subsequent operation of natural selection (Manica *et al.*, 2007). Even more funda-mentally, a proper re-conceptualization of evolution reveals that drift is in fact the *default* state of biological systems, rather than a *ceteris paribus* addendum to selection theory (Brandon, 2006). All else being equal, biological systems will tend to deviate from optimal character states. These are strong reasons not to equate evolution with natural selection, or to assume that selection is the dominant evolutionary mechanism.

But even if (i) were true, and selection was the only significant process acting on biological systems, there are a number of reasons why (i) does not logically or empirically imply (ii). First, simply because natural selection has acted on a trait does not entail that the trait is optimal. "Adaptation" in the most uncontroversial sense refers to the *etiology* of a trait – namely, that it *arose* and *came* to fixation (with emphasis on the past tense) as a result of natural selection. On the contrary, "optimality" refers to the *current* function of a trait and (perhaps) its contribution to reproductive fitness, *irrespective* of its selective history. This distinction is important; it shows that we cannot assume that the same forces that originally selected for a trait are the ones which currently maintain it. A trait that evolved due to its ability to solve a design problem in the distant past may persist long after that initial design problem is gone, due either to a shift in function ("exaptation") or to various evolutionary impediments to extinguishing it (see sections 4, 6, 9–10). Second, even if the evolutionary history of a trait is dominated by selection, this does not imply that selection has the reflexes (so to speak) to keep up with the shifting ecological sands of time. Environments can fluctuate stochastically and sometimes too rapidly for selection to track.

The transience of optimality is nicely illustrated by the so-called "Red Queen" hypothesis. The biologist Leigh Van Valen (1973) found that the probability of extinction for a given lineage is always independent of its age. Because lineages tend to optimize their adaptations over time, this surprising finding suggests that lineage survival does not co-vary with adaptive optimality. The dominant interpretation of this finding is that an organism's selective environment is constantly crumbling beneath its evolutionary feet, with the result being that it must run in place (i.e. adapt) merely to remain where it is (i.e. in existence). The decaying nature of the selective environment is due in part to the strategic interaction among co-evolving species (which generates evolutionary arms races), and in part to the supervenience of fitness on stochastically fluctuating abiotic factors, such as climate change and tectonic activity. Contrary to proponents of the MEA argument, existing traits (including our own) do not represent the adaptive apex of eons of exacting selection. Extant evolutionary forms are by no means superior in adaptive design to those that litter the fossil beds. They are just another step on the unrelenting treadmill of UGM.

As we shall argue later, there are good reasons to be cautious about IGM, but the fear of disrupting an organism's "delicate balance" or perfect adaptation to "the" envi-ronment is not one of them. The notions of "delicate balance" and "perfect adaptation" both assume a degree of environmental and functional stability that simply does not exist in nature.

(4) Evolutionary "hangovers" On most accounts, to say that X is an adaptation is to say that X is the product of an historical selective regime (Brandon, 1990). As we have just emphasized, since the environment and the design problems it poses are constantly in

flux, organisms can never be perfectly adapted to their environment. Thus, many of the traits that were fitness-enhancing in early hominid evolution may be either neutral or maladaptive today. This is not surprising, given that the origin and evolution of the human genus predates the modern condition by nearly a million years. Such "Pleistocene hangovers" may include traits like the predilection toward sweets and fatty foods, stepchild abuse, and xenophobic aggression. Evolutionary psychologists believe that many of our contemporary psychological disorders, such as depression, anxiety, and attention deficit disorder, stem from the difficulties associated with the psychological adjustment of hunter-gathering *homo sapiens* to a sedentary, monotonous, indoor existence. A similar diagnosis applies to many of the disorders observed in canine companion animals, who with equal difficulty are forced to adjust from a roaming pack life to the confines of the living room sofa.

Some hangovers are more severe in their constraining effects than others; evolutionarily speaking, the "Cambrian hangover" is perhaps the most profound. This phrase refers to the overarching parameters of the vertebrate body plan that have been entrenched (or developmentally locked in place) for some 500 million years. Vertebrate architecture has been tugged and contorted in countless directions by selection over the history of life. For instance, the vertebrate body plan designed for swimming was (in some lineages) reconfigured to accommodate terrestrial walking, and then (in a number of those lineages) transformed once again in order to re-assume a fully aquatic life. Hence there is no reason to believe that the parameters of the vertebrate body plan approach perfection. Natural selection is a *bricoleur*, not an engineer, much less a master engineer – that is, it tinkers with organisms in response to immediate need, co-opting existing structures in ad hoc fashion to meet new functional demands. Selection rarely creates things de novo, and it *never* plans ahead.

(5) The origination and fixation of mutations One obvious limitation on UGM relates to the origin and spread of beneficial mutations, a process which can take thousands or even millions of years, depending on mutation rates, population structure, and the type of the adaptation in question. Although the strength of selection pressures is an inherently difficult thing to measure, there is no question that the stronger the selection, the faster the rate of adaptive fixation (*ceteris paribus*). This would make strong selection pressure a desirable thing, if only it did not require the lamentable Malthusian scenario where there are far more births than environmental resources can support. For instance, in ancestral human populations, enormous death rates from smallpox and bubonic plague were associated with strong bouts of episodic selection leading to the fixation of pathogen-resistance (Galvani & Slatkin, 2003). The end result may be agreeable, but the process leading up to it can be nasty, brutish, and *long*.

For example, suppose (as has already proved to be the case with respect to resistance to some strains of HIV) we learn that some desirable gene or complex of genes already exists, but only in a small number of humans. Waiting for this genotype to proliferate throughout the human population through UGM would be not only empirically problematic, but morally catastrophic (Bostrom & Sandberg, 2008). Selection for the trait might not be sufficiently strong so as to result in its proliferation; and even if it were, chance events could intervene (e.g. a flu pandemic or a war could destroy the critical population of humans); and even if they didn't, the process might take thousands of years, during which time millions of people who lacked the genotype would die or suffer serious illness. Suppose also that it were possible to ensure the much more rapid proliferation of the genotype by administering an injection into the testes or, more radically, by inserting genes into embryos in the context of *in vitro* fertilization. Surely, the fact that IGM could not only realize the same beneficial results that UGM is capable of achieving, but that it can do so much more reliably, quickly, and with far less human carnage should count morally in its favor. IGM technology can also safeguard valuable genotypes much as early humans cradled fire, protecting the source of survival for current and future generations.

(6) Linkage, epistasis, and the inaccessibility of macromutation The blind and incremental nature of natural selection not only places severe constraints on how quickly natural selection can accomplish a given adaptive feat, but also on which adaptive feats can be accomplished at all. Mutation and recombination, which together provide the raw materials for natural selection in sexual organisms, impose severe constraints on what selection can work with and how it can do so. For example, when fitness-enhancing genes are located on the chromosome close to neutral or maladaptive genes (a ubiquitous phenomenon known as *linkage disequilibrium*), they will be bound together in the recombinatory shuffle and jointly destined to enter the next generation, despite the latter's detrimental effects on the phenotype. This assumes, of course, that the net gain in fitness associated with the beneficial gene outweighs the net cost from its being linked to a deleterious gene. If the benefits do not outweigh the costs of linkage, then selection will be unable to favor (i.e. differentially produce) the salutary gene. Analogous constraints are entailed by pleiotropism (where genes code for multiple unrelated functions), and by complex (epistatic) interactions between genes where the developmental state of one gene affects the function of another. Moreover, because natural selection is a blind and incremental process, it faces insurmountable hurdles when confronted with a design problem that requires hundreds or even thousands of *simultaneous* mutations to solve. Similarly, the probability of realizing any particular mutational trajectory is the product of its constituent mutations. As the number of requisite mutations grows, the chance of their contiguous or simultaneous realization decreases exponentially.

In sum, many mutational trajectories (and hence beneficial mutations) will be off-limits to natural selection, due to linkage, pleiotropy, epistasis, and the astronomically small probability of macromutation. In contrast, what is an astronomically improbable feat for natural selection can be a relatively simple task for an engineer, let alone a *master* engineer. Macromutations are well within the ambit of IGM, which is not limited to acting blindly and incrementally. The point here is not merely that IGM can usher in sweeping genetic change at a much faster pace than UGM (which it can), but that IGM can accomplish what are otherwise impossible adaptive solutions.

Thus, IGM could be an invaluable resource – literally a matter of life or death for the species – in the case where humans are confronted with an imminent design problem, the solution to which is either completely inaccessible to incremental selection, or else only achievable over vast stretches of evolutionary time. For example, IGM might enable us to alter the body's capacity for thermal regulation as an adaptive response to global warming, or to increase our resistance to emerging infectious diseases or environmental toxicity. Furthermore, by tapping into embryonic regulation, IGM has the potential to go well beyond trait *enhancement* to the wholesale *transformation* of developmental organization. As beings who can recursively reflect on the mechanisms and circumstances of their own origin, humans could learn to transform the evolutionary process in ways not possible for UGM.

(7) The absence of "lateral" gene transfer in the ugm of animals The vertical transmission of desirable mutations in complex multicellular animals is laborious, given long generation times and the fact that reproduction and gene transfer are inextricably linked (DNA transmitted between animal lineages by viruses may be an exception). This is in stark contrast to bacterial life forms, which have both rapid generation times and horizontal (lateral) modes of gene transfer. Lateral gene transfer enables organisms to exchange genes outside of sexual reproduction, allowing for the much more efficient proliferation of fitness-enhancing traits. However, IGM can act in complex multicellular species as lateral gene transfer does in prokaryotes, greatly increasing the speed and versatility with which salutary mutations can spread through the population. Through IGM, we could combine and integrate the genes of human beings who are not members of the same lineage, as well as genes from other species and those artificially created via synthetic biology. IGM-based lateral gene transfer is essentially the biological version of non-vertical cultural transmission. Like cultural exchange between members of the same generation or between different reproductive lineages in a population, lateral transfer via IGM comes with attendant risks, such as the more rapid spread of deleterious variants. Nevertheless, IGM promises to put the pace of biological evolution back on par with its cultural counterpart.

(8) Species extinction and the irrevocable loss of genes In UGM, when species go extinct, their distinctive genes are lost forever. Extinction is an absorbing boundary in nature – it is by definition irreversible, particularly in the case of the genetic basis of complex phenotypic traits, whose iterated independent origin is highly improbable. In contrast, human-initiated gene banks (akin to the Global Seed Vault which recently debuted in Norway) can be maintained in both analog and digital form long after extinction in the wild, and genetic information can even be resurrected from ancient fossil materials. To this extent, IGM can stave off and even reverse natural extinction events that would otherwise be inevitable or irrevocable. Ironically, then, the common criticism that IGM ought to be banned because it might result in irreparable mistakes applies with even greater force to UGM, which will often result in the irrevocable loss of potentially valuable genetic material.

The worry that IGM could result in irreparable mistakes is a serious one, but it deserves further scrutiny than it usually receives. The technology is already available for switching off modified genes (that is, blocking their expression) and for inserting them into the organism in a dormant state, requiring the administration of a drug to switch them back on. Hence, even if an intentional genetic modification turned out to be an error, it does not follow that it would be irremediable. To think so is to be taken by the fallacy of genetic determinism – that is, to confuse the genotype with the phenotype, or the presence of a gene with its (invariable) expression.

(9) Optimization of one trait is not improvement overall Even if one trait is "optimized" by natural selection, this does not preclude it from having detrimental consequences for other traits, so long as the selection pressure or fitness benefit associated with the former is strong enough to compensate for the damage done to the latter. In other words, UGM (via natural selection) permits damage to the organism so long as there are sufficient compensating benefits. For instance, in early hominid evolution, there was a strong selection for bipedalism, due in part to the scattering of resources and the inefficiency of knuckle-walking as a mode of locomotion. Apparently, the fitness benefits from bipedalism were so great that they outweighed the substantial costs associated with the reconstruction of the hominid skeleton in order to accommodate this new form of locomotion, including some of the highest rates of neonatal and maternal birth mortality in the animal kingdom, not to mention a susceptibility to debilitating joint and back problems. On top of this, human medical technology has greatly reduced the incidence of child mortality (through, for example, Caesarean section), relaxing selection pressure for additional (beneficial) modifications of the pelvis. If a master engineer were to design a bipedal mammal with a brain large enough for high levels of intelligence, it certainly would not have these features. Ligament tears and birth complications are not the necessary side effects of bipedalism (after all, it probably wasn't common that T-Rex tore a knee ligament), but rather they are the unfortunate consequences of a hastily assumed and highly constrained evolutionary tradeoff. IGM may be the only way to ameliorate situations in which human technology has essentially stabilized a suboptimal adaptive configuration.

(10) The inability to break out of stable local optima Even if we assume that natural selection is the dominant evolutionary force and that the selective environment remains stable over long periods of time, obstacles to optimization remain. The degree of optimality that can be achieved in nature is highly contingent on the topography of the *adaptive landscape*. This refers to a pictorial representation of the functional relationship between individual genotype/phenotypes and the environment. Where a lineage initially finds itself in the fitness landscape is largely a matter of historical contingency. If the landscape is composed of numerous fitness peaks and valleys, then selection will cause a population to climb the nearest fitness peak, even if that peak is not the highest one in the landscape. It will henceforth be stranded on this globally suboptimal peak, since to navigate to a higher one would entail that it cross a region of low fitness, which stabilizing selection will not permit. Thus, what appears to be an optimal solution from a local vantage point may be highly suboptimal when viewed panoramically – a perspective that is well beyond the limits of mechanistic evolution.

With regard to human beings in particular, there is no reason to believe that their current location in the fitness landscape is globally optimal, and in fact there are many reasons to think it is not (see sections 1, 2, 4, 6 and 9 above). With a bird's eye view of the adaptive landscape, however, IGM could prevent a population from drifting from or being locked into a local optimality. It could do this in part by identifying the highest peak, circumventing natural (spatiotemporal) barriers to gene flow, and coordinating the assembly and fixation of complex adaptations from the component traits of disparate populations.

This leads us to a crucial point: in many instances, adaptive suboptimality persists *because of* – not despite – natural selection. It is powerful stabilizing selection which resists downhill excursions in the fitness landscape, and which prohibits the evolutionary tweaking of "upstream" developmental networks that would otherwise permit the sweeping reorganization of organismic architecture. Nevertheless, even local optimality is far from guaranteed, as populations may permanently deviate from their local peak as a result of drift, mutation, linkage disequilibrium, migration, in-breeding, pleiotropy, and many other non-selective factors that can drive evolutionary change.

(11) Optimality is context-dependent Some authors have argued that if natural selection is the dominant force in evolution, then evolution should lead to optimal function, since selection tends to maximize fitness (Orzack & Sober, 1994). However, the link between adaptation and optimality remains empirically and philosophically tenuous (Brandon & Rausher, 1991). Even if there is a link, it does not support the MEA argument. Simply because a trait has been "optimized" by natural selection does not mean that it cannot be improved upon. To conflate "optimal" here with "unimprovable" is to misunderstand the nature and role of optimality in evolutionary theory. Any optimality analysis in evolutionary biology must take into account the relevant genetic, developmental, anatomical, and functional parameters that act as "engineering" constraints, just as the materials available for a construction project constrain the universe of viable engineering designs. Actually, the very notion of optimality is unintelligible when abstracted from these constraints (Sansom, 2003).

To say that a trait is optimal only entails that no further *incremental* changes in the genotype can significantly improve on the function of the trait, *given the relevant set of developmental and evolutionary parameters*. Optimality does *not* preclude, however, that non-incremental changes can result in a trait that is represented by a higher fitness peak in the overall landscape. Even if all traits are currently optimal, this is fully consistent with the possibility of an IGM-induced "leap-frog" to a higher fitness peak. The more expansive our view of the adaptive landscape, the better we will be at identifying the highest peaks; and it is only by developing IGM that we are ever likely to get there. Given the context-dependency of optimality, we should view IGM as expanding the range of the possible, rather than threatening an impeccable masterpiece of natural selection (Buchanan, 2009).

(12) The most profound constraint of all: UGM selects for traits based on fitness, not their tendency to promote human good Richard Dawkins (1986) has famously likened the process of natural selection to the work of a blind watchmaker. The idea that the watchmaker is blind does something to convey the fact that evolution does not know what it is doing, but the metaphor is misleading so far as it suggests intention. There is a more basic flaw in the analogy, however. A watchmaker, be she blind or sighted, builds something to satisfy human desires and needs; natural selection, in contrast, only "aims" at reproductive fitness; and reproductive fitness is not the same as human good.

To say that a particular trait tends to increase reproductive fitness, is just to say that it increases the probability that the genes of the organism bearing the trait will be passed on to future generations, either through the organism's own reproduction or through that of its kin. Even if every extant human trait contributes to reproductive fitness and does so in a reliable way, and even if any IGM-based change would therefore be detrimental to reproductive fitness, it would *still* not follow that any effort to improve us is likely to make us *worse off*, for the simple reason that human well-being is not the same as reproductive fitness. If we plot the desirability of traits against their contribution to inclusive fitness, there may be significant overlap between the curves, but they will not perfectly map onto one another. This is because maximizing the number of genes the current generation passes on is not the only thing of value, if it is of value at all, either for individual human beings, or for humanity collectively.

It might turn out that to maximize the number of genes the current generation passes on, the best strategy would be to increase the human population up to the Malthusian breaking point – that is, to have as many offspring as possible, even if this meant that all should be merely subsisting in conditions of dire poverty, deprived of most of what makes for a good human life. The point is that fitness only concerns the expected *number* of viable offspring – it remains totally insensitive to either the parent or the offspring's *quality of life*. Moreover, one person's conception of the good may be to crank out as many offspring as they can in their short time on earth; for others, having fewer (or no) offspring enables them to pursue other sorts of projects that make their life meaningful; and yet still others may choose to forego reproduction altogether in order to adopt the children of others who are in need of care.

The blind watchmaker analogy obscures the most profound constraint on UGM – namely, its effectiveness as a means of achieving human good – because it encourages a fundamentally mistaken view of what natural selection is about. It is not about human improvement. When UGM, operating through natural selection, produces what is valuable for human beings, it does so by sheer coincidence. And it would be unwise to wager the prospects of human survival, much less the prospects for improvement, on sheer coincidence.

The threads of the argument thus far can now be pulled together. Appeals to the wisdom of nature are frequently couched as if they either offer conclusive reasons to forego IGM, or at least constitute a strong presumption against it. In nonreligious contexts, the opponents of IGM typically cash out the idea of the wisdom of nature by likening UGM, operating through natural selection, to the work of a master engineer. On the basis of this analogy, they conclude that IGM is likely to worsen, not improve, the human condition. The picture of IGM that this analogy conveys is that of a blundering child damaging the "delicately balanced," completed work of a master engineer who has produced a product that admirably serves human ends.

We have argued that the MEA is so flawed that it cannot serve as an adequate basis for prohibiting IGM or even as a strong presumption against it. The current human organism is not a stable, completed product and the forces that have shaped it are not directed toward the human good. UGM does not engineer and re-engineer until it produces "optimal" organisms, henceforth sustaining them in a "delicate balance." On the contrary, optimization is imperfectly approximated, fleeting, and always relative to a set of constraints. Moreover, UGM is compatible with human beings having any number of features, from the propensity toward cancer during the post-reproductive years to high mortality during the birth process, that are eminently undesirable from the standpoint of human good. The appropriate move, therefore, is to discard the MEA and with it the view that nature's wisdom cautions against IGM.

A better analogy would be this: UGM is like the work of a morally blind, fickle, and tightly shackled tinkerer. The tinkerer is *morally blind* in a twofold sense: he does not have human well-being as a goal and he shows no scruples in his choice of means for achieving his ends. If a (transient) adaptation is achievable only by massive death and suffering, that is no concern of his. He is a *tinkerer*, not a master engineer, because he does not produce objects according to a plan conceived in advance; furthermore, he is fickle and always destroys his handiwork eventually, often before he has achieved his extraordinarily limited goals (i.e. producing solutions to immediate design problems without regard to long-term consequences). He is *tightly shackled* in the sense that he operates under severe constraints – potentially useful tools lie all about him, but he cannot reach them because he is tethered in a small corner of a vast workshop. The proposal to intervene in the work of a morally blind, tightly shackled tinker looks far more promising than the proposal to manipulate the work of a master engineer.

A Better Way to Think Responsibly about Intentional Genetic Modification

Thus far we have argued (i) that the unintentional genetic modification (UGM) that occurs through evolution as understood in Darwinian theory is quite unlike the work of a master engineer and that consequently (ii) attempts to argue against IGM on the basis of this faulty analogy are unconvincing. We have not merely shown that the analogy is imperfect– that would make the mistake of demanding that an analogy be an identity. Rather, we have argued that the MEA is seriously flawed as an analogy designed to provide guidance regarding IGM, because it conveys a grossly distorted view of UGM and thereby encourages a very unfavorable comparison between the two. We have argued that once the inadequacy of UGM as a process for protecting and promoting human well-being is appreciated, and once the profligate moral costs of the process are duly considered, the prospect of IGM looks more favorable. For IGM has the potential to overcome the severe constraints under which UGM operates, and can be used in such a way as to reduce or avoid the death and suffering that results from whatever improvement in the human condition UGM might happen to achieve.

We have *not* argued that IGM poses no serious risks. Indeed, everything we have said so far is compatible with the conclusion that IGM in humans ought not to be undertaken. We have shown only that the attempt to ground a prohibition or strong presumption against IGM fails *insofar as it is grounded in the deeply flawed MEA*. This is compatible with there being other weighty reasons for caution about IGM.

We now want to suggest that instead of appealing to the wisdom of nature or the genius of the master engineer of evolution, it would be better to focus more directly on the risk that intentional genetic modifications (like other human actions) can have unintended bad consequences, and then develop strategies for attempting to reduce this risk. Framing the matter of due caution regarding IGM as a matter of risk reduction is appropriate, given the fact that IGM has the potential to promote human good more effectively and at lower moral cost than UGM. Given the good that might be attained by and *only* by IGM, some risk may be worth bearing.

The inadequacy of adaptationist cautionary heuristics

We noted earlier that Bostrom and Sandberg, two philosophers who reject any prohibition or strong presumption against IGM, nonetheless take the MEA seriously and assume that it provides a sound basis for caution about the use of IGM. To their credit, instead of resting with the platitude that we should "go slow" or "proceed with caution" in the use of IGM, these philosophers go on to offer a set of more contentful cautionary heuristics, based, as they see it, on an appreciation of evolutionary theory. The difficulty is that their view of evolution, and hence their cautionary heuristics, presuppose an increasingly discredited understanding of evolution – namely, "Strong Adaptationism," a view which postulates the inexorable tendency of natural selection to overcome developmental constraints that would otherwise lead to adaptive suboptimality (Amundson & Lauder, 1994). But even if Strong Adaptationism were the correct view of evolution, their approach to cautionary heuristics would still be defective, because it focuses on adaptation, rather than upon the risk that IGM will disrupt what might be called "benign causal interdependencies" and in so doing produce bad unintended consequences.

Bostrom and Sandberg (2008) advocate a heuristic for intervention which they call the "evolutionary optimality challenge" (EOC). The EOC places the burden of proof on IGM proponents to meet the following adaptationist test: "If the proposed intervention would result in an enhancement, why have we not already evolved to be that way?" The authors propose this optimality criterion because they feel that it reflects the kernel of truth in the MEA argument.

The EOC can be based on either or both of the following claims: (i) if X is an adaptation, then X will tend to be optimal from an evolutionary and/or moral standpoint; (ii) if X is an adaptation, then manipulating its genetic underpinnings will tend to produce negative phenotypic consequences. (i) is clearly false, as the above discussion demonstrates. Placing themselves squarely in the increasingly discredited Strong Adaptationist tradition, Bostrom and Sandberg proceed as if natural selection is the only important cause of biological traits, and that traits, being adaptive, tend to be optimal. As we have seen, neither is the case. (ii) makes no claims about optimality (the EOC moniker notwithstanding). It is simply the reasonable assertion that caution is needed in modifying parts of the genome that code for complex phenotypic adaptations. The nonlinear interactions between genes and gene networks certainly counsel against the willy nilly manipulation of sequences coding for highly integrated functions. But so too should it caution against cavalier alterations of *non-adaptive* or *neutral* segments of the genome, which can have comparable (or even more serious) collateral effects. Due to "epistasis," or the interaction between genetic loci in relation to their effect on the phenotype, the manipulation of neutral alleles can alter the causal-selective regime of their non-neutral counterparts.

There is of course nothing wrong with issuing caution about IGM in the context of adaptive traits; the problem with Bostrom and Sandberg's heuristic, however, is that it focuses perilously on the *wrong set of facts*. As a result, it can lead IGM seriously astray by suggesting looser standards for the modification of maladaptive or non-adaptive segments of the genome.

There is no question that genetic perturbations, especially early in ontogeny, can wreak havoc on biological function; but this is true *whether or not the target of intervention is an adaptation.* What matters for the purposes of assessing the potential negative consequences of IGM is not whether the target of intervention is related to an adaptation (i.e. a trait with a selective etiology), but rather *how the target genes are causally connected with other genes and gene products in the ontogenetic unfolding of the organism.* In other words, our best guess as to the probable effects of IGM should always rest on an assessment of current causal capacities – not events in the distant past. Strong Adaptationism, which adheres to a purely etiological conception of function, sheds little light on this question.

To see why this is so, consider that there are two conceptual approaches to function in biology. The most popular is the "etiological" or "selected effects" version of biological function, which attributes a trait's function to its particular selective history (Wright, 1973). The "causal role" version of function, on the other hand, is concerned not with the genealogy of a trait, but rather its current causal properties (Amundson & Lauder 1994). Now for the crucial point: in the context of IGM, the current causal properties of the target render any adaptive etiology statistically irrelevant with respect to the unintended negative consequences of intervention. This is not to say that adaptive etiology cannot provide some basic clues about the risks associated with intervention; but a sufficient understanding of current causal capacities (or the co-variance structure between genes and phenotypic traits) renders information about genealogy moot. If I wanted to figure out what my college roommate was up to nowadays, I would give him a call or ask his neighbors; I would most certainly not dig up our college correspondence in an effort to reconstruct the past, merely to make an educated guess at what he might be doing in the present. And yet this is precisely what the EOC would have us do.

At this point, Bostrom and Sandberg might argue that given our current epistemic limitations regarding both the general nature and fine-grained details of complex causal networks, we should focus instead on selected effects which are easier to determine than current causal capacities. Were this in fact true, it would at least provide some basis for their adaptationist heuristics. But it is simply not the case that selected effects functions are easier to ascertain than causal role functions; in fact the reverse is probably true. "Just-so stories" may in some cases be easier to concoct than hypotheses regarding proximate causal dynamics, but this does not make them any more likely to succeed in helping us to avoid the negative consequences of intervention. In contrast, mathematical simulations have been used to model nonlinear developmental networks, allowing for specific predictions regarding the effects of mutation, genetic modification, or perturbation in non-genetic factors on the ontogeny of complex traits (see e.g. Nijhout, 2003).

The EOC is also ill-equipped to deal with the fact that many potential targets of intervention are the incidental byproduct of other unrelated adaptations – or what Gould and Lewontin (1979) called "spandrels" (in analogy to the structural byproduct of contiguous arches). Although in the world of architecture the nonfunctional spaces between neighboring arches may be decorated however one sees fit, it is not the case that simply because a trait is not an adaptation – but rather the spandrel of an adaptation – that one can manipulate it with reduced fears of negative consequences. For one thing, in the technical sense of the term, there are no "genes for" spandrels, since they are by definition structural byproducts of adaptations. An example is the human chin, which has no adaptive function but rather is formed as the product of two growth fields. In order to modify a spandrel, we would have to manipulate the genes that shape the adaptations on which it supervenes (in the case of the chin, the alveolar and mandibular growth fields).

In sum, the EOC is problematic in that it ignores the potential developmental harm that could be done by modifying both spandrels and neutral products of drift. To make matters worse, sexual selection can act powerfully on traits that are not by any obvious measure adaptations. In humans (and unlike peacocks), it is notoriously difficult to tell which traits are under sexual selection pressure. Modifying traits that are under sexual selection can have effects on fitness that are comparable to interfering with adaptations under ordinary selection pressures.

At this point, the heuristic value of the EOC is almost completely effaced. We shall nevertheless make a final but obvious point: While it is true that the vast majority of natural mutations are either maladaptive or neutral, the very point of IGM is that it does *not* mimic stochastic mutational processes. Instead, its purpose is to produce targeted, nonrandom variation in the service of some identifiable goal. The fact that natural genetic perturbations are unlikely to be beneficial supports rather detracts from the value of IGM.

Bostrom and Sandberg are right to explore the idea of contentful, cautionary heuristics that steer a course between a blanket prohibition on IGM and the vagueness of an admonition to "go slow." They are also correct in their assumption that the needed heuristics must be informed by evolutionary biology. Where they go wrong is in assuming, presumably on the basis of a Strong Adaptationist understanding of evolution, that the key question to ask is whether a trait targeted for IGM is an adaptation. Not all traits are adaptive, not all modifications of adaptations will have negative consequences, and not all modifications of non-adaptive traits will be benign in their effects. In each case, what matters is not adaptive etiology, but the causal relationship between the target trait/gene and other ontogenetic factors, including those features of the organism that we value and wish to preserve.

Cautionary heuristics grounded in a focus on causal relationships

Our purpose in this chapter is not to develop a thorough-going account of the implications of a sound understanding of contemporary evolutionary theory for intentional genetic modification of humans, but to expose the distorting effects of appeals to a faulty understanding of evolution on the debate about genetic modification. Nevertheless, before concluding we wish to offer an admittedly incomplete list of cautionary heuristics, focusing not on adaptation, but on causal relationships. These rules of thumb are not offered as necessary or sufficient conditions for the permissibility of UGM. Instead, they are an attempt to translate the correct but unhelpfully vague admonition to "go slow" in order to reduce the risk of unintended bad consequences into something more capable of providing concrete guidance for determining whether to pursue a particular proposed genetic modification for the sake of increasing human well-being. They are intended only to help reduce the risk of what might be called *biological damage*. They do not address the possibility that IGM might produce unintended bad social or moral consequences. They are not offered as anything approaching a comprehensive guide to decisions concerning IGM. We believe that, taken together, they reflect a proper concern for the risk of unintended biological consequences arising from genetic intervention into a highly complex organism, while avoiding the misconceptions that the master engineer analogy encourages. The more of these seven conditions a proposed intervention satisfies and the more fully it satisfies them, the more confident we can be that the risk of unintended bad (biological) consequences has been taken seriously. How serious the failure to satisfy one or more of the seven conditions is will depend upon a number of factors, including, of course, how valuable the intended effects of the genetic modification are and how likely it is that the intervention will produce them.

1. The intervention targets genes at shallower ontogenetic depths, ones that lie "downstream" in development. Such interventions are less likely to have cascading negative consequences for the phenotype.

2. The intervention, if successful, would not produce an enhancement that exceeds the upper bound of the current normal range of the trait in question. The idea here is that if there are existing, well-functioning individuals who already possess the trait whose frequency one is trying to increase, then this provides some assurance that the modification will not disrupt benign causal interdependencies. Thus, for example, IGM to increase some aspect of cognitive function for those at the lower end of the current normal distribution would be preferable to interventions aimed at raising the upper bound of the normal (other things being equal).

3. The intervention's effects are containable to a particular organism. In other words, if there turns out to be bad unintended consequences, the damage will be limited to the individual(s) in which the intervention occurs.

4. The intervention is containable intra-organismically – that is, it involves modifications in a highly modularized system or subsystem of the organism. Such a modification is less likely to produce unintended spillovers into other systems or subsystems.

5. The intervention's effects are reversible. If this condition is satisfied, then it will be possible to avoid ongoing damage.

6. The intervention does not require major morphological changes. The intuitive idea here is that major morphological changes are more likely to have significant consequences on phenotypic development, including unintended bad ones.

7. If the goal of the intervention is to eliminate a trait, then the *causal role* functions of the trait and of the genes that are the target of the intervention should be well understood. This heuristic reflects a recognition of the fact that even "bad" traits may have some benign consequences, and that the price of eliminating a bad trait may be prohibitive, depending on its causal connections to other genes and how they affect the phenotype.

Each of these heuristics is designed to reduce the risk of unintended bad consequences in the right way: that is, by focusing on causal relationships, rather than on the etiology of the trait targeted for intervention.

Conclusion

In relying on the idea that humans are "delicately balanced" products of "eons of exacting evolution," with "finely integrated" functions and characteristics, the harshest critics of intentional genetic modification imply that the human organism is somehow *complete* or *optimal* in the sense that efforts to improve it are almost certain to make it worse. On this view, which is guided by the notion that natural selection is a like a master engineer, the human species is regarded as an immutable, finished product of evolution, rather than an inherently unstable, flawed work in progress.

Entirely missing from this picture is the ever-changing environment in which organisms struggle to persist, and in which they are active participants. As biologists have long recognized, adaptations are not to ecological niches as keys are to locks (Lewontin, 1982). Rather, organisms engage in a reciprocal, co-constructing and co-defining relationship with their selective environment (Odling-Smee *et al.*, 2003). Humans are niche-constructors par excellence. Given the geologically recent inventions of agriculture and the modern state, and given the rapid pace of cultural evolution, it is not surprising that our biology has had little chance to catch up with our furious rate of niche construction. IGM can help human beings adjust to the new design problems that we create for ourselves.

In its most extreme form, the worry about upsetting the "delicate balance" supposedly created by the engineering genius of evolution boils down to a concern for survival. But as we have shown, survival is contingent on *change*, not *stasis*, since adaptive optimality is spatially local and temporally fleeting. IGM, as any other product of evolution, is simply one more way in which a lineage (in this case the human species) can buffer itself against the perennially decaying selective environment. Even if we had good reason to believe that IGM would reduce our prospects of survival (although we have argued that the opposite is true), it would not follow that we should refrain from IGM. For individuals and for humanity collectively, some risk of death may be worth taking, if the gains are great enough. (Everyone who drives a car, or flies in a plane, or for that matter, takes a shower, recognizes this at the level of individual survival.)

Thus, the idea that IGM is likely to upset a "delicate balance" in the evolved human organism and thus rarely to result in improvement, rests on a distorted view of natural selection as a master engineer, and either a confusion between reproductive fitness and human well-being, or the mistaken assumption that human well-being reduces to maximizing the chances of survival. On the contrary, evolutionary theory gives us good reason to believe that unless we do something radically different from what other organisms have done in the past, our chances of survival in the long run are virtually nil. Given the severe biological and moral limitations of "unassisted" evolution, and given that intentional genetic modification has the potential to avoid some of these limitations, we have good reason to develop the capacity for IGM. But evolutionary theory also helps us appreciate the causal complexity of the human organism and hence the seriousness of the risk that IGM, undertaken without sufficient knowledge of how the organism works, could result in the unwitting disruption of developmental processes. The right place to begin making decisions about using or refraining from IGM is a proper appreciation of the limits of UGM, and a frank acknowledgment of the current limits of our knowledge regarding causal interdependencies – not with a distorted picture of evolution that stacks the deck against UGM.

Notes

1. Here and throughout this chapter, by "genetic modification" we mean germline changes, that is, modifications of genes in embryos or gametes (sperm or eggs) that are expected to be passed on to the next generation, rather than somatic cell genetic modifications (as occurs, for example, when genes are inserted into bone marrow for therapeutic purposes).
2. For a critical examination of appeals to nature and the natural in the debate about the ethics of biomedical enhancements, see Buchanan (2009).
3. The nature and use of teleological language in biology has been the subject of controversy since Darwin's time. While T.H. Huxley proclaimed that "teleology…had received its deathblow at Mr. Darwin's hands," Asa Gray lauded "Darwin's great service to natural science in bringing it back to teleology" (quoted in Ruse, 2003, p.91).
4. It is an "axiom" of cancer research that tumor formation is driven by both oncogenes (dominant growth-enhancing genes) and mutations in growth-inhibitory genes, hundreds of which have thus far been discovered.

References

Amudson, R. & Lauder, G.V. (1994). Two concepts of constraint: Adaptationism and the challenge from developmental biology. *Philosophy of Science*, **61**, 556–78.
Bostrom, N. & Sandberg, A. (2008). The wisdom of nature: an evolutionary heuristic for human enhancement. In J. Savulescu & N. Bostrom (eds.), *Enhancing Humans.* Oxford: Oxford University Press.
Brandon, R.N. (1990). *Adaptation and Environment.* Princeton, NJ: Princeton University Press.
Brandon, R.N. (2006). The principle of drift: Biology's first law. *Journal of Philosophy*, **103**(7), 319–35.
Brandon, R.N. & Rausher, M.D. (1991). Testing adaptationism: A comment on Orzack and Sober. *American Naturalist*, **148**, 189–201.
Buchanan, A. (2009). Enhancement and human nature. *Bioethics*, **23**(3), 141–50.
Dawkins, R. (1986). *The Blind Watchmaker.* New York: W.W. Norton.
Dawkins, R. (2003). *A Devil's Chaplain: Reflections on Hope, Lies, Science, and Love.* Mariner Press.
Galvani, A.P. & Slatkin, M. (2003). Evaluating plague and smallpox as historical selective pressures for the CCR5-Delta 32 HIV resistance allele. *Proceedings of the National Academy of Sciences USA*, **100**, 15276–9.
Gould, S.J. & Lewontin, R.C. (1979). The spandrels of San Marco and the Panglossian paradigm: A critique of the adaptationist programme. *Proceedings of the Royal Society of London, B, Biological Sciences*, **205**(1161), 581–98.
Lewontin, R.C. (1982). Organism and environment. In H. Plotkin (ed.), *Learning, Development, Culture* (pp. 151–70) New York: John Wiley & Sons, Inc.

Manica, A., Amos, W., Balloux, F., & Hanihara, T. (2007). The effect of ancient population bottlenecks on human phenotypic variation. *Nature*, **448**, 346–8.

Nijhout, H.F. (2003). The control of growth. *Development*, **130**(24), 5863–7.

Odling-Smee, J.J., Laland, K.N. & Feldman, M.W. (2003). *Niche Construction: The Neglected Process in Evolution*. Princeton, NJ: Princeton University Press.

Orzack, S.H. & Sober, E. (1994). How (not) to test an optimality model. *Trends in Ecology and Evolution*, **9**, 265–7.

President's Council on Bioethics (2003). *Beyond Therapy: Biotechnology and the Pursuit of Happiness*. New York: Regan Books.

Raup, D.M. (1991). *Extinction: Bad Genes or Bad Luck?* New York: W.W. Norton.

Ruse, M. (2003). *Darwin and Design: Does Evolution Have A Purpose?* Cambridge, MA: Harvard University Press.

Sansom, R. (2003). Constraining the adaptationism debate. *Biology and Philosophy*, **18**, 493–512.

Schroeder, T. *et al.* (2007). Hormonal regulators of muscle and metabolism in aging (HORMA): Design and conduct of a complex, double masked multicenter trial. *Clinical Trials*, **4**(5), 560–71.

Tang, Y.P. *et al.* (1999). Genetic enhancement of learning and memory in mice. *Nature*, **401**, 63–66.

Van Valen, L. (1973). A new evolutionary law. *Evolutionary Theory*, **1**, 1–30.

Weinstein, I.B. (2002). Addiction to oncogenes – The Achilles heel of cancer. *Science*, **297**, 63–4.

Wright, L. (1973). Functions. *Philosophical Review*, **82**, 139–68.

Part II
Cognitive Enhancement

5

Cognition Enhancement: Upgrading the Brain

Anders Sandberg

Introduction

Cognition enhancement (CE) may be defined as the amplification or extension of core capacities of the mind, using augmentation or improvements of our information-processing systems. Cognition can be defined as the processes an organism uses to organize information. This includes acquiring information (perception), selecting (attention), representing (understanding) and retaining (memory) information, and using it to guide behavior (reasoning and coordination of motor outputs). Interventions to improve cognitive function may be directed at any one of these core faculties.

As cognitive neuroscience has advanced, the list of prospective internal, biological enhancements has steadily expanded (Farah *et al.*, 2004; Sandberg & Bostrom, 2006). Yet to date, it is progress in computing and information technology that has produced the most dramatic advances in our ability to process information. External hardware and software supports now routinely give humans beings effective cognitive abilities that in many respects far outstrip those of our biological brains.

An intervention that is aimed at correcting a specific pathology or defect of a cognitive subsystem may be characterized as *therapeutic*. An *enhancement* is an intervention that improves a subsystem in some way other than repairing something that is broken or remedying a specific dysfunction. In practice, the distinction between therapy and enhancement is often difficult to make, and it could be argued that it lacks practical significance. For example, CE of somebody whose natural memory is poor could leave that person with a memory that is still worse than that of another person who has retained a fairly good memory despite suffering from an identifiable pathology, such as early-stage Alzheimer's disease. A cognitively enhanced person, therefore, is not necessarily somebody with particularly high (let alone superhuman) cognitive capacities. A cognitively enhanced person, rather, is somebody who has benefited from an intervention that improves the performance of some cognitive subsystem without correcting some specific, identifiable pathology or dysfunction of that subsystem.

Enhancing Human Capacities, edited by Julian Savulescu, Ruud ter Meulen and Guy Kahane.
© 2011 Blackwell Publishing Ltd

Enhancement Methods

General notes

CE exists within a broad spectrum of practices, some of which have been practiced for thousands of years. The prime example is education and training, where the goal is often not only to impart specific skills or information, but also to improve general mental faculties such as concentration, memory, and critical thinking. Other forms of mental training, such as meditation and creativity courses, are also in common use. Many people use drugs such as caffeine, sugar, nicotine, energy drinks, and herbal supplements every day explicitly to improve their mental functioning.

Education and training, as well as the use of external information-processing devices, may be labeled as "conventional" means of enhancing cognition. They are often well established and culturally accepted. By contrast, methods of enhancing cognition through "unconventional" means, such as ones involving deliberately created nootropic drugs, gene therapy, or neural implants, are nearly all to be regarded as experimental at the present time. Nevertheless, these unconventional forms of enhancements deserve serious consideration for several reasons:

- They are relatively new, and consequently there does not exist a large body of "received wisdom" about their potential uses, safety, efficacy, or social consequences.
- They could potentially have enormous leverage (consider the cost–benefit ratio of a cheap pill that safely enhances cognition compared to years of extra education).
- They are sometimes controversial.
- They currently face specific regulatory problems, which may impede advances.
- They may eventually come to have important consequences for society and even, in the longer run, for the future of humankind.

Such means are under rapid, broad development. Many remain highly experimental or have small effect sizes, making the present scientific literature a weak guide to their eventual usefulness (Ioannidis, 2005). Findings need to be repeated in multiple studies and larger clinical trials before they can be fully trusted. It is likely that many enhancement techniques will in the long run prove less efficacious than their current promoters claim. At the same time, the sheer range of enhancement methods suggests that it would be very unlikely that all current methods are ineffective or that future advances will fail to produce an increasingly potent toolbox for enhancing cognition.

Conventional methods

Conventional methods have many significant benefits. Longer education reduces the risks of substance abuse, crime and many illnesses while improving quality of life, social connectedness, and political participation (Johnston, 2004), as well as IQ (Winship & Korenman, 1997). Enriched rearing environments have been found to increase dendritic arborization and to produce synaptic changes, neurogenesis, and improved cognition in animals (Nilsson *et al.*, 1999). Enriched environments also make brains more resilient to stress and neurotoxins. While analogous controlled experiments cannot easily be done for human children, it is very likely that similar effects would be observed. Exercise (Tomporowski, 2003; Vaynman & Gomez-Pinilla, 2005) and improving general health (Schillerstrom *et al.*, 2005) also has cognition-enhancing effects. General mental activity – "working the brain muscle" – can improve performance (Nyberg *et al.*, 2003) and long-term health (Barnes *et al.*, 2004), while relaxation techniques can help regulate the activation of the brain (Nava *et al.*, 2004). Mental training and visualization techniques are widely practiced in elite sport (Feltz & Landers, 1983) and rehabilitation (Jackson *et al.*, 2004), with apparently good effects.

Less traditional, computer games have been developed for training working memory in children with ADHD; it was found that the improvement carried over to a complex reasoning task (Klingberg *et al.*, 2002). Playing video games also appears to produce changes in visual attention and the ability to itemize (instantly count) sets of objects (Green & Bavelier, 2006).

The classic form of CE is learned strategies to memorize information. Such methods have been used since antiquity with much success (Patten, 1990; Yates, 1966). The early memory arts were often used as a substitute for written text or to memorize speeches. Today, memory techniques tend to be used in service of everyday needs such as remembering door codes, passwords, shopping lists, and by students who need to memorize names, dates, and terms when preparing for exams. In general, it is possible to attain high memory performance on specific types of material using memory techniques (Ericsson, 2003).

Drugs

Stimulant drugs such as nicotine and caffeine have long been used to improve cognition. In the case of nicotine a complex interaction with attention and memory occurs (Rusted *et al.*, 2005), while caffeine reduces tiredness (Tieges *et al.*, 2004). Lashley (1917) observed that strychnine facilitates learning in rats. In more recent years, a wide array of drugs have been developed that affect cognition, in particular long-term memory (Farah *et al.*, 2004). They include stimulants (Lee & Ma, 1995), nutrients (Meikle *et al.*, 2005; Winder & Borrill, 1998) and hormones (Gulpinar & Yegen, 2004), cholinergic agonists (Freo *et al.*, 2005; Power *et al.*, 2003), the piracetam family (Mondadori, 1996), ampakines (Lynch, 1998), and consolidation enhancers (Lynch, 2002).

Diet, and dietary supplements, can affect cognition. In order to maintain optimal functioning, the brain requires a continuous supply of glucose, its major energy source (Fox *et al.*, 1988). Increases in glucose availability, from the ingestion of sugars or the release of acute stress hormones improve memory (Foster *et al.*, 1998; Wenk, 1989) with the effects being particularly pronounced in demanding tasks (Sunram-Lea *et al.*, 2002). Creatine, a nutrient that improves energy availability, also appears to benefit overall cognitive performance (Rae *et al.*, 2003) and reduce mental fatigue (McMorris *et al.*, 2006; Watanabe *et al.*, 2002). Besides being an energy source, food can contribute to cognition by providing amino acids needed in the production of neurotransmitters, which is particularly important during periods of stress or sustained concentration (Banderet & Lieberman, 1989; Deijen *et al.*, 1999; Lieberman, 2003).

There is also some evidence that micronutrient supplementation increases nonverbal intelligence in some children. This effect might be due to correction of occasional deficiencies rather than a general enhancing action (Benton, 2001).

Advances in the scientific understanding of memory has enabled the development of drugs with more specific actions, such as drugs stimulating the cholinergic system that gates attention and memory encoding. Current interest is focused on intervening in the process of permanent encoding in the synapses, a process which has been greatly elucidated in recent years and is a promising target for drug development.

Pharmacological agents might be useful not only for increasing memory retention but also for unlearning phobias, trauma, and addictions (Hoffmann *et al.*, 2006; Ressler *et al.*, 2004). Potentially, the combination of different drugs administered at different times could give users a more fine-grained control of their learning processes, perhaps even the ability to deliberately select specific memories that they want to retain or get rid of.

Working memory can be modulated by a variety of drugs. Drugs that stimulate the dopamine and acetylcholine systems have demonstrated effects (Barch, 2004). The stimulant Modafinil has been shown to enhance working memory in healthy test subjects, especially at harder task difficulties and for lower-performing subjects (Muller *et al.*, 2004). (Similar findings of stronger improvements among low performers were also seen among the dopaminergic drugs, and this might be a general pattern for many cognitive enhancers.) Modafinil has been found to increase forward and backward digit span, visual pattern recognition memory, spatial planning, and reaction time/latency on different working memory tasks (Turner *et al.*, 2003). The mode of action of this drug is not yet understood, but part of what seems to happen is that Modafinil enhances adaptive response inhibition, making the subjects evaluate a problem more thoroughly before responding, thereby improving performance accuracy. The working memory effects might thus be part of a more general enhancement of executive function.

Modafinil was originally developed as a treatment for narcolepsy, and can be used to reduce performance decrements due to sleep loss with apparently small side effects and little risk of dependency (Myrick *et al.*, 2004). The drug improved attention and working memory in sleep-deprived physicians (Gill *et al.*, 2006) and aviators (Caldwell *et al.*, 2000), as well as humor appreciation (Kilgore *et al.*, 2006). While naps are more effective in maintaining performance than Modafinil and amphetamine during long (48h) periods of sleep deprivation, naps followed by a Modafinil dose may be more effective than either one on its own (Batejat & Lagarde, 1999). These results, together with studies on hormones like melatonin that can control sleep rhythms (Cardinali *et al.*, 2002), suggest that drugs can enable fine-tuning of alertness patterns to improve task performance under demanding circumstances or disturbed sleep cycles.

There also exist drugs that influence how the cerebral cortex reorganizes in response to damage or training. Noradrenergic agonists such as amphetamine have been shown to promote faster recovery of function after a brain lesion when combined with training (Gladstone & Black, 2000), and to improve learning of an artificial language (Breitenstein *et al.*, 2004). A likely explanation is that higher excitability increases cortical plasticity, in turn leading to synaptic sprouting and remodeling (Goldstein, 1999; Stroemer *et al.*, 1998). An alternative to pharmacologic increase of neuromodulation is to electrically stimulate the neuromodulatory centers that normally control plasticity through attention or reward. In monkey experiments this produced faster cortical reorganization (Bao *et al.*, 2001).

In brains that have already been damaged, e.g. by lead exposure, nootropics may alleviate some of the cognitive deficits (Zhou & Suszkiw 2004). It is not always clear whether they do so by curing the damage or by amplifying (enhancing) capacities that compensate for the loss, or whether the distinction is even always meaningful. Comparing chronic exposure to cognition-enhancing drugs with an enriched rearing environment, one study in rats found that both conditions improved memory performance and produced similar changes in the neural matter (Murphy *et al.*, 2006). The improvements in the drug-treated group persisted even after cessation of treatment. The combination of drugs and enriched environment did not improve the rats' abilities beyond the improvement provided by one of the interventions alone. This suggests that both interventions produced a more robust and plastic neural structure capable of learning more efficiently.

TMS

Transcranial magnetic stimulation (TMS) can increase or decrease the excitability of the cortex, thereby changing its level of plasticity (Hummel & Cohen, 2005). TMS of the motor cortex improved performance in a procedural learning task (Pascual-Leone *et al.*, 1999). TMS in suitable areas has also been found beneficial in a motor task (Butefisch *et al.*, 2004), motor learning (Nitsche *et al.*, 2003), visuo-motor coordination tasks (Antal *et al.*, 2004), working memory (Fregni *et al.*, 2005), classification (Kincses *et al.*, 2004), and even declarative memory consolidation during sleep (Marshall *et al.*, 2004). Snyder *et al.* claim to have demonstrated how TMS inhibiting anterior brain areas could change the drawing style of normal subjects into a more concrete style and improve spell-checking abilities, presumably by reducing top-down semantic control (Snyder *et al.*, 2004). While TMS appears to be quite versatile and non-invasive, there are risks of triggering epileptic seizures, and the effects of long-term use are not known. Moreover, individual brain differences may necessitate much adjustment before it can be used to improve specific cognitive capacities and the effect sizes are very small.

Genetic modifications

Genetic memory enhancement has been demonstrated in rats and mice. Tang *et al.* (1999) modified mice to overexpress the NR2B subunit of the NMDA receptor. The mice showed improved memory performance, in terms of both acquisition and retention. This included unlearning of fear conditioning, which is believed to be due to the learning of a secondary memory (Falls *et al.*, 1992). The modification also made the mice more sensitive to certain forms of pain, suggesting a nontrivial tradeoff between two potential enhancement goals (Wei *et al.*, 2001).

Increased amounts of brain growth factors (Routtenberg *et al.*, 2000) and the signal transduction protein adenylyl cyclase (Wang *et al.*, 2004) have also produced memory improvements. These modifications had different enhancing effects on different memory systems and unlearning (Tan *et al.*, 2006). These enhancements may be due to changes in neural plasticity during the learning task itself, or to ontogenetic changes in brain development that promote subsequent learning or retention.

The cellular machinery of memory appears to be highly conserved in evolution, making interventions demonstrated to work in animal models likely to have close counterparts in humans (Bailey *et al.*, 1996). Genetic studies have also found genes in humans whose variations account for up to 5% of memory performance (de Quervain & Papassotiropoulos, 2006). These include the genes for the NMDA receptor and adenylyl cyclase that were mentioned above, as well as genes involved in other stages of the synaptic signal cascade. These are obvious targets for enhancement.

Given these early results, it seems likely that there exist many potential genetic interventions that would directly or indirectly improve aspects of memory. If it turns out that the beneficial effects of the treatments are not due to changes in development, then presumably some of the effects can be achieved by supplying the brain with the substances produced by the memory genes without resorting to genetic modification.

Studies of the genetics of intelligence suggest that there is a large number of genetic variations affecting individual intelligence, but each accounting for only a very small fraction (<1%) of the variance between individuals (Craig & Plomin, 2006). This would indicate that genetic enhancement of intelligence through direct insertion of a few beneficial alleles is unlikely to have a big enhancing effect. It is possible, however, that some alleles that are rare in the human population could have larger effects on intelligence, both negative and positive.[1]

Prenatal enhancement

A notable form of chemical enhancement is pre- and perinatal enhancement. Administering choline supplementation to pregnant rats improved the performance of their pups, apparently as a result of changes in neural development (Mellott *et al.*, 2004). Given the ready availability of choline supplements, such prenatal enhancement may already (inadvertently) be taking place in human populations. Supplementation of a mother's diet during late pregnancy and three months postpartum with long chained fatty acids has also been shown to improve cognitive performance in human children (Helland *et al.*, 2003). Deliberate changes of maternal diet might be regarded as part of the CE spectrum. At present, recommendations to mothers are mostly aimed at promoting a diet that avoids specific harms and deficits, but the growing emphasis on boosting "good fats" and the use of enriched infant formulas point towards enhancement.

Brain–computer interfaces

Direct control of external devices through brain activity has been studied with some success for the last 40 years, although it remains a very low bandwidth form of signaling (Wolpaw *et al.*, 2000).

The most dramatic potential internal hardware enhancements are brain–computer interfaces. Development is rapid, both on the hardware side, where recordings from more than 300 electrodes permanently implanted in the brain are currently state of the art, and on the software side, with computers learning to interpret the signals and commands (Carmena *et al.*, 2003). Early experiments on humans have shown that it is possible for profoundly paralyzed patients to control a computer cursor using just a single electrode (Kennedy & Bakay, 1998) implanted in the brain, and experiments by Patil *et al.* have demonstrated that the kind of multielectrode recording devices used in monkeys to control robotic limbs would most likely function in humans too (Patil *et al.*, 2004). Experiments in localized chemical release from implanted chips also suggest the possibility of using neural growth factors to promote patterned local growth and interfacing (Alteheld *et al.*, 2004).

Cochlear implants are already widely used, and there is ongoing research in artificial retinas (Alteheld *et al.*, 2004) and functional electric stimulation for paralysis treatment (Weiser, 1991). These implants are intended to ameliorate functional deficits and are unlikely to be attractive for healthy people in the foreseeable future. But the digital parts of the implant could in principle be connected to any kind of external software and hardware. This could enable enhancing uses such as access to software tools, the internet, and virtual reality applications. In a demonstration project, a healthy volunteer has been enabled to control a robotic arm using tactile feedback, both in direct adjacency and remotely, and to perform simple direct neural communication with another implant (Weiser, 1991). Non-disabled people, however, could most likely achieve the essentially same functionality more cheaply, safely, and effectively through eyes, finger, and voice control.

External hardware and software

Some approaches in human–computer interaction are explicitly aimed at CE (Weiser, 1991). External hardware is of course already used to amplify cognitive abilities, be it pen and paper, calculators, or personal computers. Many common pieces of software act as cognition-enhancing environments, where the software helps display information, keep multiple items in memory, and perform routine tasks. Data mining and information visualization tools process and make graspable enormous amounts of data that our perceptual systems cannot handle. Other tools such as expert systems, symbolic math programs, decision support software, and search agents amplify specific skills and capacities.

What is new is the growing interest in creating intimate links between the external systems and the human user through better interaction. The software becomes less an external tool and more of a mediating "exoself." This can be achieved through mediation, embedding the human within an augmenting "shell" such as wearable computers (Weiser, 1991) or virtual reality, or through smart environments in which objects are given extended capabilities. An example is the vision of "ubiquitous computing," in which objects would be equipped with unique identities and given ability to communicate with and actively support the user (Weiser, 1991). A well-designed environment can enhance proactive memory (Sellen *et al.*, 1996) by deliberately bringing previous intentions to mind in the right context. Remembrance agents are software that acts as a vastly extended associative memory (Rhodes & Starner, 1996): The agents have access to a database of information such as a user's files, e-mail correspondence etc., which they use to suggest relevant documents based on the current context.

Given the availability of external memory support, from writing to wearable computers, it is likely that the crucial form of memory demand on humans in the future
will increasingly be the ability to link information into usable concepts, associations,
and skills rather than the ability to memorize large amounts of raw data. Storage and
retrieval functions can often be offloaded from the brain, while the knowledge,
strategies, and associations linking the data to skilled cognition cannot so far be
outsourced to computers. This will put a premium on some cognitive abilities.

Collective intelligence

Much of human cognition is distributed across many minds. Such distributed cognition
can be enhanced through the development and use of more efficient tools and methods
of intellectual collaboration. The World Wide Web and e-mail are among the most
powerful kinds of CE software developed to date. Through the use of such social
software, the distributed intelligence of large groups can be shared and harnessed for
specific purposes (Surowiecki, 2004).

Connected systems allow many people to collaborate in the construction of shared
knowledge and solutions. Usually, the more individuals that connect, the more
powerful the system becomes (Drexler, 1991). The information in such systems is
stored not just in individual documents but also in their interrelations. When such
interconnected information resources exist, automated systems such as search engines
(Kleinberg, 1999) can often radically improve our ability to extract useful information
from them.

Lowered coordination costs enable larger groups to work on common projects.
Groups of volunteers with shared interests, such as amateur journalist "bloggers" and
open source programmers, have demonstrated that they can successfully complete large
and highly complex projects, such as online political campaigns, the Wikipedia
encyclopedia, and the Linux operating system. Systems for online collaboration can
incorporate efficient error correction (Giles, 2005; Raymond, 2001), enabling incremental improvement of product quality over time.

One powerful technique of knowledge aggregation is prediction markets (also
known as "information markets" or "idea futures markets"). In such a market,
participants trade in predictions of future events. The prices of these bets tend to
reflect the best information available about the probability of whether the events will
occur (Hanson *et al.*, 2003). Such markets appear to be self-correcting and resilient,
and have been shown to outperform alternative methods of generating probabilistic
forecasts, such as opinion polls and expert panels (Hanson *et al.*, 2006).

New senses

The spectral range of the human eye can be extended slightly into the ultraviolet by
removing the UV-blocking lens. The result is that patients lacking lens (aphakia) or
having an UV-transparent lens can perceive near UV (down to 314 nm) as "whiteish
blue" (Griswold & Stark, 1992; Stark & Tan, 1982).

People expressing more than three photopigments appear to have a slightly richer
visual experience in terms of number of color bands they experience in a spectrum

(Jameson *et al.*, 2001). Depending on which extra opsin gene they have they experience two versions of the same fundamental color (www.rmki.kfki.hu/~lukacs/TETRACH .htm). Genetic interventions into mice have demonstrated that extra photopigments can be inserted and produce broader color vision (Jacobs *et al.*, 2007).

An interesting demonstration of a simple new sense is magnetic sensitivity. By inserting a small permanent magnet into a fingertip a person became able to sense magnetic fields due to their effect on the magnet (Laratt, 2004). The result was an extended perception of magnetic fields in the environment. Static fields were experienced as pressures while oscillating fields such as from electric motors were more noticeable vibrating sensations. Although intended more as a conceptual tool than a useful enhancement it demonstrates an entirely new sense.

Notes on technology

At present most biomedical enhancement techniques represent modest improvements of performance, as a rule of thumb about 10–20% improvement on a particular task. So far no general CE intervention has enhanced performance outside the normal human range. More dramatic results can be achieved using training and human–machine collaboration, techniques that are less ethically controversial at present. "Mental software" can achieve 1000% or more improvement of specific tasks (e.g. digit span (Ericsson *et al.*, 1980)). However, such enhancements are task-specific unlike the broad effects of e.g. increased alertness.

While schooling and mental training can have profound effects, the costs are often high. Pharmacological enhancement may be cost-effective in improving performance, especially for particular tasks or limited periods. TMS, genetic interventions, brain–computer interfaces and new senses are highly experimental and unlikely to be important over the next 15 years (but may in the long run have profound effects). External tools are on the other hand expanding rapidly. Many of the concerns about enhancement are nonspecific to the tools used to achieve it, which means that enhancement–ethic scrutiny should also apply to nonbiological external enhancements.

Ethical Issues

Safety

Safety concerns tend to focus on medical risks of internal biological enhancements. Yet risks accompany any intervention, not just biomedical procedures. External software enhancements raise safety issues such as privacy and data protection. Education can enhance cognitive skills and capacities, but it can also create fanatics, sophistic arguers, or selfishly calculating minds.

Nevertheless, it is in the area of medical enhancement that safety issues are likely to be most salient. Since the current medical risk system is based on comparing treatment risk with the expected benefit of reduced morbidity risk from successful treatment, it is strongly risk averse in the case of enhancements that do not reduce morbidity risk and whose utility to the patient may be entirely non-therapeutic, highly subjective, and context dependent. Yet precedents for a different risk model can be found, for example in use of cosmetic surgery. The consensus is that patient autonomy overrides at least minor medical risks even when the procedure does not reduce or prevent morbidity. A similar model could be used in the case of medical CEs, with the user being allowed to decide whether the benefits outweigh the potential risks, based on advice from medical professionals and her own estimates of how the intervention might affect her personal goals and her way of life.

The development of cognitive enhancers may also face problems in terms of acceptable risk to test subjects. The reliability of research is another issue, since many of the cognition-enhancing interventions show small effect sizes. This may necessitate very large epidemiological studies, possibly exposing large groups to unforeseen risks.

Purpose of medicine

One common concern about enhancements in the biomedical sphere is that they go beyond the purpose of medicine. The debate over whether it is possible to draw a line between therapy and enhancement, and if so where, is extensive. Regardless of this, it is clear that medicine does encompass many treatments not intended to cure, prevent, or ameliorate illness, such as plastic surgery and contraceptive medication, which are accepted. There are also many forms of enhancement that do not fit into the medical framework, such as psychological techniques and diet, but which nevertheless produce medical effects. Even if a boundary between therapy and enhancement could be agreed, it is unclear that it would have any normative significance.

Quick fixes

A related concern is that resort to medical or technological "fixes" will become a displacement for efforts to confront deeper social of personal problems. This concern has surfaced particularly with regard to Ritalin and other ADHD medications. These medications can function as cognitive enhancers in healthy subjects, but their widespread use in the school-aged population in the United States has sparked fierce debates, with some arguing that these medications are often used to paper over the failings of the education system by making rowdy boys calmer instead of developing teaching methods that can accommodate a wider range of individual learning styles and needs. However, if modern society requires much more study and intellectual concentration than was typical for our species in its environment of evolutionary adaptation, then it is unsurprising that many people today struggle to meet the demands of the school or the workplace. Technological self-modification and the use of CE methods can be seen as an extension of the human species' ability to adapt to its environment (Bostrom & Sandberg, 2008).

Human well-being can be improved through altering the natural environment, the social environment, psychology and biology, but they all act on the same phenotype. Hence it is rational to choose the kind of intervention that work most effectively in a given situation for a given person rather than automatically exclude one or more categories as suspect. From a practical standpoint this requires understanding of their relative strengths and weaknesses to judge their cost-effectiveness in improving well-being.

Procreative choice and eugenics

Some enhancements do not increase the capacity of any existing being but rather cause a new person to come into existence with greater capacities than some other possible person would have had who could have come into existence instead. This is what happens in embryo selection (Glover, 1984). At present, preimplantation genetic diagnosis is used mainly to select out embryos with genetic disease, and occasionally for the purpose of sex selection. In the future, however, it might become possible to test for a variety of genes known to correlate with desirable attributes, including cognitive capacity. Genetic engineering might also be used to remove or insert genes into a zygote or an early embryo. In some cases, it might be unclear whether the outcome is a new individual or the same individual with a genetic modification.

The debate over the ethics of procreative choice is extensive, with positions ranging from that parents have an obligation to select the children they judge would have the best prospects of having a good life (Savulescu, 2001) to views that "designer babies" will corrupt parents, who will come to view their children as mere products rather than unconditionally loved (Kass, 2002). Some have argued that genetic selection and enhancement would constitute a kind of "tyranny of the living over the unborn" (Jonas, 1985). Others have responded that a child is no freer if her genes are determined by chance than if they are determined by parental choice. Furthermore, some enhancements would increase the offspring's capacity for autonomous agency.

However, genetic interventions for CE purposes are likely to be rare compared to interventions for other purposes in the foreseeable future as there are few clearly advantageous targets. Most selection is going to be negative selection against deleterious genes. However, prenatal nutrition can cause changes in genetic expression which ought to be regarded as nearly as profound as genetic change.

Authenticity

The issue of authenticity has many sides. One is the idea that native or achieved excellence has a higher worth than talent that is bought. If cognitive abilities are for sale, in the form of a pill or some external aid, would that reduce their value and make them less admirable? Would it in some sense make the abilities less genuinely *ours*? Related to this, one might think that if excellence is achieved mostly through hard work, then genetic differences and parental class play a smaller role in determining success. But if there were shortcuts to excellence then access to such shortcuts would instead become the determining factor of success and failure.

In many cases, however, shortcuts to excellence are tolerated. We do not denounce athletes for wearing protective (and performance enhancing) shoes, since they enable the athletes to concentrate on interesting talents rather than on developing thick soles. In many elementary schools, calculators are disallowed in mathematics lessons, where the goal is to understand basic arithmetic, but they are allowed and increasingly necessary in the higher grades. The basics have by then been mastered, and the goal becomes to understand more advanced topics. These examples illustrate that CE aimed at extending and completing a person's talents may promote authenticity by offloading irrelevant, repetitive, or boring tasks and enabling a person to concentrate on more complex challenges that relate in more interesting ways to her goals.

Another side of the authenticity issue is the extent to which our "free choices" are manipulated by advertisers or are slavishly bound to reigning fashions by our desire to conform. If enhancements are added to the "must-haves" of a modern consumer, does that mean that our bodies and minds would come even more directly under the dominion of external and therefore "inauthentic" drivers than is currently the case? Some critics see human enhancement in general as expressive of a technocratic mindset, which threatens to "flatten our souls," sap our moral fiber, lower our aspirations, weaken our loves and attachments, lull our spiritual yearnings, undermine our dignity, and as likely to lead to trite consumerism, homogenization, and a Brave New World (President's Council on Bioethics, 2003). While these fears appear to triggered less by the prospect of CE than by other possible forms of human enhancement or modification (e.g. of mood and emotion), they do reflect a general unease about making "the essence of human nature" a project of technological mastery (Kass, 2002).

To some extent, these are cultural, social, and political issues rather than purely ethical ones. A blinkered pursuit of shallow or misguided ends is not the only way in which enhancement options could be used. If there were a widespread tendency to use the options in that way, then the problem would probably lie in our culture. The criticism is a criticism of mediocrity and bad culture rather than of enhancement. Many of the negative consequences of enhancement may be avoided or changed in different social contexts. Critics could argue that we have to look at the culture we have, not some ideal alternative, or that there are particular attributes of the technologies which will inevitably promote the erosion of human values.

Again, however, CEs have the potential to play a positive role. Insofar as CEs amplify the capacities required for autonomous agency and independent judgment, they can help a person lead a more authentic life by enabling her to base her choices on more deeply considered beliefs about her unique circumstances, her ideals, and the options available to her.

Hyper-agency, playing God, and the status quo

The concern about "hyper-agency" is in a sense opposite to the concern about authenticity. Here, the issue is that as human beings become more able to control their lives and themselves, they also become more responsible for the results and less constrained by traditional limits. The "playing God" objection asserts that human wisdom is insufficient to manage this freedom. Whether hyper-agency is a problem or not depends on both an analysis of the ethical implications of increased agency (such as the burden of responsibility for previously uncontrollable events, and the potential for increased autonomy) and the psychological and sociological question of how humans would in fact react to their increased degrees of freedom, power, and responsibility.[2] The policy challenge might be to ensure that there are adequate safeguards, regulations, and transparency to support a society of increasingly cognitively resourceful individuals, and also to moderate unrealistic expectations of infallibility.

Another version of the playing God argument asserts that it is sometimes better to respect "the Given" than to try to better things using human abilities (Sandel, 2003, 2004; but see also a critique in Kamm, 2006). The claim that we should stick with the status quo can be based on a religious sensibility, the idea that we literally risk offending God if we overstep our mandate here on Earth. It can also be based on a less theologically articulated feeling that the proper approach to the world is one of humility and that enhancement would upset the moral or practical order of things; or, alternatively, on an explicitly conservative vision according to which the existing state of affairs has, due to its age, acquired some form of optimality. Since human agency is already interfering with the natural order in many ways that are universally accepted (for example, by curing the sick), and since society and technology have always been changing and often for the better, the challenge for this version of the playing God argument is to determine which particular kinds of interventions and changes would be bad.

One recent paper has examined the extent to which opposition to CE is the result of a status quo bias, defined as an irrational or inappropriate preference for the status quo just because it is the status quo. When this bias is removed, through the application of a method which the authors call "the Reversal Test," many consequentialist objections to CEs are revealed to be highly implausible (Bostrom & Ord 2006).

Cheating, positional goods, and externalities

On some campuses it is now not uncommon for students to take Ritalin when preparing for exams (not to mention caffeine and energy drinks). Does this constitute a form of cheating akin to illicit doping in the Olympics? Or should students be positively *encouraged* to take performance enhancers (assuming they are safe and efficacious) for the same reasons that they are encouraged to take notes and to start revising early?

Whether an action constitutes cheating depends on the agreed game rules for different activities. To pick up the ball with one's hands is cheating in golf and soccer, but not in American football. If school is to be regarded as a competition for grades, then enhancers would arguably be cheating if not everyone had access to enhancements or if they were against the official rules. If school is viewed as having primarily a social function, then enhancement might be irrelevant. But if school is seen as being significantly about the acquisition of information and learning, then CEs may have legitimate role to play.

A positional good is one whose value is dependent on others not having it. If CEs were purely positional goods, then the pursuit of such enhancements would be a waste of time, effort, and money. People might become embroiled in a cognitive "arms race," spending significant resources merely in order to keep up with each other. One person's gain would produce an offsetting negative externality of equal magnitude, resulting in no net gain in social utility to compensate for the costs of the enhancement efforts.

Most cognitive functions, however, are not purely positional goods (Bostrom 2003). They are also intrinsically desirable: their immediate value to the possessor does not entirely depend on other people lacking them. Having a good memory or a creative mind is normally valuable in its own right, whether or not other people also possess similar excellences. Furthermore, many cognitive capacities also have instrumental value, both for individuals and for society. We face many pressing problems which we would be better able to solve if we were smarter or more creative. An enhancement that enables an individual to solve some of society's problems would produce a positive externality: in addition to benefits for enhanced individual, there would be spillover benefits for other members of society.

Nevertheless, competitive aspects of enhancements should be taken into account when we assess the impact they might have on society. An enhancement may be entirely voluntary and yet become difficult to avoid for those who do not desire it. It has been suggested that many people would prefer to fly with airlines or go to hospitals where the personnel take alertness-enhancing drugs. Such preferences could expand employment opportunities for those willing to enhance themselves. Economic competition might eventually force people to use enhancements on pain of rendering themselves ineligible for certain jobs (Chatterjee, 2004).

The case might be compared to that of literacy, which is also forced upon citizens in modern societies. For literacy, the enforcement is both direct, in the form of mandatory basic education, and indirect, in the form of severe social penalties for failure to acquire reading and writing skills. The dominant cooperative framework (Buchanan *et al.*, 2001) of our society has developed in such a way that an illiterate person is excluded from many opportunities and unable to participate in many aspects of modern life. Despite these enormous and partially coercive pressures, and despite the fact that literacy profoundly changes the way the brain processes language (Petersson *et al.*, 2000), literacy is not deemed to be problematic. The costs of illiteracy are placed on the individual who deliberately avoids education. As social acceptance of other enhancements increases, and if these are available at a reasonable price, it is possible that social support for people who refuse to take advantage of enhancements will diminish.

Inequality

Concern has been voiced that CEs might exacerbate social inequality by adding to the advantages of elites, or undermine the fundamental equality of people (Fukuyama, 2002; Silver, 1998).

In order for an enhancement to promote elite formation it needs to be either expensive or give a strong positional advantage. To assess this concern one would have to consider whether future CEs would be expensive (like good schools) or cheap (like caffeine). Other relevant factors include the speed of technology diffusion, the need for training to achieve full utilization of an enhancement, regulatory approach, and accompanying public policies. Public policy and regulations can either contribute to inequality by driving up prices, limiting access, and creating black markets; or reduce inequality by supporting broad development, competition, public understanding, and perhaps subsidized access for disadvantaged groups.

Given that the price of drugs and gadgets tend to fall dramatically over time as more people use them, the technology develops and the temporary monopolies created by intellectual property lapse, it does not appear unlikely that most such enhancements could be well within the reach of everyday consumers after a few years of introduction. Service-based enhancements such as surgical treatment or schooling will not drop in price as quickly and may be more socially problematic. However, as universal schooling demonstrates, many societies are willing to spend significant efforts to enhance its citizens. An analogy might be drawn to public libraries and basic education (Hughes, 2004).

Of the enhancements we have studied none appears to have clear elite-forming properties. It may be that enhancements of health may be more elite-forming than enhancements of cognition. It has been argued that very powerful enhancements (if and when they appear) could be placed within a regulatory framework for leveling the playing field if the objective is seen as important enough (Mehlman, 2000), but whether the political will to do so will be forthcoming remains to be seen.

The Ends of Enhancement

Current regulatory frameworks are inadequate for CE. There is no room for enhancement within the regulations surrounding the pharmaceutical industry. Hence enhancement drugs are developed as a "side effect" of therapeutic research, spurring medicalization of everyday conditions and a gray market for enhancer drugs. The question is not whether society should reject CE (since many forms of enhancement are widely accepted already) but how to select what kinds of enhancement are acceptable or cost-effective.

Many "ethical" criticisms in the public discourse are often more criticisms of contemporary culture than real attempts to analyze the moral status of different projects. Rather than take aim at the means it may be more productive to actually discuss the ends for which enhancement is used.

At present, for example, the enhancements discussed are mainly seen as relating to professional work, biasing the discussion towards the assumption that work is the goal of enhancement. But work has little value in itself; it is only valuable as an instrument for developing human well-being. Similarly, the moral obligation to treat or prevent disease is driven by the goodness of health. Nevertheless health itself is not what matters. Health enables us to implement our life projects while disease prevents us from doing what we want and what is good. People often trade health for well-being when they engage in risky but rewarding activities such as sport or travel. Hence it is well-being rather than health that would drive a moral obligation to enhance, or at the very least accepting some enhancements.

Notes

1. A possible example is suggested in Cochran *et al.* (2006), where it is predicted that heterozygoticity for Tay–Sachs disease should increase IQ by about 5 points.
2. "In my view, the fear of hyper-agency is misplaced; society as a whole seems always to return to the reasonable use of new knowledge. . . . Just as most people don't drink all the liquor in their liquor cabinet...our society will absorb new memory drugs according to each individual's underlying philosophy and sense of self" (Gazzaniga, 2005).

References

Alteheld, N., Roessler, G. *et al.* (2004). The retina implant new approach to a visual prosthesis. *Biomedizinische Technik*, **49**(4), 99–103.

Antal, A., Nitsche, M.A. *et al.* (2004). Direct current stimulation over V5 enhances visuomotor coordination by improving motion perception in humans. *Journal of Cognitive Neuroscience*, **16**(4), 521–7.

Bailey, C.H., Bartsch, D. *et al.* (1996). Toward a molecular definition of long-term memory storage. *Proceedings of the National Academy of Sciences of the USA*, **93**(24), 13445–52.

Banderet, L.E. & Lieberman, H.R. (1989). Treatment with tyrosine, a neurotransmitter precursor, reduces environmental-stress in humans. *Brain Research Bulletin*, **22**(4), 759–62.

Bao, S.W., Chan, W.T. *et al.* (2001). Cortical remodelling induced by activity of ventral tegmental dopamine neurons. *Nature*, **412**(6842), 79–83.

Barch, D.M. (2004). Pharmacological manipulation of human working memory. *Psychopharmacology*, **174**(1), 126–35.

Barnes, D.E., Tager, I.B. *et al.* (2004). The relationship between literacy and cognition in well-educated elders. *Journals of Gerontology Series A, Biological Sciences and Medical Sciences*, **59** (4), 390–5.

Batejat, D.M. & Lagarde, D.P. (1999). Naps and modafinil as countermeasures for the effects of sleep deprivation on cognitive performance. *Aviation Space and Environmental Medicine*, **70**(5), 493–8.

Benton, D. (2001). Micro-nutrient supplementation and the intelligence of children. *Neuroscience and Biobehavioral Reviews*, **25**(4), 297–309.

Bostrom, N. (2003). Human genetic enhancements: A transhumanist perspective. *Journal of Value Inquiry*, **37**(4), 493–506.

Bostrom, N. & Ord, T. (2006). The reversal test: Eliminating status quo bias in applied ethics. *Ethics*, **116**(4), 656–80.

Bostrom, N. & Sandberg, A. (2008). The wisdom of nature: An evolutionary heuristic for human enhancement. In N. Bostrom& A. Sandberg (eds.), *Enhancing Humans*. Oxford: Oxford University Press.

Breitenstein, C., Wailke, S. *et al.* (2004). D-amphetamine boosts language learning independent of its cardiovascular and motor arousing effects. *Neuropsychopharmacology*, **29**(9), 1704–14.

Buchanan, A., Brock, D.W. *et al.* (2001). *From Chance to Choice*. Cambridge: Cambridge University Press.

Butefisch, C.M., Khurana, V. *et al.* (2004). Enhancing encoding of a motor memory in the primary motor cortex by cortical stimulation. *Journal of Neurophysiology*, **91**(5), 2110–16.

Caldwell, J.A., Jr., Caldwell, J.L. *et al.* (2000). A double-blind, placebo-controlled investigation of the efficacy of modafinil for sustaining the alertness and performance of aviators: A helicopter simulator study. *Psychopharmacology (Berlin)*, **150**(3), 272–82.

Cardinali, D.P., Brusco, L.I. *et al.* (2002). Melatonin in sleep disorders and jet-lag. *Neuroendocrinology Letters*, **23**, 9–13.

Carmena, J.M., Lebedev, M.A. *et al.* (2003). Learning to control a brain-machine interface for reaching and grasping by primates. *PLOS Biology*, **1**(2), 193–208.

Chatterjee, A. (2004). Cosmetic neurology – The controversy over enhancing movement, mentation, and mood. *Neurology*, **63**(6), 968–74.

Cochran, G., Hardy, J. *et al.* (2006). Natural history of Ashkenazi intelligence. *Journal of Biosocial Science*, **38**(5), 659–93.

Craig, I. & Plomin, R. (2006). Quantitative trait loci for IQ and other complex traits: Single-nucleotide polymorphism genotyping using pooled DNA and microarrays. *Genes Brain and Behavior*, **5**, 32–7.

de Quervain, D.J.F. & Papassotiropoulos, A. (2006). Identification of a genetic cluster influencing memory performance and hippocampal activity in humans. *Proceedings of the National Academy of Sciences of the USA*, **103**(11), 4270–4.

Deijen, J.B., Wientjes, C.J.E. *et al.* (1999). Tyrosine improves cognitive performance and reduces blood pressure in cadets after one week of a combat training course. *Brain Research Bulletin*, **48**(2), 203–9.

Drexler, K.E. (1991). Hypertext publishing and the evolution of knowledge. *Social Intelligence*, **1**(2), 87–120.

Ericsson, A.K. (2003). Exceptional memorizers: Made, not born. *Trends in Cognitive Science*, 7 (6), 233–5.

Ericsson, K.A., Chase, W.G. *et al.* (1980). Acquisition of a memory skill. *Science*, **208**(4448), 1181–2.

Falls, W.A., Miserendino, M.J.D. *et al.* (1992). Extinction of fear-potentiated startle – Blockade by infusion of an NMDA antagonist into the amygdale. *Journal of Neuroscience*, **12**(3), 854–63.

Farah, M.J., Illes, J. *et al.* (2004). Neurocognitive enhancement: What can we do and what should we do? *Nature Reviews Neuroscience*, **5**(5), 421–5.

Feltz, D.L. & Landers, D.M. (1983). The effects of mental practice on motor skill learning and performance – A meta-analysis. *Journal of Sport Psychology*, **5**(1), 25–57.

Foster, J.K., Lidder, P.G. & Sunram, S.I. (1998). Glucose and memory: fractionation of enhancement effects? *Psychopharmacology*, **137**(3), 259–70.

Fox, P.T., Raichle, M.E. *et al.* (1988). Nonoxidative glucose consumption during focal physiologic neural activity. *Science*, **241**(4864), 462–4.

Fregni, F., Boggio, P.S. *et al.* (2005). Anodal transcranial direct current stimulation of prefrontal cortex enhances working memory. *Experimental Brain Research*, **166**(1), 23–30.

Fukuyama, F. (2002). *Our Posthuman Future: Consequences of the Biotechnology Revolution*. New York: Farrar, Strauss and Giroux.

Freo, U., Ricciardi, E. *et al.* (2005). Pharmacological modulation of prefrontal cortical activity during a working memory task in young and older humans: A PET study with physostig-mine. *American Journal of Psychiatry*, **162**(11), 2061–70.

Gazzaniga, M.S. (2005). *The Ethical Brain*. New York: Dana Press.

Giles, J. (2005). Internet encyclopaedias go head to head. *Nature*, **438**(7070), 900–1.

Gill, M., Haerich, P. *et al.* (2006). Cognitive performance following modafinil versus placebo in sleep-deprived emergency physicians: A double-blind randomized crossover study. *Academic Emergency Medicine*, **13**(2), 158–65.

Gladstone, D.J. & Black, S.E. (2000). Enhancing recovery after stroke with noradrenergic pharmacotherapy: A new frontier? *Canadian Journal of Neurological Sciences*, **27**(2), 97–105.

Glover, J. (1984). *What Sort of People Should There Be?* London: Penguin.

Goldstein, L.B. (1999). Amphetamine-facilitated poststroke recovery. *Stroke*, **30**(3), 696–7.

Green, C.S. & Bavelier, D. (2006). Enumeration versus multiple object tracking: The case of action video game players. *Cognition*, **101**(1), 217–45.

Griswold, M.S. & Stark, W.S. (1992). Scotopic spectral sensitivity of phakic and aphakic observers extending into the near ultraviolet. *Vision Research*, **32**(9), 1739–43.

Gulpinar, M.A. & Yegen, B.C. (2004). The physiology of learning and memory: Role of peptides and stress. *Current Protein & Peptide Science*, **5**(6), 457–73.

Hanson, R., Polk, C. *et al.* (2003). The policy analysis market: an electronic commerce application of a combinatorial information market. ACM Conference on Electronic Commerce 2003.

Hanson, R., Opre, R. *et al.* (2006). Information aggregation and manipulation in an experimental market. *Journal of Economic Behavior and Organization*, 60(4), 449–59.

Helland, I.B., Smith, L. *et al.* (2003). Maternal supplementation with very-long-chain n-3 fatty acids during pregnancy and lactation augments children's IQ at 4 years of age. *Pediatrics*, 111(1), 39–44.

Hoffmann, S.G., Meuret, A.E. *et al.* (2006). Augmentation of exposure therapy with D-cycloserine for social anxiety disorder. *Archives of General Psychiatry*, 63(3), 298–304.

Hughes, J. (2004). *Citizen Cyborg: Why Democratic Societies Must Respond to the Redesigned Human of the Future*. Boulder, CO: Westview Press.

Hummel, F.C. & Cohen, L.G. (2005). Drivers of brain plasticity. *Current Opinion in Neurology*, 18(6), 667–74.

Ioannidis, J.P.A. (2005). Why most published research findings are false. *PLOS Medicine*, 2(8), 696–701.

Jackson, P.L., Doyon, J. *et al.* (2004). The efficacy of combined physical and mental practice in the learning of a foot-sequence task after stroke: A case report. *Neurorehabilitation and Neural Repair*, 18(2), 106–11.

Jacobs, G.H., Williams, G.A. *et al.* (2007). Emergence of novel color vision in mice engineered to express a human cone photopigment. *Science*, 315(5819), 1723–5.

Jameson, K.A., Highnote, S.M. *et al.* (2001). Richer color experience in observers with multiple photopigment opsin genes. *Psychonomic Bulletin and Review*, 8(2), 244–61.

Johnston, G. (2004). Healthy, wealthy and wise? A review of the wider benefits of education. *New Zealand Treasury Working Paper*.

Jonas, H. (1985). *Technik, Medizin und Ethik: Zur Praxis des Prinzips Verantwortung*. Frankfurt am Main: Suhrkamp.

Kamm, F. (2006). What is and is not wrong with enhancement? KSG Working Paper RWP06-020, John F. Kennedy School of Government.

Kass, L. (2002). *Life, Liberty, and Defense of Dignity: The Challenge for Bioethics*. San Francisco: Encounter Books.

Kennedy, P.R. & Bakay, R.A.E. (1998). Restoration of neural output from a paralyzed patient by a direct brain connection. *Neuroreport*, 9(8), 1707–11.

Kilgore, W.D.S., McBride, S.A. *et al.* (2006). The effects of caffeine, dextroamphetamine, and modafinil on humor appreciation during sleep deprivation. *Sleep*, 29(6), 841–7.

Kincses, T.Z., Antal, A. *et al.* (2004). Facilitation of probabilistic classification learning by transcranial direct current stimulation of the prefrontal cortex in the human. *Neuropsychologia*, 42(1), 113–17.

Kleinberg, J.M. (1999). Authoritative sources in a hyperlinked environment. *Journal of the ACM*, 46(5), 604–32.

Klingberg, T., Forssberg, H. *et al.* (2002). Training of working memory in children with ADHD. *Journal of Clinical and Experimental Neuropsychology*, 24(6), 781–91.

Laratt, S. (2004). The gift of magnetic vision. *Body Modification Ezine*.

Lashley, K.S. (1917). The effects of strychnine and caffeine upon rate of learning. *Psychobiology*, 1, 141–69.

Lee, E.H.Y. & Ma, Y.L. (1995). Amphetamine enhances memory retention and facilitates norepinephrine release from the hippocampus in rats. *Brain Research Bulletin*, 37(4), 411–16.

Lieberman, H.R. (2003). Nutrition, brain function and cognitive performance. *Appetite*, 40(3), 245–54.

Lynch, G. (1998). Memory and the brain: Unexpected chemistries and a new pharmacology. *Neurobiology of Learning and Memory*, **70**(1–2), 82–100.

Lynch, G. (2002). Memory enhancement: The search for mechanism-based drugs. *Nature Neuroscience*, **5**, 1035–8.

Marshall, L., Molle, M. *et al.* (2004). Transcranial direct current stimulation during sleep improves declarative memory. *Journal of Neuroscience*, **24**(44), 9985–92.

McMorris, T., Harris, R.C. *et al.* (2006). Effect of creatine supplementation and sleep deprivation, with mild exercise, on cognitive and psychomotor performance, mood state, and plasma concentrations of catecholamines and cortisol. *Psychopharmacology*, **185**(1), 93–103.

Mehlman, M.J. (2000). The law of above averages: Leveling the new genetic enhancement playing field. *Iowa Law Review*, **85**(2), 517–93.

Meikle, A., Riby, L.M. *et al.* (2005). Memory processing and the glucose facilitation effect: The effects of stimulus difficulty and memory load. *Nutritional Neuroscience*, **8**(4), 227–32.

Mellott, T.J., Williams, C.L. *et al.* (2004). Prenatal choline supplementation advances hippo-campal development and enhances MAPK and CREB activation. *FASEB Journal*, **18**(1), 545–7.

Mondadori, C. (1996). Nootropics: Preclinical results in the light of clinical effects, Comparison with tacrine. *Critical Reviews in Neurobiology*, **10**(3–4), 357–70.

Muller, U., Steffenhagen, N. *et al.* (2004). Effects of modafinil on working memory processes in humans. *Psychopharmacology*, **177**(1–2), 161–9.

Murphy, K.J., Foley, A.G. *et al.* (2006). Chronic exposure of rats to cognition enhancing drugs produces a neuroplastic response identical to that obtained by complex environment rearing. *Neuropsychopharmacology*, **31**(1), 90–100.

Myrick, H., Malcolm, R. *et al.* (2004). Modafinil: preclinical, clinical, and post-marketing surveillance – A review of abuse liability issues. *Annals of Clinical Psychiatry*, **16**(2), 101–9.

Nava, E., Landau, D. *et al.* (2004). Mental relaxation improves long-term incidental visual memory. *Neurobiology of Learning and Memory*, **81**(3), 167–71.

Nilsson, M., Perfilieva, E. *et al.* (1999). Enriched environment increases neurogenesis in the adult rat dentate gyrus and improves spatial memory. *Journal of Neurobiology*, **39**(4), 569–78.

Nitsche, M.A., Schauenburg, A. *et al.* (2003). Facilitation of implicit motor learning by weak transcranial direct current stimulation of the primary motor cortex in the human. *Journal of Cognitive Neuroscience*, **15**(4), 619–26.

Nyberg, L., Sandblom, J. *et al.* (2003). Neural correlates of training-related memory improvement in adulthood and aging. *Proceedings of the National Academy of Sciences of the USA*, **100**(23), 13728–33.

Pascual-Leone, A., Tarazona, F. *et al.* (1999). Transcranial magnetic stimulation and neuroplasticity. *Neuropsychologia*, **37**(2), 207–17.

Patil, P.G., Carmena, L.M. *et al.* (2004). Ensemble recordings of human subcortical neurons as a source of motor control signals for a brain-machine interface. *Neurosurgery*, **55**(1), 27–35.

Patten, B.M. (1990). The history of memory arts. *Neurology*, **40**(2), 346–52.

Petersson, K.M., Reis, A. *et al.* (2000). Language processing modulated by literacy: A network analysis of verbal repetition in literate and illiterate subjects. *Journal of Cognitive Neuroscience*, **12**(3), 364–82.

Power, A.E., Vazdarjanova, A. *et al.* (2003). Muscarinic cholinergic influences in memory consolidation. *Neurobiology of Learning and Memory*, **80**(3), 178–93.

President's Council on Bioethics. (2003). *Beyond Therapy: Biotechnology and the Pursuit of Happiness*. New York: Regan Books.

Rae, C., Digney, A.L. *et al.* (2003). Oral creatine monohydrate supplementation improves brain performance: a double-blind, placebo-controlled, cross-over trial. *Proceedings of the Royal Society of London Series B, Biological Sciences*, **270**(1529), 2147–50.

Raymond, E.S. (2001). *The Cathedral and the Bazaar*. O'Reilly.

Ressler, K.J., Rothbaum, B.O. *et al.* (2004). Cognitive enhancers as adjuncts to psychotherapy – Use of D-cycloserine in phobic individuals to facilitate extinction of fear. *Archives of General Psychiatry*, **61**(11), 1136–44.

Rhodes, B. & Starner, T. (1996). Remembrance agent: A continuously running automated information retrieval system. The First International Conference on the Practical Application of Intelligent Agents and Multi Agent Technology (PAAM 96).

Routtenberg, A., Cantallops, I. *et al.* (2000). Enhanced learning after genetic overexpression of a brain growth protein. *Proceedings of the National Academy of Sciences of the USA*, **97**(13), 7657–62.

Rusted, J.M., Trawley, S. *et al.* (2005). Nicotine improves memory for delayed intentions. *Psychopharmacology (Berlin)*, **182**(3), 355–65.

Sandberg, A. & Bostrom, N. (2006). Converging cognitive enhancements. *Progress in Convergence: Technologies for Human Wellbeing*, **1093**, 201–7.

Sandel, M.J. (2003). What's wrong with enhancement. In President's Council on Bioethics. (ed.), *Beyond Therapy: Biotechnology and the Pursuit of Happiness*. New York: Regan Books.

Sandel, M.J. (2004). The case against perfection: What's wrong with designer children, bionic athletes, and genetic engineering? *The Atlantic Monthly*, **293**(4), 51–62.

Savulescu, J. (2001). Procreative beneficence: Why we should select the best children. *Bioethics*, **15**(5–6), 413–26.

Schillerstrom, J.E., Horton, M.S. *et al.* (2005). The impact of medical illness on executive function. *Psychosomatics*, **46**(6), 508–16.

Sellen, A.J., Louie, G. *et al.* (1996). What brings intentions to mind? An in situ study of prospective memory. *Rank Xerox Research Centre Technical Report* EPC-1996-104.

Silver, L. (1998). *Remaking Eden*. Harper Perennial.

Snyder, A. *et al.* (2004). Concept formation: "object" attributes dynamically inhibited from conscious awareness. *Journal of Integrative Neuroscience*, **3**(1), 31–46.

Stark, W.S. & Tan, K.E.W.P. (1982). Ultraviolet-light – Photosensitivity and other effects on the visual-system. *Photochemistry and Photobiology*, **36**(3), 371–80.

Stroemer, R.P., Kent, T.A. *et al.* (1998). Enhanced neocortical neural sprouting, synaptogenesis, and behavioral recovery with D-amphetamine therapy after neocortical infarction in rats. *Stroke*, **29**(11), 2381–93.

Sunram-Lea, S.I., Foster, J.K. *et al.* (2002). Investigation into the significance of task difficulty and divided allocation of resources on the glucose memory facilitation effect. *Psychopharmacology*, **160**(4), 387–97.

Surowiecki, J. (2004). *The Wisdom of Crowds: Why the Many Are Smarter Than the Few and How Collective Wisdom Shapes Business, Economies, Societies and Nations*. Doubleday.

Tan, D.P., Liu, Q.Y. *et al.* (2006). Enhancement of long-term memory retention and short-term synaptic plasticity in CBL-B null mice. *Proceedings of the National Academy of Sciences of the USA*, **103**(13), 5125–30.

Tang, Y.P., Shimizu, E. *et al.* (1999). Genetic enhancement of learning and memory in mice. *Nature*, **401**(6748), 63–9.

Tieges, Z., Richard Ridderinkhof, K. *et al.* (2004). Caffeine strengthens action monitoring: Evidence from the error-related negativity. *Brain Research and Cognitive Brain Research*, **21**(1), 87–93.

Tomporowski, P.D. (2003). Effects of acute bouts of exercise on cognition. *Acta Psychologica*, **112**(3), 297–324.

Turner, D.C., Robbins, T.W. *et al.* (2003). Cognitive enhancing effects of modafinil in healthy volunteers. *Psychopharmacology*, **165**(3), 260–9.

Vaynman, S. & Gomez-Pinilla, F. (2005). License to run: Exercise impacts functional plasticity in the intact and injured central nervous system by using neurotrophins. *Neurorehabilitation and Neural Repair*, **19**(4), 283–95.

Wang, H.B., Ferguson, G.D. *et al.* (2004). Overexpression of type-1 adenylyl cyclase in mouse forebrain enhances recognition memory and LTP. *Nature Neuroscience*, 7(6), 635–42.

Watanabe, A., Kato, N. *et al.* (2002). Effects of creatine on mental fatigue and cerebral hemoglobin oxygenation. *Neuroscience Research*, **42**(4), 279–85.

Wei, F., Wang, G.D. *et al.* (2001). Genetic enhancement of inflammatory pain by forebrain NR2B overexpression. *Nature Neuroscience*, **4**(2), 164–9.

Weiser, M. (1991). The computer for the twenty-first century. *Scientific American*, **265**(3), 94–110.

Wenk, G. (1989). An hypothesis on the role of glucose in the mechanism of action of cognitive enhancers. *Psychopharmacology*, **99**, 431–8.

Winder, R. & Borrill, J. (1998). Fuels for memory: The role of oxygen and glucose in memory enhancement. *Psychopharmacology*, **136**(4), 349–56.

Winship, C. & Korenman, S. (1997). Does staying in school make you smarter? The effect of education on IQ in The Bell Curve. In B. Devlin, S.E. Fienberg & K. Roeder (eds.), *Intelligence, Genes, and Success: Scientists Respond to The Bell Curve* (pp. 215–34). New York: Springer.

Wolpaw, J.R., Birbaumer, N. *et al.* (2000). Brain–computer interface technology: A review of the first international meeting. *IEEE Transactions on Rehabilitation Engineering*, **8**(2), 164–73.

Yates, F. (1966). *The Art of Memory*. Chicago: University of Chicago Press.

Zhou, M.F. & Suszkiw, J.B. (2004). Nicotine attenuates spatial learning lead deficits induced in the rat by perinatal exposure. *Brain Research*, **999**(1), 142–7.

6

The Social and Economic Impacts of Cognitive Enhancement

Anders Sandberg and Julian Savulescu

Introduction

The possibility of enhancing human abilities often raises public concern about equality and social impact. In a U.S. focus group study, many members were concerned that reproductive genetic technologies would only be acceptable to white and wealthy, producing disparities of health, advantage, and ability. As stated by a participant (Kalfoglou *et al.*, 2002):

> [I]t's not the poor families in Africa that are going to be doing this, it's going to be the very affluent who are going to at first have healthier children. . .and then it becomes the slippery slope, they will have stronger, faster, smarter children. . . Then you've got these two very disparate classes.

Similarly, in the "Meeting of Minds across Europe: European Citizens' Deliberation Initiative on Brain Science" similar concerns were expressed (King Baudouin Foundation & Rathenau Institut, 2004):

> Many workshop attendees made a plea for proactive reflection on the societal impacts of, specifically, cognitive enhancement. Cognitive enhancement will cause society to change incrementally. If the level of "normal" cognitive performance rises, but only one section of the population has the resources to attain this new performance level, then this would reinforce social pressures and set new societal norms.

The movie *Gattaca* (see Winship & Korenman, 1997) depicts the extreme version of this fear: a future society where people's enhancement status determines their careers, marriage prospects, and social status. Perhaps the "classic"[1] example in the literature of such extreme divisions caused by the use of biotechnology is found Lee Silver's *Remaking Eden* (1998), where he proposes that differences in access to genetic

Enhancing Human Capacities, edited by Julian Savulescu, Ruud ter Meulen and Guy Kahane.
© 2011 Blackwell Publishing Ltd

enhancement technology combined with assortive mating in a future America will lead to a division into two different human species.

But concerns over social division need not be based on heritable changes. A concern is whether "compounding" (in Nigel Cameron's words) can occur: the enhanced will become better, earning more, and hence becoming even more able and motivated to enhance themselves. Meanwhile high prices and competition keeps the unenhanced outside, producing an inevitable drift towards a stratified society. As argued by Gregor Wolbring (2006), "The more forms of enhancement become available, the bigger the ability divide will become."

Other socioeconomic concerns about enhancement include the potential risks of economic competition forcing people to use enhancers to stay competitive, the promotion of maladaptive cultural behaviors (less respect for hard earned skills, more last-minute cramming, medicalization), use in children, reduction of diversity, and possibly adverse cultural affects such as gerontocracy or the commodification of humans (Anon, 2003; Fukuyama, 2002; Kass, 2003; President's Council on Bioethics, 2003).

This chapter does not aim to analyze the full social impact of enhancement technology, but aims at one particular group of technologies, cognitive enhancement, and one particular fear, that enhancement will create social divisions and possibly expanding inequalities.

To assess this concern fully, one would have to consider whether future cognitive enhancements would be expensive (like good schools) or cheap (like caffeine). One would also have to take into account that there is more than one dimension to inequality. For example, in addition to the gap between the rich and the poor, there is also a gap between the cognitively gifted and the cognitively deficient. One should also have to consider under what conditions society might have an obligation to ensure universal access to interventions that improve cognitive performance. An analogy might be drawn to public libraries and basic education (Hughes, 2004). Other relevant factors include the speed of technology diffusion, the need for education to achieve full utilization of an enhancement, regulatory approach, and accompanying public policies. Public policy and regulations can either contribute to inequality by driving up prices, limiting access, and creating black markets; or reduce inequality by supporting broad development, competition, public understanding, and perhaps subsidized access for disadvantaged groups.

In this chapter, we will argue that cognitive enhancements could offer significant social and economic benefits. Whether these are realized, or whether one of the feared dystopias becomes a reality, will depend on how enhancements are distributed and employed. But the potential benefits for all, we will argue, are real and profound.

Types of Cognitive Enhancement and Effects

Cognitive enhancement may be defined as the amplification or extension of core capacities of the mind through improvement or augmentation of internal or external information-processing systems. As cognitive neuroscience has advanced, the list of prospective internal, biological enhancements has steadily expanded (Farah *et al.*, 2004; Sandberg & Bostrom, 2006). The basic forms of internal cognitive enhancement technologies foreseen today are pharmacological modifications, genetic interventions, transcranial magnetic stimulation, and neural implants. In addition various external enhancements exist, such as schooling, writing, software, ultra-portable computers, memory arts etc.

"Conventional" means of cognitive enhancement, such as education, mental techniques, neurological health, and external systems, are largely accepted, while "unconventional" means – drugs, implants, direct brain–computer interfaces – tend to evoke moral and social concerns. However, the demarcation between these two categories is blurred. It might be the newness of the unconventional means and the fact that they are currently still mostly experimental which is responsible for their problematic status rather than any essential problem with the technologies themselves. As we gain more experience with currently unconventional technologies, they may become absorbed into the ordinary category of human tools.

Biomedical enhancement techniques typically produce modest performance improvement (at most 10–20% improvement on test tasks). Less controversial techniques such as human-machine collaboration and mental training can allow dramatic improvements in particular domains. In narrow domains such as specific memorization tasks (Ericsson *et al.*, 1980) mental training techniques can achieve 1000% or more improvement. While pharmacological cognitive enhancements do not produce dramatic improvements on specific tasks, their effects are often quite general, enhancing performance across a wide domain, such as all tasks making use of working memory or long-term memory. External tools and cognitive techniques such as mnemonics, in contrast, are usually task-specific, producing potentially large improvements of relatively narrow abilities. A combination of different methods can be expected to do better than any single method, especially in everyday or workplace settings where a wide variety of tasks have to be performed.

Can sizable cognitive enhancement be done using conventional means? This appears relatively likely. An additional year of education is estimated to increase adult IQ by 1.8–2.7 points (Winship & Korenman, 1997). David Armor (2003) has argued that simultaneously avoiding risk factors and optimizing early development factors such as better nutrition (including breastfeeding and nutritional supplementation), reduced exposure to environmental toxins (such as lead, mercury, and mold), parasites and childhood illness, cognitive stimulation, increased parental education and income, more stable and small families etc. could achieve a 10-point increase. While appealing, early environmental interventions might have somewhat short-lived effects (Brody, 2004). However, cognitive enhancement may possibly help make effects more long-lasting.

In brains that have already been damaged, e.g. by lead exposure, cognition-enhancing drugs may alleviate some of the cognitive deficits (Zhou & Suszkiw, 2004). It is not always clear whether they do so by curing the damage or by amplifying (enhancing) capacities that compensate for the loss, or whether the distinction is even always meaningful. Comparing chronic exposure to cognition-enhancing drugs with an enriched rearing environment, one study in rats found that both conditions improved memory performance and produced similar changes in the neural matter (Murphy *et al.*, 2006). The improvements in the drug-treated group persisted even after cessation of treatment. Both interventions produced a more robust and plastic brain capable of learning more efficiently. However, the combination of drugs and enriched environment did not improve the rats' abilities beyond the improvement provided by one of the interventions alone. It may turn out that in humans cognition enhancement can compensate for impoverished upbringing, but will be less effective for already enriched individuals.

There is some evidence that enhancer drugs such as Modafinil are less effective in high-performing individuals than in low-performing individuals (Muller *et al.*, 2004), as well as in high-IQ vs. low-IQ individuals (Randall *et al.*, 2005). This has important implications for the social impact: if enhancement is self-limiting, there is less risk for compounding. Spreading enhancement widely might improve equality rather than reduce it.

While at present enhancements are modest in effect, understanding of brain plasticity and development is likely to yield enhancements that if given early in life, could have profound changes in learning, for example, in knowledge or language acquisition.

Economic Benefits of Enhancement

What is the economic value of better cognition? Cognitive enhancements can influence the economy through reduction of losses, individual economic benefits, and society-wide benefits.

Reduction of losses

Failures of cognition likely cause significant losses individually and collectively. General numbers are hard to find, but some examples illustrate the situation. One study claimed Britons lose £500 million a year due to forgotten keys, through locksmiths, break-ins, insurance premiums etc. (Halifax Home Insurance, 2005). Another survey found that almost half of the people surveyed didn't know exactly how much they were paying each month by direct debit and standing order or to whom, producing a national cost in the United Kingdom of over £400 million a month, and an average cost of £53 a month to the forgetful (Lyons, 2005). More minor forms of forgetfulness, like lost passwords, extra trips to fetch forgotten items or the need for a refresher course, are even more common and likely to be costly in terms of time, effort, and money.

Memory and attention lapses are often a component of accidents, costing lives and money. Performance decrements of 30–40% can occur during the first night of sleep deprivation, and 50–70% the following (Angus & Heslegrave, 1985), with obvious consequences for surgeons, truck drivers, pilots, etc. It is significant that U.S. pilots in Iraq regularly use Modafinil and Ritalin to improve performance. Sleepiness causes 15–20% of U.K. road accidents (as well as work-related accidents, iatrogenic illness etc). Much research is directed at reducing fatigue-related problems in shift work, medicine (Gill *et al.*, 2006), and the military (Caldwell *et al.*, 2000) using enhancers.

Higher intelligence is likely correlated with lower accident rates, and certainly with better health and longer lives, reducing the losses from premature death (Gottfredson, 2007). While non-cognitive factors play a major part in accidents, an increase in cognitive ability would likely have significant positive effects individually and collectively. These effects are non-positional and benefit both the individuals involved and society.

As an example, if 600–800 traffic deaths per year in the U.K. are due to sleepiness, widespread enhancement of wakefulness that reduced them by just 10% would save 60–80 lives each year. While an information campaign against driving when tired could likely be both cheaper and more effective, it would only prevent traffic deaths. More alert people would also avoid work-related risks, such as medical mistakes. It hence seems likely that a wakefulness enhancer with small side effects (like caffeine) could produce benefits across a broad range of situations. Similarly a memory enhancer would again produce a reduction in losses across the board, not just for keys and accounts.

Individual economic benefits

Cognition is both a consumption good – it is often desirable and happiness-promoting to have well-functioning cognition – and a capital good that reduces risks, increases earning capacity, and forms a key part of human capital. Enhancing cognition increases human capital or the potential to acquire human capital.

There is no link between higher cognitive ability and more (or less) happiness (Gow *et al.*, 2005;Hartog & Oosterbeek, 1998; Sigelman, 1981).[2] However, the findings are consistent in that lower cognitive ability correlates with unhappiness. Low cognitive ability makes people vulnerable, hinders education, and reduces the range of jobs which they can select. Higher intelligence appears to prevent a wide array of social and economic misfortunes (Gottfredson, 1997, 2004) and to promote health (Batty *et al.*, 2007;Whalley & Deary, 2001) and educational achievement. While there is certainly a positive feedback between an enriched, well-off environment, education and cognitive ability, sibling studies within the heritability of intelligence controversy have also produced data that support the claim that cognition itself, other factors being equal, increases life chances (Bound *et al.*, 1986; Murray, 2002; Neisser *et al.*, 1996; Rowe *et al.*, 1998).

There is a link between general intelligence and professional performance, especially in terms of trainability and ability to manage complex situations. While this might be less important in some occupations, the increasingly complex nature of society may put a premium on cognition (Gottfredson, 1997).

Characteristics most valued by recruiters at a job interview include relevant experience (58% of recruitment agencies ranked it as very important), dynamic personality (38%), communications skills (30%), high IQ (30%), ability to learn (27%), academic qualifications (21%), IT skills (13%), language aptitude (8%).[3] While cognitive ability itself is not strongly valued it is strongly linked with both ability to learn and academic qualifications, and a review of personnel selection methods suggest that cognitive ability plus a work sample or an interview is the best predictor of work performance (Schmidt & Hunter, 1998). Enhancements of personality and communications ability may also be possible in the future, further improving job chances for the enhanced.

Individual cognitive capacity (imperfectly estimated by IQ scores) is positively correlated with income (Rowe *et al.*, 1998). There might be a less strong correlation between IQ and accumulated wealth (0.16 rather than 0.3 for income) (Zagorsky,

2007).[4] While cognitive ability is not the only or even largest factor predicting income, it has a significant effect especially in white collar work (Cawley *et al.*, 1997).

Herrnstein and Murray (1994) estimate that a population level 3 point IQ increase would:

Poverty rate	− 25%
Males in jail	− 25%
High school dropouts	− 28%
Parentless children	− 20%
Welfare recipiency	− 18%
Out-of-wedlock births	− 15%

These benefits are individual, but they also contribute across society by reducing overall social costs and increasing productivity.

What use is enhancing the top part of the cognitive distribution? It could be that having more than a certain minimum level of ability does not confer any advantage. However, a study of the top 1% academic performers (as found by scholastic tests at age 13) found that the top quartile has an advantage compared to the bottom quartile of this distinguished group (Wai *et al.*, 2005). There was a significantly higher rate of gaining doctorates, achieving tenure at a top-50 U.S. university, and a higher probability of an above-median income for the top quartile. While these measures may represent successful competition with less gifted peers, patent production does not appear to be a competitive endeavor but rather a sign of real creativity and wealth production. The study found a doubling of the number of patents in the top quartile compared to the bottom quartile (corresponding to about 7.5 and 3.8 times the base rate of the population). This suggests that not only do the top performers do well professionally but they also add more per capita to the economy.

Societal economic benefits

While having a richer society is not valuable itself, it is instrumentally useful in many ways. Richer societies have more resources to provide for their members than poor societies. This includes both direct help for poorer or weaker members of the society and indirect enrichment of everybody through public goods such as infrastructure, education, and culture. In case of disasters, it is nearly always the poor who suffer the most, simply because they lack the economic buffers and resources providing resilience. Rich societies appear far better at handling disasters both as a whole and in terms of individual outcomes.

At a societal level, the consequences of many small individual enhancements may be profound, as the data from Weiss above suggest. A relatively small upward shift of the distribution of intellectual abilities would substantially reduce the incidence of learning problems that prevent many from flourishing, and would help large "average" groups to perform better. Such a shift would also likely have important effects on technology, economy, and culture arising from improved performance among more cognitively able groups.

Economic models of the loss caused by small intelligence decrements due to toxins in drinking water predict significant individual and social effects of even a few points change (Muir & Zegarac, 2001; Salkever, 1995), and it is plausible that a small *increment* would have positive effects of a similar magnitude. One study estimated the increase in income from one additional IQ point to 1.763% (Schwartz, 1994) while a later study found 2.1% for men and 3.6% for women (Salkever, 1995). The annual gain per IQ point (for the United States) would be on the order of US$55–65 billion, 0.4–0.5% GDP.

Another approach to estimating the collective benefit of cognition is to compare with technology. The productivity effects of computers and information technology in industry have been widely studied and found to be positive and nontrivial (Brynjolfsson & Hitt, 1998; Brynjolfsson & Yang, 1996; Stiroh, 2001). Given that the productivity increase appears to be a sizable part of the total factor productivity (Fernald & Ramnath 2003) and that GDP growth appears to track productivity growth this means that the economic gains from IT technology in the U.S. economy would be on the order of a few hundred billion dollars each year. Part of this gain would be due to the cognition-enhancing abilities of software. Arguably, a significant proportion of increase in GDP over recent years has been the result of external cognitive enhancement: the computing and IT revolutions. Add to this the recognition that human capital, itself heavily cognition-dependent, contributes a sizable fraction of economic growth (Denison, 1985), suggesting a considerable value to society of cognitive enhancement

Another, more controversial method, is to directly compare different countries economically and cognitively. Lynn and Vanhanen calculated "national IQ" based on combining test scores from different countries (Lynn & Vanhanen, 2002). Their data is highly controversial due to the use of dubious sources (small studies, conversion to IQ from other test) and problematic uses of interpolation (between countries, assuming a steady Flynn effect of secular IQ increase), but it is so far the only readily available dataset. Follow-up analysis has shown that the conclusions are robust when truncating the lowest scoring countries (Whetzel & McDaniel, 2006), excluding OECD countries (Jones & Schneider, 2006) and when compared to international educational tests (Hunt & Wittmann, 2007). Fitting "national IQ" to GDP shows an exponential relationship with moderate correlation, suggesting that a 5-point IQ increase is worth a 40% GDP increase (1 point = 8.2% GDP) (Dickerson, 2006). Fitting economic product to IQ estimated from educational testing in different U.S. states also shows a similar relationship (Kanazawa, 2006).

Demonstrating causation is problematic, since it is clear that better nutrition, schooling and health likely will tend to increase IQ scores (Daley *et al.*, 2003; Winship & Korenman, 1997), possibly confounding the results. One study tried regressing various robust growth indicators (such as equipment investment, rule of law, school enrollment etc.) together with "national IQ" and found that IQ was statistically significant as an indicator practically regardless of what other indicators were used (Jones & Schneider, 2006).[5] If IQ had just been a result of education and other societal factors it would have been far less significant when they were included. This study found 1 point of IQ to be worth 0.11% annual increase in GDP per capita. At the very least, IQ as measured by tests appears to be a reliable indicator of an important form of human capital, and it outperforms primary school enrollment as a predictor of economic growth.

While these numbers must be taken with a grain of salt, they seem to support that IQ enhancements on order of the Flynn effect (2 points increase per decade) can have enormous economic impact.

Technology diffusion

Wolbring (2006) makes the claim that the growth of ability divides would follow the pattern of divides introduced by other technologies, and that trickle-down effects would be insufficient. However, the general pattern of technological divides has usually been one of spread and falling prices. When new technology is introduced, it is costly and affordable only to select groups, but over time it falls in price and becomes a mass market. Examples of this include electric light, cars, and cell phones. Trickle down is nearly invariable but it may not happen fast enough for critics.

An illuminating example is the spread of information technology. Despite concerns over a "digital divide" between computer/internet haves and have-nots, the U.S. has done relatively little to reduce it. Still, market-driven diffusion within the society has led to a marked reduction of the original divide of the mid-1990s, both between different ethnic groups and between rich and poor.[6] On the other hand, the international digital divide did not reduce during this time, due to low penetration growth rates in non-OECD countries. Part of this difference appears to be due to differences in liberalization, the lack of pre-existing infrastructure to build on, weak public institutions, lack of education, but also a generally lower economic level.

If enhancement were to spread in a similar pattern, we would expect it to become increasingly common throughout OECD countries, as well as some other countries like China. Initially very large differences in usage would exist; followed by a growth period of exponentially increasing penetration until a sizable fraction of society were using enhancement. In the final slowdown phase the number of unenhanced would decline towards an asymptotic (but nonzero) number. In the meantime the number of enhanced in non-OECD countries would increase at a slow rate.

This can be modeled using a technology diffusion model. Early adopters adopt a new technology, and as it is proven people imitate other users leading to an S-shaped curve of penetration (Rogers, 2003). This model is based on the rate of adoption, the rate of imitation and the upper limit of penetration, although it can be extended into more complex models.

What is the speed of adoption and growth of enhancement technology? Cheaper technologies have a higher speed of adoption as more people can test it. Hence cognitive enhancement based on medications may have a higher rate of adoption than ones requiring training or surgery. Technologies with network effects, where the utility of the technology increases with the number of other users, have a higher growth rate. If enhancement is seen as a competitive advantage we should expect a higher growth rate as more people are motivated to acquire it. The number of potential adopters would also be higher. If enhancement is instead seen as a lifestyle decision with less competitive importance the growth rate would be slower, unless other social factors created a fashion effect. If views on the utility or ethics of enhancement remains divided (e.g. for religious reasons) the diffusion will only occur within the group approving of enhancement, with a fraction of society not participating in the diffusion process.

Obtaining model parameter values for a new technology in general requires making analogies with past technologies for which adoption data are available. These should ideally be similar in terms of environmental context (socioeconomic and regulatory environment), market structure (barriers to entry, number and type of competitors), buyer behavior (buying situation, attributes contributing to choice), marketing and characteristics of the innovation (relative advantage over existing products, complexity) (Thomas, 1985).

Cognitive enhancement will likely be provided through a number of techniques, both medical (drugs, TMS, genetic interventions, implants) and nonmedical (such as software, personal electronics, and training). The regulatory overhead of medical enhancement is significantly larger than the nonmedical enhancements. The market structure will be different for different kinds of enhancement, as well as dependent on political decisions.

Enhancements will be in the form of consumables (e.g. drugs), durables (e.g. software) and services (e.g. medical services, training).

Calculators or personal computers have had a fairly high rate of adoption and average (compared to other products) growth rate (Lilien *et al.*, 1999) (e.g., see Figure 6.1). Presumably enhancements similar to these that can cheaply be put into direct use would follow this behavior. This would imply them becoming widespread in society within a decade of introduction. If they are also less dependent on infrastructure they would also spread at a far higher rate than infrastructure dependent enhancements (like the internet) in poorer countries. The spread of the relatively infrastructure-light cell phone in non-OECD countries is an example of this.

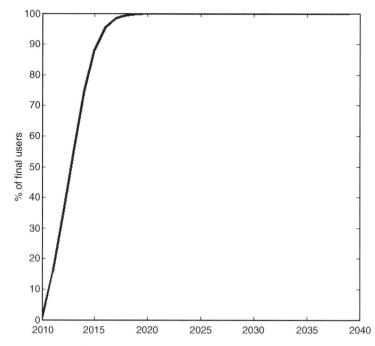

Figure 6.1   Fraction of the eventual number of users using a hypothetical calculator-like technology as a function of time, based on typical past sales data fitted to the Bass diffusion model with high innovation, low imitation

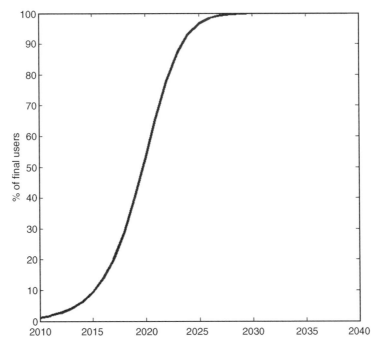

Figure 6.2   Model of adoption of a medical innovation. High imitation, low innovation

Medical innovations in general have a higher coefficient of imitation than consumer durables, producing a faster growth once they become common (Sultan *et al.*, 1990) (e.g. see Figure 6.2). However, the more complex regulatory situation and limited funding in most countries often delay introduction. Drug price and usage are for example strongly controlled by prescription rules and patents; in principle most drugs could be very cheap, but their prices are artificially increased by limited access. This also increases risks of international differences.

Services are limited by the availability of skilled personnel, making their cost dependent on their salaries (e.g. see Figure 6.3). Hence prices will come down if salaries decrease, more skilled personnel becomes available, or the process can be made more efficient through automation or other improvements.

Diffusion occurs at different rates and in different ways in different countries. A study comparing diffusion of consumer products found that the average penetration potential for developing countries is around one-third of that for developed countries, and that sales peak after 17.9% longer time (19.25 vs. 16.33 years) (Talukdar *et al.*, 2002). Poverty, illiteracy, and ethnic diversity had a negative effect on diffusion. Thus even cheap enhancements may spread slowly in developing countries, producing an enhancement difference both between the developed world and the developing, and within developing countries. But the study also noted that increases in international trade or urbanization increase the penetration potential. Since these statistics are generally rapidly increasing in developing countries the diffusion speed is likely to increase significantly over the coming decades.

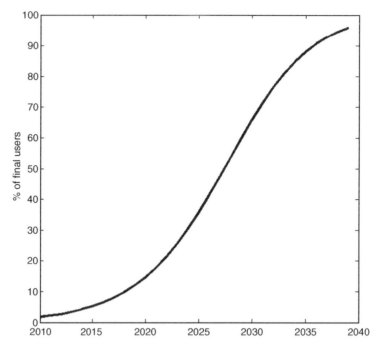

Figure 6.3   Model of adoption of a hypothetical service. High imitation, slow cost decrease

Costs of enhancement

Rough estimates of enhancement costs can be gained by examining current enhance-ments or enhancement-like activities.

A brief and informal look at online pharmaceutical prices suggest that taking 100 mg Modafinil daily today would cost about £60 per month, about 3% of the current U.K. median salary (somewhat less than smoking). This is a noticeable cost to many but not an extreme cost. If enhancements were more widespread this price would likely go down, especially since the online price reflects a gray market – 50 mg caffeine pills would cost about £2 per month, showing that pharmaceutical enhancement already exists in a very low price range.

A typical example of a medical service is in vitro fertilization (IVF), which would be necessary for genetic enhancements (together with preimplantatory testing or hybrid-ization). The mean cost of an IVF cycle in 2002 was $9,547 in the United States and $3,518 in 25 other countries (Collins, 2002). This price does not appear to have decreased since the 1980s, and it does appear to reduce the total demand.

Enhancing implants would likely have costs corresponding to major surgery plus a period of training. For example, current deep brain stimulation surgery for Parkinson's disease costs $37,000 with an additional $3,000 cost for calibration, nursing, and physician time (Tomaszewski & Holloway, 2001). In general we should expect brain implants to be at least on the order of $50,000 (Hooper & Whittle, 2003). These prices would make them relatively rare. From a medical efficiency perspective they might also have a hard time meeting demands of cost-effectiveness: the improvement in quality of life from an enhancement is likely smaller than the improvement in quality of life from a reduction of disability. Under most priority-based health care systems this would limit the amount of enhancement implants, moving them almost completely into a limited private market.

A high level of quality control tends to raise prices, especially if the quality control is service-based (i.e. requires limited, accredited certifiers) rather than automated equipment. Costs of development, risk management, and taxation will be baked into the overall enhancement cost. Especially in jurisdictions where the risk of lawsuits due to side effects or lack of effect are a concern, the cost of enhancement will include embedded legal costs.

Enhancement and Employment

How would occupations be affected by enhancement? At present we do not know how enhancement may affect different professions. Possible effects include:

- Applicants or employees in professions with strong competition have strong incentives to enhance themselves (regardless of whether the enhancement affects measurable performance or is just a symbol of work loyalty). An example is athletes.
- Occupations with high risk or high stress may benefit from enhancement. This would include soldiers, but also people working at great heights, the oil industry, and pilots.
- Shift work or occupations with need for occasional extended awareness can cause mental or physical problems. Control of diurnal rhythms or level of awareness can ameliorate this. Examples would be shift workers, nurses, and drivers.
- Enhancement may be seen as an obligation in high responsibility professions. Examples would be doctors and pilots.
- Enhancement may also make more people able to meet the necessary entry standards, which will either lead to a rise of standards (and increase in competition) or higher diversity of applicants (in professions where the number of applicants are limited in comparison to employment possibilities). This might be relevant in the most specialized scientific or technical occupations.
- New abilities may both enable new occupations or extensions of old occupations.
- People with low cognitive abilities have fewer possible occupations to choose from than people with high abilities. Enhancement would increase their range of choice, and conversely more people with higher abilities would be found in traditional low ability occupations.

Injustice[7]

As we discussed earlier, perhaps the strongest objection to the introduction of any enhancement technology is that it will create inequality, injustice, and unfairness (Annas, 2003; Fukuyama, 2004; McKibben, 2003). There is one way in which enhancement could easily create injustice. If limited resources are directed to developing or buying enhancements, at the expense of other technologies such as medical technologies, which improve well-being more, then that is a violation of distributive justice. So when considering limited community resources, then the benefit of cognitive enhancement must be weighed against the benefits to public health, or security, or widespread social justice, of deploying those resources elsewhere. Of course, where enhancements are purchased or developed with private funds in a legal and legitimate way, there would be no such violation of distributive justice. If certain enhancements provide significant increments in well-being, for example by providing greater impulse control or significantly better memory, and these are greater than the benefits of certain medical treatments or other uses of community resources, then they should have priority. To not provide such enhancements would be as unjust as failing to provide basic level education or health care.

Opponents also have another sense of injustice in mind. What they fear is a private market for enhancement where the rich get smarter, and the smart rich get richer, or derive other social benefits. It is no doubt true that enhancement technologies might create such inequality and injustice if available only through the market. But their use may also *reduce* inequality, injustice, and unfairness if market mechanisms were not used to distribute them.

Libertarians would support a market in enhancements. The rich may buy enhancements which the poor cannot afford provided that their assets have been justly and legally acquired. Those with the highest levels of well-being and privilege will be able to buy even greater happiness and opportunity. This, according to some, is unfair. It is worth stressing that on libertarian accounts of justice, like that of Nozick (1974), this is not unfair.

But let us for a moment grant that it is unfair that the rich get richer or at least happier and better off, and the poor get poorer. Is enhancement *inevitably* or *necessarily* unfair in this sense? To answer this question, we must understand what these theories of justice require. When we understand the nature of justice, we see that justice and fairness may require enhancement.

Theories of justice include utilitarianism, egalitarianism, Rawl's maximin (or justice as fairness) and prioritarianism (Savulescu, 2006).

According to utilitarianism, goods such as enhancements should be distributed to maximize the good or increase in well-being, that is, to bring about what Jeremy Bentham famously said was the "greatest good to the greatest number." Utilitarianism employs a principle of equality, as Bentham put it: "Everybody to count for one, nobody for more than one." That is, provided that enhancements are allocated strictly to maximally promote well-being, with no eye to existing social privilege, status, wealth or other irrelevant consideration, the resulting distribution is just (Savulescu, 2003).

According to egalitarianism, the proper ground for distribution of resources is need (Williams, 1962). "Equal treatment for equal need." Enhancements should be provided to alleviate need in individuals as much as possible. The greater a person's need, the greater that person's entitlement to resources.

According to Rawls' justice as fairness, we should distribute enhancements so that the worst off in society are as well off as they can be (Rawls, 1971). According to prioritarians (Parfit, 1997), we should give priority to those who are worst off, but we should also aim to maximize well-being of all members of society.

If enhancements were distributed according to such principles, they would *promote* equality and justice. If injustice is a concern, then cognitive enhancements should only be provided according to some principle of justice.

Which view of justice we accept does not matter for the purposes of this argument. Let us consider one to illustrate the point. John Mackie once suggested, against utilitarians, that everyone has a "right to a fair go" (Mackie, 1984). This is an attractive principle. According to a maximizing version of this principle, we should give as many people as possible a decent (reasonable) chance of having a decent (good) life. This has also been called "sufficientarianism."

A fair go entails that each person has a legitimate claim to some enhancement or medical intervention when that intervention provides that person with reasonable chance of reasonable extension of a reasonable life and/or a reasonable improvement in its quality. Comparable legitimate claims are those referring to similar needs. Provided as many comparable legitimate claims are being satisfied as possible, there should be equality of access.

On this view of justice, if we judged that a current IQ of, say, 100 was necessary for an adequate range of social and employment opportunities, enhancements should be provided to the 50% of the population who have IQs less than 100 ensuring as many people as possible have IQs of what today would be 100 or more. Such a distribution would likely have fewer economic benefits than providing enhancements to everyone, but it would be more fair. It is up to society to balance the value of fairness with other values, such as well-being or economic prosperity.

Enhancement would not necessarily result in injustice or unfairness. If managed the right way, it could reduce natural inequality, injustice, and unfairness. However, sometimes it is claimed that we should alter society to improve people's lives, and not employ enhancement technologies that are owned by or affect individuals. Firstly, many enhancements such as advances in nanotechnology or information technology could change the structure of society. Secondly, when we are considering cognitive enhancements, whether we should permit individuals to access these or alter social structures depends on whether there are good reasons to prefer social rather than biological interventions. Such reasons might be, for example:

- if they are safer;
- if they are more likely to be successful;
- if justice requires them (based on the limitations of resources);
- if there are benefits to others or less harm.

However, if reason favors biological rather than social enhancement, we should employ the biological. It may be that early postnatal interventions accelerate learning in a more effective way than enhanced educational programs. If this were so, we should employ them.

We have seen that nature allots advantages and disadvantages with no regard to fairness, and that enhancement improves people's lives. The best way to protect the disadvantaged from the inequalities that bioconservatives like McKibben (2003) believe will follow from enhancement is not to prevent enhancement, but to ensure that the social institutions we use to distribute enhancement technologies work to protect the least well off and to provide everyone with a fair go. People have disease and disability, and egalitarian social institutions and laws against discrimination are designed to make sure everyone, regardless of natural inequality, has a decent chance of a decent life. Enhancement to benefit the worst off would be an effective way of achieving a laudable aim.

Obstacles to Development

While there are clear economic and social benefits to cognitive enhancement, there exist a number of obstacles to its development and use. One obstacle is the present system for licensing drugs and medical treatments. This system was created to deal with traditional medicine which aims to prevent, diagnose, cure, or alleviate disease. In this framework, there is no room for enhancing medicine. For example, drug companies could find it difficult to get regulatory approval for a pharmaceutical whose sole use was to improve cognitive functioning in the healthy population. To date, every pharmaceutical on the market that offers some potential cognitive enhancement effect was developed to treat some specific pathological condition (such as ADHD, narcolepsy, and Alzheimer's disease). The cognitive-enhancing effects of these drugs in healthy subjects are a serendipitous unintended effect. Progress in this area might be accelerated if pharmaceutical companies could focus directly on developing nootropics for use in non-diseased populations rather than having to work indirectly by demonstrating that the drugs are also efficacious in treating some recognized disease.

One of the perverse effects of the failure of the current medical framework to recognize the legitimacy and potential of enhancement medicine is the trend towards medicalization and "pathologization" of an increasing range of conditions that were previously regarded as part of the normal human spectrum. If a significant fraction of the population could obtain certain benefits from drugs that improve e.g. concentration, it is currently necessary to categorize this segment of people as having some illness – in this case ADHD – in order to get the drug approved and prescribed to those who could benefit from it. This disease-focused medical model is increasingly inadequate for an era in which many people will be using medical treatments for enhancement purposes.

The medicine-as-treatment-for-disease framework creates problems not only for pharmaceutical companies but also for users ("patients") whose access to enhancers is often dependent on being able to find an open-minded physician who can prescribe the drug. This creates inequities in access. People with high social capital and good information get access while others are excluded.

The current rise of personalized medicine results both from improved diagnostic methods that provide a better picture of the individual patient, and from the availability of a wider range of therapeutic options which make it necessary to select the one that is most suitable for a particular patient. Many patients now approach their physicians armed with detailed knowledge about their condition and possible treatments. Information can be easily obtained from Medline and other internet services. These factors are leading to a shift in the physician–patient relationship, away from paternalism to a relationship characterized by teamwork and a focus on the customer's situation. Preventative and enhancing medicine are often inseparable, and both will likely be promoted by these changes and by an increasingly active and informed health care consumer who insists on exercising choice in the medical context. These shifts suggest the need for important and complex regulatory change.

Given that all medical interventions carry some risk, and that the benefits of enhancements may often be more subjective and value-dependent than the benefits of being cured of a disease, it is important to allow individuals to determine their own preferences for tradeoffs between risks and benefits. It is highly unlikely that one size will fit all. At the same time, many will feel the need for a limited degree of paternalism, to protect individuals from at least the worst risks. One option would be to establish some baseline level of acceptable risk in allowable interventions, perhaps by comparison to other risks that society allows individuals to take, such as the risks from smoking, mountain climbing, or horseback riding. Enhancements that could be shown to be no more risky than these activities would be allowed (with appropriate information and warning labels when necessary). Another possibility would be enhancement licenses. People willing to undergo potentially risky but rewarding enhancements could be required to demonstrate sufficient understanding of the risks and the ability to handle them responsibly. This would both ensure informed consent and enable better monitoring. A downside with enhancement licenses is that people with low cognitive capacity, who may have the most to gain from enhancements, could find it hard to get access if the license requirements were too demanding.

Public funding for research does not yet reflect the potential personal and social benefits of many forms of cognitive enhancement. There is funding (albeit perhaps at inadequate levels) for research into education methods and information technology, but not for pharmacological cognitive enhancers. In view of the potentially enormous gains from even moderately effective general cognitive enhancements, this area deserves large-scale funding. It is clear that much research and development are needed to make cognitive enhancement practical and efficient. As discussed above, this requires a change of the view that medicine is only about restoring, not enhancing, capacities, and concomitant changes in the regulatory regime for medical trials and drug approval.

The evidence on prenatal and perinatal nutrition suggests that infant formulas containing suitable nutrients may have a significant positive lifelong impact on cognition. Because of the low cost and large potential impact of enriched infant formula if applied at a population level, it should be a priority to conduct more research to establish the optimal composition of infant formula. Regulation could then be used to ensure that commercially available formula contains these nutrients. Public health information campaigns could further promote the use of enriched formula that promotes mental development. This would be a simple extension of current regulatory practice, but a potentially important one.

There is a wider cultural challenge of destigmatizing the use of enhancers. At present, the taking of medicine is regarded as a regrettable condition, and use of non-therapeutic medication is seen as suspect, possibly misuse. Attempts to enhance cognition are often construed as expression of a dangerous ambition. Yet the border between accepted therapy and suspect enhancement is shifting. Pain relief is now seen as unproblematic. Plastic surgery enjoys ever-wider acceptance. Millions of people ingest nutrient supplements and herbal remedies for enhancing purposes. Self-help psychology is very popular. Apparently, the cultural constructions surrounding the means of enhancement are more important for their acceptance than the actual enhancement ability of these means. To make the best use of our new opportunities, we need a culture of enhancement, with norms, support structures, and a lay understanding of enhance- ment that takes it into the mainstream cultural context. Consumers also need better information on risks and benefits of enhancers, which suggests a need for reliable consumer information and for more studies to determine safety and efficacy.

Testing of cognitive enhancers would ideally be done not only in the lab but also in field studies that investigate how an intervention works in everyday life. The ultimate criterion of efficacy would be various forms of life success rather than performance in narrow psychological lab tests. Such "ecological testing" would require new kinds of experiment, including monitoring of large sample populations. Advances in wearable computers and sensors may allow unobtrusive monitoring of behavior, diet, use of other drugs, etc. Data mining of collected materials could help determine the effects of enhancers. Such studies, however, would pose major challenges, including cost, new kinds of privacy concerns (monitoring may accumulate information not only about the consenting test subjects but also about their friends and family), and problems of unfair competition if enhancers experience beneficial effects but others cannot get access to the enhancements due to their experimental nature.

While access to medicine is currently regarded as a human right constrained by cost concerns, it is less clear whether access to all enhancements should or would be regarded as a positive right.[8] The case for at least a negative right to cognitive enhancement, based on cognitive liberty, privacy interests, and the important interest of persons to protect and develop their own minds and capacity for autonomy, seems very strong.[9] Banning enhancements would create an incitement for black markets as well as limit socially beneficial uses. Legal enhancement would promote development and use, in the long run leading to cheaper and safer enhancements. Yet without public funding, some useful enhancements may be out of reach for many of the people who would benefit the most from them. Proponents of a positive right to enhancements could argue for their position on grounds of fairness or equality, or public interest in the promotion of the capacities required for autonomous agency. The societal benefits of effective cognitive enhancement may even turn out to be so large and clear that it would be Pareto optimal to subsidize enhancement for the poor just as the state now subsidizes education.

Notes

1. Although Aldous Huxley's *Brave New World* is often cited, that society was deliberately planned into a caste society rather than an unintentional product of technology and culture, concerns over genetic or cognitive class divisions are moot when the government (or society as a whole) is promoting them.
2. However, see also Newson, 2000, for some more subtle ways intelligence might bring happiness.
3. www.bibbyfinancialservices.com.
4. This paper also makes the claim that higher intelligence increases the probability of financial distress. However, this is likely an artifact of using third-degree curve fitting and not a real effect.

5. The study also excluded some of the more problematic data and controlled for possible cultural bias by excluding the OECD countries as a control.
6. Compare the data in "Falling Through the Net: A Survey of the "Have Nots" in Rural and Urban America." Washington, DC: U.S. Department of Commerce, July 1995, at www.ntia.doc.gov/ntiahome/fallingthru.html with "A Nation Online: How Americans are Expanding their Use of the Internet." Washington, DC: U.S. Department of Commerce. 2002.
7. This section draws on Savulescu, 2006, 2009.
8. For an argument that it should, see Hughes, 2004.
9. It can certainly be argued as a negative right, cf. Boire, 2001 and Sandberg, 2003.

References

Anon. (2003). TetraTab – Cognitive Enhancement Gone Wrong. *Lancet Neurology*, **2**(8), 451.

Angus, R.G. & Heslegrave, R.J. (1985). Effects of sleep loss on sustained cognitive performance during a command and control simulation. *Behavior Research Methods Instruments & Computers*, **17**(1), 55–67.

Annas, G. (2003). Cell division. www.geneticsandsociety.org/article.php?id=164.

Armor, D. (2003). *Maximizing Intelligence*. Transaction Publishers.

Batty, G.D., Deary, I.J. & Gottfredson, L.S. (2007). Premorbid (early life) IQ and later mortality risk: Systematic review. *Annals of Epidemiology*, **17**(4), 278–88.

Boire, R.G. (2001). On cognitive liberty. *Journal of Cognitive Liberties*, **2**(1), 7–22.

Bound, J., Griliches, Z. & Hall, B.H. (1986). Wages, schooling and IQ of brothers and sisters - Do the family factors differ? *International Economic Review*, **27**(1), 77–105.

Brody, N. (2004). Book review: *Maximizing Intelligence*. *Intelligence*, **32**(3), 317–18.

Brynjolfsson, E. & Hitt, L.M. (1998). Beyond the productivity paradox. *Communications of the ACM*, **41**(8), 49–55.

Brynjolfsson, E. & Yang, S. (1996). Information technology and productivity: A review of the literature. *Advances in Computers*, **43**, 179–214.

Caldwell, J.A., Jr., Caldwell, J.L., Smythe, N.K. & Hall, K.K. (2000). A double-blind, placebo-controlled investigation of the efficacy of Modafinil for sustaining the alertness and performance of aviators: A helicopter simulator study. *Psychopharmacology (Berlin)*, **150**(3), 272–82.

Cawley, J., Conneely, K., Heckman, J. & Vytlacil, E. (1997). Cognitive ability, wages and meritocracy. In B. Devlin, S. Fienberg, D. Resnick & K. Roeder (eds.), *Intelligence, Genes, and Success: Scientists Respond to the Bell Curve* (pp. 179–92). New York: Springer Verlag.

Collins, J.A. (2002). An international survey of the health economics of IVF and ICSI. *Human Reproduction Update*, **8**(3), 265–77.

Daley, T.C., Whaley, S.E., Sigman, M.D., Espinosa, M.P. & Neumann, C. (2003). IQ on the rise – The Flynn effect in rural Kenyan children. *Psychological Science*, **14**(3), 215–19.

Denison, E. (1985). *Trends in American Economic Growth, 1929–1982*. Washington, DC: Brookings Institution.

Dickerson, R.E. (2006). Exponential correlation of IQ and the wealth of nations. *Intelligence*, **34**(3), 291–5.

Ericsson, K.A., Chase, W.G., & Faloon, S. (1980). Acquisition of a memory skill. *Science*, **208**(4448), 1181–2.

Farah, M. J., Illes, J., Cook-Deegan, R., Gardner, H., Kandel, E., King, P. *et al.* (2004). Neurocognitive enhancement: What can we do and what should we do? *Nature Reviews Neuroscience*, **5**(5), 421–5.

Fernald, J. & Ramnath, S. (2003). Information technology and the U.S. productivity acceleration. *Essays on Issues,* The Federal Reserve Bank of Chicago, Number 193, September.

Fukuyama, F. (2002). *Our Posthuman Future: Consequences of the Biotechnology Revolution.* New York: Farrar, Strauss and Giroux.

Fukuyama, F. (2004). Transhumanism. *Foreign Policy,* **144**: 42–4; www.foreignpolicy.com/story/files/story2667.php.

Gill, M., Haerich, P., Westcott, K., Godenick, K.L. & Tucker, J.A. (2006). Cognitive performance following Modafinil versus placebo in sleep-deprived emergency physicians: A double-blind randomized crossover study. *Academic Emergency Medicine,* **13**(2), 158–65.

Gottfredson, L.S. (1997). Why g matters: The complexity of everyday life. *Intelligence,* **24**(1), 79–132.

Gottfredson, L.S. (2004). Life, death, and intelligence. *Journal of Cognitive Education and Psychology,* **4**(1), 23–46.

Gottfredson, L.S. (2007). Innovation, fatal accidents, and the evolution of general intelligence. In M.J. Roberts (Ed.), *Integrating the Mind: Domain General versus Domain Specific Processes in Higher Cognition* (pp. 387–425). Hove, UK: Psychology Press.

Gow, A.J., Whiteman, M.C., Pattie, A., Whalley, L., Starr, J. & Deary, I.J. (2005). Lifetime intellectual function and satisfaction with life in old age: Longitudinal cohort study. *British Medical Journal,* **331**(7509), 141–2.

Halifax Home Insurance. (2005). Halifax Home Insurance unlocks the nation's key disasters: Over 1.2 million UK adults will lose their keys at least once this year. June 21, 2005. Retrieved June 8, 2007, from www.hbosplc.com/media/pressreleases/articles/halifax/2005-06-21-halifaxhom.asp.

Hartog, J. & Oosterbeek, H. (1998). Health, wealth and happiness: Why pursue a higher education? *Economics of Education Review,* **17**(3), 245–56.

Herrnstein, R.J. & Murray, C. (1994). *The Bell Curve.* New York: Free Press.

Hooper, J. & Whittle, I. R. (2003). Costs of thalamic deep brain stimulation for movement disorders in patients with multiple sclerosis. *British Journal of Neurosurgery,* **17**(1), 40–5.

Hughes, J. (2004). *Citizen Cyborg: Why Democratic Societies Must Respond to the Redesigned Human of the Future.* Boulder, CO: Westview Press.

Hunt, E. & Wittmann, W. (2008). National intelligence and national prosperity. *Intelligence,* **36**(1), 1–9.

Jones, G. & Schneider, W.J. (2006). Intelligence, human capital, and economic growth: A Bayesian Averaging of Classical Estimates (BACE) approach. *Journal of Economic Growth,* **11**(1), 71–93.

Kalfoglou, A., Suthers, K., Scott, J., & Hudson, K. (2002). *Reproductive Genetic Testing: What America Thinks.* Washington, DC: Genetics and Public Policy Center.

Kanazawa, S. (2006). IQ and the wealth of states. *Intelligence,* **34**(6), 593–600.

Kass, L. (2003). Ageless bodies, happy souls: Biotechnology and the pursuit of perfection. *The New Atlantis,* **Spring**, 9–28.

King Baudouin Foundation & Rathenau Institut. (2004). Connecting Brains and Society: The Present and Future of Brain Science: What is Possible, What is Desirable? European Workshop, Proceedings and Synthesis Report. April 22 and 23. Amsterdam, The Netherlands.

Lilien, G., Rangaswamy, A. Van den Bulte. C. (1999). Diffusion Models: Managerial Applications and Software, ISBM Report 7-1999, Institute for the Study of Business Markets, Pennsylvania State University.

Lynn, R. & Vanhanen, T. (2002). *IQ and the Wealth of Nations.* Westport, CT: Praeger.

Lyons, W. (2005). "Forgotten direct debits" costing billions. *The Scotsman,* January 20.

Mackie, J. (1984). Rights, utility and universalization. In R.G. Frey (ed.), *Utility and Right* (pp. 86–105). Minneapolis: University of Minnesota Press.

McKibben, B. (2003). Designer genes. *Orion* (May–June). www.orionsociety.org/pages/om/03-3om/McKibben.html.

Muir, T. & Zegarac, M. (2001). Societal costs of exposure to toxic substances: Economic and health costs of four case studies that are candidates for environmental causation. *Environmental Health Perspectives*, **109**, 885–903.

Muller, U., Steffenhagen, N., Regenthal, R. & Bublak, P. (2004). Effects of Modafinil on working memory processes in humans. *Psychopharmacology*, **177**(1–2), 161–9.

Murphy, K.J., Foley, A.G., O'Connell, A.W. & Regan, C.M. (2006). Chronic exposure of rats to cognition enhancing drugs produces a neuroplastic response identical to that obtained by complex environment rearing. *Neuropsychopharmacology*, **31**(1), 90–100.

Murray, C. (2002). IQ and income inequality in a sample of sibling pairs from advantaged family backgrounds. *American Economic Review*, **92**(2), 339–43.

Neisser, U., Boodoo, G., Bouchard, T.J., Boykin, A.W., Brody, N., Ceci, S.J. *et al.* (1996). Intelligence: Knowns and unknowns. *American Psychologist*, **51**(2), 77–101.

Newson, A. (2000). Is being intelligent good? Addressing questions of value in behavioural genetics. Paper presented at the 5th World Congress of the International Association of Bioethics, London.

Nozick, R. (1974). *Anarchy, State and Utopia*. New York: Basic Books.

Parfit, D. (1997). Equality or priority? *Ratio*, **10**(3), 202–21.

President's Council on Bioethics. (2003). *Beyond Therapy: Biotechnology and the Pursuit of Happiness*. New York: Regan Books.

Randall, D.C., Shneerson, J.M. & File, S.E. (2005). Cognitive effects of Modafinil in student volunteers may depend on IQ. *Pharmacology Biochemistry and Behavior*, **82**(1), 133–9.

Rawls, J. (1971). *A Theory of Justice*. Cambridge, MA: Harvard University Press.

Rogers, E. (2003). *Diffusion of Innovation* [1st edition 1962]. New York: Free Press.

Rowe, D.C., Vesterdal, W.J. & Rodgers, J.L. (1998). Herrnstein's syllogism: Genetic and shared environmental influences on IQ, education, and income. *Intelligence*, **26**(4), 405–23.

Salkever, D.S. (1995). Updated estimates of earnings benefits from reduced exposure of children to environmental lead. *Environmental Research*, **70**(1), 1–6.

Sandberg, A. (2003). Morphologic freedom. www.nada.kth.se/~asa/Texts/Morphological-Freedom.htm.

Sandberg, A. & Bostrom, N. (2006). Converging cognitive enhancements. *Annals of the New York Academy of Science*, **1093**, 201–7.

Savulescu, J. (2003). Bioethics: Utilitarianism. In D. Cooper (ed.), *Nature Encyclopedia of the Human Genome*. New York: Nature Publishing Group.

Savulescu, J. (2006). Justice, fairness and enhancement. In W. Sims Bainbridge & M.C. Roco (eds.), Special Issue: Progress in Convergence: Technologies for Human Wellbeing. *Annals of the New York Academy of Sciences*, **1093**, 321–38.

Savulescu, J. (2009). Enhancement and fairness. In P. Healey & S. Rayner (eds.), *Unnatural Selection: The Challenges of Engineering Tomorrow's People* (pp. 177–87). London: Earthscan.

Schmidt, F.L. & Hunter, J.E. (1998). The validity and utility of selection methods in personnel psychology: Practical and theoretical implications of 85 years of research findings. *Psychological Bulletin*, **124**(2), 262–74.

Schwartz, J. (1994). Societal benefits of reducing lead-exposure. *Environmental Research*, **66**(1), 105–24.

Sigelman, L. (1981). Is ignorance bliss? *A Reconsideration of the folk wisdom. Human Relations*, **34**(11), 965–74.

Silver, L. (1998). *Remaking Eden*. Harper Perennial.

Stiroh, K.J. (2001). Investing in information technology: Productivity payoffs for U.S. industries. *Current Issues in Economics and Finance*, 7(6).

Sultan, F., Farley, J.U. & Lehmann, D.R. (1990). A meta-analysis of diffusion models. *Journal of Marketing Research*, **27**, 70–77.

Talukdar, D., Sudhir, K. & Ainslie, A. (2002). Investigating new product diffusion across products and countries. *Marketing Science*, **21**(1), 97–114.

Thomas, R.J. (1985). Estimating market growth for new products: An analogical diffusion models approach. *Journal of Product Innovation Management*, **2**, 45–55.

Tomaszewski, K.J. & Holloway, R.G. (2001). Deep brain stimulation in the treatment of Parkinson's disease. *A cost-effectiveness analysis. Neurology*, **57**(4), 663–71.

Wai, J., Lubinski, D. & Benbow, C.P. (2005). Creativity and occupational accomplishments among intellectually precocious youths: An age 13 to age 33 longitudinal study. *Journal of Educational Psychology*, **97**(3), 484–92.

Whalley, L.J. & Deary, I.J. (2001). Longitudinal cohort study of childhood IQ and survival up to age 76. *British Medical Journal*, **322**(7290), 819–22.

Whetzel, D.L. & McDaniel, M.A. (2006). Prediction of national wealth. *Intelligence*, **34**(5), 449–58.

Williams, B. (1962). The idea of equality. In P. Laslett & W.G. Runciman (eds.), *Philosophy, Politics and Society* (pp. 121–2). Oxford: Basil Blackwell.

Winship, C. & Korenman, S. (1997). Does staying in school make you smarter? The effect of education on IQ in The Bell Curve. In B. Devlin, S.E. Fienberg & K. Roeder (eds.), *Intelligence, Genes, and Success: Scientists Respond to The Bell Curve* (pp. 215–34). New York: Springer.

Wolbring, G. (2006). The unenhanced underclass. In P. Miller & J. Wilsdon (eds.), *Better Humans? The Politics of Human Enhancement and Life Extension* (Vol. **21**). London: Demos.

Zhou, M.F. & Suszkiw, J.B. (2004). Nicotine attenuates spatial learning lead deficits induced in the rat by perinatal exposure. *Brain Research*, **999**(1), 142–7.

7

Cognitive Enhancing Drugs: Neuroscience and Society

Charlotte R. Housden, Sharon Morein-Zamir, and Barbara J. Sahakian

The use of pharmacological agents to improve aspects of cognition is now common-place. Cognitive-enhancing drugs are prescribed to patients with psychiatric disorders, such as attention deficit hyperactivity disorder (ADHD) and Alzheimer's disease, to treat cognitive deficits. However, if these drugs are used by healthy individuals, therapy becomes enhancement proper. This chapter discusses the use of pharmacological agents to improve the cognition of both those with cognitive impairments and of the general population, as well as some of the benefits, risks, and ethical issues associated with the use of cognitive-enhancing drugs.

Cognition

Cognitive skills are information-processing mental functions carried out by the human brain, including perception, attention, memory, comprehension, use of speech, and executive functions such as planning, problem solving, and self-monitoring. While attending a lecture, a student requires some of the following cognitive skills: selective attention (the ability to screen out irrelevant stimuli), working memory (the ability to hold task-relevant information while it is being processed), and response inhibition (the ability to avoid making automatic responses to incorrect stimuli). Everyday mental activity and behavior relies on the various cognitive skills. Consequently, improvements in cognitive skills, in both the cognitively impaired and the healthy, can increase both an individual's quality of life and ability to contribute to society (Beddington et al., 2008).

Given that problems relating to cognition occur in many neuropsychiatric and neurodegenerative disorders (Chamberlain et al., 2006), specific cognitive domains are important targets for pharmacological intervention. However, drugs importantly cannot target cognition itself, but rather chemicals in the brain that modulate

Enhancing Human Capacities, edited by Julian Savulescu, Ruud ter Meulen and Guy Kahane.
© 2011 Blackwell Publishing Ltd

cognition. These chemicals, called neurotransmitters, relay, amplify, or influence signals sent between neurons in the brain. They are released from a neuron into the synaptic cleft (the space between two adjacent neurons), and bind to receptors on the membrane of an adjacent neuron. Drugs can modulate these signals in different ways: they can, for instance, mimic or boost the release of neurotransmitters, increasing binding to post-synaptic receptors and thereby amplifying the effect of the neuro-transmitter. Drugs can also decrease the ability of the neurotransmitter to bind to the post-synaptic membrane, reducing its effect. Other drugs block the function of enzymes that break down neurotransmitters, thereby increasing the concentration of the latter in the synaptic cleft. Furthermore, most cognitive-enhancing drugs improve only specific aspects of cognition such as attention or memory, which are mediated differently by various systems in the brain. Although the effects that have so far been documented range from small to moderate, even small increments in cognitive performance can lead to significant improvements in functional outcome; a 10% improvement in a memory score could lead to an improvement in an A-level grade or degree class (Academy of Medical Sciences, 2008). While the generalization of enhancement from the controlled environment of the laboratory to daily life is controversial, several factors are contributing to an increasing understanding of the neural mechanisms that underlie cognition and how to target specific aspects of cognition using drugs. These include the development of sophisticated neuropsycho-logical tests, which tap into particular areas of cognition, and the routine inclusion in research studies of multiple, converging behavioral and brain-imaging measures, allowing the relationship between brain regions, neurotransmitters, and cognition to be determined.

One valuable method of testing the effects of cognitive enhancers on cognition is double-blind placebo control studies where participants undergo a battery of objective cognitive tests which measure various facets of cognition, including memory and attention. For example, in the Cambridge Neuropsychological Test Automated Battery (CANTAB) Spatial Working Memory (SWM) task, a number of colored boxes are shown on the screen (Owen *et al.*, 1990). The aim of this task is that, by touching the boxes and using a process of elimination, the subject should find one blue "token" in each of a number of boxes. Once a blue token is found in a box another one is never put in that box again, so the participant has to remember where tokens have been found and to not look in those boxes again. The number of boxes is gradually increased, until it is necessary to search a total of eight boxes. SWM is a test of the subject's ability to retain spatial information and to manipulate remembered items in working memory. It is a self-ordered task, which also assesses heuristic strategy. This test is sensitive to dysfunction in the front part of the brain, called the frontal lobe, and impairments are seen in children and adults with ADHD (Kempton *et al.*, 1999; McLean *et al.*, 2004; Mehta *et al.*, 2004).

Cognitive tasks such as SWM can be used to investigate the effects of drugs on cognition, in patient groups and healthy people. One drug that has been investigated in this way and which demonstrates this methodology is methylphenidate, a neurosti-mulant commonly called Ritalin and routinely prescribed for ADHD. Methylphenidate improves SWM performance both in children and adult patients with ADHD: patients make less task-related errors when on methylphenidate (Mehta *et al.*, 2004; Turner *et al.*, 2005). The neural substrates mediating SWM task performance have been examined using imaging techniques such as positron emission topography (PET) and indicate that the dorsolateral and mid-ventrolateral prefrontal cortex are particularly recruited (Mehta *et al.*, 2000). Studies using PET and contrasting [(11)C] raclopride binding on versus off methylphenidate have further indicated that methylphenidate influences dopamine (a neurotransmitter) function, particularly in a part of the brain called the striatum (Montgomery *et al.*, 2007). The striatum has an intimate anatomical relationship with the cortex in the form of cortico-striatal "loops" (Alexander *et al.*, 1986). Therefore, methylphenidate could be increasing the efficacy of receptors in the frontal cortex. Methylphenidate has been found to improve both performance and efficiency in the spatial working memory neural network involving the dorsolateral prefrontal cortex and posterior parietal cortex in healthy volunteers (Mehta *et al.*, 2000). There are five different kinds of dopamine receptor in the frontal lobes, with stimulation of the D1 receptor being critical for working memory. Poor functioning of the D1 receptors are associated with ADHD, schizophrenia, and aging (Arnsten *et al.*, 1994; Hirvonen *et al.*, 2006; Levy, 2008). Therefore, development of drugs that have an affinity to the D1 receptor, would improve treatments and cognitive enhancement potential. However, developing drugs such as these poses a challenge to the pharmaceutical industry and research. Indeed, as our understanding of specific receptor types, neural circuits, neurotransmitter systems, and their interactions grows through investigation, new directions for drug development can be established.

Cognitive Enhancement as a Potential Treatment

Many diseases, including neurodegenerative disorders, lead to impairments in cognitive ability. Alzheimer's disease, for example, is one such condition, and is becoming increasingly prevalent in the aging population. Alzheimer's disease is characterized by a loss of memory of recent events, but over time there is a decline in a number of cognitive functions. Currently, six million Europeans suffer from Alzheimer's disease and other forms of dementia: however, it is predicted that by 2040 over 11 million Europeans will suffer from dementia (World Health Organization). Indeed, by 2040 neurodegenerative diseases will overtake cancer to become the world's second-leading cause of death, after cardiovascular disease. This increase in prevalence will lead to greater expenditure, with the total cost of care services for the elderly with cognitive impairment rising from £4.6 billion, to around £10.9 billion in 2031 (Comas-Herrera *et al.*, 2007). In the UK, the number of people in residential care is expected to rise from 224,000 in 1998 to 365,000 in 2031. A treatment that would reduce severe cognitive impairment in the elderly by just 1%, would cancel out all the estimated increases in long-term care costs due to the aging population (Report commissioned by the Alzheimer's Research Trust in Cambridge, UK:(Comas-Herrera et al. 2007)). Drugs for neuro-protection, which slow down or compensate for the decline in cognitive function, will benefit these individuals. Such drugs would enable people to stay in work for longer, if they wished, and to live independently for a greater period of time.

There is a relationship between the functional loss of the neurotransmitter acetylcholine and memory loss (Shimohama *et al.*, 1986). This loss of acetylcholine production in the brain can be compensated for by cholinesterase inhibitors, which are drugs that stop the breakdown of acetylcholine in the synapse by the enzyme cholinesterase. Cholinesterase inhibitors have been shown to stabilize cognitive function in Alzheimer's patients at a steady level during a one-year period in approximately 50% of patients and to improve their ability to perform daily activities (Rogers *et al.*, 1998). It has also been shown that cholinesterase inhibitors improve working memory in healthy adults (Sahakian *et al.*, 1988).

Drugs that improve facets of cognition may also be beneficial for disorders for which they are not yet routinely prescribed. For instance, although it is common knowledge that people with schizophrenia typically suffer from hallucinations and delusions, it is the long-term cognitive impairments that often impede everyday function and reduce quality of life for many patients. 24 million people worldwide suffer from schizophrenia, mostly in the age group 15–35 (World Health Organization). The young age of onset of this disorder means that many individuals will need support for much of their lives. In the United States, direct and indirect costs were estimated at over $60 billion in the year 2002, with unemployment being the largest component of annual costs (Wu *et al.*, 2005). It has been suggested that even small improvements in cognitive functions could help patients make the transition to independent living.

The exact pattern of cognitive deficits experienced as a result of schizophrenia varies between individual patients, although spatial working memory, planning, and attentional set-shifting have been shown to be affected (Elliott *et al.*, 1995). Spatial working memory impairments have been shown to be associated with increased symptom levels, whereas attentional set-shifting impairments seem to represent a more stable, trait-like impairment (Barnett *et al.*, 2005). Deficits in attentional set-shifting, a kind of cognitive flexibility, have been detected in both high and low functioning schizophrenics (Barnett *et al.*, 2005). For example, when responding to a set of stimuli that are all in the same perceptual dimension, new learning is impaired in schizophrenic patients when they are no longer rewarded for responding to stimuli in that dimension, and a previously unrewarded stimuli dimension is now rewarded. The CANTAB intradimensional/extradimensional (IDED) task (Owen *et al.*, 1991) lends itself to the study of attentional set-shifting in schizophrenia, because subjects progress through different stages in which responses can be modified by feedback. These include learning to change responses when stimuli are no longer relevant (reversal learning) and shifting attention to a different stimulus dimension when the current dimension is no longer fruitful (attentional set-shifting). Schizophrenic patients find it hard to switch category, or shift their attention from one set of stimuli to another (Pantelis *et al.*, 1999). Currently, schizophrenic patients are treated with anti-psychotic medications, which have been shown to improve psychotic symptoms and some cognitive symptoms (Weickert *et al.*, 2003). A cognitive-enhancing drug, Modafinil, has been shown to improve attentional set-shifting and short-term verbal memory in schizophrenic patients (Turner *et al.*, 2004b), suggesting it may be of therapeutic use.

But it is not only adults suffering from neuropsychiatric disorders that benefit from cognitive-enhancing drugs. ADHD affects 3–7% of all children worldwide, and is the most prevalent neuropsychiatric disorder in children. ADHD is a highly heritable and disabling condition characterized by core cognitive and behavioral symptoms of impulsivity, hyperactivity, and/or inattention. It has important implications for education provision, long-term social outcomes, and economic impact. For example, long-term studies indicate that it is associated with increased educational dropout, job dismissal, criminal activities, substance abuse, other mental illness, and increased accident rates (Barkley *et al.*, 2006). The annual excess cost of ADHD in the United States in 2000 was estimated to be $42.5 billion (Pelham *et al.*, 2007).

As well as methylphenidate, discussed earlier, other drugs such as Modafinil and Atomoxetine can improve performance in some tasks of executive functioning in ADHD patients. Modafinil has been found to improve spatial planning and response inhibition in ADHD patients (Turner *et al.*, 2004a). Likewise, administration of an acute dose of Atomoxetine has been found not only to improve response inhibition in ADHD patients, but also in healthy adults (Chamberlain *et al.*, 2007). Using functional magnetic resonance imaging (fMRI), the brain mechanisms by which Atomoxetine exerts its effects in healthy volunteers has been examined in a double-blind placebo-controlled study (Chamberlain *et al.*, 2009). Atomoxetine led to increased activation in the right inferior frontal gyrus when participants attempted to inhibit their responses. Inhibitory motor control has been shown previously to depend, at least in part, on the function of this brain region (Aron *et al.*, 2003).

Non-Therapeutic Uses of Cognitive-Enhancing Drugs

With the popularization of the notion of cognition improvement, pharmacological interventions are being seen as a means not only to compensate for existing deficits, but also to prevent decline before its onset, and even to enhance normal functioning. The use of cognitive-enhancing drugs has gone up over recent years, although many individuals who take them do not suffer from neuropsychiatric disorders.

Who takes cognitive-enhancing drugs and why?

Drugs which appear to be increasingly used in healthy populations are neurostimulants such as methylphenidate (discussed earlier in relation to ADHD) and Modafinil, a novel cognitive enhancer originally developed for use in patients with narcolepsy. Individuals taking these drugs range from students to working professionals. Evidence for increased use can be seen in trends suggesting that between 1993 and 2001 there was a clear increase in the 12-month prevalence rates of nonmedical use of prescription drugs in college students (National Institute on Drug Abuse, 2005). In the United States, studies indicate that up to 16% of students on some college campuses use stimulants, while 8% of university undergraduates report having illegally used pre-scription stimulants (Babcock & Byrne, 2000). There is also a trend for increasingly younger students to use such drugs with one report indicating 2.5% of eighth graders (13–14 years) abused methylphenidate as did 3.4% of tenth graders (National Institute in Drug Abuse, 2005). The trends are also not reserved solely for the United States, as prescription rates for stimulants in England have been rising steadily from 220,000 in 1998 to 418,300 in 2004 (Parliamentary Office of Science and Technology, 2007).

The rise in prescription rates is perhaps linked to the rise in the illicit use of stimulant drugs, as a survey has shown that students obtain these drugs from peers and family more often than from the internet (McCabe & Boyd, 2005). A recent survey of 1,000 students conducted by the University of Cambridge student newspaper, *Varsity*, found that 10% of students interviewed had taken stimulant drugs such as methylphenidate, or other cognitive-enhancing drugs such as Modafinil. The most commonly reported motives for drug use are to aid concentration, to help study, and to increase alertness. Academic staff, as well as students, are taking cognitive-enhancing drugs, as reported by an informal survey, to counteract the effects of jet lag, to enhance productivity or mental energy, and to deal with demanding and important mental challenges (Sahakian & Morein-Zamir, 2007). Furthermore, the use of cognitive-enhancing drugs is not restricted to academic use, as is illustrated by the U.S. sprinter Kelli White who received a two-year ban in 2004 for using Modafinil when competing in the world championships and other U.S. national events.

One can presume that improvements in cognitive skills such as memory would also be appealing to middle-aged and elderly people who are facing a decline in memory functions. Further research is required to investigate the current use of cognitive-enhancing drugs in this population, and to find out this demographics' views on the issue of enhancing cognition. Individuals may also choose to take drugs such as Modafinil that minimize the need for sleep, while maintaining cognitive function because they have to work under sleep-deprived conditions. Surgeons, shift workers, and the military are examples of this group. In the United States, the Defense Advanced Research Projects Agency (DARPA) has invested in sleep reduction experiments, with the aim of preventing bad decisions due to sleep deprivation on the battlefield. According to DARPA's Defenses Science Officer, they are investigating pharmacological ways of preventing changes in the brain caused by sleep deprivation, optimizing memory, reversing the adverse effects of sleep deprivation, and developing "sleep resistance" (Moreno, 2004). As job demands increase, greater numbers of people may find themselves considering using drugs to boost their cognitive skill and to help them cope with sleep deprivation.

The increased use of cognitive-enhancing drugs could also be due to their wider availability, particularly on the internet. Indeed, a recent survey identified 159 sites offering drugs for sale, only two of which were regulated and 85% not requiring a doctor's prescription from the patient (The National Centre on Addiction and Substance Abuse (CASA) at Columbia University, 2008). This raises concerns about the purity and safety of the drugs that can be obtained. Increased media coverage can also make people aware of the possible benefits of taking pharmacological agents to boost certain aspects of cognition, making them more likely to try the drugs. The popular media has reported at length on studies about improved performance in healthy individuals and on the rising use of drugs that enhance cognition in healthy individuals. Some journalists have reported on their experiences while taking Modafinil, both in newspapers (*The Sunday Times*) and on the television (BBC). Furthermore, the results from our laboratory on Modafinil were reported in the media, including newspapers, magazines, and radio. Publications ranging from *The Guardian* newspaper (London) to *The New Yorker* and *Nature*, as well as the BBC, have discussed their potential for widespread use.

Limitations and risks

Experimental research has shown that drugs used to treat cognitive impairments do indeed have the potential to enhance cognitive skills in healthy individuals. For example, Modafinil produces improvements in performance in a group of healthy volunteers on tests of spatial planning, response inhibition, visual recognition, and short-term memory (Turner *et al.*, 2003). Administration of an acute dose of Atomoxetine has been found not only to improve response inhibition in ADHD patients, but also in healthy adults (Chamberlain *et al.*, 2009).

In some studies, although Modafinil had an effect on the mood of young, non-sleep deprived adults, it did not affect cognition (Randall *et al.*, 2005a; Randall *et al.*, 2005b). Furthermore, although improvements have been seen in the laboratory, it has yet to be determined how these drug-induced enhancements in cognition translate to the real world. Indeed, research has currently been confined to investigating the acute effect of these drugs on cognition, so the long-term efficacy of these drugs for healthy people is not known.

However, despite advances in our understanding of these drugs and cognition, the exact mechanism of some cognitive-enhancing drugs, such as Modafinil, has yet to be completely understood. Modafinil has been shown to have robust effects on several different chemical systems in the brain (catecholamines, serotonin, glutamate, gamma amino-butyric acid, orexin, and histamine), affecting the relationships between cortical structures that control higher cognitive processing, and more "primitive" limbic structures (Minzenberg *et al.*, 2008). Furthermore, an imaging study has shown that Modafinil blocks dopamine transporters and increased dopamine in the human brain, including an area called the nucleus accumbens (Volkow *et al.*, 2009). Because drugs that increase dopamine in the nucleus accumbens have the potential for abuse, and considering the increasing use of Modafinil, these results highlight the need for heightened awareness about potential abuse of and dependence on Modafinil. These results indicate that using drugs to enhance cognition could involve risks. As well as the potential for addiction, it should also be kept in mind that most cognitive-enhancing stimulants also have side effects; taking Modafinil, for instance, may result in headaches, nausea, and diarrhea. More worryingly, some evidence has suggested that methylphenidate may have detrimental effects on the developing brain (Moll *et al.*, 2001). Furthermore, there are apparent reductions in normal growth rates in children with ADHD who are taking stimulant medication (Rao *et al.*, 1998). Self-medication of cognitive-enhancing drugs can also be harmful if individuals are taking medications or other cognitive-enhancing drugs, as drugs can interact with each other, potentially causing side effects, or nullifying the effects of medication. Long-term effects of taking drugs such as Modafinil, in addition to the short-term side effects mentioned above, also need to be investigated further. Based on this, an evidence-based approach to the risks involved in taking these drugs is required, and then this information needs to be made easily available to the public.

Furthermore, enhancing some aspect of cognition may not always be advantageous. Enhancing memory, for example, could make memories of traumatic events stronger (Carlezon *et al.*, 2005). Moreover, enhancing some areas of cognition may lead to impairments in others.

Do Cognitive Enhancing Drugs Affect Everyone Equally?

The degree of enhancement caused by cognitive-enhancing drugs varies between individuals.

Baseline performance

The effect of different cognitive enhancers seems to depend on an individual's baseline performance. For example, individuals with a low working memory capacity improve on memory tasks when they are administered drugs that mimic the neurotransmitter dopamine. In contrast high-functioning individuals are either not affected by the drug, or may get worse (Mehta *et al.*, 2001). This pattern has been found for a variety of different cognitive skills, and different drugs (Mehta *et al.*, 2000; Vijayraghavan *et al.*, 2007).

It has been suggested that these findings may reflect ceiling effects, where the neuropsychological tasks are not difficult enough to detect change in high-functioning individuals. But this does not explain why some high-functioning individuals can get worse on some cognitive tasks after taking neurostimulants such as methylphenidate (Mehta *et al.*, 2000).

Inverted U effect

The "inverted U effect" is one way of explaining why cognitive-enhancing drugs are not as effective for those who already do well. Performance on cognitive tasks that are related to the prefrontal cortex seem to be optimal when dopaminergic stimulation is intermediate, and impairment occurs when stimulation is too high or too low. The pre-frontal cortex is critical for many cognitive functions, including working memory.

Individual differences in systems can be related to, among other things, variations in baseline levels of neurotransmitters, receptor signaling, enzymes, and re-uptake transporters. These differences are determined in part by genetics, as there are variations of genes that code for proteins, and can lead to differences in baseline levels of stimulation (Diaz-Asper *et al.*, 2006). Thus, if someone with naturally lower levels of dopaminergic stimulation in the prefrontal cortex takes a drug to further increase dopamine concentration in the synaptic cleft, cognition associated with dopamine, such as working memory, will be enhanced. Conversely, if someone with naturally high levels of dopaminergic stimulation takes a drug to further increase dopamine concentration in the synaptic cleft, cognition associated with dopamine may become worse. Genes have a diverging pathway of influence from biology to behavior as variations of genes will most likely have a functional impact on the cellular and molecular pathways associated with a gene (Hariri & Weinberger, 2003). In turn, the resulting subtle cellular and molecular alterations may produce biases at a systems level, which may or may not impact on overt behavior. However, with the development of human pharmacogenetics, cognitive enhancers may be matched to individuals that might benefit from them the most.

Dose response

The dose of a drug will also determine its effect on cognition. It has been found that some drugs have a linear dose-dependent relationship with cognition: as the dose increases, improvements are seen. Some drugs have an inverted-U dose response, cognitive skill gets better as the dose increases, but at higher doses impairments in cognitive skill are seen. This inverted-U dose response has been observed in rats, monkeys, and humans performing cognitive tasks (Cai & Arnsten, 1997; Gibbs & D'Esposito, 2005; Zahrt *et al.*, 1997).

Some drugs have simultaneous linear and inverted-U effects on cognition. For example, in children with ADHD, as the dose of methylphenidate is increased, performance on sustained attention tasks improves in a linear fashion. However, at high doses, response inhibition is worse than at low doses (Konrad *et al.*, 2004). This poses practical problems for the use of cognitive-enhancing drugs.

Some Ethical Issues

The idea of enhancing cognition is not a new one; we have all enhanced our cognitive skills through education and learning. There are other non-pharmacological ways to boost cognition: exercise, nutrition, and sleep have all been shown to induce beneficial neural changes. Training specific cognitive skills by increasing blood to certain neural networks through cognitive problem solving may also be beneficial to overall cognitive function. However, although there has been much public and media interest in "brain training" of this kind, there remains a dearth of empirical data. Some cognitive stimulants which influence neurotransmitters in the brain are also already widely used (e.g. caffeine). Indeed, some neuroscientists do not believe there is a great difference between taking methylphenidate or Modafinil and drinking coffee (Chan & Harris, 2006). Therefore, the idea of enhancing cognition in healthy people is not a new one, and using pharmacological tools is certainly not the only way to achieve improvements in cognitive skill.

It is important to consider the views of the general public, as well as neuroscientists, on pharmacology and cognitive enhancement. A survey run by the journal *Nature*, which was prompted by a commentary by the authors of this chapter, asked readers for their views on the issues surrounding cognitive enhancement. Almost all of the respondents thought that individuals with psychiatric disorders should have access to cognitive-enhancing drugs. Furthermore, four-fifths of respondents thought that healthy adults should be able to take cognitive-enhancing drugs if they want to. With regard to pharmacological cognitive enhancement in children, most respondents (86%) said that use of these drugs by children should be restricted. However, interestingly, one-third of respondents said they would feel pressurized to give their children cognitive-enhancing drugs if other children were taking them. This reflects concerns that have been raised over *coercion*, and the worry that some people may feel pressured into taking cognitive-enhancing drugs in order to keep up with their peers. Other concerns that have been raised include erosion of character, as some people view the use of cognitive-enhancing drugs as "*cheating*" or being dishonest to themselves. Others feel that there are many factors making up one advantage over another, and that thus taking a drug would only have a small overall part to play. This also raises the issue of *authenticity*. Does the use of an external aid make our abilities less ours? (Bostrom & Sandberg, 2009). What makes the external aid of a cognitive-enhancing drug, as opposed to a private tutor, cheating? Furthermore, these drugs only have the potential to enhance certain aspects of cognition: they will not guarantee success in exams or career advancement. Another concern that has been raised is that the use of cognitive-enhancing drugs will widen the *gap* between classes and opportunities, as those who are better off will be able to afford drugs, which others may not be able to obtain. It can be seen that the ethical issues surrounding the use of cognitive-enhancing drugs are complex and require discussion among different groups. Indeed, the Academy of Medical Sciences in a report of a work group on brain science, addiction, and drugs discussed at length the use of cognitive-enhancing drugs, and also their potential use by healthy people. Forums also need to be created to engage the public in debates on these issues, as their views should be heard. Furthermore, engagement with the public on issues regarding medicine and science will allow the development of policies that are collaborations between the views of society, medical professionals, neuroscientists, educators, and regulators.

Future Directions

These concerns need to be addressed by policy makers, to support fairness, protect individuals from coercion, and minimize socioeconomic disparities. Safety and responsible use of cognitive-enhancing drugs should also be monitored, but this can only happen with the development of consistent regulations for cognitive-enhancing drugs. Training is also required for neuroscientists and physicians working in this field, allowing them to communicate with the public and to help them deal with issues arising from their work. Indeed, there has been a call for neuroscientists working in this rapidly developing field to be given teaching on neuroethics (Sahakian & Morein-Zamir, 2009). In addition, the Neuroethics Society (www.neuroethicssociety.org/) aims to promote the developments and responsible application of neuroscience through research, education, and public engagement for the benefit of all peoples.

With the development of new drugs and methods of enhancing cognition, such as brain stimulation, the need for further research and discussion is likely to become more pressing. Numerous novel cognitive enhancers, many of which are aimed at improving memory and learning, are currently under development. For example, ampakines, which work by enhancing a receptor's response to glutamate, improve cognition in healthy aging volunteers. Novel compounds such as nicotinic alpha-7 receptor agonists are now in phase 2 of clinical trials in Alzheimer's disease and schizophrenia (e.g., MEM 3454 Memory Pharmaceuticals/Roche). Further research is also required into the cognitive-enhancing drugs that are already widely used, to ensure their long-term safety and efficacy. It is possible that drugs used to enhance one aspect of cognition could also affect abilities in other areas of cognition or other domains, such as emotional intelligence. The profile of cognitive effects of each drug on specific populations should be mapped, along with its potential for harms. This will facilitate ethical and regulatory discussion about each pharmacological substance. Nonetheless, the development of tailored, cognitive-enhancing treatments for a wide range of neuropsychiatric disorders, as well as for normal function, holds much future promise.

References

Academy of Medical Sciences (UK Working Group Report on Brain Science, Addiction and Drugs (2008). Chapter 8, Cognition Enhancers, pp. 143–60.

Alexander, G.E., DeLong, M.R. & Strick, P.L. (1986). Parallel organization of functionally segregated circuits linking basal ganglia and cortex. *Annual Review of Neuroscience*, **9**, 357–81.

Arnsten, A.F., Cai, J.X., Murphy, B.L. & Goldman-Rakic, P.S. (1994). Dopamine D1 receptor mechanisms in the cognitive performance of young adult and aged monkeys, *Psychopharmacology (Berlin)*, **116**, 143–51.

Aron, A.R., Fletcher, P.C., Bullmore, E.T., Sahakian, B.J. & Robbins, T.W. (2003). Stop-signal inhibition disrupted by damage to right inferior frontal gyrus in humans. *Nature Neuroscience*, **6**, 115–16.

Babcock, Q. & Byrne, T. (2000). Student perceptions of methylphenidate abuse at a public liberal arts college. *Journal of American College Health*, **49**, 143–5.

Barkley, R.A., Fischer, M., Smallish, L. & Fletcher, K. (2006). Young adult outcome of hyperactive children: adaptive functioning in major life activities. *Journal of the American Academy of Child and Adolescent Psychiatry*, **45**, 192–202.

Barnett, J.H., Sahakian, B.J., Werners, U., Hill, K.E., Brazil, R., Gallagher, O. *et al.* (2005). Visuospatial learning and executive function are independently impaired in first-episode psychosis. *Psychological Medicine*, **35**, 1031–41.

Beddington, J., Cooper, C.L., Field, J., Goswami, U., Huppert, F.A., Jenkins, R. *et al.* (2008). The mental wealth of nations. *Nature*, **455**, 1057–60.

Bostrom, N. & Sandberg, A. (2009). Cognitive enhancement: methods, ethics, regulatory challenges. *Science and Engineering Ethics*, **15**, 311–41.

Cai, J.X. & Arnsten, A.F. (1997). Dose-dependent effects of the dopamine D1 receptor agonists A77636 or SKF81297 on spatial working memory in aged monkeys. *Journal of Pharmacology and Experimental Therapeutics*, **283**, 183–9.

Carlezon, W.A., Jr., Duman, R.S. & Nestler, E.J. (2005). The many faces of CREB. *Trends in Neuroscience*, **28**, 436–45.

Chamberlain, S.R., Del Campo, N., Dowson, J., Muller, U., Clark, L., Robbins, T.W. & Sahakian, B.J. (2007). Atomoxetine improved response inhibition in adults with attention deficit/hyperactivity disorder. *Biological Psychiatry*, **62**, 977–84.

Chamberlain, S.R., Hampshire, A., Muller, U., Rubia, K., Del Campo, N., Craig, K. *et al.* (2009). Atomoxetine modulates right inferior frontal activation during inhibitory control: a pharmacological functional magnetic resonance imaging study. *Biological Psychiatry*, **65**, 550–5.

Chamberlain, S.R., Muller, U., Robbins, T.W. & Sahakian, B.J. (2006). Neuropharmacological modulation of cognition. *Current Opinions in Neurology*, **19**, 607–12.

Chan, S. & Harris, J. (2006). Cognitive regeneration or enhancement: The ethical issues. *Regenerative Medicine*, **1**, 361–6.

Comas-Herrera, A., Wittenberg, R., Pickard, L. & Knapp, M. (2007). Cognitive impairment in older people: Future demand for long-term care services and the associated costs. *International Journal of Geriatric Psychiatry*, **22**, 1037–45.

Diaz-Asper, C.M., Weinberger, D.R. & Goldberg, T.E. (2006). Catechol-O-methyltransferase polymorphisms and some implications for cognitive therapeutics. *NeuroRx*, **3**, 97–105.

Elliott, R., McKenna, P.J., Robbins, T.W. & Sahakian, B.J. (1995). Neuropsychological evidence for frontostriatal dysfunction in schizophrenia. *Psychological Medicine*, **25**, 619–30.

Gibbs, S.E. & D'Esposito, M. (2005). Individual capacity differences predict working memory performance and prefrontal activity following dopamine receptor stimulation. *Cognitive, Affective, & Behavoral Neuroscience*, **5**, 212–21.

Hariri, A.R. & Weinberger, D.R. (2003). Imaging genomics. *Britsh Medical Bulletin*, **65**, 259–70.

Hirvonen, J., van Erp, T.G., Huttunen, J., Aalto, S., Nagren, K., Huttunen, M. *et al.* (2006). Brain dopamine d1 receptors in twins discordant for schizophrenia. *American Journal of Psychiatr*, **163**, 1747–53.

Kempton, S., Vance, A., Maruff, P., Luk, E., Costin, J. & Pantelis, C. (1999). Executive function and attention deficit hyperactivity disorder: Stimulant medication and better executive function performance in children. *Psychological Medicine*, **29**, 527–38.

Konrad, K., Gunther, T., Hanisch, C. & Herpertz-Dahlmann, B. (2004). Differential effects of methylphenidate on attentional functions in children with attention-deficit/hyperactivity disorder. *Journal of the American Academy of Child and Adolescent Psychiatry*, **43**, 191–8.

Levy, F. (2008). Pharmacological and therapeutic directions in ADHD: Specificity in the PFC. *Behavioral and Brain Functions*, **4**, 12.

McCabe, S.E. & Boyd, C.J. (2005). Sources of prescription drugs for illicit use. *Addictive Behaviors*, **30**, 1342–50.

McLean, A., Dowson, J., Toone, B., Young, S., Bazanis, E., Robbins, T.W. & Sahakian, B.J. (2004). Characteristic neurocognitive profile associated with adult attention-deficit/hyperactivity disorder. *Psychological Medicone*, **34**, 681–92.

Mehta, M.A., Goodyer, I.M. & Sahakian, B.J. (2004). Methylphenidate improves working memory and set-shifting in AD/HD: Relationships to baseline memory capacity. *Journal of Child Pyschology and Psychiatry*, **45**, 293–305.

Mehta, M.A., Owen, A.M., Sahakian, B.J., Mavaddat, N., Pickard, J.D. & Robbins, T.W. (2000). Methylphenidate enhances working memory by modulating discrete frontal and parietal lobe regions in the human brain. *Journal of Neuroscience*, **20**, RC65.

Mehta, M.A., Swainson, R., Ogilvie, A.D., Sahakian, J. & Robbins, T.W. (2001). Improved short-term spatial memory but impaired reversal learning following the dopamine D(2) agonist bromocriptine in human volunteers. *Psychopharmacology (Berlin)*, **159**, 10–20.

Minzenberg, M.J., Watrous, A.J., Yoon, J.H., Ursu, S. & Carter, C.S. (2008). Modafinil shifts human locus coeruleus to low-tonic, high-phasic activity during functional MRI. *Science*, **322**, 1700–2.

Moll, G.H., Hause, S., Ruther, E., Rothenberger, A. & Huether, G. (2001). Early methylphenidate administration to young rats causes a persistent reduction in the density of striatal dopamine transporters. *Journal of Child and Adolescent Psychopharmacology*, **11**, 15–24.

Montgomery, A.J., Asselin, M.C., Farde, L. & Grasby, P.M. (2007). Measurement of methylphenidate-induced change in extrastriatal dopamine concentration using [11C]FLB 457 PET. *Journal of Cerebral Blood Flow & Metabolism*, **27**, 369–77.

Moreno, J.D. (2004). DARPA on your mind. *Cerebrum*, **6**, 91–9.

National Institute on Drug Abuse. (2005). *Prescription Drugs: Abuse and Addiction* (NIH Publication Number 05-4881). U.S. Department of Health and Human Services. Washington, DC: U.S. Government Printing Office.

Owen, A.M., Downes, J.J., Sahakian, B.J., Polkey, C.E. & Robbins, T.W. (1990). Planning and spatial working memory following frontal lobe lesions in man. *Neuropsychologia*, **28**, 1021–34.

Owen, A.M., Roberts, A.C., Polkey, C.E., Sahakian, B.J. & Robbins, T.W. (1991). Extra-dimensional versus intra-dimensional set shifting performance following frontal lobe excisions, temporal lobe excisions or amygdalo-hippocampectomy in man. *Neuropsychologia*, **29**, 993–1006.

Pantelis, C., Barber, F.Z., Barnes, T.R., Nelson, H.E., Owen, A.M. & Robbins, T.W. (1999). Comparison of set-shifting ability in patients with chronic schizophrenia and frontal lobe damage. *Schizophrenia Research*, **37**, 251–70.

Pelham, W.E., Foster, E.M. & Robb, J.A. (2007). The economic impact of attention-deficit/hyperactivity disorder in children and adolescents. *Journal of Pediatric Psychology*, **32**, 711–27.

Parliamentary Office of Science and Technology (2007). *Better Brains*. (Publication Number 285). London.

Randall, D.C., Shneerson, J.M. & File, S.E. (2005a). Cognitive effects of modafinil in student volunteers may depend on IQ. *Pharmacology Biochemistry and Behavior*, **82**, 133–9.

Randall, D.C., Viswanath, A., Bharania, P., Elsabagh, S.M., Hartley, D.E., Shneerson, J.M. & File, S.E. (2005b). Does modafinil enhance cognitive performance in young volunteers who are not sleep-deprived? *Journal of Clinical Psychopharmacology*, **25**, 175–9.

Rao, J.K., Julius, J.R., Breen, T.J. & Blethen, S.L. (1998). Response to growth hormone in attention deficit hyperactivity disorder: effects of methylphenidate and pemoline therapy. *Pediatrics*, **102**, 497–500.

Rogers, S.L., Doody, R.S., Mohs, R.C. & Friedhoff, L.T. (1998). Donepezil improves cognition and global function in Alzheimer's disease: a 15-week, double-blind, placebo-controlled study. Donepezil Study Group. *Archives of Internal Medicine*, **158**, 1021–31.

Sahakian, B.J. & Morein-Zamir, S. (2007). Professor's little helper. *Nature*, **450**, 1157–9.

Sahakian, B.J. & Morein-Zamir, S. (2009). Neuroscientists need neuroethics teaching. *Science*, **325**, 147.

Sahakian, B.J., Morris, R.G., Evenden, J.L., Heald, A., Levy, R., Philpot, M. & Robbins, T.W. (1988). A comparative study of visuospatial memory and learning in Alzheimer-type dementia and Parkinson's disease. *Brain*, **111**, 695–718.

Shimohama, S., Taniguchi, T., Fujiwara, M. & Kameyama, M. (1986). Biochemical characterization of alpha-adrenergic receptors in human brain and changes in Alzheimer-type dementia. *Journal of Neurochemistry*, **47**, 1295–301.

The National Centre on Addiction and Substance Abuse at Columbia University (2008). "You've got drugs!" V: Prescription Drug Pushers on the Internet. New York.

Turner, D.C., Blackwell, A.D., Dowson, J.H., McLean, A. & Sahakian, B.J. (2005). Neuro-cognitive effects of methylphenidate in adult attention-deficit/hyperactivity disorder. *Psychopharmacology (Berlin)*, **178**, 286–95.

Turner, D.C., Clark, L., Dowson, J., Robbins, T.W. & Sahakian, B.J. (2004a). Modafinil improves cognition and response inhibition in adult attention-deficit/hyperactivity disorder. *Biological Psychiatry*, **55**, 1031–40.

Turner, D.C., Clark, L., Pomarol-Clotet, E., McKenna, P., Robbins, T.W. & Sahakian, B.J. (2004b). Modafinil improves cognition and attentional set shifting in patients with chronic schizophrenia. *Neuropsychopharmacology*, **29**, 1363–73.

Turner, D.C., Robbins, T.W., Clark, L., Aron, A.R., Dowson, J. & Sahakian, B.J. (2003). Cognitive enhancing effects of modafinil in healthy volunteers. *Psychopharmacology (Berlin)*, **165**, 260–9.

Vijayraghavan, S., Wang, M., Birnbaum, S.G., Williams, G.V. & Arnsten, A.F. (2007). Inverted-U dopamine D1 receptor actions on prefrontal neurons engaged in working memory. *Nature Neuroscience*, **10**, 376–84.

Volkow, N.D., Fowler, J.S., Logan, J., Alexoff, D., Zhu, W., Telang, F. *et al.* (2009). Effects of modafinil on dopamine and dopamine transporters in the male human brain: clinical implications. *Journal of the American Medical Association*, **301**, 1148–54.

Weickert, T.W., Goldberg, T.E., Marenco, S., Bigelow, L.B., Egan, M.F. & Weinberger, D.R. (2003). Comparison of cognitive performances during a placebo period and an atypical antipsychotic treatment period in schizophrenia: critical examination of confounds. *Neuropsychopharmacolog*, **28**, 1491–500.

Wu, E.Q., Birnbaum, H.G., Shi, L., Ball, D.E., Kessler, R.C., Moulis, M. & Aggarwal, J. (2005). The economic burden of schizophrenia in the United States in 2002. *Journal of Clinical Psychiatry*, **66**, 1122–9.

Zahrt, J., Taylor, J.R., Mathew, R.G. & Arnsten, A.F. (1997). Supranormal stimulation of D1 dopamine receptors in the rodent prefrontal cortex impairs spatial working memory performance. *Journal of Neuroscience*, **17**, 8528–35.

8

Cognitive Bias and Collective Enhancement

Steve Clarke

Biased Individuals

Ordinary cognition is subject to the influence of a variety of systematic distortions or biases (Gilovich & Griffin, 2002). For example, the majority of participants in a study of the lay understanding of risk information considered that a cancer that was described as causing the death of "1,286 out of 10,000 people" posed a greater threat than one that was described as causing the death of "24.14 out of 100 people" (Yamagishi, 1997). The majority of participants in this study are demonstrably in error and a very plausible explanation for their error is that they suffer from the bias of "base-rate neglect" (Tversky & Kahneman, 1974). It seems that when many people compare two fractions they have a tendency to make a direct comparison of the two numerators in question and to lose sight of the fact that these are supposed to be understood in relation to two very different denominators. 1,286 is a much larger number than 24.14, so, being guided by a "directly compare the numerators" heuristic, or rule of thumb, many reason that because 1,286 is a larger number than 24.14, 1,286 out of 10,000 must be a larger fraction than 24.14 out of 100.

Starting with the work of Amos Tversky and Daniel Kahneman in the 1960s and 1970s, an increasing number of examples of ordinary judgments that seem deficient have been identified by scholars working in the "heuristics and biases" tradition. Such deficiencies are explained by these scholars as resulting from biases of cognition that accompany our use of simplifying heuristics in the formation of ordinary judgments (Gilovich & Griffin 2002; Kahneman *et al.*, 1982). Some of these heuristics, such as base-rate neglect, are biases of omission, but many are biases of commission, where additional information that is liable to distort ordinary judgment is introduced. An example of a bias of commission is caused by the widespread use of the "availability heuristic" to assess lay risks. When people are asked to estimate the risk of a dangerous event occurring, such as a terrorist attack in their own county, an accident at a nuclear power plant or a major earthquake, they tend to equate the magnitude of that risk with

Enhancing Human Capacities, edited by Julian Savulescu, Ruud ter Meulen and Guy Kahane.
© 2011 Blackwell Publishing Ltd

the ease with which they are able to bring to mind particular examples of the dangerous event in question (Schwartz & Vaughn, 2002). If, for example, a lay reasoner has recently watched a documentary on terrorism, then terrorism will seem much more familiar to that lay reasoner than it had been hitherto, and her assessment of the likelihood of a future terrorist attack will tend to increase dramatically. But there is no evidence that the broadcasting of documentaries about terrorism has a dramatic effect on the actual rate of occurrence of terrorist attacks, so it looks like the use of the availability heuristic has led to biased reasoning, in this case.

To describe a piece of reasoning as biased, and do so justifiably, we must be able to appeal to a standard of correct reasoning that it diverges from. When standards of correct reasoning are generally accepted, as they are in almost all areas of mathematics, it is uncontroversial to describe reasoning that diverges from these standards as biased. It is not in dispute that the majority of subjects in Yamagishi's (1997) study of base-rate neglect reasoned in a biased manner because it is not in dispute among those who are even minimally competent in mathematics that 24.14 out of 100 is a larger fraction than 1,286 out of 10,000. However, when standards of good reasoning are in dispute the charge of bias is much harder to sustain. Affective states make a significant difference to our assessments of certain risks. Roughly, the feeling that some activity is bad is liable to increase our assessment of the magnitude of risk associated with that activity (Alhakami & Slovic, 1994). Evidence that states of affect are liable to alter our perceptions of risk is usually taken to be evidence, *mutatis mutandis*, of the existence of an affect bias which distorts lay assessments of risks (Slovic *et al.*, 2002). But not all will agree. If, like Roeser (2007) you think that the appropriate way for people to conduct a complete risk assessment includes consulting their moral emotions, then you will be inclined to see what others see as evidence of bias as evidence of good reasoning.

As well as those who will dispute the charge of bias in particular cases, there are commentators who are skeptical about the generalizability of the charge of bias to commonplace examples of ordinary judgment. Gigerenzer and Todd (1999) accept that the use of heuristics in everyday reasoning is very widespread, but argue that the use of such heuristics mostly leads to accurate judgments about the various real-world circumstances that we are likely to find ourselves in; and is only liable to lead to systematically inaccurate judgments in very unusual circumstances. Proponents of the generalizability of cognitive bias reject Gigerenzer and Todd's (1999) line of reasoning and point to the sheer volume of studies illustrating bias, as well as the breadth of contexts in which evidence of cognitive bias has been found, to substantiate their case (Gilovich & Griffin 2002, pp.11–12).

Lay reasoning which is rendered significantly less susceptible to the influence of cognitive bias than is normally the case, through our interventions, is reasoning that is improved or enhanced beyond levels that could ordinarily be obtained. Procedures that return impaired human capacities to normal levels of functioning are often thought of as instances of therapy and procedures that raise human capacities above levels that could normally be obtained are often thought of as instances of enhancement. At any rate this is how Bostrom and Roache (2007) construe the enhancement–therapy distinction (while allowing that the notion of a normal healthy state is somewhat problematic). So on their view, which we will follow, procedures that significantly ameliorate the ordinary instances of cognitive bias that pervade lay reasoning are considered to be forms of enhancement.

But can we significantly reduce cognitive bias and thereby enhance ordinary reasoning? There are many who are optimistic about our ability to correct for biases given the identification of instantiations of those biases and the application of ordinary will power (e.g. Liao, 2008, p.259). On this optimistic view, cognitive enhancement via the amelioration of bias is reasonably easily to come by. However, there are several reasons to be pessimistic about the propensity and indeed the ability of individuals to correct actual instances of cognitive bias (Wilson & Brekke, 1994). One problem is that while people find it easy enough to identify biased reasoning when others are doing the reasoning, they are often unable to identify situations in which they themselves are utilizing biased reasoning and they are often unable to accept the charge of bias when it is directed at them by others.

A further problem is that it is often very difficult to identify the degree to which one is biased. If I am biased against students from the Torres Strait Islands then I will be biased against those students to a particular degree. If I only know about the direction of my bias but do not know about the magnitude of my bias then I will be unable to correct reliably for that bias. Does the Torres Strait Islander student who I gave a C really deserve a B or an A? If I correct her mark and now give her a B when she really deserves an A then my correction has not overcome my bias (although it has reduced my bias). If I give her an A when she really deserves a B then I have overcorrected and have ended up being biased in favor of the student from the Torres Strait Islands. But it is difficult to acquire accurate information about the magnitude of particular biases in individuals and even if we are able to acquire such reliable information we may be unable to exert sufficient self-control to accurately correct for those biases.

In the remainder of this chapter we will consider an approach to the amelioration of cognitive bias that is very different from the approach of asking individuals to directly correct for their biases. We will consider ways in which individual cognitive biases may be corrected at the group level. Group-level corrections that ameliorate cognitive bias fill a small but significant segment of what Bostrom and Roache (chapter 9, this volume) refer to as the "spectrum of enhancement methods," which includes general education, specific mental training techniques, the use of drugs, direct interventions into the brain and the supplementation of cognition with external hardware and software. As Bostrom and Roache note, some of the most powerful techniques that we have developed to improve cognition are techniques of "collective cognition." In this chapter we look at the use of some collective cognition techniques to correct for individual cognitive bias. We will proceed as follows. In the next section the possibility of group-level corrections to cognitive bias is introduced and the problem of biases that emerge at the group level is raised. In the subsequent section some examples of the use of the internet to create corrections to cognitive biases is discussed. Then the possibility of institutions engineering solutions to individual cognitive biases is considered. The last section contains concluding remarks.

Groups

In his *The Wisdom of Crowds*, James Surowiecki (2004) recounts the story of a visit to the annual West of England Fat Stock and Poultry Exhibition by the famous statistician and eugenicist Francis Galton. Intent on demonstrating the incompetence of ordinary non-expert judgment Galton (1907) examined 800 tickets submitted to a weight-judging competition. The lay weight estimators made various partially informed and uninformed guesses. Although most of the guesses were off the mark, the median of all of the guesses was within 1% of the correct result and the mean was extremely close to the correct result, forecasting that the fat ox would weigh 1,197 pounds after it had been slaughtered and dressed. In actual fact it weighed 1,198 pounds. How could the partially informed and the uninformed collectively arrive at such an accurate result? Surowiecki's explanation is that because the group of individual estimators was sufficiently diverse and independent and because individual errors that the participants in the competition made were distributed more or less randomly, they tended to cancel one another out, leaving an accurate result (2004, p.10–11). This does seem to be a case in which group processes can enhance our ability to make accurate judgments, provided that we know how to interpret the outcome of those group processes. Surowiecki (2004) makes a further assumption which is that the individuals in the group in question have, on average, some information which informs some of their judgments. If they have no information at all then, even if their collective errors cancel one another out perfectly, they will be left with nothing more than an average random guess.

Larger groups will tend to produce more accurate judgments than smaller groups. This propensity can be explained by the Condorcet Jury Theorem. According to the Condorcet jury theorem (Janis, 1982, pp.7–9; Sunstein, 2006, pp.25–9) groups will tend to produce more accurate majority judgments than individuals whenever the probability of individual members of the group being correct, given a choice between two possible outcomes, is greater than 50%. As the group increases in size the accuracy of the majority judgment increases until it approximates to 100% accuracy. But this does not mean that we should always prefer the judgment of larger groups to the judgment of smaller groups (and individuals). In circumstances where the judgment of the average individual within the group is liable to produce judgments that are less than 50% likely to be correct, in a choice between two possible outcomes, the majority judgment of the group will tend to be less accurate than that of the average individual and as the group increases in size the inaccuracy of the majority judgment will tend to increase, to the point at which the probability of the majority judgment being accurate approximates to 0%.

The ability of group processes to enable enhanced judgmental accuracy depends *inter alia* on the accuracy of the judgment of the individuals who make up those groups. The accuracy of the judgment of individuals is hindered by the various cognitive biases that affect the reasoning of those individuals and, unfortunately, it is also hindered by various biases that are caused by interactions between members of groups. One well-known example of such a bias is group polarization. It is well established that the individual biases of group members are often made more extreme by the process of deliberation within a group (Brown, 2000, pp.193–225). A deliberating group that is predominantly conservative is liable to derive collective conclusions that are even more conservative than those that one would expect given the average political dispositions of its members before deliberation. And the same holds for liberal groups that deliberate. Groups who share common assumptions often fail to subject these to appropriate scrutiny and often fail to consider alternative points of view. Unfortunately, ordinary social pressures make it difficult for members of such groups to air concerns that are liable to lead to group disapproval. Sufficiently like-minded groups can make disastrous decisions. Famous examples include the decisions within NASA that lead to the 1986 Challenger disaster (Feynman 2001, pp.165–6), and the decision making within the U.S. intelligence community that informed the 2003 invasion of Iraq (Drogin, 2007).

The experience of feeling social pressure to avoid airing views that a group will disapprove of should be familiar to most everyone. However, there are also more subtle factors that can bias group deliberations. One such effect is the effect of the opinions voiced earlier by others in a group. Suppose that I am asked to provide my opinion to a group regarding a particular issue about which I lack a strong opinion. If I hear another member of the group state their opinion then I will be more likely to agree with them than I would be otherwise. In part this is because of social pressure to conform, but it is also, in part, because their testimony counts as evidence for me, and it can be rational to update my opinion in response to the testimony that has been provided. But if I also announce that I agree with the opinion of the person who voiced an opinion before me then my making that announcement adds further pressure on the next person who is due to speak and can appear to count as further independent testimony on behalf of the view which is now gaining more support. If this process continues then an "information cascade" is set up, and a preference that is announced early on in a group discussion can have a much larger effect on group deliberation than it would otherwise, just because it was announced early (Sunstein, 2006, pp.88–91).

One reason why the wisdom of the crowd was exhibited in Galton's weight-judging trial was that for the most part members of the crowd did not deliberate much. Perhaps some of them talked to others about the likely weight of the ox, but the weight estimators were not particularly placed under social pressure to make guesses that would meet with the approval of others in the group. Because they wrote their answers down independently of one another there was no serious danger of an information cascade occurring. The independence of decision makers within the group helps prevent the influence of group biases from distorting the group's overall judgment. But independence is bought at a cost. For the most part it seems that our decisions are independent of those of others when we do not deliberate with them. However, deliberation can also serve to improve group decisions. Deliberating with others helps individuals to identify errors of judgment and enables those individuals to adopt new perspectives that in turn enables them to make better judgments. In many cases we are faced with a dilemma. We can have the benefits of group deliberation but only at the cost of allowing ourselves to be susceptible to the effects of group biases. If we are to immunize ourselves from the influence of group-level biases then we are also deprived of the benefits of deliberation.

Perhaps because of the complicated nature of interactions between biased individual reasoners and group processes which can reduce bias, increase bias and introduce entirely new biases, there is no straightforward general answer to be had to the question of whether deliberating groups produce more accurate judgments than individuals or not (Kerr *et al.*, 1996). It depends on particular circumstances and on particular types of judgment. In the discussion that follows we look at some artificial contexts in which deliberation is largely avoided and which seem to enable the production of group judgments that are superior to individual judgments.

The Internet

The development of the internet has enabled many more people to communicate with many more people faster and more efficiently than could have happened previously. It has also enabled people to locate other people with particular interests rapidly and efficiently. Cannibals are extremely rare, at least in Western societies, and people who have the desire to be eaten are rarer still. Before the rise of the internet it would have been vanishingly unlikely that a cannibal would be able to meet a willing victim. However, in 2002, a German man with cannibalistic tendencies was able to use the internet to locate someone who was willing to be eaten by him (Boyes, 2002). Because the internet can be used to bring people together rapidly and efficiently it can be used to form groups and to exploit the power of groups to enhance cognition. In what follows I discuss three significant ways in which the internet has, so far, been used to enhance cognition. These are: (i) the aggregation of judgments; (ii) prediction markets; and (iii) wikis. No doubt there are also other ways worth considering, and very probably people will devise new powerful ways to use the internet to enhance cognition in the future.

Amalgamation

As we saw in the example of Galton's ox weight-estimating competition, the aggregation of the judgments of groups of suitably diverse participants operating independently is capable of producing more accurate judgments than those of almost all individuals. The internet is a natural host for polls and surveys that aggregate individual judgments. It is easy to set up voting functions that large numbers of people can access, and easy enough to check that participants in polls and surveys are deciding independently and comprise a suitably diverse information base (assuming that such participants are generally willing to answer elementary questions about themselves honestly). The internet can also be used to combine traditional polls, surveys, and other judgments to give us the average judgment of a virtual group with larger numbers of participants than its constituents. According to the Condorcet jury theorem this should enable more accurate forecasts than those produced by smaller groups. A website where such an amalgamation has been conducted very effectively is "Pollyvote" (see: www.forecastingprinciples.com/PollyVote/), which combines forecasts from traditional polls, expert opinions, a prediction market, and a number of quantitative models to produce amalgamated election result forecasts that have so far proven to be extremely accurate.

Prediction markets

In ordinary markets people trade in commodities, shares, insurance policies, and so on. In prediction markets they trade in judgments on future outcomes. Prediction markets are now flourishing on the internet. On Intrade (see: www.intrade.com/) and on the

Iowa Electronic Markets (see: www.biz.uiowa.edu/iem/) anyone can "put their money where their mouth is" and trade on a variety of forecasts. If I think that there is a significant chance that Sarah Palin will formally announce a run for President of the United States then I may want to buy that forecast on Intrade. I can sell it later on at profit, or at loss depending on how the market values the forecast in the future. Intrade suggests that there is currently (as of August 6 2010) a 62.3% chance that Sarah Palin will formally announce a run for President before the end of 2011. It also suggests that there is a 17% chance that the Higgs boson will be found before the end of 2011 and a 9% chance that the United States will conduct overt military action against North Korea before the end of March 2011.

Famously, Friedrich Hayek (1988) argued that markets reveal tacit dispersed information about prices held by the trading community. In other words they reveal the "wisdom of crowds." He further argued that because planned economies lacked access to this crucial information they can never function as effectively as market economies. Market can be viewed as a generally reliable source of information about circumstances in which individuals make largely rational, mostly independent decisions about purchases and sales. This tends to happens much of the time, because when we buy or sell the stakes are generally raised for us, and so we are motivated to make careful decisions; and careful decisions are more likely to be superior decisions than careless ones. We generally care about profit and loss and so we are generally disposed to make the best decisions we can when our money is at stake.

As we saw earlier, the Condorcet jury theorem tells us that when the chance that individuals make accurate decisions is above 50%, the accuracy of group decisions will exceed that of individuals, so the wisdom of prediction markets should generally result in accurate judgments (Hahn & Tetlock, 2005; Hanson, 1999; Sunstein, 2006). The evidence that is in, about the accuracy of prediction markets, appears to support this view. For example, the Iowa Electronic Market has been used to predict the results of presidential elections with a higher degree of accuracy than most polls (Snee, 2008), and prediction markets persistently outperform experts in forecasting the results of many sporting events (Sauer, 1998).

Wikis

The Vienna Circle positivist philosopher Otto Neurath was the driving force behind an early twentieth-century project to create an exhaustive, updateable *International Encyclopedia of Unified Science*. He saw this as the key component of an ambitious plan (with a distinctly socialist hue) to improve the lives of ordinary people by providing reliable easily accessible scientific information to the entire population (Nemeth & Stadler, 1996). Neurath's international encyclopedia was never completed. Surprisingly, however, the project is being replicated in a sense, from the bottom up, as a result of the creation in 2001 (by Jimmy Wales and Larry Sanger) of Wikipedia. Wikipedia is a free online encyclopedia, currently available in 262 languages, which anyone can edit. It has grown rapidly and in September 2007 the English language Wikipedia became the largest encyclopedia in the world. Hundreds of new entries are added and thousands of existing entries are updated every day (Lih, 2009). Wikipedia is only one of many wikis – websites that can be updated by any user. Although Wikipedia is growing at a remarkable rate, that rate of growth appears to be sustainable (Spinellis & Louridas, 2008). If Wikipedia is a generally reliable source of information then clearly it is of great benefit to humanity, potentially providing a non-socialist variant of Neurath's *International Encyclopedia of Unified Science.*

Can Wikipedia be a reliable source, given that it can be updated by anyone and everyone? It can if the average correction tends to make entries more rather than less accurate and if there are sufficiently many corrections. Some entries are well intended but amateurish, others contain hoaxes, and others are the subjects of ongoing controversy. However, all of these problems can be addressed. Amateur entries are often improved, hoaxes often identified and corrected for, and the existence of material in entries that is the subject of ongoing controversy is indicated on Wikipedia by a statement that "the neutrality of this article is disputed" (currently accompanied by an icon representing a pair of unbalanced scales). While many academics are quick to condemn appeals to Wikipedia in student writing, assuming that its lowly origins mean that Wikipedia will be unreliable (e.g. Jakubovitz & Paul, 2006) a study of Wikipedia conducted by *Nature* found that it is surprisingly accurate, at least in the sciences. *Encyclopedia Britannica* is generally regarded as a repository of very high standard expert judgments across a wide range of topics. Nevertheless, science entries in *Encyclopedia Britannica* contain an average of three inaccuracies (Giles, 2005). Surprisingly, the average science entry in Wikipedia comes close to meeting this very high standard. Science entries in Wikipedia contain an average of four inaccuracies (Giles, 2005). It seems plausible to think that sufficiently well-edited Wikipedia entries are an expression of the wisdom of crowds and are, for the most part, far more reliable than ordinary, non-expert judgment.

Institutions

Contemporary organizations such as large corporations, schools, and government agencies can contain thousands of members. One perennial problem that prevents organizations from functioning as well as they might is that the knowledge held by some members of the organization is not readily available to other members of that organization. In particular, the "collective wisdom" of members of organizations is often not available to the leadership structure of those organizations. Increasingly, contemporary organizations are utilizing strategies that have been used on the internet, which we have already discussed, to ensure that information is shared effectively within organizations and that the collective wisdom of the members of those organizations is utilized effectively. Wikis that can be edited by approved members of organizations have been utilized by a variety of corporations including Eastman Kodak, Walt Disney, and Oxford University Press (Sunstein, 2006, p.163). Prediction markets have been used internally by several major corporations including Google, Hewlett Packard, and Microsoft to provide forecasts that help guide corporate planning (Sunstein, 2006, pp.113–16).

As well as trying to benefit from the wisdom of crowds, organizations can adopt another approach to ameliorating the effects of individual bias and improve overall organizational performance, which is to use our knowledge of cognitive biases to introduce changes into the environment in which choices are typically made so as to reduce the deleterious effects of individual biases. This approach is known as "choice architecture" and has recently been championed by Richard Thaler and Cass Sunstein (2008). When choosing food at a cafeteria people are much more likely to choose items that are at eye level than items that are placed above or below eye level. Knowing this, organizations such as schools that are concerned about the health of their members, can arrange the food sold at their cafeterias so that more healthy food choices are placed at eye level and are therefore more likely to be selected (Thaler & Sunstein, 2008, p.1). Similarly, the propensity of men using urinals to fail to pay attention to where they are aiming can be ameliorated by providing them with a target. In the urinals of Schiphol airport in the Netherlands an image of a fly is to be found. Men using these urinals tend to aim at the image of the fly and as a consequence spillage has been reduced by 80% (Thaler & Sunstein, 2008, p.4). Again, an environmental change has been made which restructures individual choices making it more likely that the choices individuals make will be ones that suit the purposes of institutions.

Individual biases have been reduced by groups in the above examples, but not by being cancelled at the group level. Instead organizations have learned how to manipulate the contexts in which individual choices are made, making it more likely that individuals will make choices that are in accord with the needs of the group. This approach to the amelioration of individual bias seems vulnerable to the accusation of paternalism. Thaler and Sunstein (2008) plead guilty to the charge of paternalism but argue that their approach involves a very mild unobjectionable form of paternalism which they refer to as "libertarian paternalism." They argue that the paternalism they are defending is of a libertarian flavor, because the uses of choice architecture that they defend do not involve denying anyone any choices and do not depend on deception. Choice architecture can still be effective when people are aware that the context in which their choices are being made has been deliberately structured in a particular way to promote particular choices.

Concluding Remarks

We have learned how to ameliorate some of the cognitive biases that affect individuals by utilizing group processes and choice architecture. To the extent that we have been successful we may be said to have enhanced individual cognition. Our ability to enhance individual cognition in these ways is currently limited. There is much we do not know about the interaction of individual cognitive biases, group processes, group-level biases, and the contexts in which choices are made. It may be that in the future we will be able to refine the techniques that we currently use to make them more effective; and it may be that we will be able to develop even more powerful techniques to overcome more individual cognitive biases.

Acknowledgments

Thanks to Guy Kahane, S. Matthew Liao, and Ruud ter Meulen for helpful comments on an earlier version of this chapter.

References

Alhakami A.S. & Slovic, P. (1994). A psychological study of the inverse relationship between perceived risk and perceived benefit. *Risk Analysis*, **14**, 1085–96.

Bostrom, N. & Roache, R. (2007). Ethical issues in human enhancement. In J. Ryberg, T.S. Petersen& C. Wolf (eds.), *New Waves in Applied Ethics*. Basingstoke: Palgrave Macmillan. www.timesonline.co.uk/tol/news/world/article801599.ece (accessed April 6, 2009).

Brown, R. (2001). *Group Processes: Dynamics Within and Between Groups*, 2nd edition. Oxford: Blackwell.

Drogin, B. (2007). *Curveball*. London: Random House.

Feynman, R. (2001). *What Do You Care What Other People Think?* London: W.W. Norton.

Galton, F. (1907). Vox populi. *Nature*, **75**, 450–1.

Gigerenzer, G. & Todd, P.M. (1999). Fast and frugal heuristics: The adaptive toolbox. In G. Gigerenzer, P.M. Todd & ABC Research Group (eds.), *Simple Heuristics that Make Us Smart* (pp. 3–34). New York: Oxford University Press.

Giles, J. (2005). Internet encyclopedias go head to head. *Nature*, **438**, 900–1.

Gilovich, T. & Griffin, D. (2002). Introduction – Heuristics and biases: then and now. In T. Gilovich, D. Griffin & D. Kahneman (eds.), *Heuristics and Biases: The Psychology of Intuitive Judgement* (pp. 1–18). Cambridge: Cambridge University Press.

Hahn, R.W. & Tetlock, P.C. (2005). Using information markets to improve public decision making. *Harvard Journal of Law and Public Policy*, **29**, 213–89.

Hanson, R. (1999). Decision markets. *IEEE Intelligent Systems*, **14**, 16–19.

Hayek, F. (1988). *The Fatal Conceit: The Errors of Socialism*. Chicago: University of Chicago Press.

Jakubovitz, J. & Paul, D. (2006). Wide world of Wikipedia. See www.emorywheel.com/detail .php?n=17902 (accessed April 7, 2009).

Janis, I.L. (1982). *Groupthink*, 2nd edition. Boston: Houghton Mifflin.

Kahneman, D, Slovic, P. & Tversky, A. (2002). *Judgement under Uncertainty, Heuristics and Biases*. Cambridge: Cambridge University Press.

Kerr, N.L., MacCoun, R.J. & Kramer, G.P. (1996). Bias in judgment: Comparing individuals and groups. *Psychological Review*, **103**, 687–719.

Liao, S.M. (2008). A defense of intuitions. *Philosophical Studies*, **240**, 247–62.

Lih, A. (2009). *The Wikipedia Revolution: How a Bunch of Nobodies Created the World's Greatest Encyclopedia*. New York: Hyperion.

Nemeth, E. & Stadler, F. (eds.). (1996). *Encyclopedia and Utopia: The Life and Work of Otto Neurath (1882–1945)* Dordrecht: Kluwer.

Roeser, S. (2007). Ethical intuitions about risks. *Safety Science Monitor*, **11**, 1–30.

Sauer, R.D. (1998). The economics of wagering markets. *Journal of Economic Literature*, **36**, 2021–64.

Schwartz, N. & Vaughn, L. A. (2002). The availability heuristic revisited: Ease of recall and content of recall as distinct sources of information. In T. Gilovich, D. Griffin & D. Kahneman (eds.), *Heuristics and Biases: The Psychology of Intuitive Judgement* (pp. 103–19). Cambridge: Cambridge University Press.

Slovic, P., Finucane, M., Peters, E. & d MacGregor, D.G. (2002). The affect heuristic. In T. Gilovich, D. Griffin & D. Kahneman (eds.), *Heuristics and Biases: The Psychology of Intuitive Judgement* (pp. 397–420). Cambridge: Cambridge University Press.

Snee, T. (2008). IEM within half a percentage point in presidential race prediction. University of Iowa Media Release: http://tippie.uiowa.edu/news/story.cfm?id=2058 (accessed April 7, 2009)

Spinellis, D. & Louridas, P. (2008). The collaborative organization of knowledge. *Communications of the ACM*, **51**, 68–73.

Sunstein, C. (2006). *Infotopia: How Many Minds Produce Knowledge*. Oxford: Oxford University Press.

Surowiecki, J. (2004). *The Wisdom of Crowds*. New York: Doubleday.

Thaler, R.H. & Sunstein, C. (2008). *Nudge: Improving Decisions about Health, Wealth and Happiness*. New Haven: Yale University Press.

Tversky, A. & Kahneman, D. (1974). Judgement under uncertainty: Heuristics and biases. *Science*, **185**, 1124–31.

Wilson, T.D. & Brekke, N. (1994). Mental contamination and mental correction: Unwanted influences on judgements and evaluations. *Psychological Bulletin*, **116**, 117–42.

Yamagishi, K. (1997). When a 12.86% mortality is more dangerous than 24.14%: Implications for risk communication. *Applied Cognitive Psychology*, **11**, 495–506.

9

Smart Policy: Cognitive Enhancement and the Public Interest

Nick Bostrom and Rebecca Roache

Background

Definition

Cognitive enhancement is the amplification or extension of core capacities of the mind through improvement or augmentation of internal or external information-processing systems. Cognition refers to the processes an organism uses to organize information. These include acquiring (perception), selecting (attention), representing (understanding) and retaining (memory) information, and using this information to guide behavior (reasoning and coordination of motor outputs). Interventions to improve cognitive function may be directed at any of these core faculties.

Biomedical enhancement as part of a wider spectrum of enhancement methods

Such interventions may take a variety of forms, many of them age-old and mundane. The prime example is education, where the goal is often not only to impart specific skills or information but also to improve general mental faculties such as concentration, memory, and critical thinking. Other forms of mental training, such as yoga, martial arts, meditation, and creativity courses are also in common use. Caffeine is widely used to improve alertness. Herbal extracts reputed to improve memory are popular, with sales of Ginkgo biloba alone on the order of several hundred million dollars per year in the United States (van Beek, 2002). In an ordinary supermarket or health food store we can find a veritable cornucopia of energy drinks and similar preparations, vying for consumers hoping to turbo-charge their brains.

Enhancing Human Capacities, edited by Julian Savulescu, Ruud ter Meulen and Guy Kahane.
© 2011 Blackwell Publishing Ltd

As cognitive neuroscience has advanced, the list of prospective biomedical enhance-ments has expanded (Bostrom & Sandberg, 2009a; Farah *et al.*, 2004). Yet, to date, the most dramatic advances in our effective cognitive performance have been achieved through non-biomedical means. Progress in computing and information technology has vastly increased our ability to collect, store, analyze, and communicate information. External hardware and software supports now routinely give humans beings effective cognitive abilities that in many respects far outstrip those of our biological brains. Another important area of progress has been in "collective cognition" – cognition distributed across many minds. Collective cognition has been enhanced through the development and use of more efficient tools and methods for intellectual collaboration. The World Wide Web and e-mail are among the most powerful kinds of cognitive enhancement developed to date. Non-technological approaches to enhancing collec-tive cognition have also made important advances: it is possible to view institutions, such as academic peer-reviewed journals, and social conventions, such as limitations on the use of *ad hominem* arguments in discussions, as part of the cognitive enhancement spectrum.

It is useful to bear in mind this wider perspective on the various forms that cognitive enhancement can take. Such a perspective helps us see just how important advances in cognitive and epistemic functioning are to individuals and to modern societies. It also helps us avoid a myopic fixation on biological paths to enhancement to the exclusion of other ways of achieving similar goals, which in many cases may be more practicable. Nevertheless, biomedical forms of cognitive enhancement are worthy of serious consideration, not only because of their novelty but also because they could eventually offer enormous leverage. Consider, for example, the cost–benefit ratio of a cheap, safe, cognition-enhancing pill compared to that of years of extra education: in terms of improving cognition, both could achieve similar results, yet the biomedical route would do so using a tiny fraction of the time and resources demanded by the educational route.[1]

In this chapter, we concentrate mainly on biomedical cognitive enhancements, but many of our remarks apply equally to enhancements that work on non-cognitive capacities, and to non-biomedical means of enhancement.

Assessment

Protecting and promoting cognition as accepted goals in current practice

There are many laws and regulations instituted with the purpose of protecting and improving cognitive function. Regulation of lead in paints and in tap water; require-ments of boxing, bicycle, and motorcycle helmets; bans on alcohol for minors; mandatory education; folic acid fortification of cereals; legal sanctions against mothers taking drugs during pregnancy: these all serve to safeguard or promote cognition. To some extent, these efforts may be motivated by a concern to control behavior and promote health and well-being, generally conceived; yet greater efforts appear to be made when cognitive function is at risk. Such regulations seem implicitly to recognize the value of cognition. By contrast, we are unaware of any public policy intended to limit or reduce cognitive capacity. One may also observe that mandated information duties, such as labeling of food products, were introduced to give consumers access to more accurate information in order to enable them to make better choices. Given that sound decision making requires not only reliable information, but also the cognitive ability to retain, evaluate, and use this information, one would expect that enhancements of cognition will also promote rational consumer choice.

Feasibility of biomedical enhancement of cognition: narrow vs. wide enhancement targets

At present, biomedical enhancement techniques produce at best modest gains in cognitive performance. Reported improvements of 10–20% in some test tasks are typical. It remains unclear to what extent such improvements in a laboratory setting would translate into performance gains on real-world tasks. The sustainability of any short-term gains is also often unclear. For example, although stimulants can temporarily reduce the need for sleep and improve performance in sleep-deprived subjects, it is unclear whether the long-term use of such drugs would improve work capacity.

More dramatic results can be achieved through training and human–machine collaboration. Mental techniques (e.g. mnemonic tricks) can achieve upwards of 1000% improvement in narrow domains such as specific memorization tasks (Ericsson *et al.*, 1980). However, while biomedical enhancements do not produce dramatic improvements on specific tasks, their effects are typically broad. A drug might, for instance, enhance performance on all tasks that rely heavily on working memory, or on long-term memory. External tools and cognitive techniques such as mnemonics, by contrast, are usually task-specific, producing potentially huge improvements in relatively narrow abilities. To evaluate the value of some enhancement, one must consider not only the degree to which some capacity is enhanced, but also how general and useful this capacity is. The broader the target capacity, the greater the potential positive effects of even a small degree of enhancement.

Correlates and consequences of higher cognitive ability

General cognitive capacity of individuals – imperfectly measured by IQ scores – is positively correlated with a number of desirable outcomes. It reduces the risk of a wide array of social and economic misfortunes (Gottfredson, 2004), such as bad health (Batty *et al.*, 2009a; Pavlik *et al.*, 2003; Whalley & Deary, 2001), accidents (Batty *et al.*, 2009b), and even being the victim of homicide (Batty *et al.*, 2008), while reducing overall mortality (Batty *et al.*, 2007) and improving educational outcomes. In prisoner's-dilemma type experiments people with higher cognitive abilities cooperate more often and appear to have a stronger future orientation (Jones, 2008), something that appears to promote economic success (Burks *et al.*, 2009). While many non-cognitive factors also play large roles in determining professional and life success, cognitive capacity is part of an important feedback loop of human capital acquisition.

At a societal level, the sum of many individual enhancements may have an even more profound effect. Economic models of the loss caused by small intelligence decrements due to lead in drinking water predict significant effects of even a few points change

(Muir & Zegarac, 2001; Salkever, 1995). Correspondingly significant *benefits* can be expected if a similarly small amount of intelligence were gained instead of lost (Bostrom & Ord, 2006). It may therefore be worth seriously considering the possibility that improving cognition could have benefits not only for individuals, but also cultural and economic benefits for society.

It is important to remain aware when weighing evidence about the efficacy of pharmacological enhancers that such drugs are typically tested within a laboratory setting for particular tasks. While this enables more exact measurement and elimination of confounders, its relevance to real-life situations is debatable. One could imagine, for example, that some drug increases performance on one kind of task, while subtly decreasing performance on various other tasks that were not included in the test battery. Alternatively, some drug might give a short-term benefit but its efficacy might degrade with use over longer periods than those used in testing (some stimulant drugs, for example, might fit this pattern). Or a drug might improve some particular capacity yet fail to produce meaningful improvements in key outcomes variables such as academic performance, economic productivity, or life satisfaction. Furthermore, people's values and lifestyles might lead them to use enhancement technologies in non-prescribed ways, with unexpected and possibly undesirable results. There is scant data at the current time on such "ecological effects" of cognitive enhancers.

Ethical concerns

The prospect of enhancement often evokes ethical concerns. Generally speaking, only certain types of enhancement give rise to discussion of such concerns. "Conventional" means of cognitive enhancement such as education, mental techniques, neurological health initiatives, external information technology, and epistemic institutions are quite uncontroversial. "Unconventional" means such as drugs, implants, direct brain–computer interfaces, and genetic engineering are more likely to evoke moral concerns. The boundary between these two categories, however, may increasingly blur. For instance, neurological "health" objectives such as maintaining full cognitive performance into old age, or remedying specific cognitive deficits such as a concentration and memory problems, are likely to become increasingly hard to distinguish from enhancement objectives as the range of available biomedical interventions expands.

We suspect that the controversy surrounding unconventional means of cognitive enhancement (with the possible exception of germ-line genetic therapy) is largely due to the fact that they are currently novel and experimental rather than to any problem inherent in the technologies themselves. As we learn, through research and practical experience, about the strengths and weaknesses of these unconventional methods for improving cognitive performance, our acceptance of them is likely to increase. This is what has happened with many once-controversial technologies such as oral contraceptives, IVF, and even the telescope. The debate about cognitive enhancement might then become absorbed into the ordinary discussions about the merits and demerits of various kinds of tools, technologies, medicines, and practices.

Opinions about the value of enhancements are also influenced by the fact that enhancements aim to effect deviations from the status quo – that is, from what we regard as "normal." Allowing status quo bias to affect our attitudes towards enhancement could result in our missing out on valuable goods. One of us has outlined a method for reducing the influence on our judgments of status quo bias (Bostrom & Ord, 2006).

A more specific concern about biomedical cognitive enhancement has recently hit the headlines (Henderson, 2008). Following reports that some students use currently available drugs like Modafinil and Ritalin to improve examination performance, some worry that use of such "smart drugs" constitutes cheating (Rose, 2005; Sahakian & Morein-Zamir, 2007; Schermer, 2008; Warren *et al.*, 2009). The accusation of cheating is figurative: an activity constitutes cheating if it allows participants to gain an advantage by violating a rule, but currently no rules prohibit using smart drugs. Those who claim that use of smart drugs constitutes cheating, then, are best understood as claiming that such drugs enable users to gain an unfair advantage, and that therefore the rules ought to be changed so as to prohibit them. Assessing whether they ought to be banned in educational institutions requires addressing questions about the value of education and our attitudes towards other more familiar methods of improving examination performance, such as working hard or hiring a private tutor (Roache, 2008).[2] A more nuanced approach to the issue could assess enhancements on a case-by-case basis, taking the context into account, and considering factors such as the health risks of different enhancers, their cost and availability, the feasibility of detecting illicit use, and whether individual rights would be infringed by a prohibition. If a smart drug could be proven sufficiently safe and effective, then instead of being forbidden, its use could be encouraged for the same reasons that students are now encouraged to eat and sleep well, to revise, and to take notes in preparation for exams.

Related to the worry about cheating, it is sometimes desirable to discourage the pursuit of what the economist Fred Hirsch has called "positional goods": those goods whose value to those who have them depends on others not having them. The collective pursuit of positional goods is a waste of time and resources: as Hirsch remarked, "if everyone stands on tiptoe, no one sees better" (Hirsch, 1977). If the value of cognitive enhancement rested solely on its ability to enable one to compete better than others, it would fall into this category. However, we have already noted that improved cognitive function brings valuable non-positional benefits, and so cognitive enhancement cannot be condemned as a purely positional good. Certain other types of enhancement may bring purely positional benefits, though, and their use should arguably be discouraged. This is the attitude that the World Anti-Doping Agency adopts towards physical enhancement in sport; although others have argued that doping should be permitted (Savulescu *et al.*, 2004).

If enhancement could really deliver great benefits, should we consider the possibility that there is there a right to enhance? While access to medicine is commonly regarded as a human right constrained by cost concerns, it is less clear whether access to all enhancements should be regarded as a positive right. The case for at least a negative right to cognitive enhancement based on cognitive liberty, privacy interests, and the interest of persons in protecting and developing their own minds and capacity for autonomy, seems very strong (Boire, 2001; Sandberg, 2003). Proponents of a positive right to (publicly subsidized) enhancements could argue their case on grounds of fairness or equality, or on grounds of a public interest in the promotion of the capacities required for autonomous agency. The societal benefits of effective cognitive enhancement may turn out to be so large and unequivocal that it would be economically efficient to subsidize enhancement for the poor, just as the state now subsidizes education.

Policy Issues

Drug approval criteria

One major obstacle to the development of safe and effective biomedical enhancers is the present system for licensing drugs and medical treatments. This system was created to deal with medicine that aims to prevent, detect, cure, or mitigate diseases. In this framework, there is no room for enhancing medicine. Drug companies seeking regulatory approval for a pharmaceutical useful solely for improving functioning in the healthy population would face an uphill struggle without major changes to the current licensing framework.

To date, every licensed pharmaceutical on the market that offers some potential cognitive enhancement effect was developed to treat some specific disease condition, such as attention-deficit hyperactivity disorder (ADHD), narcolepsy, or Alzheimer's disease. The enhancing effect of these drugs in healthy subjects is a serendipitous unintended benefit. It seems likely that progress in developing biomedical enhancements would be accelerated if pharmaceutical corporations could focus directly on developing nootropics for use in non-diseased populations rather than having to work indirectly by demonstrating that the drugs are efficacious in treating some recognized disease.

One of the perverse effects of the failure of the current medical framework to embrace the potential of enhancement medicine is the trend towards the pathologization of an increasing range of conditions previously regarded as part of the normal human spectrum. If, for example, a significant fraction of the population could obtain certain benefits from drugs that improve concentration, it is currently necessary to categorize these people as having some disease – in this case ADHD – in order to allow them access to the drugs in question via the usual channels, such as prescription by a doctor. This disease-focused medical model is increasingly inadequate in an era in which many people will be using medical treatments for purposes of modification or enhancement.

Research funding

One consequence of the disease framework for drug regulation is to discourage investment in development of cognitive enhancers. Pharmaceutical firms can be expected to focus on investing in the development and testing of those drugs for which they expect to obtain regulatory approval. Given the difficulties associated with obtaining approval for purely enhancing drugs, such companies have little incentive to focus directly on developing them, unless they stand to profit significantly from encouraging off-label use of enhancers.

Academic research is also hampered by the disease framework, since researchers find it difficult – even impossible – to secure funding to study potential cognitive enhancers except in contexts where the study can be linked to some recognized pathology.[3] As a result, public funding for research into biomedical cognitive enhancement does not yet reflect the potentially vast personal and social benefits that could be realized through the development of safe and effective enhancers. A case could be made that even on purely economic grounds, the field deserves large-scale funding, since the limited available evidence suggests large potential economic gains from increased cognitive abilities.[4]

Regulation of access to enhancers

The medicine-as-treatment-for-disease paradigm creates problems not only for pharmaceutical companies and academic researchers, but also for individual users whose access to enhancers is often dependent on being able to find an open-minded physician who will prescribe the drug. This creates inequities in access. People with high social capital and good information get access while others are excluded.

Any novel technology poses risks, and biomedical cognitive enhancement is no exception. Assessing the seriousness of the potential risks, and deciding how to respond to them, requires taking into account not only what harms might accrue from irresponsible use of such technology, but also the potentially great benefits offered by enhancement. Some opponents of enhancement ignore its potential benefits and focus only on the risks, leading to an overly pessimistic attitude towards enhancement (Fukuyama, 2002; Kass, 2003; Sandel, 2004): a result, perhaps, of the sort of status quo bias mentioned in the previous section. A more constructive approach would focus not only on anticipating potential harms and benefits, but also on identifying potential supporting policies and practices that can alter the balance for the better.

As cognitive enhancement technology grows more sophisticated, so must legislation to promote cognitive function. In part, it is likely that this will be due to the practical challenge of deciding which cognitive capacities to enhance, which may at least sometimes entail a tradeoff between different cognitive abilities. For example, staying awake by using stimulants prevents the memory consolidation that occurs during sleep, meaning that enhanced wakefulness may not be possible without paying a price in terms of a reduction in memory functioning. It may not always be possible to predict in advance where such tradeoffs are likely to occur: while our biology and evolutionary history gives us some important clues (Bostrom & Sandberg, 2009b), new enhancement drugs may give rise to unexpected effects, some of which might be subtle and take a long time to manifest.

This raises the point that a "one size fits all" approach is unlikely to be suitable for enhancement. While the value of being cured of some disease is often similar across individuals who have the disease, the benefit to an individual of some particular enhancement will often depend sensitively on his or her personal values, preferences, and idiosyncratic context. This suggests that in many cases individuals will be best placed to decide for themselves whether and how to enhance.

At the same time, many will feel the need for a limited degree of paternalism that would protect individuals from the worst health risks. How, then, can a policy approach best be determined?

One option would be to establish some baseline level of acceptable risk in approved interventions. This could be done through comparison with other risks that society allows individuals to take (merely for fun or on any personal whim or preference), such as risks from smoking, mountain climbing, or horseback riding. Enhancements that could be shown to be no more risky than these activities would be allowed, with appropriate information and warning labels when necessary.

Another possibility would be "enhancement licenses". People willing to undergo potentially risky but rewarding enhancements could be required to demonstrate sufficient understanding of the risks and the ability to handle them responsibly. This would ensure informed consent and enable better monitoring. However, it would discriminate against poorly educated individuals. In particular, those of low cognitive capacity, who may have the most to gain from some enhancements, could find it hard to gain access if license requirements were demanding.

The increasing popularity of cosmetic surgery[5] highlights an important area of risk that may also arise in the case of cognitive enhancement. As more cosmetic procedures of different types become available, there arises the problem that some new procedures may not be covered by extant legislation. As a result, the public may believe that cosmetic procedures are strictly regulated even though some types of procedure "slip through the net" and can be offered by practitioners who have undergone only minimal training (British Association of Cosmetic Doctors, 2009). The result is that the public may feel overconfident about undergoing inadequately regulated procedures. Something similar could happen with cognitive enhancement. Regulation of such drugs would need to be continuously reviewed in order to ensure that the public is protected from the worst harms of irresponsible enhancement use.

Low-hanging fruits

Special attention should be given to areas in which relatively easy, inexpensive, and low-tech approaches are likely to be able to achieve comparatively big results.

One such approach might involve ensuring that infant formula contains the nutrients required for optimal neurological development. Evidence on prenatal and perinatal nutrition suggests that the composition of infant formulas and maternal nutrition can have a significant lifelong impact on cognition. Recent studies have indicated that children's IQ can be improved by increasing maternal docosahexaenoic acid (DHA) intake during pregnancy (Cohen *et al.*, 2005), by supplementing infant formula with DHA (Birch *et al.*, 2007; Scott *et al.*, 1998), and by increasing the period for which the infant is breastfed (Horwood & Ferguson, 1998). Good infant nutrition can increase a child's IQ by as much as 5.2 points in cases where low birth weight infants are fed human milk (Anderson *et al.*, 1999). Because of the low cost and extremely large potential impact of enriching infant formula with the nutrients needed to ensure optimum cognitive functioning if applied at a population level, it should be a priority to conduct more research to establish the optimal composition of infant formula in order to maximize cognitive ability in bottle-fed children. Regulation could then be put in place to ensure that commercially available formula contains these nutrients. Public health information campaigns could further promote the use of enriched formula or breast-feeding practices. This would be a simple extension of current regulatory practice, but potentially a highly effective one.

Another easy and cheap approach to increasing cognitive functioning is to treat the two billion people worldwide suffering from iodine deficiency, the world's most common cause of preventable mental impairment (Zimmermann *et al.*, 2008). Those worst affected by iodine deficiency are found in inland areas of sub-Saharan Africa, South Asia, and Central and Eastern Europe/Commonwealth of Independent States (Horton *et al.*, 2008). Iodine deficiency adversely affects health in a number of ways, and its specific effect on cognition is severe: iodine deficient populations average between 12.5 and 13.5 IQ points less than normal populations (Qian *et al.*, 2005). The deficiency can be easily treated by supplementing food with iodized salt; an intervention costing about $0.05 per person per year (Horton *et al.*, 2008). The cost of such an intervention is dwarfed by the cost to the developing world of iodine deficiency: it has been estimated that iodine supplementation would avert specifically cognitive losses with a benefit–cost ratio of 30:1 (Horton *et al.*, 2008), and losses to general health with a benefit–cost ratio of 70:1 (Horton, 2006). When we factor in the less quantifiable benefits to sufferers and their communities of improved cognitive function – in terms, for example, of well-being, choices, quality of life, and personal relationships – the ratios increase further still. It is morally and prudentially scandalous that this problem has not already been solved.

Given the scale and adverse effects of iodine deficiency compared with the relative ease of treating it, this final example powerfully illustrates that cognitive enhancement policy need not center on preparing the ground for sophisticated, yet-to-be-realized technologies. "Smart policy" should, rather, take as its starting point the recognition that effective cognition is not only subjectively valuable to individuals, but also delivers significant social, cultural, financial, and scientific benefits. Maximizing these benefits need not be difficult, risky, controversial, or expensive.

Recommendations

- Conceptualize biomedical cognitive enhancers as part of a wider spectrum of ways of enhancing the cognitive performance of groups and individuals.
- Modify the disease-focused regulatory framework for drug approval into a well-being-focused framework in order to facilitate the development and use of pharmaceutical cognitive enhancement of healthy adult individuals.
- Assess risks by balancing against benefits rather than against the status quo, and by allowing individuals to determine risk acceptability where appropriate.
- Provide public funding for academic research into the safety and efficacy of cognitive enhancers, for the development of improved enhancers, and for epidemiological studies of the broader effects of long-term use.
- Increase public funding for research aimed at determining optimal nutrition for pregnant women and newborns to promote brain development.
- Address the problem of iodine deficiency as a global priority.
- Bear in mind that enhancement regulation may need to be continuously reviewed in order to keep in step with progress.[6]

Notes

1. Although education, of course, can often bring benefits in addition to its effect on cognition, such as social, technological, and artistic skills.
2. One of us has argued elsewhere that, following such consideration, the use of smart drugs ought not to be viewed as akin to cheating, since there is no significant general difference between using smart drugs and, say, hiring a private tutor (Roache, 2008).
3. Danielle Turner and Barbara J Sahakian, personal communication.
4. Economic models of the loss caused by small intelligence decrements due to lead in drinking water predict significant effects of even a few points change (Muir & Zegarac, 2001; Salkever, 1995). Correspondingly significant benefits can be expected if a similarly small amount of intelligence were gained instead of lost (Bostrom & Ord, 2006). For a detailed discussion of the social and economic benefits of cognitive enhancement, see Sandberg and Savulescu, chapter 6, this volume.
5. In 2007, 32,453 cosmetic procedures were carried out in the UK, compared to 28,921 in 2006, 22,041 in 2005, and 16,367 in 2004 (British Association of Aesthetic Plastic Surgeons, 2008, available at: www.baaps.org.uk/content/view/280/62/, accessed July 15, 2009).
6. We are grateful to Anders Sandberg for research collaboration.

References

Anderson, J.W., Johnstone, B.M. & Remley, D.T. (1999). Breast-feeding and cognitive development: A meta-analysis. *American Journal of Clinical Nutrition*, 70, 525–35.

Batty, G.D., Deary, I.J. & Gottfredson, L.S. (2007). Premorbid (early life) IQ and later mortality risk: Systematic review. *Annals of Epidemiology*, 17(4), 278–88.

Batty, G.D., Gale, C.R., Tynelius, P., Deary, I.J. & Rasmussen, F. (2009b). IQ in early adulthood, socioeconomic position, and unintentional injury mortality by middle age: A cohort study of more than 1 million Swedish men. *American Journal of Epidemiology*, 169(5), 606–15.

Batty, G.D., Mortensen, L.H., Gale, C.R. & Deary, I.J. (2008). Is low IQ related to risk of death by homicide? Testing a hypothesis using data from the Vietnam Experience Study. *Psychiatry Research*, 161, 112–15.

Batty, G.D., Shipley, M.J., Dundas, R., Macintyre, S., Der, G., Mortensen, L.H. & Deary, I.J. (2009a). Does IQ explain socio-economic differentials in total and cardiovascular disease mortality? Comparison with the explanatory power of traditional cardiovascular disease risk factors in the Vietnam Experience Study. *European Heart Journal*, doi:10.1093/eurheartj/ehp254.

Birch, E.E., Garfield, S., Castañeda, Y., Hughbanks-Wheaton, D., Uauy, R. & Hoffman, D. (2007). Visual acuity and cognitive outcomes at 4 years of age in a double-blind, randomized trial of long-chain polyunsaturated fatty acid-supplemented infant formula. *Early Human Development*, 83(5), 279–84.

Boire, R.G. (2001). On cognitive liberty. *Journal of Cognitive Liberties*, 2(1), 7–22.

Bostrom, N. & Ord, T. (2006). The reversal test: Eliminating status quo bias in applied ethics. *Ethics*, 116(4), 656–80.

Bostrom, N. & Sandberg, A. (2009a). Cognitive enhancement: Methods, ethics, regulatory challenges. *Science and Engineering Ethics*, 15(3), 311–41.

Bostrom, N. & Sandberg, A. (2009b). The wisdom of nature: An evolutionary heuristic for human enhancement. In J. Savulescu & N. Bostrom (eds.), *Human Enhancement*. Oxford: Oxford University Press.

British Association of Cosmetic Doctors (2009). Statement from British Association of Cosmetic Doctors warning against "Discount Injectables. *Medical News Today*. Available at: www.medicalnewstoday.com/articles/134617.php (accessed July 15, 2009).

Burks, S.V., Carpenter, J.P., Goettec, L. & Rustichini, A. (2009). Cognitive skills affect economic preferences, strategic behavior, and job attachment. *Proceedings of the National Academy of Sciences USA*, **106**(19), 7745–50.

Cohen, J.T., Bellinger, D.C., Connor, W.E. & Shaywitz, B.A. (2005). A quantitative analysis of prenatal intake of n-3 polyunsaturated fatty acids and cognitive development. *American Journal of Preventative Medicine*, **29**(4), 366.

Ericsson, K. A., Chase, W.G. & Faloon, S. (1980). Acquisition of a memory skill. *Science*, **208**(4448), 1181–2.

Farah, M.J., Illes, J., Cook-Deegan, R., Gardner, H., Kandel, E., King, P. *et al.* (2004). Neurocognitive enhancement: What can we do and what should we do? *Nature Reviews Neuroscience*, **5**(5), 421–5.

Fukuyama, F. (2002) *Our Posthuman Future*. New York: Farrar, Straus and Giroux.

Gottfredson, L.S. (2004). Life, death, and intelligence. *Journal of Cognitive Education and Psychology*, **4**(1), 23–46.

Henderson, M. (2008). Academy of Medical Sciences suggests urine tests to detect smart drugs. *The Times*, May 22.

Hirsch, F. (1977). *Social Limits to Growth*. London: Routledge & Kegan Paul.

Horton, S. (2006). The economics of food fortification. *Journal of Nutrition*, **136**, 1068–71.

Horton, S., Alderman, H. & Rivera, J.A. (2008) *Copenhagen Consensus 2008 Challenge Paper: Hunger and Malnutrition*. Copenhagen: Copenhagen Consensus Center.

Horwood, L.J. & Fergusson, D.M. (1998). Breastfeeding and later cognitive and academic outcomes. *Pediatrics*, **101**(1), e9.

Jones, G. (2008). Are smarter groups more cooperative? Evidence from prisoner's dilemma experiments, 1959–2003. *Journal of Economic Behavior and Organization*, **68**(3–4), 489–97.

Kass, L. (2003). Ageless bodies, happy souls: Biotechnology and the pursuit of perfection. *The New Atlantis*, Spring, 9–28.

Muir, T. & Zegarac, M. (2001). Societal costs of exposure to toxic substances: Economic and health costs of four case studies that are candidates for environmental causation. *Environmental Health Perspectives*, **109**, 885–903.

Pavlik, V.N., Alves de Moraes, S., Szklo, M., Knopman, D.S., Mosley, T.H. & Hyman, D.J. (2003). Relation between cognitive function and mortality in middle-aged adults. *American Journal of Epidemiology*, **157**(4), 327–34.

Qian, M., Wang, D., Watkins, W.E, Gebski, V., Yan, Y.Q., Li, M. & Chen, Z.P. (2005). The effects of iodine on intelligence in children: A meta-analysis of studies conducted in China. *Asia Pacific Journal of Clinical Nutrition*, **14**(1), 32–42.

Roache, R. (2008). Enhancement and cheating. *Expositions*, **2.2**, 153–6.

Rose, S. (2005). *The Future of the Brain*. Oxford: Oxford University Press.

Sahakian, B. & Morein-Zamir, S. (2007). Professor's little helper. *Nature*, **450**, 1157–9.

Salkever, D.S. (1995). Updated estimates of earnings benefits from reduced exposure of children to environmental lead. *Environmental Research*, **70**(1), 1–6.

Sandberg, A. (2003). Morphologic freedom. *Eudoxa Policy Studies*. Available at: www.eudoxa.se/content/archives/2003/10/eudoxa_policy_s_3.html (accessed July 15, 2009).

Sandel, M. (2004). The case against perfection. *The Atlantic*, April, 1–11.

Savulescu, J., Foddy, B. & Clayton, M. (2004). Why we should allow performance enhancing drugs in sport. *British Journal of Sports Medicine*, **38**, 666–70.

Schermer, M. (2008). On the argument that enhancement is "cheating." *Journal of Medical Ethics*, **34**, 85–8.

Scott, D.T., Janowsky, J.S., Carroll, R.E., Taylor, J.A., Auestad, N. & Montalto, M.B. (1998). Formula supplementation with long-chain polyunsaturated fatty acids: Are there developmental benefits? *Pediatrics*, **102**(5), e59.

van Beek, T.A. (2002). Chemical analysis of Ginkgo biloba leaves and extracts. *Journal of Chromatography A*, **967**(1), 21–55.

Warren, O., Leff, D., Athanasiou, T., Kennard, C. & Darzi, A. (2009). The neurocognitive enhancement of surgeons: An ethical perspective. *Journal of Surgical Research*, **152**, 167–72.

Whalley, L.J. & Deary, I.J. (2001). Longitudinal cohort study of childhood IQ and survival up to age 76. *British Medical Journal*, **322**(7290), 819–22.

Zimmermann, M.B., Jooste, P.L. & Pandav, C.S. (2008). Iodine-deficiency disorders. *The Lancet*, **372**(9645), 1251–62.

Part III
Mood Enhancement

10

Scientific, Ethical, and Social Issues in Mood Enhancement

Ron Berghmans, Ruud ter Meulen,
Andrea Malizia, and Rein Vos

Introduction

Since the introduction of Prozac (fluoxetine), a number of so-called selective serotonin reuptake inhibitors (SSRIs) – the "new antidepressants" – have been developed and introduced. Originally developed for the treatment of major depression and other affective and anxiety disorders where disability, morbidity, and distress indicate the presence of (mental) illness, such mood enhancers presently are also, and increasingly, prescribed for people whose problems are not recognized mental illnesses, whose disability and morbidity are either not documented or severe enough and where brain function may not be abnormal (President's Council on Bioethics, 2003). Some people using SSRIs who have no recognized illness feel in Kramer's words, "better than well" when taking an antidepressant (Elliott, 2003; Kramer, 1993), They report that they feel energized, more alert, more able to cope with the world, and to understand themselves and their problems (Elliott, 1999). The enhancement of mood and ability to withstand adversity for such nonclinical purposes raises different ethical and societal questions and concerns.

The first set of concerns consists of the progressive extension of the boundaries of psychiatry and psychopharmacology, leading to the further medicalization of "normal" emotional and social problems. The second set of concerns is related to less easy to articulate worries resulting from the many ways in which enhancements that alter fundamental brain function intersect with our understanding of what it means to be a person, to be healthy and whole, to do meaningful work, and to value human life in its imperfection (Farah & Wolpe, 2004). These concerns are related to our sense of self, identity, and self-understanding. Another set of concerns has to do with the political implications of mood enhancement: Is taking tablets a viable alternative to creating better communities through social and economic commitment? Is taking medicines an

---

Enhancing Human Capacities, edited by Julian Savulescu, Ruud ter Meulen and Guy Kahane.
© 2011 Blackwell Publishing Ltd

acceptable complement to poor housing, failing education, and unsafe local environments? Would these issues ever become "recognized public health problems" that would justify adding medicines to water supply as fluoride was added to prevent tooth decay? If such a medicine was available, would governments strive to suppress the aspects of affective functioning that are uncomfortable – a contemporary realization of Aldous Huxley's soma? A fourth set of concerns relates to issues of agency, justice and fairness in the access to mood-enhancing drugs. The fifth set of concerns involves conceptual problems: What do we mean by saying that mood is enhanced? What concepts of well-being, goodness, and mood are at stake?

SSRIs and Other Technologies that Improve Mood

SSRIs make an important contribution to the treatment of major depressive disorder, which is set to become the most disabling condition worldwide in the working age group by 2020. Anxiety and stress disorders are the main source of total psychiatric costs to society in terms of health care utilization and loss of productivity because of their high prevalence. Some of these disorders, e.g. chronic post-traumatic stress disorder (PTSD) or recurrent depression, have individual costs and burdens that are as high as conditions such as schizophrenia. Antidepressants are most efficacious in preventing recurrence of depressive disorders in people who suffer from such recurrent depression. SSRIs are also used for the treatment of other disorders: dysthymia (persistent mild depression of longer than two years' duration); social phobia (which some commentators argue is an extreme form of shyness and which is characterized by anxiety and disabling self-consciousness; Lane, 2007); premenstrual dysphoric disorder (a recurrent negative mood associated with PMS); and various anxiety and eating disorders respond well to SSRIs (Farah & Wolpe, 2004).

The main currently recognized effects of SSRIs is to alter the brain's handling of serotonin. Like other neurotransmitters, serotonin is released from one neuron to bind with and activate another. The brain recycles serotonin after each release, gathering it up again by means of a "reuptake system." SSRIs inhibit the serotonin reuptake system, thus increasing the concentration of serotonin available to the receiving neurons – hence the name "serotonin reuptake inhibitor." When given to patients diagnosed with mood disorders, SSRIs reverse depression or stabilize moods in most patients, presumably as a result of the increased availability of serotonin in certain crucial places in the brain. Scientists do not yet know how inhibiting the reuptake of serotonin alters the mental state or why it takes weeks for the effect to be significant; the reuptake inhibition occurs within a couple of hours of the first dose while the therapeutic effects can take up to 6–8 weeks. What serotonin does, how it functions, and even whether it is a serotonin problem that causes depression in the first place, remain largely unknown (President's Council on Bioethics, 2003). A recent meta-analysis of licensing studies has generated public concerns by claiming that the effect of SSRIs in mild depression is not significantly better than placebo (Kirsch *et al.*, 2008). While methodological and other fundamental issues make the specific conclusions debatable (Nutt & Malizia, 2008), the wide publicity that the Kirsch *et al.* paper received is testimony to public (or at least press) concerns.

The growth in sales of SSRIs clearly indicates that more people, with less severe depression, are using them (Farah, 2002; Pieters, te Hennepe & de Lange, 2002). Has the threshold for SSRI use already dropped below the line separating the healthy from the sick (Farah, 2002)? Is the increase due to better recognition of affective disorders or to injudicious prescribing? Have the goalposts moved to include self-limiting and transient phenomena? For several reasons, these questions are difficult to answer. Firstly, the line between healthy and sick is fuzzy. There is no simple discontinuity between the characteristic mood of patients with diagnosable mood disorders and the range of moods found in the general population. Secondly, diagnostic thresholds are clearly being expanded as a result of discovering that there are people who describe benefits from these very treatments. Other, less debilitating conditions than "clinical" depression are also being treated with SSRIs, such as cyclic changes in women's moods before menstruation. Thirdly, although depression is most commonly a remitting-relapsing disease with typically years between episodes, patients, whose needs for prophylaxis have not been documented, can be left on antidepressant medication for periods of 1–3 years, even when symptom-free. The dilemma here is how we ensure that people with recurrent depression where episodes come close together receive adequate and effective prophylaxis while not overprescribing for the three-quarters of people with depression who will experience only one or two episodes in their lifetime. For the first group depression, also in its early phase, is a serious disorder leading to a high risk of relapse and disability. However, prolonged prescription for the second group is unwarranted.

These changes in psychiatric practice have resulted in many people using SSRIs and other antidepressants who would not have been prescribed these drugs 10 years ago. There is no reason to predict their ranks will not continue to swell, and to include healthier and higher functioning people (Farah, 2002). Here is another dilemma, many cases of depression remain undiagnosed (Nuyen *et al.*, 2003) and an understanding and facilitating attitude as well as appropriate prescribing is warranted for these people when they consult their doctors. However, training in recognition of these disorders can result in overzealous inclusion especially when it is quicker to prescribe than to wait and support.

The effects of SSRIs on the moods of healthy people are very largely unknown. A handful of studies have assessed the effects of SSRIs on mood and personality in normal subjects over short periods of a few months or less (Knutson *et al.*, 1998; Tse & Bond, 2002). The effects are relatively selective, reducing self-reported negative affect (such as fear and hostility) while leaving positive affect (happiness, excitement) the same. To this extent a nomenclature that gets away from "mood enhancement" may be useful in the future. The drugs also increase affiliative behavior in laboratory social interactions and cooperative/competitive games played with confederates (Tse & Bond, 2002). In a small study it was found that in all subjects, after few days of SSRI treatment, emotional lability disappeared, and their emotion control and behavior were both modified (Scoppetta, Di Gennaro & Scoppetta, 2005). In a study on the effect of SSRIs on the processing of social cues, volunteers receiving citalopam detected a higher number of facial expressions of fear and happiness, with reduced response times, relative to those given the placebo. By contrast, changes in the recognition of other basic emotions were not observed. Notable differences in mood were also not apparent in these volunteers. These results suggest that even acute administration of antidepressant drugs affect neural processes involved in the processing of social information (Harmer *et al.*, 2003). A study in healthy elderly volunteers showed that SSRI use did not cause affective blunting. However, the SSRI group, but not the placebo group, demonstrated a significant drug-dependent decrease in negative affect related to negative events (Furlan *et al.*, 2004). We agree with Farah (2002) that much more research is needed to clarify the effects of SSRIs and other antidepressant agents on mood and behavior of normal subjects, but the evidence so far suggests subtle effects that may be desirable if the person taking them is not affected by the common side effects such as jitteriness, impotence, and nausea.

What risks are connected to mood-enhancing drugs? This is not an easy question to answer. Illustrative is the controversy over the use of SSRIs and the (increased) risk of suicide attempts in children, adolescents, and adults (Fergusson *et al.*, 2005; Healy, 2003; Healy & Whitaker, 2003; Simon *et al.*, 2006). The issue of SSRI safety was in the spotlight in June 2003 when Eliot Spitzer, New York Attorney General, sued GlaxoSmithKline, the manufacturer of Paxil, for concealing evidence that the drug caused suicidal behavior in young patients. What followed was a series of FDA and Congressional hearings, memorable for heart-wrenching testimony of parents whose children committed suicide while taking the medication, and an ambitious re-analysis of data from 24 clinical pediatric trials. (Trials in which, it must be noted, none of 4,400 children killed themselves.) In March 2004 the FDA warned physicians and patients of increased risk of suicide with 10 newer antidepressant drugs. In October 2004, an FDA advisory group voted 15–8 in favor of putting a "black box" warning on all anti-depressants prescribed for childhood depression (including the older ones which preceded SSRIs and that are still on the market), announcing the risk of suicidal thinking and behavior (the FDA accepted the recommendation). A black box is the strongest caution the FDA uses; the next step would be an outright ban on prescriptions à la Vioxx.

Most recently, GlaxoSmithKline announced that it had found an increase in suicidal behavior in adults taking paroxetine (Paxil/Seroxat) compared with placebo (cf. Lenzer, 2006). The researchers found that 0.32% (11/3455) of people taking paroxetine for depression attempted suicide compared with 0.05% (1/1978) of depressed patients taking placebo (odds ratio 6.7, 95% confidence interval 1.1 to 149.4; $P = 0.058$). GlaxoSmithKline said the data should be interpreted with caution and that the "overall risk-benefit of paroxetine in the treatment of adult patients with MDD [major depressive disorder] remains positive." Most often the increased risk is in the initial phase of treatment and current recommendations are that people prescribed antidepressants (including SSRIs) should be closely monitored in the initial period. This has to be balanced by the fact that most people who actually die by suicide, are not taking antidepressants and antidepressants reduce suicide risk in people with moderate to severe major depression. In recurrent severe depression the risk of suicide is up to 15% and increased prescribing of antidepressants has been associated with decreases in suicide rates. Technical advances in physics and neurochemistry have led to non-pharmaceutical methods for altering brain function creating potential mood enhance-ment tools (Farah & Wolpe, 2004). Transcranial magnetic stimulation (TMS) and, more rarely, vagus nerve stimulation and deep-brain stimulation (DBS) have already been used to improve mental function or mood in patients with medically intractable neuropsychiatric illnesses (Berghmans & De Wert, 2004; Carpenter, 2006; Castelli *et al.*, 2006; Hälbig *et al.*, 2005; Nuttin *et al.*, 2008; Schutter & Van Honk, 2006). Deep brain stimulation is still in its infancy and although over 40,000 people have had it worldwide for dystonias and Parkinson's disease, evidence for its effects is still limited. In addition, because of the nature of the procedure, it is unlikely that its effects on healthy people will ever be really known. In fact, deep brain stimulation in healthy volunteers seems very futuristic. Implantation is a surgical technique that would not be considered ethical in healthy people because of the considerable risks associated with the procedure. There are reports of mood changes emerging with DBS for Parkinson's disease but these have been successfully reversed by switching off stimulation or changing parameters and they do not seem to be qualitatively different from the effects encountered with some medications where the beneficial effects on the motor systems are always balanced by considerations of side effects. Research on the effects of non-pharmaceutical methods on brain function in normal individuals has been limited to the less invasive TMS (Farah & Wolpe, 2004).

It is probable that in the near future the combination of data from advanced biochips and brain imaging will accelerate the development of neurotechnology (Lynch, 2004). Progress in the neurosciences, enhanced by exponential advances in neurotechnologies are rapidly moving brain research and clinical applications beyond the scope of purely medical use (Sententia, 2004). So-called *neuroceuticals*, used for therapy and enhancement, and to improve different aspects of mental health, will become possible. Unlike today's psychopharmaceuticals, neuroceuticals will be efficient neuromodulators with negligible side effects. By being able to target multiple (sub)receptors in specific neural circuits, neuroceuticals will create the possibility for dynamic intracellular regulation of an individual's neurochemistry (Lynch, 2004). Other kinds of drugs are propranolol and related beta blocking agents which may prevent PTSD by detaching disastrous events like fire, traffic accidents, rape, natural disasters, death of dear ones, and violent attacks from the heavy emotions experienced in these events. These agents are seen as forerunners of a new generation of memory and mood softening and brightening drugs (President's Council on Bioethics, 2003).

Cosmetic Psychopharmacology: The Normal and the Pathological

In *Listening to Prozac*, the psychiatrist Kramer describes the potential of Prozac not so much of "restoring" the depressive patient to his or her pre-depressed state, but of "transforming" people, making them feel "better than well" (Kramer, 1993, p.xix). Prozac has the potential of altering one's sense of self: mood, self-consciousness, personality, and identity seem to become different as a result of using this SSRI. Kramer states that at the heart of his book is the following thought experiment: Imagine that we have a medication that can move a person from a normal psychological state to another normal psychological state that is more desired or better socially rewarded. He then asks: "What are the moral consequences of that potential, the one I called cosmetic psychopharmacology?" (Kramer, 2004). What, in other words, would be the consequences of an "aspirin for the mind" becoming available (Freedman, 1998)?

With this thought experiment the stage is set for a debate about the use of psychopharmacological and other means for purposes of mood enhancement. Illustrative in this respect is the medicalization of shyness (Cottle, 1999; Elliott, 2003; Healy, 2004; Lane, 2007; Moynihan & Cassels, 2005; Moynihan, Heath & Henry, 2002; Moynihan & Henry, 2006; Rose, 2003, 2005; Scott, 2006). Shyness is a relatively normal experience: many people can identify with episodic feelings of shyness that arise in certain types of situation. However, some people are not only shy but feel constantly anxious, lonely and frustrated, leading to a chronic and debilitating condition that interferes with their everyday lives. Over the past 50 years, this more extreme form of shyness has come to be seen as a mental illness: social phobia, social anxiety disorder, and avoidant personality disorder (Scott, 2006).

Obviously, this raises questions about what exactly "normal mood" and "normal anxiety" are and what "pathological mood" and "pathological anxiety" are, and what it means to have a mood which is "more desired or better socially rewarded" (as Kramer describes the *telos* and result of cosmetic psychopharmacology). Above that, it is important to be aware that historical, cultural, and societal factors play a role in the conceptualization of mood, the demarcation of psychiatric illnesses and diagnoses (i.e. depression, manic depressive disorder, anxiety disorders, social phobia, etc.), and different societal ways of dealing with suffering individuals. Is it possible to draw a clear line between "normal" and "pathological"? Is there any scientific evidence that may support such a division and is this morally relevant? How should we conceptualize the goals of psychiatry and of medicine in general? Should medicine in the future transgress its classic moral bounds, that is avoidance of premature death, preservation of life, prevention of disease and injury, promotion and maintenance of health, relief of pain and suffering, avoidance of harm, into the novel moral bound of promoting well-being (Varelius, 2006)? Does the development and use of mood brighteners overstep the moral bounds of medicine in this way (DeGrazia, 2005a, p.222)? Does the use of medicines in altering personal resilience pertain to medicine or should it be part of personal choice and available over the counter as some psychotropics already are (nicotine, alcohol, for example). And if so, does this preclude the use of such methods outside medicine and health care?

Identity, Authenticity, and Personality

A major concern raised by mood-enhancing technologies is the impact they may have on personal identity, authenticity, and personality (DeGrazia, 2005a; Elliott, 1999, 2003). According to Elliott mood-enhancing drugs and enhancement technologies in general may lead to changes in one's capacities and characteristics which are fundamental to one's identity (Elliott, 1999, p.28). To discuss the implications of mood enhancement for (personal) identity, we need to distinguish different notions of personal identity (Glover, 1988). What is personal identity, why does it matter morally, and how exactly might mood brighteners have an impact on it? Personal identity deals with questions about us *qua* people (or persons). The most common question is what it takes for us to persist from one time to another. What is necessary, and what is sufficient, for some past or future being to be *you* (Olson, 2002)? The morally important question involved in personal identity seems to be what makes you the person you are, in a time frame and in your personal history, and as compared to others. A first notion of personal identity is *numerical identity* (DeGrazia, 2005a; Olson, 2002). To say that this and that are numerically identical is to say that they are one and the same: one thing rather than two. This is different from *qualitative identity*. Things are qualitatively identical when they are exactly similar. Identical twins may be qualitatively identical – there may be no telling them apart – but they are not numerically identical, for there are two of them. A past or future person needn't be exactly like you are now in order to be you – that is, to be numerically identical with you. You don't remain qualitatively the same throughout your life: you change in size, appearance, and in many other ways (Olson, 2002). So numerical identity seems not to be really what matters when talking about mood enhancement. *Nothing* could make me a numerically different person from the one I am now. Neither is qualitative identity, as it is a fundamental fact of life that people change in many ways throughout their lives. What we care about (and what is a concern with regard to mood-enhancement technologies) is the question whether the person now (after using a mood brightener) is psychologically continuous with the person before (who has not yet used the mood brightener).

   Then two other possible notions of personal identity become relevant: *psychological identity* and *narrative identity*. The notion of psychological identity is prominently present in the approach of Parfit (1984). In a Lockean tradition, he understands personal identity in terms of psychological continuity. Although persons apparently cannot exist without bodies, personal identity over time depends on psychological relations (DeGrazia, 2005a, p.16). Two elements are essential in Parfit's approach: psychological *connectedness* and psychological *continuity*. Psychological connectedness is the holding of particular direct psychological connections, and psychological continuity is the holding of overlapping chains of strong connectedness (Parfit, 1984, p.206).

   The notion of "a narrative identity" allows one to think through the question of personal identity in a new way, taking into full account the temporal dimension (the temporality) of a being who, by existing with others in the horizon of a common world, is led to transform him(her)self in the course of a life history, that is, who is what he or she is only in the course of becoming himself or herself (Ricoeur, 1990). This notion also makes it possible for Ricoeur to distinguish two dimensions within the pseudo-unitarian notion of identity: identity as sameness (Latin: *idem*); and identity as selfhood (Latin: *ipse*) (Christman, 2004). This approach parallels the theory of personal identity which is developed by Marya Schechtman, in which she argues that the unifying element of a person's life is the narrative form of experience (Schechtman, 1996). A self understood as the author of a history (story), the one upon whom the story confers a sort of identity, is a self whose temporization shapes itself in accordance with a narrative model.

   We need an answer to the question how transformations resulting from the use of mood-enhancing technologies affect personal identity in terms of the various notions of personal identity (numerical, qualitative, psychological, and narrative). Particularly psychological and narrative conceptions of personal identity seem promising candidates to evaluate the implications of a shy and socially anxious person becoming more outgoing; an uptight one becoming more easy-going; or somebody with poor self-esteem becoming more self-confident. Relevant considerations which need to be taken into account seem to be: character, remaining true to oneself, self-creation, the place of crises. Questions which deserve attention are how mood enhancers may affect psychological and narrative identity? Does the use of mood enhancers provide reason to believe that deep psychological changes give rise to a "new identity" of the person involved? Can the changes resulting from taking mood brighteners be considered as part of the narrative history of the person? Are these changes to be seen as a form of self-creation?

Related to concerns over identity and personality is the issue of authenticity or the "authentic self." The ideal of authenticity says that if a person is not living a life as him- or herself, than he or she has missed out on what life has to offer (Elliott, 2003). This need not imply that an authentic life is a happier life; an authentic life is considered to be a higher life, because it is a life in which a person knows who she is and lives out her sense of herself. Authenticity presupposes self-discovery and self-understanding. The already-mentioned transformations which may result from mood enhancers may be seen as chemical makeovers (suggesting inauthenticity), or, alternatively, as chemical self-discoveries, which contribute to a sense of authenticity.

As Kramer reports, some users are convinced that their "true self" has come forward as a result of using Prozac. This would amount to self-discovery and not to "making over" and parallels the "restoration" taking place in depressed people using antidepressants. This raises deep questions about who we are (if we can be so altered by medication) and why the medicated self can on occasion be felt the "more true" oneself than the un-medicated self? What happens to the self of a person using mood-enhancing medications can be described in quite different terms: remodeling, remaking, reshaping, transforming or discovering of the self. How this is morally evaluated may vary with the description. The changes brought about by mood enhancers are not wholly "designed," exactly foreseeable or predictable, and sometimes they are accompanied by undesired changes (a person becoming less timid – which is desired – but at the same time more aggressive – which is not desired). Chance and luck play a role, whereas we know from history of medicine that much progress involves "mixed blessings."

Concerns about the impact of mood enhancement on personality, identity, self, and authenticity are connected to the question how individual mood enhancement influences interpersonal relationships and communication. Dominant accounts of personal identity in the analytical philosophical tradition generally take a very individualized stance and do not take into account social relationships (Daniels, 1988). It can be argued that facts about psychological connectedness and continuity are not sufficient conditions for personal identity, but that the degree of connectedness and continuity among the stages of a person's life may themselves depend on psychological facts about other persons' attitudes and beliefs concerning the person.

People have a social self (Glover, 1988). Our identity is (at least partly) socially constructed. Role theory claims that an "inner core" of a person is an illusion. But even if such an "inner core" is real, it cannot be so without taking social relationships into account. Depending on the impact the use of a particular enhancer has on the mood (and personal make up) of a particular individual, this may (and will) have repercussions for this person's relationships with others. The metaphor of "becoming another person" may imply that the person is not recognized anymore by others, which may have deep implications for personal relationships.

Potential changes in our self-understanding are connected to views regarding the good life, a just society, and to personhood and moral responsibility. Although having a happy or happier life is a goal many people will share, it is not at all clear what a happy or happier life consists of. A good or happy life at least partly seems to depend on individual striving and effort, and on being connected to other people by way of social relationships and interactions. To produce their effects, mood enhancement technologies do not depend on such strivings, efforts and human relationships, and may ultimately result in a shallower life, instead of a richer life. Such interventions may produce and reinforce social isolation and societal non-participation in individuals who lack well-being. Also, immediate short-term gratification may undermine character formation and delay of gratification, and reinforce conformist, hedonistic, and narcissistic character traits in individuals. Moreover, leading a good life and being happy seems to depend also on so-called contrast experiences. Sadness, grief, and suffering are inherently part of human life, as much as feelings of joy, happiness, and elevated mood are. They are like two sides of a coin. Trying to eliminate negatively valued experiences may ultimately and paradoxically lead to a lower level of well-being.

It is important to bear in mind that there is no agreed clear-cut definition of mood enhancement. Mostly mood enhancement is negatively defined, namely as the treatment of a lack of good mood, as in the case of DSM IV description of clinical depression "in which a person's enjoyment of life and ability to function socially and in day to day matters is disrupted by intense sadness, melancholia, numbness, or despair." "Enhancing" such a negative mood state into a more positive mood state is clearly desirable and any technology, chemical, physical or psychological, to improve such a negative mood state in a safe and effective way will be appreciated. Unlike cognition or physical fitness, emotions have both a positive and negative value. In past two decades emotions and mood states have been studied extensively and the major conclusion of this research has been that both positive and negative feelings are important for human beings, individually and socially, for survival, aspiration, achievement, prosperity, and communal life. In light of this, it is hard to make *a priori* claims about the type of mood states we should aim to "enhance."

Antidepressants do not result in feeling happy or great or whatever sort of elevated mood. Alcohol, cocaine, morphine, amphetamines, cannabis, and ecstasy all undoubtedly have immediate and short-term euphoric effects, yet none are effective antidepressants; in addition if they have a positive effect on people with depression, this is usually accompanied by quick tolerance and a disappearance of the initial beneficial modulation. Conversely, antidepressants of any sort do not have any euphoric effect and indeed have zero or almost zero street value as they are unable to produce an effect that people would recognize as mood enhancing. Further, their antidepressant action in disease takes weeks to develop and does not stop people from feeling low at times of personal distress although some people report a decrease in fear in challenging situations.

Some critics charge that the use of SSRIs promotes biopsychiatry's dubious agenda of reducing emotional and personal struggles to mechanistic terms – as if these struggles were just another form of pain to be treated with pills (DeGrazia, 2005b, p.217). Questions with regard to changes in our self-understanding have a speculative character and are at least partly of an empirical nature. Systematic research on the self-experience and self-understanding of (healthy) people using SSRIs is lacking. Is it to be expected that the use of mood brighteners will paradoxically lead to a shallower life instead of a richer life? Will it reinforce conformist, hedonist, and narcissistic character traits in individuals? Will it undermine character formation and lead to passivity regarding human striving? And how to evaluate such changes from a moral point of view?

Agency, Justice, and Human Diversity

A particular aspect of our (self-)understanding as human beings concerns our views regarding (moral) agency and moral responsibility. How might mood-brightening interventions influence these views? What defines human (moral) agency, how is this related to concepts of free will and determinism, and why and when are human agents (to be) held morally responsible for their acts and omissions (Fischer, 2005)? Another issue in this context relates to the notion of personal autonomy (Mele, 2002). Does the use of mood brighteners diminish our freedom and power for autonomous action? How does cosmetic psychopharmacology affect the control agents have over their choices and actions, or is this influence only marginal? And if yes, in how far does this influence moral responsibility and accountability. Apart from moral account-ability, how can and should the use of mood-enhancing drugs (rightly or wrongly) affect legal and criminal liability and responsibility (Eastman & Campbell, 2006; Rosack, 2001)?

Mood-enhancing technologies may not become available to all who might want to use them. This raises questions about justice. Some may be able to afford SSRIs if their insurance company will not cover this, but many less wealthy individuals cannot (DeGrazia, 2005c). Presuming everybody has access to basic health care (which is not universally the case),[1] can unequal access to mood enhancements be morally justified from a standpoint of justice? The answer to this question seems to (at least partly) depend on the benefits involved in using mood brighteners. Another justice argument is that allowing enhancement could be used to reduce natural inequality. This seems to presuppose access of all to mood-brightening drugs. Will the use of mood enhancers lead to a competitive advantage? Would opportunities for increasing welfare be unequally distributed among those who can afford to use such technologies and those who cannot afford these? Will mood-enhancing drugs reduce natural inequality?

As a result of the "natural lottery," significant genetic diversity exists within species. This relates not only to physical characteristics and appearance, but also to character, personality style, and psychological make up. As other enhancement technologies, mood enhancement may result in a reduction of human diversity. If many or most people would choose to use chemical mood enhancers, then a kind of *Gleichschaltung* might be the result. With regard to mood, the bell-curve might get flatter as the range of different individual moods would become more restricted. The first question to be addressed is whether diversity is a value. Next we must ask whether it is probable that the use of mood enhancers will reduce diversity, and in what ways.

Conclusions

The scientific, ethical, and social issues raised by mood enhancement and alteration of personal resilience require further exploration. Here a combined approach of empirical research and philosophical reflection is needed. The agenda for empirical research is not restricted to research into biological mechanisms underlying different mood-enhancement technologies, and the effects of these interventions on predefined endpoints for measuring an increase in mood. Empirical research should also cover psychological and sociological research into perceptions and experiences of individuals who have used mood-brightening drugs or other technologies and attitudes of society at large towards different aspects of the use of mood enhancers outside the medical domain. Philosophical and ethical analysis is needed to explore relevant concepts as they relate to personal identity, authenticity, and what it means to be human.

Notes

1. Unequal access to health care and the parallel development and use of enhancement technologies further divides the haves and have nots with new enhancement technologies available only to the advantaged, and would thus increase the injustice (DeGrazia, 2005c, p. 226).

References

Berghmans, R.L.P. & De Wert, G.M.W.R. (2004). Mental competence in the context of deep brain stimulation. *Ned Tijdschr Geneeskd*, **148**(28), 1373–5 (Dutch).

Carpenter, L.L. (2006). Neurostimulation in resistant depression. *Journal of Psychopharmacology*, **20**, 35–40.

Castelli, L., Perozzo, P., Zibetti, M. *et al.* (2006). Chronic deep brain stimulation of the subthalamic nucleus for Parkinson's disease: Effects on cognition, mood, anxiety and personality traits. *European Neurology*, **55**(3), 136–44.

Christman, J. (2004). Narrative unity as a condition of personhood. *Metaphilosophy*, **35**(5), 695–713.

Cottle, M. (1999). Selling shyness. How doctors and drug companies created the "social phobia" epidemic. *The New Republic*, August 2.

Daniels, N. (1988). *Am I My Parents' Keeper? An Essay on Justice between the Young and the Old.* Oxford: Oxford University Press.

DeGrazia, D. (2005a). *Human Identity and Bioethics.* Cambridge: Cambridge University Press.

DeGrazia, D. (2005b). Enhancement technologies and self-creation. In D. DeGrazia (ed.), *Human Identity and Bioethics* (pp. 203–43). Cambridge: Cambridge University Press.

DeGrazia, D. (2005c). Enhancement technologies and human identity. *Journal of Medicine and Philosophy*, **30**, 261–83.

Eastman, N. & Campbell, C. (2006). Neuroscience and legal determination of criminal responsibility. *Nature Reviews Neuroscience*, 7, 311–18.

Elliott, C. (1999). *A Philosophical Disease. Bioethics, Culture and Identity.* New York: Routledge.

Elliott, C. (2003). *Better Than Well: American Medicine Meets the American Dream.* New York: W.W. Norton.

Farah, M.J. (2002). Emerging ethical issues in neuroscience. *Nature Neuroscience*, 5(11), 1123–9.

Farah, M.J. & Wolpe, P.R. (2004). New neuroscience technologies and their ethical implications. *Hastings Center Report.* May–June, 35–45.

Fergusson, D., Doucette, S., Glass, K.C. *et al.* (2005). Association between suicide attempts and selective serotonin reuptake inhibitors: Systematic review of randomised controlled trials. *British Medical Journal*, **330**, 653.

Fischer, J.M. (2005). Free will and moral responsibility. In D. Cobb (ed.), *The Oxford Handbook of Ethical Theory* (pp. 321–355). Oxford: Oxford University Press.

Freedman, C. (1998). Aspirin for the mind? Some ethical worries about psychopharmacology. In E. Parens,(ed.), *Enhancing Human Traits. Ethical and Social Implications* (pp. 135–50). Washington DC: Georgetown University Press.

Furlan, P.M., Kallan, M.J., Have, T.T. *et al.* (2004). SSRIs do not cause affective blunting in healthy elderly volunteers. *American Journal of Geriatric Psychiatry*, 12(3), 323–30.

Glover, J. (1988). *I: The Philosophy and Psychology of Personal Identity.* London: Penguin.

Hälbig, T.D., Gruber, D., Kopp, U.A. *et al.* (2005). Pallidal stimulation in dystonia: Effects on cognition, mood, and quality of life. *Journal of Neurology, Neurosurgery & Psychiatry*, **76**, 1713–16.

Harmer, C.J., Bhagwagar, Z., Perrett, D.I. *et al.* (2003). Acute SSRI administration affects the processing of social cues in healthy volunteers. *Neuropsychopharmacology*, 28(1), 148–52.

Healy, D. (2003). Lines of evidence on the risks of suicide with selective serotonin reuptake inhibitors. *Psychotherapy & Psychosomatics*, **72**, 71–9.

Healy, D. (2004). Shaping the intimate: Influences on the experience of everyday nerves. *Social Studies of Science*, **34**(2), 219–45.

Healy, D. & Whitaker, C. (2003). Antidepressants and suicide: Risk-benefit conundrums. *Journal of Psychiatry and Neuroscience*, **28**(5), 340–7.

Kirsch, I., Deacon, B.J. *et al.* (2008). Initial severity and antidepressant benefits: A meta-analysis of data submitted to the Food and Drug Administration. *Public Library of Science Medicine*, 5, 26 February.

Knutson, B., Wolkowitz, O.M., Cole, S.W. *et al.* (1998). Selective alteration of personality and social behavior by serotonergic intervention. *American Journal of Psychiatry*, **155**, 373–9.

Kramer, P. (1993). *Listening to Prozac.* New York: Viking. [Penguin Books edition with a new afterword, 1997].

Kramer, P. (2004). The valorization of sadness. Alienation and the melancholic temperament. In C. Elliott & T. Chambers (eds.), *Prozac as a Way of Life* (pp. 48–58). Chapel Hill: University of North Carolina Press.

Lane, C. (2007). *Shyness. How Normal Behavior Became a Sickness.* New Haven: Yale University Press.

Lenzer, J. (2006). Manufacturer admits increase in suicidal behaviour in patients taking paroxetine. *British Medical Journal*, **332**, 1175.

Lynch, Z. (2004). Neurotechnology and society (2010–2060). *Annals of the New York Academy of Sciences*, 1013, 229–33.

Mele, A.R. (2002). Autonomy, self-control, and weakness of will. In R. Kane (ed.), *The Oxford Handbook of Free Will* (pp. 529–48). Oxford: Oxford University Press.

Moynihan, R., Heath, I. & Henry, D. (2002). Selling sickness: The pharmaceutical industry and disease mongering. *British Medical Journal*, **324**, 886–91.

Moynihan, R. & Cassels, A. (2005). *Selling Sickness: How Drug Companies are Turning us all into Patients*. Allen & Unwin.

Moynihan, R. & Henry, D. (2006). The fight against disease mongering: Generating knowledge for action. *Public Library of Science Medicine*, **3**(4), e191.

Nutt, D.J. & Malizia, A.L. (2008). Why does the world have such a downer on antidepressants? *Journal of Psychopharmacology*, **22**(3), 223–6.

Nuttin, B.J., Gabriëls, L.A., Cosyns, P.R. *et al*. (2008). Long-term electrical capsular stimulation in patients with obsessive-compulsive disorder. *Neurosurgery*, **62**, 966–77.

Nuyen, J., Volkers, A.C., Verhaak, P.F.M., Schellevis, F.G. *et al*. (2003). Accuracy of diagnosing depression in general practice: the impact of comorbidity. *European Journal of Public Health*, **13**(4) supplement, 76.

Olson, E.T. (2002). *Personal identity. The Stanford Encyclopedia of Philosophy* (Fall 2002 Edition), Edward N. Zalta (ed.), http://plato.stanford.edu/archives/fall2002/entries/identity-personal

Parfit, D. (1984). *Reasons and Persons*. Oxford: Oxford University Press.

Pieters, T., te Hennepe, M. & de Lange, M. (2002). *Pillen & psyche: culturele eb- en vloedbewegingen. Medicamenteus ingrijpen in de psyche*. [Pills & psyche: cultural ebb-tide and flood-tide movements. Pharmacological intervention in the psyche] Den Haag: Rathenau Instituut, Working document 87.

President's Council on Bioethics (2003). *Beyond Therapy. Biotechnology and the Pursuit of Happiness*. New York: Regan Books.

Ricoeur, P. (1990). *Soi-même comme un autre*, Éditions du Seuil, Paris [*Oneself as Another*, University of Chicago Press, Chicago, 1992].

Rosack, J. (2001). SSRIs called on carpet over violence claims. *Psychiatric News*, **36**(19), 6.

Rose, N. (2003). Neurochemical selves. *Society*, November/December, 46–59.

Rose, N. (2005). *Will Biomedicine Transform Society? The Political, Economic, Social and Personal Impact of Medical Advances in the Twenty First Century*. Clifford Barclay Lecture, 2 February 2005.

Schechtman, M. (1996). *The Constitution of Selves*. Ithaca, NY: Cornell University Press.

Schutter, D.J. & Van Honk, J. (2006). Increased positive emotional memory after repetitive transcranial magnetic stimulation over the orbitofrontal cortex. *Journal of Psychiatry and Neuroscience*, **31**, 101–4.

Scoppetta, M., Di Gennaro, G. & Scoppetta, C. (2005). Selective serotonin reuptake inhibitors prevents emotional lability in healthy subjects. *European Review for Medical and Pharmacological Sciences*, **9**, 343–8.

Scott, S. (2006). The Medicalisation Of Shyness: From Social Misfits to Social Fitness. *Sociology of Health & Illness*, **28**, 133–53.

Sententia, W. (2004). Neuroethical considerations: Cognitive liberty and converging technologies for improving human cognition. *Annals of the New York Academy of Sciences*, **1013**, 221–8.

Simon, G.E., Savarino, J., Operskalski, B. & Wang, P.S. (2006). Suicide risk during antidepressant treatment. *American Journal of Psychiatry*, **163**, 41–7.

Tse, W.S. & Bond, A.J. (2002). Serotonergic intervention affects both social dominance and affiliative behavior. *Psychopharmacology*, **161**, 324–30.

Varelius, J. (2006). Voluntary euthanasia, physician-assisted suicide, and the goals of medicine. *Journal of Medicine and Philosophy*, **31**, 121–37.

11

Reasons to Feel, Reasons to Take Pills

Guy Kahane

Almost every day, we try to control our emotions – by avoiding boring events, taking hot baths to relax, pinching ourselves to stop laughing, and in a million other ways. We live in times where it is also possible to control our emotions using biomedical means – for example by taking pills that make us feel better. If we understand enhancement to be the contrary of therapy or treatment, then the use of antidepressants in cases of severe depression is clearly not an example of enhancement. But many use antidepressants in circumstances where it is doubtful that any disorder is present, and this use of "positive mood enhancers" in order to feel "better than well" is highly controversial (Elliott, 2003).

In this chapter I want to consider one worry about the biomedical enhancement of mood. It is hardly the only worry, but it is a worry that seems to me to play an important role in more familiar objections to biomedical enhancement of mood, such as the objection that it would lead to inauthenticity. It is, however, a distinct and important worry, and deserves to be addressed directly. The worry is that the use of positive mood enhancers will corrupt our emotional lives. I will explicate this worry and what it presupposes, and then argue that although it has genuine force, it does not add up to a persuasive objection to the biomedical enhancement of mood. As will emerge, one reason why it does not add up to such an objection is that, in an important respect, our emotional lives are already awry.

Hedonic Reasons

According to rational egoists, we only have reasons to promote our own well-being. According to utilitarians, we have reasons to promote the well-being of everyone equally. According to commonsense morality, however, we have reasons of both kinds – prudential reasons to promote our own well-being, as well as moral ones to promote the well-being of others. What it is exactly we have reason to promote any of these views depends on our understanding of well-being. On hedonic theories of

Enhancing Human Capacities, edited by Julian Savulescu, Ruud ter Meulen and Guy Kahane.
© 2011 Blackwell Publishing Ltd

well-being, a person's well-being consists of the balance of pleasure over pain. On this view, our reasons to promote well-being are reasons to make people feel as good as possible, and to feel least bad. I will call these *hedonic* reasons. On such theories, these are the only reasons given by well-being. But even on most competing theories of well-being – desire-satisfaction and objective theories – we would still have such hedonic reasons, although well-being would also generate other kinds of reasons (e.g. to fulfill desires that do not have hedonic content, or, on some objective theories, to obtain important knowledge, or nurture personal relations, independently of whether these will give us pleasure).

Our hedonic reasons instruct us to generate as much pleasure as we can, and diminish pain to the minimum possible. They instruct us, for example, to take painkillers whenever possible, and to do things we will enjoy. Few would deny that we should follow such reasons to prevent or minimize physical pain. And, to a somewhat lesser extent, it is uncontroversial that we should also follow them with respect to physical pleasure (so long as we leave enough space for the pursuit and appreciation of other kinds of goods).

To the extent, then, that positive mood enhancers make us feel better, our hedonic reasons deliver a clear verdict: take the pill.[1] Many supporters of the biomedical enhancement of mood explicitly or implicitly base their case on such appeal to hedonic reasons.

Affective Reasons

But things are more complicated. For, besides hedonic reasons, we also have what I will call *affective* reasons, reasons to feel.

Let me quickly clarify the key notions of feeling, emotion, and mood. Feelings are episodes of consciousness. There is something it feels like to feel angry or sad. Emotions are broader behavioral dispositions which include dispositions to have certain feelings, as well as dispositions to behave, think, and attend in certain ways. Importantly, although to be angry at someone is, among other things, to be disposed to feel angry at the person, one can be angry even when one isn't literally *feeling* angry. Moods are even broader dispositions, dispositions that govern one's entire emotional orientation for a certain period. To be bored or elated is not to have some particular emotion but to have a general orientation to things that shapes one's various more specific emotions.

Having distinguished feelings and emotions, I will from now on, for reasons of simplicity, use these terms more or less interchangeably. The distinction between mood and emotion will, however, have some further role to play later on.

Do affective reasons really exist? Some people would find the idea surprising. After all, reason and emotion are often presented as contraries. We sometimes speak as if to be emotional is to be unreasonable, and to be reasonable is to be unemotional. But this of course can't be quite right. Emotions are not just things that happen, like headaches or itches. Some situations *call for* certain feelings, some emotions are in order, others inappropriate. As someone is struck by disease or good news arrive, as disasters unfold or a war ends, we mustn't remain impassive observers. The world around us is laden with value, and reason calls upon us to respond to it, with feeling.[2]

Why then are reason and feeling sometimes seen as contraries? This might be because *strong* emotions can disturb the operation of reason. They can make it hard for us to properly respond to our reasons. However, even strong emotions are within the scope of reason. Sometimes we have reasons to feel strong emotions – to feel very sad or angry – even though such feelings also increase the risk that we would act, feel, or believe irrationally.

There *are* reasons for feelings: reasons to feel sad, or pleased, or indignant. The existence of such affective reasons is often overlooked, and sometimes denied. Some worry, for example, that feelings are involuntary, and thus cannot be subject to reasons. But our beliefs are also involuntary, and if this worry were valid, we could not have reasons for belief either, an absurd claim.

Others admit that, in one sense, there are affective reasons, but think that these are merely *pragmatic* or *instrumental*. What matters, they think, is not how we feel but what gets done – what happens in the world. They hold that emotions are merely means to promoting certain forms of appropriate behavior. Thus, for example, moral indignation is useful because it disposes us to treat wrongdoers in certain appropriate ways. But they also think that if we could behave in those ways without feeling indignation, what we feel would not matter.

I reject this view. We often have *intrinsic* affective reasons. Think of someone who is about to die. A person in such a situation might have reasons to feel regret or satisfaction with her life, or to feel affection for or disappointment in others. She would have these reasons even if there was no way in which they could shape her future behavior.[3]

Value and Affective Reasons

If we have various feelings to feel, what, then, *ought* we to feel? Unfortunately, ethics has not yet provided a systematic answer to this question. It has largely focused on how we ought to act – or at most, on what motives should guide our acts. But one source of affective reasons is widely recognized: value often generates reasons to feel. We have reasons to respond positively to the good, and negatively to the bad. These reasons often call for certain actions – for example to take acts that would bring good things into existence. They also often call for certain emotions. We should feel good about the good, and feel bad about the bad, though what it is exactly we should feel (elation, joy, content, satisfaction, etc.) will depend on the different respects in which different things are valuable.[4]

This is just a rough statement of the relation between value and reasons for feeling. For obviously, although the world around us is teeming with value, with both good and evil, our capacity to feel is limited. We couldn't possibly feel for all the world. Thus, although value generates various *pro tanto* affective reasons, it is a separate question what, overall, we *ought* to feel at some point in time.

The Priority of Affective Over Hedonic Reasons

We have hedonic reasons to make ourselves feel good, and to avoid feeling bad. These reasons have sovereignty when it comes to physical pleasure and pain. They do not directly *govern* physical pleasure and pain, because such hedonic states do not *directly* respond to reason. Nobody can be sensibly criticized for not enjoying his meal. So hedonic reasons are reasons for *action*; for doing what it takes to *cause* ourselves to feel better.

Like physical pleasure and pain, emotions also have a hedonic dimension. Negative emotions typically feel bad, positive ones typically feel good.[5] So here our hedonic reasons come into direct competition with our affective reasons. For, at least in the case of negative emotions, the two types of reasons will often point in opposite directions. A loss gives us affective reasons to feel grief. But grief can be excruciating. So it seems we should have hedonic reasons to alleviate it.

I think it clear enough that in such cases we give priority to our affective reasons.[6] Few of us think that if a nice vacation could prevent grief at the loss of a loved one, it would be right for us to take it. To do so might make us feel better, but it would also corrupt our emotional lives. It would be to focus on how things feel like inside at the expense of a full appreciation of how things are around us – it would distort our relation to what matters in the same way that a person entering Robert Nozick's "experience machine" has lost touch with reality.

This is not to say that even in such cases we just ignore hedonic considerations. We do try to comfort others who are in deep grief – not just because of their loss, but also because of their pain. And to the extent that people feel grief for longer, or more intensely, than is reasonable, we do try to alleviate it, not just because such grief is in itself unreasonable, but because it involves needless suffering.[7]

Depression, Mood Enhancement, and What We Ought to Feel

Turn now to positive mood enhancers. Suppose someone is doing very badly. He is going through an acrimonious breakup, or has been fired from his job. He becomes increasingly unhappy and desperate. Some would think that it would be in order for such a person to start taking positive mood enhancers. This recommendation is clearly driven by what I called hedonic and pragmatic reasons. This person is suffering, and that is bad in itself. And his suffering might also prevent him from dealing with his problems, making him sink even further into despair. But what about his affective reasons? What happened to their alleged priority?

It might be replied that this complaint overlooks the point that such a person might be not just sad but *depressed*. But I have deliberately avoided referring to depression. I think that it is better if we first think of such situations in terms of affective reasons. People often tend to feel bad when they have no affective reasons to do so. Or even when they do have such reasons, they feel worse, and for longer, than they should – their emotions are disproportionate. As I noted above, in such situations we would indeed have strong hedonic and pragmatic reasons to alleviate their mental suffering. This is something we can say without referring to depression or disorder. To be sure, one common *explanation* of why people respond in such unreasonable ways might be some abnormality in the biochemistry of their brain. But, in principle such an abnormality might have made them *better respond* to their affective reasons. When we judge that such a person is depressed, and should therefore be treated, we are not making some biological or medical judgment. We are firstly making a substantive normative judgment about how their emotions measure against their affective reasons.

Suppose we judged differently. Suppose that, after reflection, we judged that this person's unhappiness is not disproportionate – that it is broadly the right affective response to the difficult situation he is in. If that person went and took a positive mood enhancer that would greatly reduce his unhappiness, he would no longer be responding to his affective reasons. He might be feeling better, which would in itself be good, but he would no longer be giving his affective reasons the priority they deserve compared to hedonic reasons. In this case, it seems wrong for him to take the pill.[8]

Two Objections to Positive Mood Enhancers

This, then, is the kind of worry about biomedical mood enhancement that I wish to consider here. My discussion of this worry will make some assumptions about the nature of positive mood enhancers. I will assume that when taken regularly they have a continuous effect on mood;[9] that this effect is fairly general, not focused on this or that particular emotion; and that positive mood enhancers tend to generally reduce negative emotion and also (though perhaps to a lesser extent) to increase positive emotion. I take it that this is a broadly accurate characterization of common antidepressants. But given the nature of the questions I want to consider, I will remain at this rather abstract level of description, and set the empirical details to one side.[10]

Now given these assumptions, two objections can be raised against the use of positive mood enhancers. First, positive mood enhancers make us feel *contrary* to reason, by making us feel good (or even just "neutral") when we should feel bad. Second, even when mood enhancers make us feel good when we *should* feel good, they prevent us from genuinely *responding* to our reasons. When we take positive mood enhancers – so the objection goes – we merely *conform* to our reasons. We feel good *when* we ought to, but not *because* we ought to. In these two ways, positive mood enhancers might be said to corrupt our emotional lives. They prevent us from properly responding to our affective reasons.

Threats to Authenticity and Spontaneity

These two objections, I believe, capture at least an aspect of the more familiar worry that biomedical enhancement of mood can compromise our authenticity.[11] If authenticity involves being true to oneself, or to one's values, then there is a sense in which, if these objections are correct, when one uses mood enhancers, one is at most conforming to one's values. Even if the exterior seems right, there is still a sense of falsity or artificiality. Similarly for the worry that the use of enhancement expresses a calculating as opposed to spontaneous attitude to one's life.[12] Again, one aspect of spontaneity seems to be the immediate and unmediated responsiveness to one's affective reasons – feeling sad when things go bad, feeling thrilled at a victory, and so forth. Spontaneity is lost if one needs to work at feeling sad.

I just wanted to highlight these apparent connections. But there may well be more to these other objections to biomedical enhancement of mood than the worry I am considering here – and vice versa. Indeed, it's an advantage of the worry about affective reasons that it makes no appeal to the controversial and perhaps obscure notions of authenticity and the true self, or to what is "natural" or "given."[13]

Conforming vs. Responding to Reasons

The example of using positive mood enhancers to overcome grief is an example of feeling *contrary* to one's affective reasons. I now want to say some more about what I mean by mere *conformity* to such reasons.

It might be useful to briefly consider a parallel problem about belief. Think of how reasons for belief work. If you have good evidence that p, then you ought to believe that p. If the question whether p is an important matter, then you have reasons to seek out relevant evidence. It is valuable to know important truths.

Suppose, however, that I form a belief about some important matter not through some normal process of gathering evidence and responding to epistemic reasons (including, importantly, testimonial reasons to believe things you were told by authoritative others), but by taking a pill. A belief formed in such a way might be true, but, it seems, it would not be justified. Such a belief would merely conform to one's epistemic reasons, but not be based on them.

The same goes for affective reasons. Even if I *should* feel happy, because things are going so well, and a mood enhancer *makes* me feel happy, this happiness merely conforms to my affective reasons. For it seems that I feel happy because of the pill, not because I am responding to the fact that things are good.

Second Best is Still Better than Nothing

I now turn to consider possible replies to this objection. Consider again the example of belief. Suppose that, although you have been provided with an overwhelming amount of evidence supporting the theory of evolution, your traditional upbringing makes it psychologically impossible for you to genuinely believe it. You are suffering from epistemic weakness of the will. Since you *can't* believe in evolution on the basis of your epistemic reasons, it might still be *better* if you believe in it by taking the pill, compared to not believing it at all. True beliefs merely in conformity with reasons might still be better than having false beliefs on the matter.

Again, the same goes for our affective reasons. If we cannot directly respond to our affective reasons, it might still be better to conform to them than not to even feel what we ought to feel. It might be best to directly feel grief in response to a loss, but if some emotional inhibition prevents this, it would still be better to feel grief by artificial means, than not to feel grief at all.

In such cases, we still are *responding* to our epistemic and affective reasons, just not *directly.* We are responding to them by taking actions that are likely to cause us to enter the right mental state.

Mere Causal Manipulation or Increased Responsiveness?

I have so far granted that positive mood enhancers can merely *cause* us to feel better. But this is by no means obvious. Recall the earlier distinction between emotion and mood. Mood enhancers change our *mood*, our general affective orientation. And it is possible that what they do is help us better *appreciate* the good things in life – they might just make it easier for us to recognize and respond to our positive affective reasons. Now whether this is really the case is, in part, an empirical question. If it can be answered it in the affirmative, then the worry about mere conformity would be misplaced.[14]

Whether We Even Know What We Ought to Feel

These two replies address the mere conformity objection. But positive mood enhancers can't be plausibly said to make us better conform – let alone be more responsive – to our *negative* affective reasons. So the first objection, that positive mood enhancers make us feel *contrary* to reason, still stands.

This objection might have force only if taken literally. For positive mood enhancers can also prevent us from responding to merely *illusory* negative affective reasons – from feeling bad when there is no reason to. And they might also *reduce* our response to negative affective reasons in ways that make our response more *proportionate*. But I'll concede here that positive mood enhancers might in some cases prevent us from responding to genuine negative affective reasons.

It might be replied that the force of this objection is limited by the fact that we do not yet have a good enough understanding of our affective reasons. That is, although we often agree on what *pro tanto* affective reasons are given by particular things, we have a far weaker grasp on how all of these different affective reasons fit together. We have a far weaker grasp on the question, What ought we to feel *overall*? Is it better to feel strongly or intensely, or should we feel only moderate and measured emotions? Should our feelings change rapidly as things around us change, or should they be lasting and stable? Should we respond at once both to the positive and to the negative – feeling bitter sweet contentment, or sadness mixed with joy – or should our feelings alternate, responding once to the bad, once to the good? But until we have answers to these and similar questions, how can we be confident that positive mood enhancers would corrupt our emotional lives?

This seems too quick. For we clearly do accept the priority of negative affective reasons over hedonic ones in many specific contexts, and if so, there should be at least a *prima facie* presumption that the use of positive mood enhancers prevents us from responding to these reasons. We do not need a systematic theory of affective reasons to know that.

The Affective Priority of Good over Bad

There is a better way to block this objection to positive mood enhancers. I now want to argue that once we reflect on what we ought to feel overall, the tentative answer that emerges doesn't only defuse the objection, but actually turns out to *support* the use of positive mood enhancers.

Think of the sheer scale of evil and misfortune in our world. When we reflect on all the suffering and wickedness around us, it can seem depraved, or a kind of moral blindness, that anyone feels happy. But if so, should we live our lives in grim, sober sadness? Many of us think that this would not be the right response. We think that we should rather maintain cheer in the face of adversity. That we should appreciate the glimmers of goodness in what is otherwise a dark landscape.

There seems to be an interesting asymmetry in our normative thinking. When it comes to action, we tend to give the prevention of evil clear priority over the promotion of good. We think that it's more important to relieve misery than to increase happiness. But when it comes to feeling, we seem to take the opposite view. We think that people should, overall, look on the bright side of things.

What explains this priority? It is certainly supported by the hedonic and pragmatic reasons we have already discussed. If we add up all our hedonic reasons (which all point in the positive directions) with our affective reasons (which point in both), perhaps the result is something skewed upwards. And there are pragmatic reasons not to feel too bad (though perhaps also not to feel *too good* either), for that would make us less able to fight evil and adversity. However, given the priority we earlier noted of affective over hedonic (and pragmatic) reasons, these suggestions couldn't be the whole story.

Indeed, it seems to me that there are *intrinsic* affective reasons in favor of orienting our lives around the good. The existence of good somehow matters *more* than that of evil – goodness is the primary notion, and evil is merely an obstacle to its full realization.[15] The idea is not that we should ignore evil, but that we should refuse to grant it equal standing.

In other words, although affective reasons have general priority over hedonic ones, there is within the affective realm priority to positive affective reasons over negative ones.[16]

To the extent that such a normative priority really holds, then positive mood enhancers, on the whole, are something to favor – something that directs our affective orientation in exactly the *right* direction.[17] This would apply most strongly if, as I suggested above, mood enhancers actually allow us to better respond to our positive affective reasons. It would apply more weakly if positive mood enhancers merely made it easier for us to conform to such reasons.[18]

Now this argument has even greater force in the case of those whose affective orientation naturally points in the opposite, negative direction. And as we shall now see, consideration of this fact – the fact that our present affective dispositions are hardly purely responsive to reason – offers even further support to the use of positive mood enhancers.

Affective Adaptation: Why Our Affective Lives are already Defective

Questions about the ethics of biomedical enhancement often require us to answer many empirical questions, questions about the possible future effects, good or ill, of various forms of enhancement. We often have little evidence to answer such questions, and can only crudely speculate. The final consideration I wish to raise also revolves around empirical claims. But these are empirical claims, not about the possible future effects of biomedical enhancement, but about how people actually happen to be, *prior* to such enhancement.

What I have in mind are two broad findings of decades of scientific research into subjective well-being. First, there is strong evidence that people's subjective well-being – a notion that is meant to be at least a rough measure of both positive feeling and subjective satisfaction – is to a significant extent rooted in innate factors that vary widely between individuals (Goldsmith, 1983; Tellegen *et al.*, 1988).

Second, there is extensive evidence that people's basic level of subjective well-being (their "hedonic set point") is largely unaffected by even the most dramatic life events. Those who are typically cheerful or grim would remain so whether or not they win the lottery, witness the death of their lifelong spouse, or lose both legs in a car accident. Although such events produce some immediate (positive or negative) effect on one's mood, it fairly quickly returns to its initial level. Our subjective well-being almost always "adapts" to changing circumstances (Brickman *et al.*, 1978; Fujita & Diener, 2005).

What does all of this mean? First, it means that to a large extent our feelings seem to be shaped by non-rational factors. If I tend to see things more pessimistically than you do, this needn't be because I am more accurately registering what really matters, but rather because of some arbitrary fact about my genes. The "state of nature" is already not one of pure responsiveness to affective reasons.

Second, the surprising fact that even, for example, bereavement or severe disability might not, in the long term, have much affect on our mood, shows that we already often fail to respond to what we take to be strong affective reasons. Most people not only expect to feel prolonged grief after the death of a loved one but also think they *ought* to feel such grief.[19] But, when they do in fact suffer such a loss, the evidence shows they are not likely to feel nearly as much grief as they expect.[20]

Third, because of their natural endowment, at least some people are naturally disposed to negative mood and find it generally difficult to appropriately respond to their positive affective reasons. The evidence about hedonic adaptation suggests that external factors will not significantly change this fact – indeed, most of the goods that many people spend their lives seeking would in fact have little effect on how they feel. Here there seem to be both strong hedonic reasons and indirect affective reasons to use mood enhancers.[21]

To summarize, this large body of empirical evidence strongly suggests that in our current state we are very far from being perfectly responsive to our affective reasons. And this means that our emotional lives were never in some pristine natural state that mood enhancers might corrupt. Many of us fail to appropriately respond to our affective reasons, and our emotions are at least partly shaped by clearly irrational factors. Thus in many (though certainly not all) cases, mood enhancement might significantly *improve* our responsiveness to our affective reasons, or at least help us better conform to them.

Alternative Forms of Mood Enhancement?

When people talk about biomedical enhancement of mood, they typically have in mind *positive* mood enhancement, and I have so far focused on this form of mood enhancement. Now if we only had hedonic reasons, then positive mood enhancement would have been the only form of enhancement worth having. However, once we consider the full range of affective reasons, other possible forms of mood enhancement come into view. I would like to end with a brief discussion of these.

Consider first *negative* mood enhancement. This may sound like an oxymoron, or some perverted invention for masochists. But to think in this way is to assume that we only have hedonic reasons. We do, however, often have strong reasons to feel *bad*, and we may be bad in responding to these reasons. When we say that someone has finally managed to grieve some childhood loss only after years of therapy, and treat this as an achievement, we implicitly recognize the value of such negative mood enhancement. Indeed some people might be endowed with a strong cheerful disposition that is inappropriate to their life circumstances. These points hold even if we take into account the overall priority of positive over negative affective reasons.

Consider next the possibility of mood enhancers that *generally* increase our responsiveness to affective reasons, both positive *and* negative. I said that it is unclear whether positive mood enhancers cause us to feel better, or rather make us more responsive to positive affective reasons we genuinely have. But such enhancers clearly work only in one direction. Might it be possible to generally increase our responsiveness to our affective reasons – both positive and negative? This is an empirical question that depends on how our cognition, valuation, and emotion are neurally wired.[22]

Furthermore, it might be possible to enhance our responsiveness to certain *kinds* of affective reasons. Take the affective reasons given by past life events. There is now some discussion of memory-erasing drugs which could be used to treat or prevent post-traumatic stress disorder. Here we are preventing people from being *over*-responsive to what are usually genuine and important affective reasons. Such treatment would be broadly motivated by hedonic reasons: these people needlessly suffer. One effect, however, might be that they would also be prevented from responding *at all* to these affective reasons. All I want to point out here is that we can also conceive of biomedical treatment that would improve autobiographical memory, and thus increase our capacity to respond to the affective reasons given by past events. Similarly, treatments that increase our foresight and awareness of the long-term consequences of our actions might also increase our responsiveness to affective reasons given by possible future events.

I do not expect that such enhancers would arrive anytime soon. People are generally more easily motivated by their hedonic reasons than by negative affective ones, and the focus of biomedical research reflects this psychological asymmetry. And, as I suggested, there might be an affective priority of good over bad. But when we discuss biomedical mood enhancement, it would nevertheless be a mistake to assume it can only take a positive form.

Conclusion

I started by noting the numerous familiar ways in which all of us try to control our feelings. When the use of biomedical enhancement is criticized, it is common to respond by pointing out its continuity with these more mundane forms of enhancement. This strategy is appropriate in the context of a dialectic – it exposes an apparent inconsistency on the part of the critic. But it often sheds little light on the underlying normative issues. For it may be that reflection on biomedical enhancement would lead us to realize that even our current ways need mending. Critique of enhancement need not be conservative in a literal sense.

In this chapter, I have tried to argue that ethical questions about the biomedical enhancement of mood are often really questions about our affective reasons, as well as about their relation to other kinds of reasons. These are difficult and, unfortunately, largely neglected questions. Those who entirely dismiss affective reasons, or at least think that negative affective reasons are extremely weak, are likely to see little problem with positive mood enhancers. Those who give great weight to negative affective reasons would see things rather differently. But this is not really a debate about the use of biomedical enhancement. It is a substantive normative debate about the form that our emotional lives should take.

Notes

1. What about the so-called "paradox of hedonism"? This is the claim that if we directly tried to maximize our pleasure, this would be self-defeating, because if we were so calculating in the pursuit of pleasure, we would enjoy life far less. But this is an empirical claim. And although it might have some truth when it comes to the active pursuit of pleasant activities, it simply has no hold when it comes to biomedical intervention. If a pill makes you feel better then, by definition, by taking it you will succeed in making yourself feel better. There is nothing self-defeating here.
2. Isn't this an over-intellectualized picture of the emotions? You might get this impression if you failed to distinguish *reasons* and *reasoning*. We of course do not usually need to engage in any kind of reasoning or inference in order to respond to our affective reasons. Which is not to say that there aren't difficult situations where finding out what we ought to feel requires careful imaginative deliberation.
3. Affective reasons can be both moral and non-moral. In what follows I will simply assume that they have intrinsic normative force. It is another question, which I will not consider, whether responding appropriately to our affective reasons also directly contributes to our well-being.
4. The tie between values and reasons for emotion is closest in the case of so-called "thick" evaluative properties such as cruelty. But it is widely agreed that value generally generates reasons to hold appropriate attitude, including feelings, towards it.
5. There are exceptions: for example, people sometimes enjoy being angry. Note also that it is, of course, not emotions *per se* but *feelings* – episodes of consciousness – that have such a hedonic dimension.
6. This is, of course, in the first instance a priority to our *negative* affective reasons – to our reasons for feeling negatively toned affect. But we can also conceive of cases where one's hedonic reasons give reasons *not* to feel some *positive* feeling, because such a feeling would lead to *lesser* overall pleasure later on. I think that even in such cases we will often see no overall reason to suppress the feeling.
7. Moreover, there might be a threshold of mental suffering beyond which we might stop giving priority to affective reasons. Think, for example, of cases where we think it right to withhold some very bad news from someone who is already unhappy.

8. Wasserman and Liao (2008) discuss somewhat different issues in connection with what they call "duties to have emotions."

9. I thus won't be considering mood enhancers that induce short-lived ecstatic effect – though the extension of the arguments of this chapter to that type of case is fairly straightforward.

10. There appears to be stronger evidence that existing antidepressants reduce negative emotion rather than directly increase positive emotion, and even this evidence is strong only with respect to more severe forms of depression. But my interest here is in substantive normative questions, not with these empirical issues – including important issues about possible harmful side effects. Notice also that for my purposes, it does not matter at all to what extent the effect of some positive mood enhancers is due to the placebo effect. This is merely a point about the mechanism that produces the affective change. What really matters to us is that there *is* such an effect, however it is produced.

11. There is no agreed definition of authenticity, and I do not intend to offer one. For discussion of the problem of authenticity in the context of biomedical enhancement, see Parens (2005).

12. I first heard this worry raised by Allan Buchanan in his 2008 Uehiro Lectures at Oxford.

13. Although the President's Council on Bioethics (2003) is often interpreted as expressing a concern about authenticity, there are many passages in it that are better read as expressing the worry I am discussing here, for example, when they write that we "desire not simply to be satisfied with ourselves and the world, but to have this satisfaction as a result of deeds and loves and lives worthy of such self-satisfaction" (p.251), or when they discuss the "danger that our new pharmacological remedies will keep us 'bright' or impassive in the face of things that ought to trouble, sadden, outrage, or inspire us – that our medicated souls will stay flat no matter what happens to us or around us" (p.255). See also their discussion of grief on pp.255–7.

14. Positive mood enhancers are often presented in an unfavorable light compared to psychotherapy. Perhaps it is assumed it is only through psychotherapy that people really develop a genuine appreciation of their positive affective reasons. My response to the "mere conformity" objection should also cast some doubt on this assumption. Indeed, it might even be the case that it is rather some forms of psychotherapy that merely cause people to feel better without improving their responsiveness to genuine positive affective reasons (for example, certain forms of cognitive therapy that focus on reducing negative thoughts might be based on repressing our capacity to respond to our negative affective reasons).

15. This idea echoes (but is not the same as) the view that evil is merely the privation of good.

16. This claim should not be understood too strongly. A permanently cheerful demeanor, smiling brightly even when one's loved ones are suffering or dying, is something we don't appreciate even in the saintly. The overall balance of positive vs. negative affective reasons ultimately depends on the circumstances we find ourselves in, and these might sometimes be just too bleak. But it seems to me that even in grief, there is reason to give space to the good – say, to fond remembrance of the good in the life of the deceased, and that exclusive focus on the badness of the loss is often mistaken.

17. Note that I am not claiming that positive mood enhancers are likely to make us *perfectly* respond (or conform) to what we ought to feel. It might indeed be that, as claimed by the objection, they would cause us to sometimes fail to respond to genuine negative affective reasons. The claim is only that, *on balance*, positive mood enhancers are likely to make many of us better respond (or conform) to our affective reasons, compared to not taking them.

18. Indeed, even if such enhancers merely reduced our responsiveness to negative affective reasons (whether genuine and illusory), and did not directly increase positive affect, this

would still shift our overall affective orientation upwards, and leave more space for positive emotions.

19.   Note I am not claiming here that, for example, people ought to feel deeply unhappy if they become severely disabled. I am only claiming that most people believe that such a condition is a grave misfortune that merits such a response. The empirical findings on adaptation at the very least show that we are not responsive to what most people *take* to be very strong affective reasons.

20.   For discussion of the implications of this particular finding see Moller (2007).

21.   Although the phenomenon of adaptation is extensive, I don't want to give the impression that it is all encompassing or insurmountable. There are negative things to which people do not adapt to – these include physical pain and continuous noise. And although people's subjective well-being does largely adapt even to severe disability, they do not always completely regain their prior levels of subjective well-being. Finally, close personal relationships and other factors do seem to have a positive long-term effect on subjective well-being. For discussion, see Diener, Lucas & Scollon (2006).

22.   Some people are made more emotional by alcohol – but being generally more emotional is not the same things as being more accurately responsive to one's affective reasons.

References

Brickman, P., Coates, T. & Janoff-Bulman, R. (1978). Lottery winners and accident victims: Is happiness relative? *Journal of Personality and Social Psychology*, **36**, 917–27.

Diener, E., Lucas, R.E. & Scollon, N.C. (2006). Beyond the hedonic treadmill: Revising the adaptation theory of well-being. *American Psychologist*, **61**(4), 305–14.

Elliott, C. (2003). *Better Than Well: American Medicine Meets the American Dream*. New York: W.W. Norton.

Fujita, F. & Diener, E. (2005). Life satisfaction set point: Stability and change. *Journal of Personality and Social Psychology*, **88**, 158–64.

Goldsmith, H.H. (1983). Genetic influences on personality from infancy to adulthood. *Child Development*, **54**, 331–55.

Moller, D. (2007). Love and death. *Journal of Philosophy*, **104**, 301–16.

Parens, E. (2005). Authenticity and ambivalence: Toward understanding the Enhancement Debate. *The Hastings Center Report*, **35**(3), 34–41.

President's Council on Bioethics (2003). *Beyond Therapy*. New York: Regan Books.

Tellegen, A., Lykken, D., Bouchard, T.J., Wilcox, K.J., Segal, N. & Rich, S. (1988). Personality similarity in twins reared apart and together. *Journal of Personality and Social Psychology*, **54**, 1031–9.

Wasserman, D. & Liao, S.M. (2008). Issues in the pharmacological induction of emotions. *Journal of Applied Philosophy*, **25**(3), 178–92.

12

What's in a Name? ADHD and the Gray Area between Treatment and Enhancement

Maartje Schermer and Ineke Bolt

Introduction

In a discussion about human enhancement it is common to make a distinction between medical treatment and enhancement. A common definition of enhancement holds that enhancements are "interventions designed to improve human form or functioning beyond what is necessary to sustain or restore good health" (Juengst, 1998). The well-known report of the President's Council on Bioethics speaks of interventions "beyond therapy" (President's Council on Bioethics, 2003).

A part of the "enhancement debate" concerns Enhancements with a capital E; enhancements that clearly go not only beyond health, but beyond what we currently understand as the "normal or naturally human." For example, giving people infrared vision, engineering them with perfect pitch, or doubling or tripling their IQ, all belong to the fantasies of the transhumanist movement and feed the nightmares of so-called bioconservatives. This is not the debate we want to join in this chapter, and it is not a debate in which it is very useful to distinguish between treatment and enhancement.

The part of the "enhancement debate" which we will be concerned with here turns on more mundane improvement or enhancements of human functioning – enhancements with a "small e." Breast implants, enhancing height by growth hormone, or improving one's personality or behavior with psychopharmacology, are examples. These are all used as paradigm cases of "enhancement" in the ethical discussion (Elliott, 2003; Parens, 1998; President's Council on Bioethics, 2003). It is in this discussion that the distinction between treatment and enhancement plays an important – if much disputed – role.

Enhancing Human Capacities, edited by Julian Savulescu, Ruud ter Meulen and Guy Kahane.
© 2011 Blackwell Publishing Ltd

The treatment–enhancement distinction

The treatment–enhancement (TE) distinction serves a number of purposes. First, it is supposed to draw the boundaries of the medical domain. Second, it is used to distinguish between interventions for which reimbursement in some collective health insurance plan is morally obligatory, and interventions for which collective reimbursement is not obligatory. As Juengst says, the treatment–enhancement distinction functions "to help define the social role of the medical profession, demarcate the proper sphere of biomedical research, and help set limits on health care payment plans" (Juengst, 1998, p.29). Finally, the TE distinction also plays a role in the discussion about the moral acceptability of biomedical interventions, about the societal effects of such interventions, and about personal decisions regarding self-improvement (Parens, 1998).

The TE distinction, however, has been discussed, criticized, and even rejected by numerous authors, because it has major flaws. First, the TE distinction requires clear concepts of health and disease but these are notoriously difficult and elusive to define. A universally accepted conception is lacking. The notion of disease is, according to many, inherently normative and includes assumptions on what is normal and abnormal, desirable and undesirable. So, if one wants to draw clear and exact lines between interventions that are treatments and interventions that are enhancements, the concept of disease is not the normatively neutral, objective arbiter it is often believed to be (Daniels, 2000).

Second, the TE distinction does not map neatly onto the moral evaluation of biomedical interventions. It does not do the moral work it is supposed to do. Daniels has argued, and many agree with him, that with regard to obligations of justice (should an intervention be reimbursed or not?) the TE distinction does not always coincide with the obligatory–non-obligatory distinction. For example, abortion and contraception are reimbursed in many health insurance plans although they are not treatments of diseases. In these cases, the moral obligation for reimbursement stems from reasons of equality of women rather than from a TE distinction. Finally, many authors agree that the TE distinction does not discriminate neatly between morally justified and morally unjustified interventions. Contraception can be taken as an example here, as can the general acceptance of cosmetic surgery.

The gray area

Despite the problems with the TE distinction, Daniels (2000) has argued that there is no reason to abandon the distinction altogether. He claims that in general, the distinction works well; we merely should not expect too much of it but use it in a "limited way." This implies that the distinction may work as long as we are faced with extreme and evident examples of treatments and enhancements, but it leaves us with unanswered questions if we are confronted with the borderlines cases in the muddy gray area between obvious treatment and obvious enhancement. These cases are not rare but occur frequently; as is shown by the adult attention deficit hyperactivity disorder (ADHD), which we will elaborate on in this chapter.

It is exactly this gray area, however, that poses the most pressing problems. It is the borderline cases that are especially problematic for medical professionals and for policy makers. They are looking for criteria or other footholds on which to base their decisions and, regardless of the philosophical critique on the TE distinction, they tend to revert to concepts of disease, health and normalcy, and to the distinction between treatment and enhancement to justify their decisions. In other words, the TE distinction still constitutes the conceptual framework that informs policy making and medical practice. Also in public debates about such issues, the TE distinction is frequently employed.

In the gray area it is not clear how biomedical interventions should be valued: as treatments or as enhancements. This difficulty in labeling interventions is directly related to the difficulty in determining whether something is a disease or a disorder, or rather a normal condition or a normal variation. It has been pointed out that the gray area can therefore easily be exploited by "disease mongerers," who have an interest in defining as many conditions as possible as diseases. Disease mongering can be defined as "the selling of sickness that widens the boundaries of illness and grows the markets for those who sell and deliver treatments" (Moynihan & Henry, 2006). This also implies that interventions that can be understood as enhancements are sold under the guise of treatment: "The manufacturers of enhancement technologies will usually exploit the blurry line between enhancement and treatment in order to sell drugs. Because enhancement technologies must be prescribed by physicians, drug manufacturers typically market the technologies not as enhancements, but as treatments for newly discovered or under-recognized disorders" (Caplan & Elliott, 2004).

It has also been pointed out that this leads to a new form of medicalization, not driven by medical profession and social movements or interest groups but by technology, the pharmaceutical industry, and an increasingly market-based medicine. According to Conrad (2005), drug companies are having increasing impact on the boundaries of the normal and the pathological. One of the reasons why this is worrisome is that such companies have commercial interests that are not always in line with the patient's best interests in rational drug prescription.

In this chapter, we will focus on this gray area, show its complexities, and ask how we can answer questions regarding the medical domain, or regarding the moral obligation for reimbursement if we cannot depend on the TE distinction. We will use the example of adult ADHD to show, first, how difficult it is to distinguish between treatment of disease and enhancement of normal function, especially given the phenomena of medicalization, disease mongering, and expanding disease definitions. Because of those difficulties, we will then argue that we should not depend on a distinction between disease and normalcy, or between treatment and enhancement, to make normative decisions with regard to access to and reimbursement of biomedical interventions. Instead, we should address the normative considerations that are involved in such decisions directly.

Adult ADHD as a Case Study

We will discuss the case of ADHD in adults as an example of a condition that lies in the gray area between disease and normal variation, and the use of methylphenidate and other psychostimulants as lying in the gray area between treatment and enhancement. Ritalin use in children has been frequently mentioned as an example in the enhancement debate (e.g. President's Council on Bioethics, 2003), but adult ADHD has not yet been studied in this context.[1] Here, we will use adult ADHD to explore the complexity and the dynamics of definitions of health and disease, normality and abnormality, and of the moral issues related to enhancement, disease mongering, and medicalization in the gray area. We will use some results of a qualitative interviews study to illustrate these issues and deepen understanding.

Attention deficit hyperactivity disorder is classified as a disorder in the DSM-IV. It is characterized by symptoms like being restless, easily distracted, having difficulty planning, and being overly impulsive and chaotic. To qualify for the diagnosis the number of symptoms and the severity of the symptoms are crucial. Symptoms must lead to "clinically significant impairment in social, academic, or occupational functioning" and be present to a degree that is "maladaptive" (DSM-IV). About 1 to 3% of the adult population is said to suffer from ADHD (Kooij, 2006) but estimates range from 0.05 to 7% (Health Council of the Netherlands 2000).

As these criteria and data already indicate, the demarcation line between ADHD and normal restlessness, impulsivity, and lack of concentration is difficult to draw. According to some, ADHD should not even be understood as a disorder but rather as a normal variation of human behavior or character. From this point of view the use of psychopharmacological substances to improve functioning is a form of enhancement rather than treatment. The variety of views and the difficulties in demarcation indicate that adult ADHD is an example of a condition that lies in the gray area between (obvious) treatment and (obvious) enhancement.

Methodology

We have conducted a qualitative study into the experiences that adults with ADHD have with their condition and with the use of medication. We have interviewed 19 adults with ADHD. The respondents were recruited via a call on the website and in the magazine of the Dutch ADHD patient association. After the first 10 interviews (on a first enrolled, first interviewed basis) we selected further respondents based on the criterion of diversity. We interviewed 9 males and 10 females; their ages ranged from 21 to 59 years and the time since being diagnosed with ADHD ranged from 3 months to 10 years. All were diagnosed in adulthood, not as children. Geographical variation covered almost the whole of the Netherlands. Education and occupational levels varied from lower professional education (nursing aide, hairdresser) to academic education (Ph.D. student, management advisor). Those with a higher education were overrepresented as compared to the normal population, and only one respondent was from an ethnic minority group. Most respondents used some form of medication, mostly Ritalin (methylphenidate) or Concerta (methylphenidate extended release); two (had) used dexamphetamine. Some also used other psychopharmacological drugs (mainly SSRIs) often because of co-morbidity such as depression and anxiety. Six deliberately used no medication at all.

The interviews lasted from one to one-and-a-half hours and were taped and transcribed before being analyzed. We used a semi-structured interview method with open questions; for every main question we had some follow-up questions and some reformulations. The main topics were: the process of getting the diagnosis, impact of the diagnosis, experience of having and living with ADHD, how to understand ADHD and medication use in relation to "self," experiences with medication, and reasons for either using or not using medication.

Experiences with ADHD

Disease vs. normal variation

From the interviews it was clear that all respondents experienced or had experienced problems because of their condition, some quite serious, others less serious.

Many of them had become "stuck" in their personal lives, or in their work; they frequently suffered from depression, anxieties, stress, or burn-out. As the "most annoying, bothersome aspects of ADHD" they mentioned things like: always being restless and stressed, even at night; being emotionally unstable (either very "high" or very "low"); being easily irritated, frustrated, or angry; being unable to order and plan things; being unable to finish things; being unable to perform at one's intellectual level; or being overly impulsive and thereby getting into trouble. These problems had often been the reason to seek professional help, which in turn had rendered the diagnosis. Many, however, had first self-diagnosed or had been "diagnosed" by friends, family, or tests on the internet and only went to see a medical professional to have this diagnosis confirmed.

When asked how they viewed ADHD, only a small minority clearly defined it as a disease. "Well, I believe that it's a stupid disease, that you have something... well too little, or too much of something, some substance, is being produced in your brain..."

Most respondents did not call ADHD a disease, but used other related words such as "a mental condition," "a disorder," "an abnormality," or "an inconvenience." Their most important arguments to see ADHD as some sort of medical condition was the fact that "you lack a certain substance in your brain." This was mentioned frequently, although in fact the exact causes of ADHD have not yet been unraveled and the exact role of neurotransmitters is not yet clear. Another related argument was that there was medication for it, or that medication worked, so that it could not be anything but a "real" medical condition.

Other respondents were more ambivalent or unclear on the topic. One said that you *could* qualify it as a disease because it was in the DSM-IV; however, the rest of the interview revealed that he did not really endorse this view himself.

A young academic, who gave an elaborate answer to the question, was very aware of the difficulties in defining disease and could not really make up his mind about how to define ADHD: "... well, a disorder, or disease, whatever you want to call it, in other words: 'there's something wrong with you' [...] it depends on how you choose to look at it, disease is difficult to describe, of course." In general, he believed that the more trouble the condition caused you, the more reason there was to call it a disease, in line with conditions like burn-out and other mental limitations or impairments. "But it depends very much on your point of view," he stressed.

Some respondents did not consider ADHD as a medical condition at all but saw it as a variation of normal human character traits: "The capacity of the human brain has a certain range that is evolutionary determined. There are a number of variables. And the mix of variables determines your cognitive capacities and all your other abilities. I believe ADHD is no more and no less than a specific mix, a certain set of variables. "[...] I do not even believe it is a disease. I do not believe it is a disorder. I believe it is a variation." And another respondent said: "I do not have a disease, this is who I am. I do not *have* ADHD, I *am* ADHD." Both considered their way of being a normal variation, one that nevertheless caused them problems in the current society. "Unfortunately, a lot of the qualities and characteristics that I have are less valued in this society. Well, so be it."

A remarkable finding, which bears on the question of whether ADHD is a medical disorder or rather a normal variation in character traits, is that most of the respondents evaluated some of their ADHD-related character traits or behavior in a very positive way. Although some saw no positive aspects at all, many said they liked being spontaneous, creative, fast-thinking, and energetic. They appreciated, and were appreciated by their friends, for having spontaneous, funny ideas, or creative plans. They also mentioned things like being able to think along different "tracks" at the same time, easily making contact with others and having a good sense of humor. For a number of respondents it was one of the downsides of the medication that it affected such traits.

This finding is remarkable, because symptoms of diseases or disorders are not generally experienced as positive. If we see these "symptoms" as a normal variation in character, however, it seems easier to understand some character traits as more and others as less positive, or to see the positive and negative sides to certain traits, for example of being "spontaneous" versus "overly impulsive."

Personality vs. disorder

We asked the respondents what they themselves believed to be the difference between being a chaotic, lively, impulsive or hyperactive person, and having ADHD. Broadly speaking, two opinions could be distinguished: one group believed that there was a clear difference, while others indicated that it was more like a continuum. Arguments from the first group were that ADHD is the lack of a substance in the brain; or that it is clearly different from a normal personality because medication works. Also, they believed that the psychiatrists who made the diagnosis had thorough tests to make the distinction.

The second group, however, indicated that the difference between a normally hyperactive person and a person with ADHD might lie in the fact that people with ADHD have a more extensive set of symptoms, or have certain traits more extremely, or that the difference depends on the degree of problems that you experience due to these character traits. The degree of trouble that their personality caused them was taken by some as a reason to understand it as a medical disorder rather than a personality trait: "those character traits, once you see that they belong to ADHD, and they are traits you would like to get rid of, but you can't, then I would tend to see it as a disease." Some respondents explicitly stated that they viewed it as a continuum, and others said that ADHD was just the end of a spectrum.

In both groups there were respondents who referred to the role of social factors that contributed to the burden of ADHD. Some mentioned the large amount of "stimuli" (like advertisements, stores, cell phones, television) in current urban environments; these were considered to be especially difficult to deal with by people with ADHD. Rural environments were seen as more relaxed and easier to cope with. Moreover, some respondents mentioned the greater social pressure on performance, especially at work or school, as something more difficult to cope with for persons with ADHD.

The Use of Medication

In light of the various views on the status of ADHD, how can the use of Ritalin or other psychostimulants be understood? When ADHD is seen as a disease or disorder, caused by the "lack of a substance," it is natural to see Ritalin or other drugs as medication compensating for that lack and thus as a treatment.

On the other hand, when ADHD is seen more in terms of a normal variation of character traits, the use of Ritalin is less easy to label. Should it be considered an enhancer? After all, it does enhance certain capacities that people feel they lack (like being able to structure things or finish things) and it does help them to function and perform better. We have asked the respondents about their views on medication, the effects, and the impact on their life.

For many respondents medication had positive effects. They reported being less muddled and chaotic, feeling calm and more peaceful, more focused and better concentrated, less impulsive or less quick-tempered. Apart from side effects such as sleep problems, headaches, and rebounds, many respondents experienced other negative effects described as feeling "flattened," being less funny, social, creative or spontaneous, and feeling unnatural or artificial. "Yes, I'm more in balance now, however, for me that is unnatural. So, now and then it's fun, that crazy impulsiveness, and that is gone now. Or that you are really, really happy ... yes, that's gone as well. That's a pity." Experiences like this gave rise to ambivalence. Although many respondents felt that medication helped them, some also felt unnatural and not themselves on medication.[2]

When asked how they viewed their medication most of the respondents described their medication as an aid, a help, or as a support. Many saw it as something that helped them to function properly, both in their work or study and in social relationships. These respondents indicated that due to ADHD they were less able to function adequately and often somehow unable to do things they believed they could do. Medication helped to improve their perceived underperformance. "I always felt there is more in me than appears" said one, "that is the pity of ADHD, that's why I am always underperforming." And another told us: "I could not do the job, while actually it should have been easy for me. I considered that as dysfunctioning."

The degree to which their functioning was improved differed among the respondents. Many indicated that medication helped them to complete a study or education where previously they had failed, to keep a job, or to relate better to family and friends. Others said that if only they had been diagnosed early in life, their life would have taken a different, better, course; schools could have been completed, careers would have gone better, marriages might have stayed intact, and their life in general would have been more in balance. In general, medication made the respondents feel better and function better, but they clearly perceived this as a kind of restoration to normal levels of functioning. "It helps me to minimize the hindrances that ADHD causes for me. It is not like 'I can do anything and want something on top of that,' no, it's one step closer to that line... So in that way it is a reparation, restoration."

While some strictly adhered to their medication treatment, others were more flexible and tinkered with the medication to make it accommodate their needs. For example, one respondent skipped his medication when he had to go to a party because otherwise he would feel somewhat detached and "miss a lot of what's going on." Another respondent, however, said she always took some extra medication before going to a party, because without it she would be "too hyper."

One respondent used medication only in case specific work-related activities required concentration and focus. For example, if he traveled to a meeting by train and had to do some work during the journey, he needed his medication to focus; however, he had decided to abstain from medication in his private life. For him, the medication was meant to help him to function properly at work, while in his private life he chose to accept "more chaos." The fact that he solely used drugs to function properly in specific job-related activities raised some difficult questions for him: "What makes me different from someone who is not diagnosed (as ADHD) but now and then needs something for his concentration?"

ADHD from the Inside and the Outside

Overall, respondents did not regard ADHD medication as an enhancement in the sense that it made them "better than well." Our respondents viewed medication mostly as an aid to normal functioning or as a "normalizer" rather than as a performance enhancer. Some regarded it as a remedy for their own perceived underperformance: it enabled them to do what they believed they were intellectually capable of, or ought to be capable of, but could not do because of ADHD-related traits. This perspective can be called the "insider's perspective.".

In contrast, from an "outsider's perspective" it seems that social norms of performance and "normal functioning" are gradually shifting and "underperformance" is seen as less and less acceptable. It is from this outsider's perspective that the sociological study of Conrad and Potter describes the expansion of ADHD as "the medicalisation of underperformance" (Conrad & Potter, 2000). They show how the criteria for ADHD have been extended over the years to include more people, and to include adults as well as children. It is only since 1994 that adult ADHD has been recognized as an official psychiatric diagnosis.

Moreover, since the demands of society and the norms for adequate functioning are changing, this may result in a shift as to what behavior is regarded as "underperformance." One of our respondents was at home on sick leave, partly because he could not handle the increasing administrative load related to his job as a salesman. He said that due to ADHD he was not very good with paperwork and administration and he could not handle the increased pressure at work. However, it was not him who had changed over the years (he might always have had ADHD, but never really noticed it), but rather his working conditions and the demands made on him.

Another respondent considered it a failure that she had not set up and finished a Ph.D. project, next to her job and children; she blamed this "underperformance" on her ADHD.

One respondent apparently recognized this process; he commented: "if more brain-workers are needed, it is to be expected that those not fitted for this kind of job will be injured. Society should make room for people who do not fit easily in."

How can we evaluate the dispute between the two perspectives on adult ADHD and psychopharmacological interventions: Is ADHD a disease and psychostimulant medication a treatment, or is it a normal variation and are psychostimulants enhancers? Where does a normal variation become a disorder? And how does the outcome of such an evaluation bear on moral issues?

We assume here that diseases are at least partly social constructions: what comes to be seen as a disease depends not only on biological factors but also on social norms and context. As many sociologists and philosophers of science have argued: "although biological and clinical factors set boundaries for which symptoms might plausibly be linked in a disease concept, social influences largely explain which symptom clusters have made it as diseases" (Aronowitz, 2001, p.808).

Sociologists concerned with medicalization theory and more recently critics of "disease mongering" have clearly described how the social construction of diseases works. The expansion of the diagnostic category of ADHD as documented by Conrad and Potter (2000) for instance is an example of such a social construction of a disorder. This kind of medicalization through the expansion of medical categories is a reason to be less optimistic than Daniels about the "objectivity" of the DSM categories and the possibility to distinguish between "medically defined deviations of normal functioning" and "unchosen constraints on personal capabilities" (Sabin & Daniels, 1994).

While medicalization can be seen as a neutral description of a social process, it is also often used in a pejorative sense. In other words, the social processes in which some conditions come to be labeled as "disorders" are criticized for various reasons (e.g. for promoting the power of the medical profession, individualizing social problems, or increasing iatrogenic damage). Still, medicalization can be understood in merely descriptive terms. Disease mongering, however, which can be understood as one of the forms that medicalization takes in the 21st century, is certainly not a neutral, descriptive term but is clearly normative (Moynihan, Heath & Henry, 2002). While medicalization is usually seen as an unintentional social process in which classifications get rearranged, disease mongering is described as an intentional process driven especially by the pharmaceutical industry and its interests. The critique on disease mongering is that because of financial interests, conditions that are basically normal are transformed into something that they are not, namely diseases or disorders. This framing presupposes, however, that the critics do know what diseases *really* are and what should *really* be understood as a disease and what not.[3] It supposes they have access to some independent criteria to determine how disease should be distinguished from normal situations and treatment from enhancement or from deception. However, if we assume a constructivist model of disease there is no independent standard that determines whether a given condition "really" is or is not a disease. We have only better or worse arguments and reasons to classify them either in terms of disorder/treatment or normal/enhancement – or to frame them in yet another way, for example as learning difficulties, to be solved by the educational system.

Treatment or enhancement – what difference does it make?

From this perspective, the question we should ask here is not so much whether it is *correct* (with reference to some independent criterion) to call ADHD either a disorder (disease, disability) or a normal variation, but rather, we should ask how desirable it is that this condition is constructed as either one of these. In other words, we could ask what the (social, political, moral) *effects* are if we call it either a disorder or a normal variation, and what *difference* it makes if we called it either way. The "gray area" between treatment and enhancement is a definitional battlefield. Classifying is not (only) a factual or descriptive activity but (also) a political one.

If we look at the effects of labeling a condition as either a disease or a normal condition, and certain drugs as either treatments or enhancements, it becomes clear that these effects depend to a large extent on our social institutions and arrangements. As long as access to psychostimulant drugs runs through the medical system, as it does in our current health care system, labeling ADHD as a disease gives people this access, while calling it a normal variation and psychostimulants an enhancement would preclude access.

A similar argument can be made for reimbursement. As long as reimbursement depends on whether something is a treatment, as it does in the current system, framing psychostimulants like Ritalin as a medical treatment means it will be reimbursed, while calling it an enhancement would mean that the community would not pay for it.

So, within a system that only provides access to psychopharmaceuticals if a condition is labeled a disease, there are certain advantages to such labeling. When the disease label also gives access to reimbursement of medication, the advantages of such a label are even bigger.

If, however, we do not take our present regulations and institutions as self-evident, but step back for a while, the question of classification – is it a disease or normal condition; a treatment or an enhancement – becomes less meaningful. Much of the importance of this classification rests on the role it plays in our social arrangements. Assuming a constructivist model of disease, these social arrangements themselves influence the classification process. So, we appear to be caught in a vicious circle. In order to escape from that, we believe we should address the normative questions (e.g. those concerning access and reimbursement) directly, and not make them dependent upon such contested and inherently normative concepts as disease, disorder, and health. In the final section we give a brief and preliminary sketch of how we could proceed.

Addressing the Issues Directly

The advance of psychopharmaceuticals and other biomedical techniques that might improve human functioning – regardless of whether they have an officially classified disease or not – presses us to discuss issues like access, regulation, and reimbursement. If we cannot depend on a clear and undisputed distinction between treatment and enhancement to guide decision making in these issues, what considerations should we depend on instead?

Access

With regard to access, one might argue that if people could benefit from a drug in some way, whether this is in the form of "treatment" or in the form of "enhancement," it would not be fair if access were precluded. From a liberal point of view, there would be little reason to prohibit the use of such drugs. Access could, for example, be arranged in a "schmocter" scheme. Schmocters have been defined by Parens as "experts at using new biotechnologies to enhance human capacities and traits" who sell their services on the market (1998, p.11). With a "schmocter" scheme we mean a situation in which medically trained "schmocters" would be allowed to practice, within the limits of some safety regulations and other legal constraints. This is comparable to the current situation in many European countries regarding cosmetic clinics. Within a "schmocter" scheme, everyone could have access to psychostimulant drugs – provided they were safe – even if these were taken to be enhancements rather than treatments. Reasons to prohibit the use of such drugs might still be found, however, in their societal effects, for example because they could stimulate a rat race society or create unfair inequalities.

Risks and side effects

One legitimate worry of the critics of disease mongerers and of medicalization alike is that the expansion of medical categories and treatment would increase iatrogenic effects, something Illich (1982) already warned about in his book *Medical Nemesis*. This is also a legitimate worry about enhancement technologies: that the costs in terms of risks and side effects would not weigh up against the advantages. Often, risks and side effects are said to be less acceptable in case a less serious disease is treated, and even less cases of enhancement of normal traits or capacities. What we should be looking at, however, is not the absolute risks and side effects, but the risks and side effects relative to the gained benefits. We should look at the *balance* between benefit and adverse effects. There is no difference in principle between making up a balance in case of treatment or in case of enhancement. Whatever it is called, it seems that the benefit–adverse effect ratio should be positive.

The important question in either case is who should assess this ratio and who should judge the acceptability of a specific risk–benefit ratio? Doctors or schmocters may have the best medical knowledge to assess a risk–benefit ratio, but they may be misguided due to the promotional activities of the industry or, in case of schmocters, may not always have the best interest of their clients as their guiding principle. Patients/clients are not always knowledgeable enough to make a good assessment and they may be influenced by social pressures or promotional activities.

Synofzik (2006) proposes a moral framework for "medicine-on-demand" that might be suitable here, building on the familiar principles of beneficence, non-maleficence, and autonomy. He proposes a continuum between a physician's firm recommendations of an intervention on the one end, to a refusal to intervene on the other end. In between, physician and patient should deliberate about risks and benefits in the light of the patient's own autonomous preferences and values. Interesting issues here concern the degree to which a physician can question the patient's values and preferences, can question their authenticity, or can impose his own or society's values on the patient. These issues are not specific for "enhancements" as opposed to treatments, although individual preferences and values may be more diverse – and therefore may play a more important role in deliberations – in the gray area than they do when a generally recognized serious illness is at stake. A framework for the assessment of benefits when these are not primarily the traditional benefits of cure or palliation of symptoms, but rather benefits in terms of improvements, is yet to be developed.

Who pays?

If reimbursement schemes would aim at fair equality of opportunity, as Daniels' influential account says it should, and if they looked more at disabilities and less at their causes, it probably would not really matter what a condition like ADHD would be called, a normal variation or a disorder. If Ritalin or a similar drug would significantly improve functioning of a significant group of people and increase equality of opportunity, we might choose to reimburse it regardless of whether it was a therapy for abnormal traits or an enhancement of otherwise normal traits, as Daniels himself admits (2000, p.320): "Our arguments would turn on the effects on equality of opportunity and on considerations of social productivity."

A proposal that turned on the effects on equality of opportunity would beg the question what we should do with those persons who already perform above average but could still benefit from Ritalin. Take, for example, the very bright young respondents who already have an academic degree and even a career, but still feel they "underperform." It might seem as if they have equal enough opportunity as it is – should they be reimbursed as well? From the point of view of social productivity, however, reimbursing them might be a very sensible thing to do. This shows that there can be a conflict between the criteria proposed by Daniels and that further discussion on this point is necessary.

Self-understanding and social position

A final point we would like to stress is that little attention has been paid to the effect that the distinction between treatment and enhancement, or between disease and normal functioning, has on the persons it concerns in terms of their self-understanding and in terms of the way they are looked upon by others. A medical label offers a number of advantages, so-called "illness gain." First, it offers an explanation for behavior that was previously considered to be strange, deviant, or incomprehensible. Many of our respondents welcomed their diagnosis, because it provided them with more self-understanding. "Some pieces of the puzzle fell into place – why I sometimes acted as I did. I could suddenly explain certain behaviors of mine: *that's* what is causing it!"

Apart from providing an explanation, a medical label can also provide an excuse for deviant behavior and for underperformance. If one's failure to perform or to behave in accepted ways can be ascribed to a medical disorder, this can free one from blame and from feelings of insufficiency. Although many respondents refused to use their ADHD label as an excuse for their present behavior or performance, some blamed their problems and failures in the past on the disorder.

Although a medical label can improve (self-)understanding and provide an excuse, a medical label, especially a psychiatric label, also has disadvantages because there is still a taboo on mental disorders. A number of respondents mentioned that other people did not understand ADHD or considered one to be "mad" if one had a psychiatric diagnosis or a mental problem. They did not tell everyone they had ADHD. In this respect, a framing in terms of "normal variation" may be easier to bear for some people. Moreover, without the medical label, one does not need to struggle with the identity question: What part of me is *me*, and what part is the disorder? Avoiding (psychiatric) disease labels may have a positive effect on a person's self-image and confidence. However, without the medical label, there is no excuse for poor performance, failure, or deviant behavior. If ADHD or similar conditions were considered to be normal variations, people would have only themselves to blame.

Perhaps understanding conditions like ADHD as normal variations would create more room for the acceptance of differences between people. However, if effective performance-enhancing drugs became available, it appears more likely that all people would eventually come to see themselves as "improvable" in some respect.

Finally, a well-known problem of medicalization is that it can individualize problems that are (also) social or political problems, thereby putting all the "blame" for the problem on the individual and overlooking or discarding solutions on a social or political level. In the case of ADHD, one could think of the social factors contributing to the problems that people with ADHD face, like the increased performance pressure at work or the increased stimulus-density of modern societies. Instead of changing these factors, people with ADHD received medication. The same would be true, however, if ADHD was considered to be a normal variation and drugs were considered enhancements, which shows that enhancement of human functioning by way of biotechnological intervention runs the same risk of individualizing socio-political issues as medicalization does.

Conclusions

To conclude, we can say that how a condition in the borderline area between treatment and enhancement is classified only really matters within a system that links both access to and reimbursement of drugs to the question of whether it concerns a "treatment" of a "medical condition" rather than a nonmedical enhancement of normal traits and functioning. Such a system will come increasingly under pressure with the advance of effective performance-improving interventions. Once we have effective means to improve functioning it will become increasingly difficult to distinguish between "normal" and "subnormal" functioning and between "normal" and "abnormal" forms of dysfunction or underperformance. Norms of "normal functioning" are dynamic and flexible and will shift due to social processes as well as technological advances. We have argued that questions concerning reimbursement and access to medication in the "gray area" should be considered separately and should not appeal to concepts such as disease, medical disorder, or medical necessity, but should rather address the normative considerations involved directly.

It seems almost inevitable in our liberal societies that at least some performance-enhancing drugs will become available for people (either self-paid or in some kind of reimbursement scheme and perhaps even as school/work supplies). Such "medicine-on-demand" might require a moral framework like Synofzik's to regulate it on an individual doctor–patient level. We believe, however, that for policy making on a societal level, we should be more aware of social pressures, disease-mongering-like practices, financial interests, and societal effects of the use of performance-enhancing drugs – like the risk of creating a rat race society or the effects on self-understanding of people – than we presently are.

Notes

1. For research on issues related to ADHD children's experiences of stimulant drug medication see Singh (2005, 2007).
2. For an analysis of effects of psychopharmacological medication on personal identity see Bolt and Schermer (2009).
3. For example, two forms of disease mongering mentioned by Moynihan *et al.* (2002) are: turning ordinary ailments into medical problems and treating personal problems as medical. However, the question is how Moynihan *et al.* know the difference between "ordinary ailments" or "personal problems" and medical problems.

References

Aronowitz, R.A. (2001). When do symptoms become a disease? *Annals of Internal Medicine,* **134**, 803–8.

Bolt, I. & Schermer, M. (2009). Psychopharmaceuticals enhancers – Enhancing identity? *Neuroethics,* **2**, 103–11.

Caplan, A.& Elliott C. (2004). Is it ethical to use enhancement technologies to make us better than well? *Public Library of Science Medicine,* **1**(3), 172–5.

Conrad, P. (2005). The shifting engines of medicalization. *Journal of Health and Social Behavior,* **46**, 3–14.

Conrad, P. & Potter D. (2000). From hyperactive children to ADHD adults: Observations on the expansion of medical categories. *Social Problems,* **47**(4), 559–82.

Daniels, N. (2000). Normal functioning and the treatment-enhancement distinction. *Cambridge Quarterly of Health Care Ethics,* **9**, 309–22.

Elliott, C. (2003). *Better Than Well. American Medicine Meets the American Dream.* New York: W.W. Norton.

Health Council of The Netherlands (2000). *Diagnosis and Treatment of ADHD.* Health Council of the Netherlands, The Hague, publication no. 2000/24.

Illich, I. (1982). *Medical Nemesis.* New York: Pantheon Books.

Juengst, E.T. (1998). What does "enhancement" mean? In E. Parens (ed.), *Enhancing Human Traits: Ethical and Social Implications* (pp. 29–47). Washington, DC: Georgetown University Press.

Kooij, S. (2006). *ADHD in adults. Clinical studies on assessment and treatment*, dissertation, Nijmegen.

Moynihan, R., Heath, I. & Henry, D. (2002). Selling sickness: The pharmaceutical industry and disease mongering. *British Medical Journal*, **324**, 886–91.

Moynihan, R. & Henry, D. (2006). The fight against disease mongering: Generating knowledge for action. *Public Library of Science Medicine*, **3**(4), e191.

Parens, E. (1998). *Enhancing Human Traits: Ethical and Social Implications.* Washington, DC: Georgetown University Press.

President's Council on Bioethics (2003). *Beyond Therapy: Biotechnology and the Pursuit of Happiness.* New York: Regan Books.

Sabin, J.E. & Daniels N. (1994). Determining "medical necessity" in mental health practice. *Hastings Center Report*, **24**(6), 5–13.

Singh, I. (2005). Will the "real boy" please behave: Dosing dilemmas for parents of boys with ADHD. *American Journal of Bioethics*, **5**(3), 34–47.

Singh, I. (2007). Clinical implications of ethical concepts: The case of children taking stimulants for ADHD. *Clinical Child Psychology and Psychiatry*, **12**(2), 167–82.

Synofzik, M. (2006). Kognition à la carte?' *Ethik in der Medizin*, **18**(1), 37–50.

13

What is Good or Bad in Mood Enhancement?

Rein Vos

Macbeth:	Canst thou not minister to a mind diseas'd,
	Pluck from the memory a rooted sorrow,
	Raze out the written troubles of the brain,
	And with some sweet oblivious antidote,
	Cleanse the stuff'd bosom of that perilous stuff
	Which weighs upon the heart?
Doctor:	Therein the patient
	Must minister to himself

Introduction

Who has not wanted to escape the clutches of oppressive and punishing memories? Or to calm the burdensome feelings of anxiety, disappointment, and regret? Or to achieve a psychic state of pure and undivided pleasure and joy? The satisfaction of such desires seems inescapable from our happiness, which we pursue by right and with passion.

This is how the President's Council on Bioethics (2003, p. 230) introduces the topic of "Happy Souls," the issue of brightening or blunting mood, or more widely the enhancing of mood. The connection between a good mood and happiness seems to be self-evident, but as many authors show after further inspection and analysis the matter is much more complicated (Chatterjee, 2006; Elliot, 2005; Farah & Wolpe, 2004; Sententia, 2004). Issues of authenticity, identity, and the nature of happiness itself are dragging issues concealing fundamental but also very different cultural views and traditions in Western societies regarding self, identity, and good life

Enhancing Human Capacities, edited by Julian Savulescu, Ruud ter Meulen and Guy Kahane.
© 2011 Blackwell Publishing Ltd

(Christman, 2004; DeGrazia, 2005; Fischer, 2005; Foster, 2006; Freedman, 1998; Olson, 2002). However, who could object to any technology which may be applied to give people better memories, ease their worries, and make them feel happier? Why should such a technology be a threat for human identity, authenticity, and personality?

In order to assess whether judgments regarding mood-enhancing technologies as good or bad are appropriate, a conceptual analysis is imperative. What do we mean by saying that it is good (or bad) to intervene in people's lives to let them have better memories, ease their worries and make them feel happier?

I want to discuss three different ways of talking about mood enhancement following the illuminating work of von Wright. First, if we do want to enhance, what is good enhancement? This is the instrumental way of proposing (or opposing) enhancement. Second, if one wants to enhance, what is the usefulness of enhancement? This is the utilitarian way of proposing (or opposing) enhancement. Third, if we want to enhance, what might be the beneficial (or harmful) effects? This is the benefactorial way of discussing enhancement.[1] It should be noted that the terms instrumental and utilitarian as used by von Wright differs from current use in ethics, but I will soon clarify in what sense these terms are intended here.

In the debate about enhancement these three ways of using the terms good and bad have to be disentangled. Once disentangled, I will discuss whether we need the concept of personal (or human) identity for judging the outcome of mood enhancement, whether an ethical judgment is required to evaluate what is meant by "good," "better," or "bad," and whether human beings have an obligation or duty to enhance their mood (Harris, 2007; Savulescu & Bostrom, 2009).

To illustrate the conceptual analysis in this chapter, two classes of drugs to enhance mood will be used. First is the class of selective serotonin reuptake inhibitors (SSRIs) – the "new antidepressants" – which are claimed by users that they feel energized, more alert, more able to cope with the world, and to understand themselves and their problems, that is "mood-improving drugs" (Elliott, 2005). Second is the class of beta blocking agents, which are claimed to be good as "memory-smoothing" drugs – memory smoothing here is defined to include the easing or reduction of bad memories, whence the comforting of worries of people, and the production of good memories provoking good feelings (Giles, 2005). In short, both classes of drugs are claimed to deliver "happy souls" (President's Council on Bioethics 2003).

Instrumental Goodness and Badness

One of the major reasons for criticizing possible uses of mood enhancement or other forms of cognitive, emotional, and behavioral enhancement is the way science might provoke the further "instrumentalization" of human beings: humans are reduced to "machines." This leads to discussions on the threat to self, identity, and authenticity of human beings. However, a painstaking analysis of what it does mean to use the notions of good and bad in terms of machines, if humans can be taken analogously as biological machines, is lacking. This we will take up in this section.

What does it mean to say that something is instrumentally good (or bad)?

Instrumental goodness is mainly attributed to instruments and tools such as knives, watches, and cars. A good knife is good *as a knife*. One can use other objects to perform the same purpose like using an ax to cut something, but it is not a *knife*. A knife is good as such when it performs the cutting well. If a knife is not doing its job well, it is a *poor* knife.

This can be applied to mood-enhancing therapies. So construed, SSRIs can be claimed to be good as mood-improving drugs or beta blocking agents can be claimed to be good as "memory-smoothing" drugs.

Then we have to distinguish between two cases. The first case is that SSRIs are good as mood-improving drugs or beta blocking agents are good as memory-smoothing drugs – that is, formally expressed, *good as a K*. The second case is that SSRIs are, as mood-improving drugs, good or, that beta blocking agents are, as memory-smoothing drugs, good – both groups of agents are, formally expressed, *as a K good*.

In the former case we imply that SSRIs are not mood-improving drugs *per se*, but are good to be used as mood-improving drugs. In the latter case it is claimed that SSRIs are mood-improving drugs *per se* and are *as such* good. Similarly, in the former case we imply that beta blocking drugs are not memory-smoothing drugs *per se*, but are good to be used as memory-smoothing drugs. In the latter case it is stated that beta blocking drugs are memory-smoothing drugs *per se* and are *as such* good.

The use of the concept "good" here refers to the idea that a thing – here a drug – serves some purpose well. However, the difference between the two cases is that in the former case some capacity is *not essentially* associated with some purpose, say mood improving or memory smoothing, whereas in the latter case it is. The simple example to illustrate this point is to say that a knife, with a thick and heavy handle, may be used to drive in nails and thus can be used *as a* hammer. But it is not a hammer. Such a knife is good as a hammer (good as a K), but not as a hammer good (not as a K good).

The current state of the art in neuroscience does not allow drawing this distinction (Berghmans *et al.*, 2007). For the time being it can only be said that SSRIs may be (good) to be used as mood-improving drugs and that beta blocking drugs may be (good) to be used as memory-smoothing drugs, that is, good as a mood-enhancing drug (good as a K), but not as a mood-enhancing drug good (not as a K good).

Sub-kinds of improving the mood or smoothing memories

Mood-improving and memory-smoothing drugs may serve different purposes, which are linked to the general purpose of improving the mood or smoothing memories. Let us take the case of mood-improving drugs. Some mood-improving drugs may be suited for becoming optimistic, others for being relieved, again others for feeling "euphoric." Then we need to distinguish between different kinds of mood-improving drugs, or sub-kinds of the mood-improving drugs, such as optimism-producing drugs, relieving drugs, and "euphoric" drugs according to the specifications of what neuroscientists consider the sub-kinds of the generic purpose of improving mood. Presumably, neuroscientists would claim that different *pathways* are involved, some leading to some purposes, some leading to other purposes. It is like saying that we have carving knives, paper knives, table knives, and razor knives, which have been designed to serve the specified purposes. Just so, this might happen during the development of mood-improving drugs. Suppose neuroscientists find out that mood improvement is a 2-tuple, 3-tuple, 4-tuple or n-tuple process, that is a "bundle" of specific mood functions and purposes of the (human) organism, then we will see "selective" profiling of mood-improving drugs, as is the case in other domains of pharmacology (Vos, 1991). The scientific drive is that "common" pathways can be disentangled, that is, cholinergic, serotinergic, dopaminergic, and other "XYZ-ergic" pathways and within these pathways a variety of sub-pathways can be separated. Neuroscientists aim to find "selective" paths in order to stimulate one function and to inhibit another. The basic assumption is that such pathways can be selectively influenced. But what if this is not possible? The prime example here is the neurological pathway leading to "risk-prone" behavior, in the one case leading to culturally valued attitudes and behaviors of being ambitious, competitive and striving, and in the other case leading to culturally de-valued attitudes and behaviors of being risky, dangerous and addictive. As long as these "common" pathways cannot be disentangled, ethical problems about how to value these biological properties (or processes) as good or bad remain at the forefront, disrupting presumed notions of what should be called "good" and "bad" in the enhancement debate. The claims of what can be considered as "good" or "bad" are more and more dependent on the technical possibilities to disentangle biological–neurological pathways.

The normative setting of the purpose

What does it mean to say that one (enhancing) drug or therapy is "better" than another? The neuroscientist might respond that one drug is better when it enhances an optimistic mood more smoothly than another drug. There are two sorts of relationship relevant. One is that the connection between the mechanistic action of the drug and its *effect*, i.e. the smoothing, mood optimistic kind of activity, is a *causal* connection. A particular drug somehow "processes" the causal pathway, say it is stretched like XYZ, in a "more fine-tuned" way than another drug does, such that it delivers a better smoothing, mood optimistic kind of activity. This connection has to be distinguished from the second one, i.e. between the smoothing effect and the goodness of the drug. The second and latter relationship is a **logical** one and not a causal connection: it is only the particular setting, wanting to have the smoothing effect, that there is a meaningful connection between the two aspects. We call this setting the *normative* setting of the purpose: namely wanting to smooth the mood-optimistic activity as much as possible.

It might be argued that this is a "vague" use of the concepts "fine-tuned-processing of pathways" and "smoothing effects." Neuroscientists have developed extensively elaborated scientific models – *in vitro* cell or tissue lines, or experimental animal models – with a set of quantitative outcome parameters being able to designate what it precisely means to say some drug processes pathway XYZ in a "more fine-tuned" way than another drug as well as to determine as exactly as possible what this delivers in terms of "smoothing" the mood-optimistic kind of activity. In such a case the "exact" scientist might accuse the ethicist of using vague terms like "good.". This is quite misleading.

Absolute terms like "fine-tuning" and "smooth" are as vague as the term "good." But the comparative terms "more fine-tuned," "smoother," and "better" are not. If the terms "more fine-tuned" and "smoother" are precisely defined in scientific terms, then the normative notion of "better" is as exact as the former "scientific" ones.

The issue here is that two senses of "good-making" properties are conflated in the debate on enhancement in general and on mood enhancement in particular, both by neuroscientists and ethicists. One way is to say that the causally relevant properties are the good-making properties. Thus, drugs which process the pathway XYZ in a more fine-tuned way are (causally) the better ones. The other way is to say that the logically relevant properties are the good-making properties, which implies the claim that the smoother working drugs are the better ones. The important thing is not to call the one exact and the other vague, but to distinguish between the two ways, the causal and the logical, in which a property of a drug can be called good. Either way, if the scientific terms are vague, the ethical term is vague, but paradoxically, if science develops, the ethical evaluation increases its sharpness. So it is not about neuroscience and ethics as separated domains or between neuroscientists and ethicists as separate breeds of academic origin or even as a conflict between cultures (the alpha and the beta – Snow, 1959). It is about causal and logical relationships *within* neuroscience, and hence within ethics as well. The one comes with the other.

Utilitarian Goodness and Badness

The second sense of the term good is *utilitarian* goodness (or badness). In this sense one can say that it is *useful* to have mood-improving drugs. In daily life, worries and bad feelings trouble people, and it would be good to be able to use mood-improving drugs. Thus, we can say that it is "good to have" something. To have something (or to be something) is like saying that this something is useful *under the circumstances* which are being considered (von Wright, 1963, p.41).[2] This also applies to states of mood, for example, to be optimistic or relieved may be useful in a variety of social situations. In all cases where states of mood are not useful, they are useless.

Now, some person might say that being calmer is useful for her, for example, because she finds herself more attractive in this way, or simply, she likes it as such or people remark that in such a mood she resembles much more like her grandfather whom she really cares for. This is different from claiming that the drug serves her purpose of becoming calm. In the former cases she can only claim that under the circumstances of her (personal) situation such a drug is useful (for her). In the latter case, if the purpose is set as "making calm" then reference to the user doesn't change the claim of the efficiency of the SSRIs, namely being drugs that can calm people. Currently SSRIs, perhaps, may be called the "best" drugs to calm people. It may be the case that in the near future other drugs appear on the scene which might then be called "better" than the SSRIs.

In all cases it is important to stress the essential difference between instrumental and utilitarian goodness (von Wright, 1963, p.43).[3] One might argue that to say that something is useful means that it is favorably relevant to some *end of action*: a mood-improving drug is useful to improve the mood, and with a view to obtaining an enhanced level of mood it is causally relevant to have mood-improving drugs. The dispute about terminology is futile here, because the word "good" in "a good mood-improving drug" does not mean the same as "useful." Even a poor mood-improving drug can, under the circumstances, be useful, like a poor knife can be useful in a threatening situation in the jungle. It follows that the opposite of "good for this purpose" (useful) is "not good for this purpose" (useless), the latter meaning that it cannot be used to serve this purpose. This is in contrast with the opposite of "serves the purpose well," i.e. "serves this purpose poorly," which means that it can be used for this purpose as even a very poor knife can be used: "nothing can serve a purpose even poorly unless it can serve it, i.e. unless it is *in a sense* good for this purpose" (von Wright, 1963, p.44).

Instrumental goodness expresses an excellence or indicates a rank or grade, which is not the case for utilitarian goodness. In the case of instrumental goodness, such as with mood-improving drugs or memory-smoothing drugs we are mostly interested in judging whether one drug (or class of drugs) is better (or less poor) than another one. In the case of usefulness, we are mostly interested to judge whether something can be used or is no good for a certain purpose. However, we do grade usefulness in many cases, for example in the case of two medicines the one less efficacious in curing illness could still be useful for restoring health. By contrast, the better of two knives for carving meat or bread, does not need to be a good carving knife.

The distinction between instrumental and utilitarian goodness and badness is helpful for understanding what is meant when it is said that mood-improving drugs or memory-smoothing drugs, hence also states of mood, such as temperance, optimism, relief, or courage, can be useful by serving other purposes or ends in human life and society, i.e. they might also carry utilitarian goodness (or badness). Optimism can be useful for stimulating other people in such a way that it promotes quality of the service of public institutions or the sales of private companies, hence the prospering of sociality and economy. Thus, mood-improving drugs can be useful for public institutions and private companies. Similarly, certain states of mood can be useful for the individuals in the circumstances considered, for example it is useful to be optimistic, conscientious, and active in learning at school. In all cases states of mood, which are judged useful, become essentially connected to some purpose. If so, then the useful kind of activity becomes judged according to its instrumental goodness.

Here lies a real threat. Scientific claims that mood-enhancing drugs are useful, generally speaking, are inapt, inadequate, and indeterminate. The usefulness always has to be assessed under the circumstances considered. We usually do make general claims about usefulness, such as (broadly speaking) it is useful to have a knife (or some other weapon) in the jungle when being threatened by some animal. Such claims do not pertain to mood enhancing, e.g. becoming calmer, without specifying some sort of general context. In school or in work it might be useful to have calm people, but that depends. Perhaps, we need more "active" people there. Certain states of "mind," say being intelligent, optimistic or active, might be called useful in a general sense. If so, some general context has to be specified such as that, for example, improving intelligence can be considered useful in the "hypercognitive" world we presently live in modern, Western liberal democratic societies (Post, 2000). This generalization seems to be more difficult in states of mind which do not have a clearly positive (or negative) tone, e.g. being introvert or extravert, calm or restless, humorous or ironic. Unlike cognitive or physical enhancement – who does not want to be more intelligent or fit? – it is unclear how to select the proper mood state for enhancing.

Benefactorial Goodness and Badness

The third sense of the term good is "benefactorial goodness." In this case the oppositional terms are beneficial and harmful. One can say that a knife may have beneficial effects on a person's life in the hands of a surgeon removing a malign and painful tumor, whereas a knife may well have harmful effects in the hands of a murderer. Medicines may in some cases be beneficial for the sick, but in other cases they may be harmful, for example in toxic doses or in a patient with an allergy. In these cases the use of the term "good" implies that something is "good for" or "does good to" a certain thing or being, whereas the term "bad" says that something is "bad for" or "does bad to" a certain thing or being.

The enhancement debate is deeply influenced by the utilitarian way of reasoning. Enhancement is about something consequentially good to individuals and society, hence profitable – we do not need to embark on the issue of what kind of "utility calculus" is used to determine the societal profit of some enhancing treatment. However, it is crucial to discuss the differences between utilitarian and "benefactorial" goodness, because these two ways of assessing (mood) enhancement are often con- flated. The logical relationship between the category of the useful and the category of the beneficial is that the latter is a sub-category of the former. As von Wright notes: "Everything beneficial is also useful, but not everything useful is also beneficial. Things which are useful without also being beneficial I shall call 'merely useful'" (von Wright, 1963, p.42).

The specific feature of the beneficial is that things which are useful are causally related to the end which may be characterized as *the good of some being*. Physical exercise is not only useful; it is in addition beneficial, because it is good for the health, health being another name for the good (welfare) of the body. As von Wright points out "Generally speaking: everything which is beneficial affects favorably the good (welfare) of some being" (von Wright, 1963, p. 42). The "recipe" to distinguish the (merely) useful from the beneficial is the following semantic procedure:

> When "good" in "be good for somebody" means "useful," then the whole phrase cannot – as when "good" means "beneficial" – be replaced by "do good to somebody." But of that which is useful, we often say that it is "good to be" or "good to have" (von Wright, 1963, p. 42).

Thus, it can be said that is it is "good to be calm"– or optimistic, active, aroused, ambitious – but this is quite distinct from saying that being calm, optimistic, active, aroused, or ambitious "does good to somebody." Suppose it can be shown that raising intelligence or increasing physical fitness – in terms of the average level in the population (Savulescu & Bostrom, 2009) – is prosperous to individuals and society, promoting living standards, work status, income, and health. In such a case, raising intelligence or increasing physical fitness is not only useful to someone or to society, but is also beneficial; in this sense one can say that a high(er) intelligence or fitness does good to someone or to society. Is this similar to raising "some mood state" in the population? This seems to me doubtful. It can be useful to be optimistic or pessimistic, egoistic or altruistic, active or passive, extrovert or introvert, cheerful or sad, and elated or quiet. But is one of the opposite terms really the candidate for doing good to someone or even to society? I think it highly unlikely. There is no reason to pick out some mood state as good or bad, which I would like to call the mood-state selection (MSS) problem. This also applies to the enhancing methods of neuroscience. It might be good to have mood-enhancing drugs when one wants to enhance mood, but this is fundamentally different from saying that such a class of drugs does good to someone, to some group or to society.

Is to Have a "Good" Mood "Good as Such"? – The Answer Must Be No!

The sense of instrumental goodness does *not* apply to mood. A good mood is not good *as such*. It is not like attributing a goodness of its kind to a thing such as in the case of a good knife or a good car or mood-enhancing drugs. A good mood is not good *as* a mood. Being optimistic or pessimistic, relieved or not relieved, euphoric or dysphoric are not good as such. Obviously, the person wanting to be optimistic – or more generally the person who wants to have a "good mood" – may possess "bad," that is poor, kinds of optimistic pathway processing capacities not well suited to become optimistic. In that sense this person trying to become optimistic is a poor "optimism striving kind of person" or to put it more precisely: the neural pathways wired in his brain are poorly equipped for becoming optimistic. The person with such a wired brain simply is the person he or she is, which might be useful or not, beneficial or harmful, either for that person or for other ones.

Good and Bad Mood Patterns – At the Core or the Periphery of Identity?

It is common usage to call some experiential state (which we will denote further on as some mood pattern) good or bad. Being dumb, stubborn, clumsy, egoistic, and hate-bearing are generally considered bad mood patterns (or states). Being intelligent, fit, altruistic, and minded can be clearly conceived as good mood patterns (or states). We need to see what kinds of mood patterns belong to the identity of an individual. Is being pessimistic, optimistic, intelligent, or dumb a quality which belongs to the deep core of someone's identity? This addresses the issue that some mood patterns might be felt to be associated so much with some people that they are taken to be something natural, a second skin so to speak, something which marks the identity of a person (or perhaps even a community). In the latter case the person would consider being pessimistic, optimistic, intelligent, or dumb not as good or bad *per se*, since it expresses something of his or her identity (or perhaps even the identity of the community to which he or she belongs, e.g. the discussion on deafness as a "cultural value" for the deaf community).

Apparently, there seems to be a decisive difference, that is the triviality which pertains to "superficial" mood patterns such as being handy, witty, or entertaining in contrast with other kinds of mood patterns such as being empathic, competitive, or risk-prone, which seem to be deeply embedded in a person's life and self-identity. This person views the latter mood patterns as so much his or her "own" way of doing things or being that probably this would not count as something good or bad, but just as "that's me." A "trivial" mood pattern seems to be something which can be thrown off just as one takes off a jacket. This defies, however, the inherent character of a mood pattern. A mood is a disposition which belongs to the individual (or group) and which shows itself in specific circumstances and particular settings. Mood may belong to the core or periphery of the identity of a person. Thus, mood states may have different effects on individuals and communities, effects which can be either beneficial or detrimental, so much so that they sustain or threaten one's selfhood or group identity. Below I will specify in what ways to apply the notions of good and bad. Here it suffices to say that there is no reason to differentiate between moods which belong to the core or periphery of a person's or group's identity. Core-identity prone or peripheral mood states are equally open for judgments of good or bad.

There is another sense in which core-identity mood states seem to be distinct from more peripheral mood states, namely that the former are considered good (or bad) *as such*. For some people a good person implies being empathic or altruistic. So construed, however, there seems equally to be a reason to label "more trivial" mood states like being handy or witty good or bad as such. If the presumed distinction is considered helpful for differentiating between the effects which shape one's identity, then the effect is gradual, not categorical. The conclusion is that there is no reason to differentiate between mood states which belong to the core or periphery of one's identity or to claim that core-identity related mood states are good (or bad) as such. What is crucial is that there is a variety in attributing goodness or badness, either in different senses or in intensities, to mood states.

The Ethical Stance: What Kind of Goodness and Badness in Mood Enhancement is Apt for an Ethical Judgment?

To disentangle the varieties of uses of the terms good and bad is helpful in analyzing when and why moods deserve judgments of goodness and badness and in what senses. Von Wright phrases the value of such a conceptual investigation as follows:

> The investigation would show, for one thing, in how many different senses something can be a "cause" of good or of evil. To observe these different senses is essential to any ethics, which measures the moral value or rightness of acts in terms of the consequences of actions. Yet it is an observation which traditional ethics has habitually neglected to make (von Wright, 1963, p.23).

In the mood enhancement literature and debate ethical judgments about whether the use of enhancing drugs and tools is appropriate, prudent, permissive or morally justified, or perhaps even necessary and obligatory, are driven by notions of good and bad. Accordingly, we think it is desirable to identify the different senses of the terms good and bad, which may be used in the mood enhancement debate. The geography of the conceptual landscape can be sketched as follows.

1. The concept of instrumental goodness only applies in a limited sense to current mood-enhancing drugs and tools. The state of the art in neuroscience is far away from being able to claim that these drugs and tools are as mood-enhancing therapies good. At most, these therapies can be claimed as (currently) the best as mood-enhancing technologies. This should constrain both proponents and opponents of mood enhancement from overstretching and exaggerating claims of goodness or badness. However expressed, modestly or extremely in the positive or negative sense, such claims cannot be moral judgments. The question whether the purpose of enhancing mood is good (or bad) requires a fundamentally different justification. Evidence-based statements about the effectiveness of mood-enhancing drugs or tools aim to provide such a justification. However, these only show the evidence for the causal relationship between the agents serving the purpose of mood enhancing, not the logical relationship. The normative setting of wanting and expecting prosperous effects of enhancing the mood has to be legitimized on different grounds.

2. The concept of utilitarian goodness does apply to mood enhancement. However, concepts of usefulness and uselessness have to be clearly delineated from claims about beneficial or harmful effects, either on individuals or groups, communities, and society at large. In many social settings, such as school, work or private life, certain mood states may be useful (or not), but that is far away from claiming that such effects should be considered as doing good to someone or to society. Furthermore, it is quite difficult to specify social settings in a general way such that one specific "mood state" can be picked out as the most useful (or not). In very specific cases, such as extreme forms of shyness or aggressiveness, one can find a ground for claiming badness, but most certainly in such cases harmful effects are being considered, which is quite different from labeling a mood state as (very) useful or (very) useless.

3. The concept of benefactorial goodness certainly applies to mood enhancement and mood disorders. However, we have to be careful. At this stage the state of the art in neurosciences does not provide much evidence in this respect. The principal issue is whether there are reasonable grounds to select one specific mood state – or perhaps one specific "mix" of mood states – as doing good to somebody or to society. In cases of intelligence or fitness it seems to be reasonable to say that more of it seems to be doing good to someone or society – in terms of performing well at school, work, and social life. Even in such cases one should be careful, since any human intervention comes with a cost, physically, psychologically, and socially. It is too early to justify a definitive judgment. Nevertheless, the argument is made here that in case of mood enhancement a fundamentally different issue is at stake, which I have called above the mood-state selection (MSS) problem.

4. Instrumental and utilitarian goodness or badness – the assessment of capacities and the usefulness of the consequences – are not apt for moral judgment. In both cases we may use the terms good or bad (more precisely good versus poor and useful versus not useful), but there is no inherent moral loading of these judgments. Only

beneficial or harmful consequences, either for individuals or groups, communities or society at large, are apt for moral judgment. However, such judgments are only possible to a limited extent considering the problems and the present state of the art in neuroscience as discussed above. Additionally two problems have to be noted. One is that certain mood states may have mixed blessings and the other is that certain mood states may be differently – personally or culturally – appreciated. The mood state of being ambitious may have beneficial effects for that person (causing hedonistic pleasure) but in certain circumstances it may have harmful effects on other people. The mood of wanting to be helpful might have harmful effects, for example, helping thieves in the British Museum to carry away the Van Gogh paintings, or parents or partners helping their children so much that they stifle their development. The decisive source for normatively evaluating mood patterns in a consequential way of reasoning in ethics is the nature of the behavioral consequences of these mood patterns: calling these good in cases of beneficial effects, calling these bad in cases of harmful effects, and being normatively "neutral" when these activities do not carry beneficial and/or harmful effects.

Considering the conceptual landscape regarding the use of good and bad in mood enhancement as sketched above, it can be noted that there is ample space for using the evaluative terms good and bad, but there is not – as yet – much room for ethical judgments, neither in terms of endangering identity, authenticity and personality nor in terms of obligations or duties. One exception, though, seems to be unequivocal. That is, mood states which generate clearly bad effects are to be prevented or interfered with in an ethically sound way. This counts for all diseases, syndromes or disorders, which deeply affect or disrupt people's lives. There is no need to draw the distinction between therapy and enhancement here, since it is the suffering and the social disruption which can be easily noted, either in (officially medical declared) disease states or in other personal and social states, which fall outside medical classifications of disease, invalidity, and disability.

Conclusion

Three different ways of using the terms "good" or "bad" are shown to be in play in mood enhancement, and these are conflated in the current enhancement debate. This pluralistic approach to goodness and badness challenges the received view that there is a deep, self-evident connection between mood enhancement and its necessary goodness, whence critics and opponents self-evidently have to refer to its obvious badness. The connection between good or bad in enhancement inherently assumes an ethical stance leading to discussions whether one has an obligation or perhaps even a duty to "enhance." In the (mood) enhancement debate it is presumed that there is a deep connection between "good mood" and happiness or well-being or pleasure, leading to the conclusion that it is ethically permissible, desirable, or even obligatory to pursue the end of mood enhancement (cf. Harris, 2007; Savulescu & Bostrom, 2009). For the same reason critics or opponents of mood enhancement have to accept this black and white picture and therefore have to stress that intrinsically mood enhancement is morally wrong (cf. Elliot, 2005; Healy, 2004). However, it is argued in this chapter that only one kind of goodness (or badness) is open for moral judgment, namely the well-being of the individuals involved or society at large. Good mood (or bad) mood is not good (or bad) as such. Useful consequences are useful and not useful consequences are not useful, nothing more. Only consequences for the well-being of persons or society are morally relevant. In many, if not most or perhaps all cases in mood enhancement – excluding the domain of psychiatric diseases, disorders, and syndromes – there is no reason to appeal to any further ethical stance, let alone to speak about an ethical responsibility, obligation, or duty to enhance oneself or others. This moral basis is sufficient and for that reason we do not really need the "thick" concept of identity and authenticity or the "thick" concepts of obligation or duty to judge forms of mood enhancement as good or bad.

Notes

1. Von Wright does not use the term "benefactorial goodness," because it is a sub-category of utilitarian goodness. However, this sub-category is treated by von Wright as a separate notion. For reasons of presentation we use the term "benefactorial goodness" as a separate term for this specific sense of goodness (and badness).
2. Other terms to express that something is useful are "advantageous" and "favorable"; these three sister-categories von Wright calls "utilitarian goodness," but he uses the term "useful" as a common name for the three sister-categories and "usefulness" as a synonym for "utilitarian goodness."
3. In fact as von Wright argues, many philosophers would actually reserve the term "instrumental goodness" for the category of the useful.

References

Berghmans, R., ter Meulen, R., Malizia, A. & Vos, R. (2007). Feeling better – Scientific, ethical and social issues in mood enhancement. *Journal of Medical Ethics*, **33**, 560–3.

Chatterjee, A. (2006). The promise and predicament of cosmetic neurology. *Journal of Medical Ethics*, **32**, 110–13.

Christman, J. (2004). Narrative unity as a condition of personhood. *Metaphilosophy*, **35**(5), 695–713.

DeGrazia, D. (2005). *Human Identity and Bioethics*. Cambridge: Cambridge University Press.

Elliot, C. (2005). The tyranny of happiness: Ethics and cosmetic psychopharmacology. In E. Parens (ed.), *Enhancing Human Traits. Ethical and Social Implications* (pp. 177–88). Washington, DC: Georgetown University Press.

Farah, M.J. & Wolpe, P.R. (2004). New neuroscience technologies and their ethical implications. *Hastings Center Report*, **34**(3), 34–45.

Fischer, J.M. (2005). Free will and moral responsibility. In D. Cobb (ed.), *The Oxford Handbook of Ethical Theory* (pp. 321–55) Oxford: Oxford University Press.

Foster, K.R. (2006). Engineering the brain. In J. Illes (ed.), *Neuroethics. Defining the Issues in Theory, Practice and Policy* (pp. 186–99) Oxford: Oxford University Press.

Freedman, C. (1998). Aspirin for the mind? Some ethical worries about psychopharmacology. In E. Parens (ed.), *Enhancing Human Traits. Ethical and Social Implications* (pp. 189–99) Washington, DC: Georgetown University Press.

Giles, J. (2005). Beta-blockers tackle memories of horror. *Nature*, **436**, 448–9.

Harris, J. (2007). *Enhancing Evolution: The Ethical Case for Making Better People*. Princeton, NJ: Princeton University Press.

Healy, D. (2004). Shaping the intimate: influences on the experience of everyday nerves. *Social Studies of Science*, **34**(2), 219–45.

Olson, E.T. (2002). Personal Identity. In E.N. Zalta (ed.), *The Stanford Encyclopedia of Philosophy* (Fall 2002 Edition), http://plato.standord.edu/arhives/fall2002/entries/identity-personal.

Post, S.G. (2005). The concept of Alzheimer's disease in a hypercognitive society. In P.J. Whitehouse, K. Maurer& J.F. Ballenger (eds.), *Concepts of Alzheimer's Disease – Biological, Clinical and Cultural Perspectives* (pp. 245–56). Baltimore: Johns Hopkins University Press.

President's Council on Bioethics (2003). *Beyond Therapy – Biotechnology and the Pursuit of Happiness*. New York: Regan Books.

Savulescu, J. & Bostrom, N. (eds.) (2009). *Human Enhancement*. Oxford: Oxford University Press.

Sententia, W. (2004). Neuroethical considerations: Cognitive liberty and converging technologies for improving human cognition. *Annals of the New York Academy of Sciences*, **1013**, 221–8.

Snow, C.P. (1959). *The Two Cultures and the Scientific Revolution*. Cambridge: Cambridge University Press.

von Wright, G.H. (1963). *Varieties of Goodness*, London: Routledge and Kegan Paul.

Vos, R. (1991). *Drugs Looking for Diseases. Innovative Drug Research and the Development of the Beta Blockers and the Calcium Antagonists*. Dordrecht: Kluwer Academic.

14

Asperger's Syndrome, Bipolar Disorder and the Relation between Mood, Cognition, and Well-Being

Laurens Landeweerd

Introduction

Many drugs and therapies currently under development in neuroscience and biotechnology can be used to enhance human capacities. In the near future we "may see biotechnologies with such potential being applied to make people think better, feel happier or to improve their physical skills in sports or to extend their lifespan" (ter Meulen, 2005). Proponents of such enhancement technologies often adhere to "well-being" as a generic ethical term with which one would be able to assess in which cases their introduction would be justified. As Bostrom and Roache state:

> [...] it has been argued that decisions about what would make people's lives go best – and also, therefore, what is in their best interests – should be guided not by whether a treatment will cure a disease or heal an injury, but by whether it will increase well-being. [...] since it is acceptable to treat diseases or injuries in those who are unable to give consent, it is also acceptable to treat non-disease states in such people if the treatment would increase well-being, provided that the level of well-being we expect them to achieve is not likely to be outweighed by any stress or risks associated with the treatment (Bostrom & Roache, 2007).

In effect, enhancement technologies are a means to increasing our well-being. Or as Julian Savulescu suggests:

> When enhancement is understood as an intervention which increases the chances of a person having a good life, it is hard to see how there could be any objections to trying to make people's lives go better. Indeed, the fact that enhancements increase well-being provides a strong moral obligation based on beneficence to provide them (Savulescu, 2006).

Enhancing Human Capacities, edited by Julian Savulescu, Ruud ter Meulen and Guy Kahane.
© 2011 Blackwell Publishing Ltd

The enhancement of any state, one's physical abilities, one's mood or one's cognitive abilities, is supposed to have direct influence on one's well-being. But is this assumption that there is an inherent relationship between enhancement and well-being correct? Is it the case that by enhancing mood or cognition, one also enhances well-being? What should we think of enhancing therapies which do improve mood but have negative effects on cognition or vice versa? It seems these intriguing questions are currently overlooked in the enhancement debate. This urges for a more detailed analysis of that connection.

Let us start with the stipulative definition of enhancement that Savulescu uses: enhancement includes the increase of a capability, "to enhance any state of a person's biology or psychology which increases the chance of leading a good life in circumstances C" (Savulescu, 2006, p.325). To put it another way: "to enhance is to increase in value," which in the case of human beings means "to increase the value of a person's life." This defense of enhancement technologies on the basis of their supposed contribution to people's overall well-being holds an implicit presumption that well-being can be used as a generic term, as a master value: all other things are only valuable in so far as they contribute to it. Such a conceptualization of well-being holds several disadvantages in its use as a guiding concept for practical moral action.

The American philosopher Tim Scanlon criticizes the use of well-being on the basis of the following thought experiment: suppose someone wanted to become an artist, or a labor organizer, even though this may lead to a lower level of well-being overall for this person. From the perspective of well-being as a master value, such career moves and life choices should not be pursued or supported. Nonetheless, there are quite justified reasons to help someone to pursue such careers: it might be that someone feels a deeper need than individual well-being to become an artist; a friend may have justified reasons to want to help this person in pursuing such a career in spite of the expected decrease of well-being (Scanlon, 1998, p.135). Broadening the concept of well-being does not seem to help clarify why making such choices or helping a person to make such choices can be justified.

In this chapter I will highlight the complexity of the relationship between enhancement of mood and cognition on the one hand and the improvement of people's well-being on the other. To do so, I will present two psychiatric conditions: Asperger's syndrome and bipolar disorder (manic depression). Although these syndromes are taken to be disorders (both are classified in psychiatry as diseases), the effect of these syndromes on people's well-being is not clear: some people are incapacitated; others are enabled by these disease states to develop brilliant careers. Intriguingly, these two syndromes have differential effects on what people are able to think and feel: for some these syndromes have positive effects on mood and negative effects on cognition, for others it is the reverse. A worthwhile life might therefore very well be a life with less-than-average well-being. Someone who is ill may lead a worthwhile life, not in spite of but because of his or her illness. An examination of these two cases may help shed light on the central questions of this chapter: *Is it the case that by enhancing mood or cognition, someone's well-being is necessarily improved? And if not, are there not tradeoffs between improving mood and worsening cognition – or vice versa – lessening the well-being of the person involved? And if so, is this reason not to promote the improvement of mood, or the improvement of cognition?* In other words: *Is well-being a useful concept in the ethical assessment of enhancement technologies?*

Rather than advancing into the question area in the traditional philosophical fashion of presenting cases and the arguments for and against, I would like to study the various ways people speak about autism spectrum disorders and bipolar disorder. This means I do not aim to study the coherence and scientific validity of current definitions of autism spectrum disorders. Instead I would like to look at how neuroscientists and people with a milder form of autism and with a bipolar disorder talk about these disorders in order to construct the language which governs our way of thinking about these two syndromes. Such accounts bear a high degree of relevance to the issue of enhancement of mood, cognition, and well-being.

Asperger's, Mood, and Cognition: Advantage Or Disadvantage?

Asperger's syndrome is one of the so-called "autism spectrum disorders." The word "autism" was first used in 1912[1] but a formal classification of autism was not given until 1943, when psychiatrist Leo Kanner introduced the label "early infantile autism." He suggested "autism" from the Greek word for self, to describe the lack of interest in others shown by 11 children he had under his supervision. When adult, two of these children seemed to function quite normally in spite of their earlier diagnosis (Kanner *et al.*, 1972). Almost simultaneously, in 1944, the Austrian doctor Hans Asperger observed four children in his practice he referred to as "little professors," because of their technical language use and their social impairments. He referred to the syndrome as "autistic psychopathy" (Asperger, 1944).

Asperger's work did not receive much attention outside of the German-speaking countries until, in 1980, Lorna Wing used his name to describe what would later be seen as a mild form of autism (Wing, 1997). Although the children Asperger observed clearly had several handicaps, they also seemed more conscious of their environment than one might expect, given the severity of their social dysfunction. This has something seemingly paradoxical to it: on the one hand, these children are very much socially handicapped, but on the other, they seem to have a sense of everything around them that is better developed than generally is the case. The social disability seems to be combined with a perceptual and intellectual super-ability:

> In the best cases, this ability [...], offers the potential for a career perspective, determines the special achievements of these people, which others do not have. The ability to abstract thought is of course an advantage for scientific achievements. And indeed, under important scientists, there are many autistic personalities. The helplessness that comes from such a social disorder in practical life, which characterises the "professor," and makes him such an immortal cartoon figure, is enough proof for that (Asperger, 1944, pp.117–18).

To have Asperger's syndrome need not be considered as a harm in all respects. The disorder in question can be the basis, for example, for a brilliant scientific career that might even border on genius. Suppose there was a way to determine by precon-ception or preimplantation genetic diagnosis whether a child would have Asperger's syndrome, would this then constitute "a good" or not? This depends on how one ranks the traits associated with Asperger's syndrome. But the ranking of these traits is highly dependent on how they are perceived within a specific sociocultural context.

A cultural shift in perspective has occurred where mild autism spectrum disorders, previously perceived as something negative, are being seen in a more positive light, due to media representations of the syndrome such as the movie *A Beautiful Mind*, about John F. Nash, a brilliant mathematician who suffered from paranoid schizophrenia, portrayed as a loner to the point of autism. Lorna Wing stated:

> Asperger's syndrome seems to exert a fascination for the lay public, even those not personally involved. The evidence for this is the appearance of characters with Asperger's syndrome in movies such as "'Mercury Rising", television plays, including episodes in popular series and literary fiction. The recent novel titled "'The Curious Incident of the Dog in the Night-Time", in which the narrator is a teenager with the syndrome, has achieved remarkable general popularity in the UK, even to the extent of being the subject of a question in a radio quiz show. Such characters were depicted in fiction long before the syndrome was named. [...] Sherlock Holmes was the perfect example. The enduring popularity of characters of this kind is further proof of the fascination that the syndrome exerts, which has probably been enhanced by giving it a name (Wing, 2005, p.197).

Often, Asperger-like traits are associated with the socially inept, "nerd"-type of scientist. One account is given by Oliver Sacks, in his article on the scientist Henry Cavendish (1731–1810):

> Many of the characteristics that distinguished Cavendish are almost pathognomic of Asperger's syndrome [...] Many of these are the very traits he used so brilliantly in his pioneering scientific research, and we are perhaps fortunate that he also happened to have the means and opportunity to pursue his "eccentric" interests despite his lack of worldliness.

Although it is true that genius may have a devouring or isolating capacity of its own, and that genius may be (though by no means must be) associated with profound neurosis [...] the case of Cavendish seems to present an entirely different situation. There has been some tendency recently to claim Einstein, Wittgenstein, Bartok, and others as exemplars of autism, claims that seem very thin at best. But in the case of Cavendish, the evidence gathered by his biographer is almost overwhelming [...] (Sacks, 2001, p.1347).

The traits exhibited by people diagnosed with Asperger's syndrome appeal intuitively to the larger public. But although the negative aspects are often ignored or under-represented in media representations, the type of personality portrayed in the media does coincide with several aspects of the professional perception of the syndrome:

> Professor Fitzgerald said the number of people being diagnosed with Asperger's had significantly increased as doctors had become more aware of the condition. He came to his conclusion after comparing the behaviour of his patients with that described in the biographies of the famous. He believes the author Lewis Carroll, the poet W.B. Yeats and former Irish Prime Minister Eamon de Valera also showed signs of autism disorders (Medical News Today, 2008).

The prevalence of autism in the Silicon Valley community may serve as a striking example. Rather than speaking of an autism epidemic, one should remember that the positive traits associated with "milder" forms of autism such as Asperger's syndrome can actually prove to be an advantage:

> It's a familiar joke in the industry that many of the hardcore programmers in IT strongholds like Intel, Adobe, and Silicon Graphics – coming to work early, leaving late, sucking down Big Gulps in their cubicles while they code for hours – are residing somewhere in Asperger's domain. Kathryn Stewart, director of the Orion Academy, a high school for high-functioning kids in Moraga, California, calls Asperger's syndrome "the engineers' disorder." Bill Gates is regularly diagnosed in the press: His singleminded [sic] focus on technical minutiae, rocking motions, and flat tone of voice are all suggestive of an adult with some trace of the disorder.... In *Microserfs*, novelist Douglas Coupland observes, "I think all tech people are slightly autistic" (Silberman, 2008).

And, as Baron-Cohen – a recognized expert in autism spectrum disorders – states:

> [...] one would predict higher rates of AS in the children of couples living in environments which function as a niche for individuals with superior folk-physics abilities (e.g. "Silicon Valley," MIT, Caltech) compared to environments where no such niche exists. Our recent survey of scientists in Cambridge University showing increased familiality [sic] of autism spectrum conditions is a first such clue that such effects may be operating (Baron-Cohen, 2000).

Having a mild form of autism can be a handicap in an average social environment. Chances are that one would find oneself in a position of social isolation and this indeed often leads to depression for the people who exhibit the symptoms of the disorder. This might not be the case in an environment where most have a similar ineptness in social interaction. In that case, to have a mild form of autism might be a cognitive advantage, while not necessarily being a social disadvantage. This is not to open the question whether Asperger's syndrome is a disorder or not. The semantic jungle that came into being around the term autism may seem to justify this, but the described dysfunction can indeed be a handicap for both the persons diagnosed with it and their environment. Still, to allow for preimplantation genetic diagnosis to specify a milder form of autism in the offspring of couples in Silicon Valley might not be unjustified given that specific context. If it were up to Microsoft, society would probably be allowed to pre-select on these "milder" forms of autism.

The list of people associated with Asperger's syndrome post-factually is growing. It includes people that seem to have been socially awkward to a certain degree and many of them are famed for their "touch of genius" in different areas and disciplines. This of course builds on the notion of Asperger's syndrome as super-ability rather than disability. It serves to create a history or even a culture for mild autism. Still, even with the added value of Asperger's syndrome, not all people embrace the idea that these people were "suffering" from the condition: "For fans of Warhol, however, the suggestion that their hero's view of the world was impaired by a mental disorder is upsetting. It undermines the idea that he knowingly shaped our understanding of pop art" (Thorpe, 2008).

Apart from what the general audience thinks of Asperger's syndrome and other milder forms of autism, people with the syndrome also have their own perspective on the dysfunction. People with a milder form of autism, or another personality (disorder) associated with autism, often do not agree with or accept the idea that they are suffering from an affliction. Although they will acknowledge that in several aspects of their existence they do show a handicap, or a form of lesser functioning, they also describe their condition as advantageous. For example, Anna Hayward, a mother diagnosed with Asperger's syndrome, states:

> I make mistakes, and more when I'm stressed, since every conversation requires maximal concentration: and mistakes mean people get irritated and offended by me. The more this happens, the more stressed I get, and so the more it happens, in a vicious circle. The result is social isolation: no one to baby-sit, no one to visit when the kids are getting me down, no one to compare notes with, no visitors to the house... (Hayward, 2008).

But in her opinion, this is not the only aspect of her affliction. She also states:

> I have been told that my children have exceptional abilities to communicate their feelings and needs, possibly to compensate for my inability to "read" them, like other mothers. Alice stunned a psychologist when she was two by saying, in the middle of a tantrum, "I do not know why, but I cannot stop crying!" Emma, at six years old, is a playground politician and diplomat, with amazing social insight (Hayward, 2008).

It appears an unforeseen side effect of Hayward's Asperger's syndrome is actually that her children compensated for her social handicap, therefore being more overt, understanding, and conscious of social contexts than children of their age normally are. Although on an individual level, Hayward experiences her Asperger's syndrome as a difficult disorder to live with, within the social context of her family, the fact that she suffers from Asperger's syndrome actually proved to have secondary benefits.

Having Asperger's syndrome can also have more immediate positive effects as well, as the following self-report, by Laurence Benjamin Arnold, suggests:

> I believe that because I am the divergent thinker that I am, I have been able to take a sideways look at the world and come up with new and innovative ways of doing things. I am a visual thinker. An essential quality in a graphic designer/photographer and this is an advantage that is conferred upon me by my "disability" (Arnold, 2008).

Oliver Sacks describes a case that supports this view. In his 1995 book *An Anthropologist on Mars* (Sacks, 1995) a high-functioning autistic author by the name of Temple Grandin speaks about her disorder. In her case, her direct perception of the world is not a disability but rather a different form of mental processing. This alternative way of perceiving the world is described as "visual thinking." According to her, visual thinkers process images rather than ideas. For example, when addressing the subject of, say, boats, she would see a boat in her mental eye, rather than a concept of boat. Depending on the context, this can also be an advantage[2].

Many people with a milder form of autism seem to be doing well and do not experience a lesser form of well-being, although their social ineptness might sometimes tempt "us normals" to think otherwise. Some milder forms of autism are associated with a more than average cognitive ability, but this ability obviously is not directly connected to functioning well in a broader sense of the word. Having a higher degree of intelligence than average is often directly associated with having had an enhancement that promoted one's well-being. But in the case of milder forms of autism there seems to be a higher degree of intelligence involved while the syndrome is intrinsically linked to having a lower ability to experience and understand the emotional. Nobody would link this to a higher degree of well-being. In spite of this, many individuals with a mild form of autism would not want to be rid of it.

A Parallel Case: Bipolar Disorder, Creativity, and Mood

There is a dual nature to bipolar disorders. People with a bipolar disorder express the tendency to go through periods of high exaltation and through periods of deep depression. Next to the negative aspects of both the manic and the depressive phases of the disorder, there are also positive side effects. During a manic phase, people feel more energetic, euphoric, experience a rise in their sexual abilities, and need less sleep. Some even associate bipolarity with "creative genius":

> Though this psychopathology is not for one to wish [sic], one interesting association with bipolar disorder is the creativity of those afflicted. This is not the normal creativity experienced by the above-average people (on the scale of creativity). This creativity is the creative genius, which is so rare, yet an inordinate percentage of the well-known creative people were/are afflicted with manic depression. Among the lengthy list are: (writers) F. Scott Fitzgerald, Ernest Hemingway, Sylvia Plath; (poets) William Blake, Sara Teasdale, Walt Whitman, Ralph Waldo Emerson; (composers) Rachmaninoff, Tchaikovsky (Krishna, 1998).

It seems that a similar list of famous people is often recycled by different mental disability interest groups, Einstein being the main trophy every mental disorder community claims as their's. But one cannot diagnose the dead without jeopardizing the neutrality of that diagnosis. Still, there has been research on the living as well:

> In the 1970s, Nancy C. Andreasen of the University of Iowa examined 30 creative writers and found 80% had experienced at least one episode of major depression, hypomania, or mania. A few years later Kay Redfield Jamison studied 47 British writers, painters, and sculptors from the Royal Academy. She found that 38% had been treated for bipolar disorder [...] The additive results of these studies provide ample evidence that there is a link between bipolar disorder and creative genius. The question now is not whether or not there exists a connection between the two, but why it exists. (Krishna, 1998)

Similar to milder forms of autism, bipolar disorders are not merely associated with dysfunction. Even if one were to describe bipolar disorder in biological language, one will find positive aspects to the condition.

> [...] the manic state is physically alert. That is, it can respond quickly and intellectually with a range of changes (i.e. emotional, perceptual, behavioral). The manic perception of life is one without bounds. This allows for creativity because the person feels capable of anything.

It is as if the walls, which inhibit the general population, do not exist in manic people, allowing them to become creative geniuses. They understand a part of art, music, and literature which normal people do not attempt (Krishna, 1998).

A similar opinion is often expressed by people with a bipolar disorder. Actor Stephen Fry, for example, was diagnosed with a bipolar disorder. In an interview about his documentary *The Secret Life of the Manic Depressed*, he stated:

I approach it from the point of view of one who suffers, according to a psychiatrist at least, from cyclothymia which is sometimes called "bipolar light." I take that to mean I have most of the benefits of hypomania, a slightly less psychotic form of energy, vitality and exuberance and some, one hopes, creativity. There are certainly spending sprees but happily very little promiscuity. That's just my good fortune in this regard (Fry, 2008).

Indeed, some individually, potentially deleterious cognitive states such as bipolar disorder might occasionally produce benefits to society as a whole through, for example, artistic creativity. Cognitive enhancements may introduce a similar situation where enhancing interventions may harm individuals but benefit society. Should one refrain from intervening in these cases for the benefit of society? A key aspect of bipolar disorder is that the so-called "highs," for many people, compensate for the lows. Although it is not easy to live with a bipolar disorder, people seem to embrace it nonetheless as an integral part of not only their personality but also of what makes their life worthwhile, that is to say, a valuable life. This is different from saying that it is "a good life." The person involved may have good reason to pursue this artistic life, even though this leads to a lower level of well-being for him or her overall because of the difficulty and discomfort that this life involves. Thus, the association with artistic genius does not mean that we should rally behind the idea of pre-selecting children for bipolarity. This may be the moral conclusion with regard to cognitive enhancements as well.

Whether bipolarity carried with it an increased or decreased sense of well-being seems to be irrelevant for many people that have been diagnosed with the disorder. We already have recreational drugs that mimic the symptoms of the highs experienced during the stage of mania and that without the lows that are part of bipolar disorders. Such a state of euphoria, however, inevitably leads to high-risk behavior, bad judgment, and lower cognitive performance. This means that the effect of enhancement of mood on well-being can be both negative and positive. One will always need to look at the specifics of a situation.

It seems well-being is too broad a notion to serve as an instrument for assessing specific and individual goals while it is too narrow in a societal setting in which other values are seen to be more important. Different individuals will hold different conceptions of what is well-being. Any societal introduction of enhancement technologies will by consequence exclude a number of interventions that are considered to be dyshancements, although some might consider these to be enhancements in their own right. Generalizing the concept of well-being to a level to make societal rules seems to render the concept void of any practical significance, while specifying it for each circumstance renders it unfit for ethical assessment.

Conclusion

Well-being might not be decreased by having a disorder. And an enhanced cognition or enhanced mood does not necessarily equal enhanced well-being. Well-being is either too subjective to define neutrally and use as an ethical assessment tool, or too broad, since to name everything people value *ipso facto* a "promoter of well-being" does not provide us with a useful criterion to discern what counts as an enhancement and what as the opposite. A valuable life or valuable experience does not necessarily mean better than average well-being. This leads to the conclusion that enhancement, well-being, and desirability of introduction (of a specific enhancement technology) are not interlinked. In discussion of enhancement technologies, the concept of well-being does little to either support or oppose the use of specific enhancement technologies. So long as we think about well-being in such a generic way, it will remain unclear under what circumstances a certain enhancement technology will be acceptable.

As we have seen, many people with a milder form of autism regard the properties that give cause to that diagnosis as something they *are*, rather than are *affected* by. Even people with more severe forms of autism do not necessarily want to be "cured" of their condition. They regard their autism as constitutive of what they are, not as an "external" defect, a problem of the machinery. In spite of the fact that the philosophical notion of an authentic self crumbled over the past four decades, in daily life, we often still cling to this idea of a true self, an authentic core of our being. For both autistic and manic depressed, the dysfunctional side of their condition is often well compensated for by the positive side of the condition:

> I do not wish to be "cured" from my autism, and many autistic persons who are able to communicate their feelings, say the same thing. Autism is not something that I have, it is something that I am. [...] You cannot talk about a person "emerging" from autism. If it were possible to remove autism from a person, you would get a different person. A person who, perhaps, fits in better with his surroundings. Maybe a person who abides by the rules of society more. A person who does not stick out. That person will look identical to the previous one, but will be a different person nonetheless (Anonymous, 2008).

Similarly, many people with a bipolar disorder also do not perceive of their bipolarity as something external to themselves, but as part of who they are. Even though there are both negative and positive aspects to Asperger's syndrome or to bipolar disorders, taking away even these negative aspects would not necessarily promote well-being. And it might be impossible to isolate the positive aspects of these disorders. An increase in specific forms of cognition might be intrinsically connected to a decrease in specific aspects of mood. A decrease in specific aspects of mood might be intrinsically connected to an increase in creativity. Neither is necessarily linked to any changes in some general form of "well-being." Van Gogh's absinthe addiction and abuse of other substances are of direct influence on his style: his yellow period is said to have been caused by an abuse-related sight defect[3] and his haunting style is often linked to his acquaintance with the notorious green fairy, who is also said to, if not have caused, have triggered or augmented his tendency to bipolarity. In such cases there seems to exist a link between an increase in creativity and a decrease in mood and mood stability.

As can be concluded from both cases, one will need to consider the trait in question in a given context and in the light of a richer understanding of well-being to be able to see what type of intervention would be acceptable. Although for some, autism or bipolar disorder is incapacitating, for others it is enabling. For many it is both at the same time, positive effects on mood and negative effects on cognition or positive effects on cognition, while having negative effects on mood, or both positive effects on mood and on cognition, but in such a way that a person's well-being is not promoted by it. It seems the field is more complex than can be tackled with a mere categorization from negative to positive.

The assumption of a direct relationship between enhancement and well-being is not supported by practice. Euphoria for example is a state of high mood that can be fatal for one's well-being. Although some conditions can be enabling for one's creativity, cognition, or mood in general, they can simultaneously have a negative effect on one's well-being. Enhancing therapies for autism might heighten people's sociability, but lower their cognitive abilities and mood-smoothening drugs for bipolarity can have negative repercussions on both one's creative abilities and one's sense of self. Although such tradeoffs between enhancing certain capacities at the expense of others might not be associated with every kind of enhancement technology, the lesson is that a richer conception of well-being is needed to assess what is at stake in enhancement, one that takes into account not only the trait in question, but also other traits it might be related to, as well as what is unique to the individual in question. In this respect it also has to be taken into account that people consciously and autonomously choose options that do not seem to promote their well-being in the generally accepted sense of the word. Some choices might be good choices even though they do not promote one's well-being in this generic sense.

Well-being is a very individually and subjectively experienced state. This is why Asperger's syndrome or bipolar disorder can actually contribute to one's well-being, in spite of the fact that they are seen as disorders. However, even if well-being would not be promoted by for example Asperger's syndrome or bipolar disorder, one cannot state these "disorders" or "dysfunctions" are not valuable in some other fashion. Choices that do not promote more subjectively or idiosyncratically defined forms of well-being that are not irrational, reprehensible, or undesirable. This forces us to accept that the horizon of morality stretches out more widely than a generic conception of well-being.

Acknowledgments

I would like to thank Rein Vos and Ron Berghmans for their critical discussions and helpful advice on elaborating and polishing the rough material that was to become this chapter.

Notes

1. At least in English, by Swiss psychiatrist Eugene Bleuler in a 1912 number of the *American Journal of Insanity*.
2. Blume, H. (2003). The culture of autism. Inward-looking autistics often display remarkable artistic gifts: What do their talents tell us about their minds-and the history of western art?

Vaccination News, www.vaccinationnews.com/DailyNews/2003/February/Culture
Autism19.htm.
3. In Arnold, W.N. and Loftus, L.S. (1991). Xanthopsia and van Gogh's yellow palette. *Eye*, **5**
(5), pp. 503–10. it is claimed van Gogh's preference for yellow may have been a result of
xanthopsia, a disorder of the eyes, causing yellow vision, which can be exacerbated by
malnutrition and substance abuse. Contrary to popular rumor, digitalis seems to be a more
likely culprit than absinthe.

References

Anonymous (2008). The mind within. blog. http://within.autistics.org/nocure.html (accessed
October 10, 2008).
Arnold, L. (2008). Neurological differences page. www.larry-arnold.info/Neurodiversity/
index.htm (accessed October 10, 2008).
Asperger, H. (1944). Die "Autistischen Psychopathen" im Kindesalter', *Archiv fur Psychiatrie
und Nervenkrankheiten*, **117**, 76–136.
Baron-Cohen, S. (2000). Is high-functioning autism/Asperger's syndrome necessarily a dis-
ability? *Development and Psychopathology*, **12**, 489–500.
Bostrom, N. & Roache, R., (2007), Ethical issues in human enhancement. In J. Ryberg (ed.),
New Waves in Applied Ethics. New York: Palgrave Macmillan.
Fry, S. (2008). Interview on "The Secret Life of the Manic Depressive." www.youtube.com/
watch?v=AQkE56eFyk4 (accessed October 10, 2008).
Hayward, W.A. (2008). Alien parenting – A mother with Asperger's syndrome. *Disability
Pregnancy and Parenthood International*, **34**, 3–5.
Kanner, L., Rodriguez, A. & Ashenden, B. (1972). How far can autistic children go in matters of
social adaptation? *Journal of Autism and Childhood Schizophrenia*, **2**(1), 9–33.
Krishna, H.K. (1998). Bipolar disorder and the creative genius. http://serendip.brynmawr
.edu/exchange/node/1726?page=1&destination=(accessed May 17, 2010).
Medical News Today (2008). Were Socrates, Darwin, Andy Warhol and Einstein autistic?
www.medicalnewstoday.com/medicalnews.php?newsid=5274 (accessed October 10,
2008).
Sacks, O. (1995). *An Anthropologist on Mars: Seven Paradoxical Tales*. New York: Alfred
A. Knopf.
Sacks, O. (2001). Henry Cavendish: An early case of Asperger's syndrome? *Neurology*, **57**,
1347–422.
Savulescu, J. (2006). Justice, fairness, and enhancement. *Annals of the New York Academy of
Sciences*, **1093**(1), 321–38.
Scanlon, T. (1998). *What We Owe to Each Other*. Cambridge: Belknap Press.
Silberman, S. (2008). The geek syndrome. www.wired.com/wired/archive/9.12/
aspergers_pr.html (accessed, October 10, 2008).
ter Meulen, R. (2005). About the Enhance Project. www.enhanceproject.org/about.html
(accessed October 10, 2008).
Thorpe, V. (2008). Was autism the secret of Warhol's art? www.guardian.co.uk/Archive/
Article/0,4273,3837088,00.html (accessed October 10, 2008).
Wing, L. (1997). The history of ideas on autism: Legends, myths and reality. *Autism*, **1**, 13–23.
Wing, L. (2005). Reflections on opening Pandora's box. *Journal of Autism and Developmental
Disorders*, **35**(2), 197–203.

15

Is Mood Enhancement a Legitimate Goal of Medicine?

Bengt Brülde

The Question

There are many different kinds of medical technologies, ranging from neurosurgery and plastic surgery to pharmaceutical and other drugs, growth hormone treatments, and radiation. The existing repertoire of interventions will most likely be expanded by e.g. genetic engineering, nanotechnologies, neural interfaces, rational drug design, transcranial magnetic stimulation, and "neuroceuticals." These biotechnologies have all been developed for "therapeutic purposes" – e.g. to cure or prevent disease, to heal injuries, to eliminate defects, or to prevent premature death – or for palliative purposes (to relieve suffering). The possible uses of these technologies are not restricted to therapy, however, e.g. they can also be used to enhance different properties or functions of healthy people. It is not impossible that our cognitive abilities will be amplified or extended, our physical fitness (e.g. strength or endurance) increased, our lifespans extended, our behavior modified, our appearances improved, and our moods enhanced.

These (remote) possibilities give rise to a number of questions, many of which are ethical in character. The perhaps most general of these questions is whether enhancement is ever a legitimate goal of medicine. Should medicine concern itself with this sort of thing? There are also more specific questions, related to specific technologies or areas of enhancement. For example, are some technologies more acceptable than others, e.g. is it ever acceptable to engage in genetic engineering (for any purpose)? And are some types of enhancement more acceptable than others, e.g. is it more acceptable to improve functioning than to improve appearance, and is it ever acceptable to improve performance in sports by medical technologies?

In this contribution, I will restrict myself to one aspect of the general question, namely whether mood enhancement is a legitimate goal of medicine. I will assume that the relevant medical resources are limited. In an imagined case where resources are unlimited, I see no reason why medicine should not do whatever it can to improve our lives. In this case, enhancement is perfectly legitimate, at least on the assumption that the risks involved are not too big. This "liberal view" might not be tenable in real life, however, where medical resources are scarce.

Enhancing Human Capacities, edited by Julian Savulescu, Ruud ter Meulen and Guy Kahane.
© 2011 Blackwell Publishing Ltd

How our question should be answered depends on how the enhancement enterprise is financed, e.g. whether it is publicly funded or not. If we assume a publicly funded health care system, the question is whether it is ever legitimate to spend tax payers' money on enhancement. If we assume a more or less free market for medical services, the question is rather how and to what extent these markets should be regulated, e.g. whether there should be a free market for enhancement services. I will not address the market issue any further. Suffice it to say that most of us have no objections to enhancement as such as long as it takes place on the market, e.g. in the case of psychotherapy or (perhaps) plastic surgery.

That is, my question is really whether enhancement is a legitimate goal of medicine when medical resources are limited and the medical enterprise is publicly funded. To be able to answer this question, we first need to know what enhancement is, e.g. what interventions should count as enhancements. We also need to know roughly what practices should count as medical, how the goals of medicine have been conceived of traditionally, and most importantly, what exactly is covered by the question of the goals of medicine. What needs to be included in a reasonably complete conception of the goals of medicine, broadly conceived? Let us take a brief look at these preliminaries.

The Notion of Enhancement

What interventions should count as enhancements? A rather common answer to this question is to contrast enhancement with treatment or therapy. On this view, a medical intervention is an enhancement if it does *not* aim at curing disease or eliminating a disability. This view is very problematic. Firstly, it makes the notion of enhancement dependent on the notion of disorder (and the highly contested issue of what conditions we have good reason to pathologize), and all the obscurities that are associated with the latter notion are incorporated into the former. Secondly, if the view is combined with the normative idea that we should give priority to treatment, it has morally unacceptable consequences. Suppose that A is in better health than B (that he is both functioning better and feeling better), but that only A suffers from an identifiable disorder. In this case, the treatment view suggests that A is more entitled to medical help than B, which is hardly reasonable.

This gives rise to another suggestion, viz. that the crucial question is where on the health scale (or the like) the (intended) improvement occurs. If an intervention aims at improving health above a certain critical level on the health scale (e.g. "normal" or "acceptable" health), then it should count as enhancement. It may well be necessary to specify the critical level in terms of normality. If we do this, we may arrive at the idea that an intervention counts as enhancement if it aims to improve e.g. the physical condition, mood level or appearance in normal and healthy individuals. Sometimes, the two suggestions are combined into one. For example, according to Tännsjö, an intervention should be regarded as negative (or curative) if it aims at curing disease or eliminating a handicap or disability, it should count as positive if it aims at improving functioning (or the like) within a natural variation, and it should be conceived of as enhancement proper if it aims to take an individual beyond normal human functioning (cf. Tännsjö, 1993).

It is somewhat unfortunate to mix different considerations in this way. Moreover, the distinction between "positive interventions" and "enhancement proper" is ethically unimportant and can be ignored. In this contribution, the term "enhancement" will be used to refer to both, i.e. "enhancement" is tentatively defined in relation to the normal functioning (mood, etc.) of the individual, not in relation to what is normal for the species. That is, to improve people's appearance through plastic surgery counts as enhancement, as does the use of gene doping to help the average athlete to make it to the top 20 on the district level.

The Traditional Conception of the Goals of Medicine: The Relevant Dimensions

It is far from obvious what should be included in medicine, i.e. what activities or practices that should be regarded as medical (cf. Nordenfelt, 2001). Traditional hospital services should of course be included, but what about nursing, palliative care, social care, rehabilitation, health education, environmental care, and legal health protection? There are several notions of medicine, some of which are more narrow than others (Nordenfelt, 2001). The fact that enhancement is not included in the most narrow notion of medicine – i.e. curing, palliation, and perhaps medical disease prevention, like inoculation – cannot be taken to imply that medicine should not engage in enhancement. What interventions that count as medical may change over time (cf. the case of monitoring the birth process), and the question can hardly be settled on semantic grounds.

Whatever we mean by "medicine," it is far too vague to claim that the legitimate goal of medicine is to cure disease. A conception of the goals of medicine needs to be far more precise than this. First, such a conception needs to tell us in what respects or dimensions (e.g. health or life expectancy) that medicine should benefit the relevant individuals, e.g. the patients. To identify the relevant dimensions is not sufficient, however, e.g. since these dimensions are common to both therapy and enhancement. A complete conception of the goals of medicine also needs to specify the relevant levels, i.e. it needs to tell us who the medical enterprise should benefit, and to what extent. The first question is not dependent on the available resources, but the second is.

In Brülde (2001), I tried to answer the first question in a comprehensive and unified way, namely by formulating a theory of the relevant dimensions in which medicine should benefit the patient. After having conducted a review of the relevant literature, I arrived at the conclusion that there are at least seven plausible goals that are irreducible to each other:

1. To promote functional ability, especially health-related functioning.
2. To maintain or improve normal structure and function (on the part level), especially by preventing disease or injury or by curing disease.
3. To promote subjective well-being, especially by relieving pain and suffering.
4. To save and prolong life, especially to prevent premature death.

In certain cases, medicine should also:

5. Help the patient cope with his or her condition.
6. Improve the external conditions under which people live, either in order to promote freedom and independence (as in the case of handicap) or in order to prevent disease or injury.
7. Promote growth and development (of children).

This list may not be complete, e.g. it is possible that medicine should also restore other biological features (like appearance or fertility), and Nordenfelt (2001) also wants to include prenatal care of the fetus and well-being of third parties (in the case of forensic psychiatry). It is worth noting that these goals are mainly dimensional, but that references to certain levels are sometimes included as well.

Now, if we eliminate all references to levels and if we restrict our attention to the sort of technologies that are of interest here (e.g. mood-enhancing drugs or deep brain stimulation), we can ignore some of these goals, e.g. to improve the environment or help people cope better. In "technological medicine," the central dimensional goals are rather: (i) to promote the functioning of the person as a whole, e.g. physically or cognitively; (ii) to promote subjective well-being, e.g. by increasing mood level; (iii) to prolong life; (iv) to improve structure and function (on the organ or cellular level); and (v) to improve appearance.[1]

Are any of these five dimensional goals "defining goals," i.e. a necessary condition of medical practice? I think not, I don't think there is any such thing. Sometimes the central aim is to improve well-being by reducing suffering (intense displeasure), sometimes the major goal is to improve functioning (e.g. rehabilitation after a stroke), and so on. There is no goal that figures in every medical activity.

It should be noted that these dimensional goals are, *as goals*, not just causally related to one another, and that they should therefore, again *as goals*, not be regarded in isolation. Instead, we should conceive of the goal of medicine in structural terms, i.e. we should think of the medical enterprise as having a *goal structure* rather than a single goal. For example, the only reason why medicine should try to improve structure and function is that this has positive effects in the other four dimensions, and it can be argued that functioning is only valuable in so far as it has positive effects on well-being.

Who Should Medicine Benefit and to What Extent? The Case of Well-Being

Now that we have specified the relevant dimensions, let us introduce the question of the relevant levels, and ask who is entitled to help, and how much (given scarce resources). For example, should medicine only benefit those who are badly off in the relevant dimensions, e.g. those who suffer and function badly? And should these people's functioning or well-being only be improved up to a certain point, e.g. to some kind of normal level? If so, how can this level be determined? In the following, I will restrict myself to the case of well-being, since this dimension is most relevant in a mood enhancement context.

Since the difference between therapy and enhancement is nothing but a matter of level (on the view defended above), this is where my central question is properly located. So, is mood enhancement ever a legitimate goal of medicine when medical resources are limited and the medical enterprise is publicly funded? For purposes of illustration, I will restrict myself to the case of mood enhancement through so-called cosmetic psychopharmaceuticals.

If we, for the time being, ignore "the how" – the question of what means are most appropriate, e.g. drugs vs. psychotherapy – and "the why" – how a person's hedonistic level should be explained, e.g. whether or not it is caused by disease – the question is really twofold. Firstly, is the entitlement to medical help dependent on where on the scale (on what level) one is located, e.g. should we always give priority to the people who suffer most? Secondly, should we (from a medical perspective) attribute the same value to a certain increase in well-being regardless of where on the scale it occurs, or should we attribute more value to a certain increase the further down the scale it occurs? Here are five possible answers to these questions:

1. We should give absolute priority to those who suffer most. For example, a slight improvement in subjective well-being (hedonistic level) on the low end of the scale has more weight than a very large improvement on the upper end of the scale.
2. We should give equal weight to all improvements in well-being, regardless of where on the scale they occur. (This view is similar to classical utilitarianism, but note that the latter is not a theory about the goals of medicine.)
3. The better a person feels, the less is the value of a certain improvement, i.e. the marginal value of subjective well-being is diminishing.
4. Once a certain level of subjective well-being (e.g. "normal" mood) has been attained, a further improvement is worth nothing from a medical perspective. Medicine should do nothing to help people beyond this level.
5. An improvement beyond normal mood still has value, but it is worth less (from a medical perspective) than an improvement below this level.[2]

Note that the second view is most compatible with the idea that medicine should engage in enhancement, but that the third and fifth views also imply that enhancement might be a good idea under certain conditions.

The first view is not plausible since it suggests that we spend all resources on those who suffer most, even if this is of little benefit. People who suffer less but who would

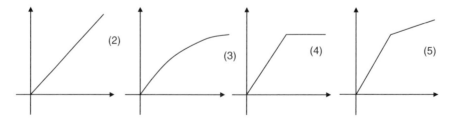

Figure 15.1   Graphical representations of positions (2)–(5). The first view cannot be represented graphically. The measure on the x-axis is subjective well-being and the measure on the y-axis is value from a medical perspective

benefit immensely from certain interventions would get nothing. This kind of dicta-torship of the worst-off is hardly plausible. The second view implies that we should always give a certain improvement in well-being the same weight, regardless of whether this improvement befalls someone who suffers intensely or whether it befalls someone who is already happy. This is a repugnant view. The fourth and fifth views both refer to a certain critical level. If this level is taken to coincide with "normal mood," these views are rather repugnant as well. The reason for this is that there is no such thing as a *common* normal level, the "normal" or "natural" variation is substantial. A number of empirical happiness studies strongly suggest that a person's average hedonistic level over time depends on her temperament, i.e. that we all have genetically determined "set points" (cf. Diener & Lucas, 1999; Heady & Wearing, 1989, 1991, 1992; Lykken & Tellegen, 1996; Tellegen *et al.*, 1988). However, we differ considerably in this regard, and it is thus unfair to refer to what is normal. If different hedonistic levels are normal to different people, this implies that there might be cases where two people are on the same hedonistic level, but where only one of them is entitled to medical help. This is also somewhat repugnant, and I therefore conclude that the third view is most plausible.

However, it can be argued that we also need to take the relevant causes ("the why") into account. A person A might suffer less (over time) than another person B, but her suffering might be health related (e.g. a symptom of a mental disorder) whereas B is perfectly healthy, i.e. her low hedonistic level is due to external or genetic factors. In this case, it might be argued that B's (long-term) suffering falls outside the scope of medicine, and that we should therefore help A. Is there any good argument for this view? It is of course possible that it is not in the power of medicine to help B feel better, and that medicine should help A for this reason. But suppose that medicine actually has the ability to help B. In this case, I suggest that medicine should give priority to B. To argue that medicine should restrict itself to health-related properties only is certainly arbitrary and ill-founded.[3]

It can also be claimed that we need to take the different types of interventions into account. For example, it might be argued that we should adopt a restrictive attitude towards medicalization, e.g. that it is better to improve well-being through psychotherapy than through pharmaceuticals or deep brain stimulation (DBS). There are at least two types of reasons for adopting a restrictive or cautious attitude on these matters. Arguments of the first type purport to demonstrate that it is better for the person herself if her well-being is improved through counseling, meditation, mental training or psychotherapy, rather than through drugs or DBS. These arguments are not just restricted to the case of enhancement; they also try to show that it is often worse for the suffering person himself if his suffering is treated with drugs rather than with psychotherapy (but this is not to deny that it is sometimes good to combat suffering with drugs, e.g. as in the case of severe and paralyzing sufferings). The arguments of the second type are not concerned with the effects that drugs have on the individual, but (rather) with the effects on society as a whole. These arguments are concerned with enhancement rather than with reduction of suffering.

In discussing this question, I will (for the sake of argument) assume that drugs work. Or more specifically, I will both assume that they can be used to eliminate or reduce different types of disorders – e.g. depression, panic anxiety, compulsiveness, obsession, eating disorders, substance abuse, attention deficit disorder – and that they can make people more socially confident and competent, more relaxed and energetic, less sensitive to rejection and loss, more outgoing and courageous, and the like. I will also (again for the sake of argument) assume that there are no undesirable side effects. So, assuming that drugs have positive direct effects that outweigh the side effects, what reasons can there be for adopting a restrictive view?

Are Mood-Enhancing Drugs Bad for the Suffering Individual?

What the arguments of the first group try to show is not so much that the long-term effects of pharmacological drug use are positively bad, but rather that such treatments make certain good things impossible, more difficult, or more unlikely (in comparison to some alternative treatment, that is, or perhaps to no treatment at all). Or alternatively put: The idea is that not all improvements on the hedonistic scale are good for a person, e.g. that the instrumental value of a certain suffering may well be large enough to outweigh its final (or "intrinsic") badness. There are several arguments of this type:

1. Certain kinds of suffering can become a "source of knowledge"; in particular, it makes self-knowledge possible, but it can (of course) also improve the understanding of the suffering of others. To eliminate suffering by means of drugs in these cases makes a certain kind of self-understanding more difficult. But how is the suffering person supposed to realize the opportunity for self-knowledge that her suffering provides? By choosing psychoanalysis instead? And why is self-knowledge good for a person, e.g. does it have final value or is it good because it makes a substantial contribution to her future happiness?
2. A closely related idea is that certain kinds of suffering can have value for a person because it contributes to her personal development, i.e. because it tends to make her a better person (this may of course happen through an improvement in self-understanding, but it may also happen in other ways). So, in what respects can a suffering person become a better person as a result of her suffering? There are several options here, e.g. one may become stronger, less self-centered, a better listener, better at living in the here and now, or more empathetic. Personal development can also be accomplished through medication, however, but such medication-induced change is often regarded as inferior to the change that takes place in psychotherapy, viz. because it is not accompanied by growth in self-understanding.
3. Another well-known idea is the idea that a certain amount of suffering is necessary for creative activity, critical thinking, or the like. A weaker version of this idea is probably more plausible, however, viz. the idea that suffering often motivates the suffering person to engage in these activities, or that it is likely that such a person is (because of his suffering) engaged in such activities to a higher extent than he would otherwise be. However, even if this is so, it is doubtful whether the negative value of the suffering in question is outweighed by the positive value that can be attributed to the increase in creativity (etc.).

4. There is also the idea that certain kinds of suffering are (like most pain) functional, i.e. that it can (and should) be viewed as an appropriate response to an untenable situation. On this view, the appropriate way to get rid of such suffering is not to medicate, but to deal with the underlying problem in a more constructive manner. And it is definitely more fruitful in the long run to solve a problem than to dissolve it temporarily, isn't it? This idea may be combined with the idea that a normal life is full of problems and challenges, e.g. in connection with major events like separating from one's parents, finding a partner, or having children. If such challenges are not met in a satisfactory way, they might give rise to different sorts of suffering, e.g. depression, anxiety, doubts, worry, or disappointment. It goes without saying that medication is, in most cases, not what is needed to solve the problem and move on to the next step in life.

5. There is also the possibility that medication should, in some cases, be avoided because it is positively bad (apart from its more immediate side effects, that is). This is an example offered by Kramer (1993): In his experience, Prozac tends to affect people's opinions about what it is to be oneself, it tends to redefine people's understanding of what is essential to them (what traits, etc. that are "me") and what is intrusive and pathological (i.e. "not-me"). "Suddenly those intimate and consistent traits are not-me, they are alien, they are defect, they are illness – so that a certain habit of mind and body that links a person to his relatives and ancestors from generation to generation is now 'other'" (Kramer, 1993, p. 19). It goes without saying that such a revision of what is "authentic" in the self might have bad consequences, and not just because of the confusion it gives rise to, but also because it tends to affect one's relationships in a negative way.

6. Another example of possible long-term negative effects is that people's personalities may sometimes change for the worse, e.g. the new personality may be "blander" and less complex than the old one, too many "character-giving wrinkles" may get "ironed out" (Kramer, 1993).

7. It might also be argued that "successful" treatment with antidepressants might be bad because it tends to constitute a threat to our desire for "internal responsibility for our lives" as well as to our desire "to find meaning in our errors" (Kramer, 1993, p. 13). The reason for this is those traits or attitudes that disappear as a result of medication (e.g. one's devotion to a certain person) tend to be viewed as merely a matter of biology. But we should regard it is an open question whether a certain anxiety is "meaningful" or "meaningless," shouldn't we?

These arguments do not show that one should abstain from using mood enhancers, but they strongly suggest that one should not take them mindlessly, e.g. that there are circumstances under which one should (for self-interested reasons) abstain from taking them. In this context, we should also note that mood enhancers may well have positive effects on the determinants of happiness, and that this would give us a good reason for taking them (in addition to their immediate effect). It has been shown that happiness has positive effects on some of its determinants, e.g. that happy people tend to be healthier and more social, that they have better relationships, and that they perform better (cf. Argyle, 2001; Layard, 2005; Oishi *et al.*, 2007). Now, the fact that "normally caused" happiness has positive effects on these determinants does not automatically imply that artificially induced mood enhancement has similar effects, but it is certainly possible. To what extent this is actually the case is an empirical question, where the answer is in part dependent on what neurophysiological mechanisms are involved (cf. Brülde, 2007).

Bad Effects on Society as a Whole?

Let us now turn to the arguments that purport to show that a widespread use of antidepressants and other mood-enhancing drugs will most likely have detrimental effects on society as a whole, compared to e.g. a widespread use of psychotherapy, or to no "treatment" at all. Why is an increase in "cosmetic psychopharmacology" regarded as bad? If we regard it as acceptable to use psychotherapy for enhancement purposes, why should we not consider it appropriate to use chemicals to modify people's personality in useful, attractive ways?

1. It might be argued that such a cosmetic use of mood-enhancing drugs would interact in unfortunate ways with certain tendencies of the broader culture. Firstly, it might reinforce perfectionist attitudes and make it harder to value human life in its imperfection, and this might actually have a detrimental effect on our happiness. Secondly, there is a risk that mood-enhancing drugs will be used to conform to certain (destructive?) social norms and values – e.g. the idea that a normal or real person is happy, outgoing, and energetic – and that it will thus reinforce these norms. (This is what Carl Elliot calls the problem of cultural complicity.) Other examples are how a widespread use of plastic surgery reinforces the norm that women with big breasts are more attractive, or that "Asian eyes" are less beautiful. Thirdly, the use of enhancement can sometimes be regarded as an expression of a certain immature or infantile attitude, namely an unwillingness or inability to accept one's own limitations, or even the human condition in general. A widespread use of "enhancement reasoning" can also reinforce these attitudes, e.g. by encouraging fantasies about eternal life or a life free from displeasure and suffering, which might be bad for us in the long run. This argument is based on the idea that a higher level of acceptance and maturity is good most for us, either in itself or because it tends to have positive effects on our long-term happiness.
2. If mood-enhancing technologies become available on the market, it is likely that the wealthy and privileged will gain an even bigger competitive advantage than they have at present, which is unfair. The competitive effects are due to the fact that an enhanced mood is not just valuable in itself: it also has positive effects on performance. For example, it is well established that happy people are more social, cooperative, agreeable, healthy, active, and that they have better relationships (cf. Argyle, 2001). Now, if everyone would have equal access to the relevant technologies, it could still be undesirable, since everyone would have to use stimulants to keep up with everybody else (what Carl Elliott calls a looping effect would be present: a new technology shapes society in a way that makes us more dependent on the very same technology).
3. There is a risk that we will permit successful medications to define what is health and what is illness. As Kramer (1993) points out, psychiatric diagnosis has already

been subject to a sort of "diagnostic bracket creep" – the expansion of categories to match the scope of the relevant medications; i.e. the idea that "if it responds to an antidepressant, it's depression" (p. 15). This means that there is a risk that less and less severe mood states (e.g. what is today regarded as an ordinary low mood) will be pathologized, and that a larger and larger sphere of human problems will be defined as medical. (This risk is most probably higher when the pharmaceutical companies operate in a market economy.) For example, certain dispositions now considered awkward or endearing, depending on taste (e.g. a romantic or decadent stance, melancholy or overseriousness), might be seen as medically correctable flaws: ailments to be pitied and, where possible, corrected. So, what is so bad about this? Well, apart from all the problems related to being labeled as ill (e.g. mentally ill), it might have detrimental effects on certain valuable practices, e.g. psycho-analysis and certain spiritual practices. Just like problems once regarded as spiritual are now widely regarded as psychological, many emotional problems might soon be regarded as medical problems.

4. The success of mood-enhancing drugs may give rise to a false view on what is and what isn't biologically determined, and to what extent. This is what Kramer writes about a woman who was successfully treated by Prozac:

> If her self-destructiveness with men and her fragility at work disappeared in response to a biological treatment, they must have been biologically encoded. Her biological constitution seems to have determined her social failures. But how does the belief that a woman who was abused as a child and later remains stuck in abusive relationships largely because of her biologically encoded temperament affect our notions of responsibility, of free will, of unique and socially determinative individual develop-ment? Are we willing to allow medications to tell us how we are constituted? (Kramer, 1993, p.18).

As it stands, this is certainly no valid argument: Of course we should be willing to hear the truth about how we are constituted. The problem is rather that it is quite tempting to simplify things in this area, e.g. that successes like the one above tend to amplify an already widespread simplistic biological determinism (a view that goes far beyond the scientific evidence, and which is partly for this reason, and partly because a widespread adoption of the view is so obviously in the interest of e.g. the pharmaceutical industry, best regarded as an ideology).

It is easy to imagine what effects the combination of a widespread biological view of man and the medicalization mentioned above might have in our contemporary culture. Suppose that someone suffers as a result of having been abused or neglected in childhood, or for structural reasons (because she belongs to an oppressed class, or the like). Here, a society which prefers to ignore certain issues, and that values economy over thoroughness in health care, is likely to medicate rather than to try to remove the roots of suffering. A widespread biological view of man might also bolster certain unfortunate individualist or antisocial tendencies, e.g. the idea that important problems need not be solved together with other people. In general, the biological view might (so to speak) undermine the value and importance of human interaction, or enhance a false view of society as consisting of a number of essentially disconnected individuals. In short, social efforts to improve our lot may become displaced by medications.

5. We may finally ask ourselves how the use of antidepressants for enhancement purposes can be distinguished from the street use of e.g. amphetamine, cocaine, or alcohol. In itself, this is not really an argument, but more of an invitation to guarantee that there is a fit between one's intuitions concerning licit drug use and those concerning illicit drug use.

What should we make of all this? Do these counter-arguments outweigh the obvious advantages that a successful use of mood-enhancing drugs might have for the individual and her loved ones? I leave it to the reader to do the balancing.

Conclusions

There are some cases where mood enhancement might be acceptable, even in a publicly funded system where resources are limited. If large improvements in mood can be achieved at very low cost, we should not object to this. Moreover, we should not forget that once new technologies are developed, there is no way to prevent them from being used for enhancement purposes. These technologies are bound to appear on the market, and it is important that we are prepared when this happens. Much reflection is still necessary on how these markets should be regulated (a question that I have deliberately avoided).

Notes

1. Nothing is gained by using the terms "health" or "disease" ("malady" or "disorder") in this context. "Health" can either be understood: (a) in terms of normal biological and physiological function (e.g. as absence of disease or impairment); (b) in terms of the physical and mental functioning of the person as a whole; (c) in terms of quality of life (or well-being); or (d) pluralistically, e.g. both in terms of functioning and well-being (Brülde 2000a, 2000b; Brülde & Tengland 2003). If we conceive of disorder as a phenomenon on the level of physiological function, we can see that the goal of combating disorder is also best regarded as a special case of (iv), i.e. the promotion of normal anatomical, biophysical or psychological structure and/our normal physiological and psychological function. Medicine should not just try to achieve this aim by combating disorder, however, but also by trying to eliminate or prevent injuries, defects, malnutrition and the like. If we, instead, conceive of disorder in symptomatic terms, the goal to combat disorder is rather as a special case of (i), (ii), and perhaps also (iii) and (v).
2. Similar views can be distinguished in the case of functioning, but this case is more complicated. The reason for this is that good functioning has instrumental rather than final value (it is good as a means rather than as an end), and that the connection between good functioning and the relevant final values (e.g. subjective well-being) is far from straightforward. In some cases, slight increases in functioning can give rise to big increases in well-being, but in other cases, big increases in functioning have no effects at all on well-being. The case of life expectancy is easier to deal with, however: A key issue here is whether we should always attribute the same "medical value" to each additional life year, i.e. whether each life year should be given the same weight, regardless of when during the life cycle it occurs. There are at least four possible answers to this question (if we ignore the view that the youngest should have absolute priority, or that a life year is worth less during infancy). (i) Each life year added is equally valuable (given a certain

acceptable level of health, etc). (ii) The older the person is, the less is the value of an additional year, i.e. the marginal value of a life is diminishing with increasing age. Medicine should work harder to prolong the lives of younger people. (iii) After a certain (high) age, an additional year is worth nothing from a medical perspective. Medicine should do nothing to save lives once a certain age has been attained. (iv) After e.g. the age of 90, an additional year still has value, but it is worth less (from a medical perspective) than it was before this age. Medicine should do less to save lives once a certain age has been attained.

3. It can also be argued that a person is less entitled to medical assistance if he is responsible for his own suffering, e.g. if his suffering is caused by an unhealthy lifestyle. There might be some plausibility in this view, but it is hardly applicable in practice, in part because it is often impossible to determine how much depends on lifestyle factors and how much depends on e.g. genetic factors.

References

Argyle, M. (2001). *The Psychology of Happiness*, 2nd edition. London: Routledge.

Brülde, B. (2000a). On how to define the concept of health: A loose comparative approach. *Medicine, Health Care and Philosophy*, **3**, 305–8.

Brülde, B. (2000b). More on the looser comparative approach to defining "health": A reply to Nordenfelt's reply. *Medicine, Health Care and Philosophy*, **3**, 313–15.

Brülde, B. (2001). The goals of medicine. towards a unified theory. *Health Care Analysis*, **9**, 1–13.

Brülde, B. (2007). Can successful mood enhancement make us less happy? *Philosophia*, **79**, 39–56.

Brülde, B. & Tengland, P.-A. (2003). *Hälsa och sjukdom – en begreppslig utredning [Health and Disorder – a conceptual analysis]*. Studentlitteratur. Lund: Studentlitteratur.

Diener, E. & Lucas R.E. (1999). Personality and subjective well-being. In D. Kahneman, E. Diener,& N. Schwarz (eds.), *Well-Being: The Foundations of Hedonistic Psychology* (pp. 213–29). New York: Russell Sage.

Headey, B. & Wearing, A. (1989). Personality, life events, and subjective well-being: Toward a dynamic equilibrium model. *Journal of Personality and Social Psychology*, **57**, 731–9.

Headey, B. & Wearing, A. (1991). Subjective well-being: A stocks and flows framework. In F. Strack, M. Argyle & N. Schwarz (eds.), *Subjective Well-Being: An Interdisciplinary Perspective* (pp. 49–73). Oxford: Pergamon Press.

Headey, B.W. & Wearing, A. (1992). *Understanding Happiness. A Theory of Subjective Well-Being*. Melbourne: Longman Cheshire.

Kramer, P.D. (1993). *Listening to Prozac: A Psychiatrist Explores Antidepressant Drugs and the Remaking of the Self*. New York: Viking.

Layard, R. (2005). *Happiness: Lessons from a New Science*. London: Allen Lane.

Lykken, D. & Tellegen, A. (1996). Happiness is a stochastic phenomenon. *Psychological Science*, **7**, 186–9.

Nordenfelt, L. (2001). On the goals of medicine, health enhancement and social welfare. *Health Care Analysis*, **9**, 15–23.

Oishi, S., Diener, E. & Lucas, R.E. (2007). The optimum level of well-being: Can people be too happy? *Perspectives on Psychological Science*, **2**, 346–60.

Tellegen, A., Lykken, D.T., Bouchard, T.J., Wilcox, K.J., Segal, N.L. & Rich, S. (1988). Personality similarity in twins reared apart and together. *Journal of Personality and Social Psychology*, **54**, 1031–9.

Tännsjö, T. (1993). Should we change the human genome? *Theoretical Medicine*, **14**, 231–47.

16

Cognitive Therapy and Positive Psychology Combined: A Promising Approach to the Enhancement of Happiness

Tony Hope

The Café Dôme in Paris was a meeting place for the literati, Sartre included, until it became popular with soldiers from the occupying forces in 1940. There is a story, probably from the 1920s, told by Geoffrey Fraser (1996).[1]

> An old man comes in, hatless, stumpy, with greyish hair and beard, fine eyes and a laughing mouth... "Who's that?" "Don't know his name – only thing I do know is he hasn't had a room these last years." "No room? Where does he sleep?" "In cafés here and there. They all know him around here."

> ...I remember once catching a glimpse of one of the world's richest men; a little, crabbed, wizened old creature, sour discontent etched on his face. And this homeless old man is radiating with happiness and love.

Some people seem to find happiness despite adverse circumstances; others born "with a silver spoon in their mouth" notice only the taste of tarnish. It would be callous to argue that circumstances don't matter, or to sideline the importance of social justice, but happiness, it seems, is as much about how we think about ourselves and the world, as it is about the world itself. For Hamlet, Denmark is a prison: "...for there is nothing either good or bad but thinking makes it so" (Shakespeare, *Hamlet,* Act 2, scene 2). In short, there is a strong cognitive component to our experiences of happiness.

A lesson from cognitive behavior therapy (CBT) is that it is possible for people to change their beliefs and attitudes in ways that enhance mood. Although the focus of CBT has of course been on helping people who have problems and disorders – people for example who are depressed – there seems no theoretical barrier to using the insights and methods of CBT to *enhance* mood. The rapidly growing field of positive psychology – the scientific exploration of happiness and human flourishing – is indeed providing support for the importance of the way people think about

Enhancing Human Capacities, edited by Julian Savulescu, Ruud ter Meulen and Guy Kahane.
© 2011 Blackwell Publishing Ltd

themselves and the world in their overall level of happiness. If we want to enhance human happiness, therefore, a promising approach is to combine the insights from positive psychology with the theory and practice of cognitive behavior therapy.

What is Cognitive Behavior Therapy?

Cognitive behavior therapy is a psychological treatment originally developed to help people suffering from depression. Over the last 40 years it has greatly expanded both in the range of psychological disorders that it addresses and in the number of techniques that it uses. It is now routinely used in the treatment of various anxiety disorders, obsessive-compulsive disorder, eating disorders, post-traumatic stress disorder, and increasingly as part of the therapy for people with psychotic illnesses. It is even used for non-psychological disorders, for example in the management of tinnitus – the unpleasant constant high-pitched ringing in the ears that some people suffer and that Smetana incorporated into his first string quartet.

The underlying theoretical basis for CBT is that the cognitive model has two main aspects:

1. The idea of causal two-way interactions between thoughts, feelings and mood, behavior, and physiology. According to this model, for example, depressed mood increases the salience of depressed thoughts (miserable memories; negative self-judgment), and depressed thoughts lead to a further lowering in mood. A vicious cycle of depressed mood and thoughts is set up each enhancing the other leading to an ever lowering of mood, or at best, the maintenance of low mood.
2. That thoughts (cognitions) are the major (although not exclusive) focus for change. Cognitive behavior therapy works mainly through helping people to replace their negative thoughts by more positive thoughts, thus reversing the vicious cycle.

Cognitive behavior therapy borrows heavily from the Western philosophical tradition of rationality. First is the idea that exploring and providing reasons is an appropriate way to the truth. The idea of client and therapist engaged in a mutual rational process comes explicitly from Plato's dialogues. Second, CBT aims to use rational methods to bring about change. Third, it puts great value on respecting client autonomy, and in its understanding of autonomy it makes use not simply of the idea of respecting capacitous choice, but the view that to respect autonomy is to respect those choices based on reasons. CBT also puts great store on the use of empirical studies (such as randomized controlled studies) to test and develop its effectiveness.

What is Positive Psychology?

Martin Seligman (2005) wrote:

> The aim of positive psychology is to catalyze a change in psychology from a preoccupation only with repairing the worst things in life to also building the best qualities...we must

bring the building of strengths to the forefront in the treatment and prevention of mental illness. . . . The field of positive psychology at the subjective level is about positive subjective experience: well-being and satisfaction (past); flow, joy, the sensual pleasures, and happiness (present); and constructive cognitions about the future – optimism, hope, and faith.

Positive psychology would include the scientific study of environmental factors that enhance mood and other aspects of human flourishing. In this chapter I will discuss mainly how the ideas from positive psychology combined with the therapeutic methods developed in CBT might provide ways of helping individuals to enhance their mood and increase happiness.

There have been some initial and tentative programs to enhance individual happiness although these predate the recent rapid expansion in research in positive psychology (Fordyce, 1977, 1983; Lichter *et al.*, 1980)[2,3], In addition, both solutions-based therapy (O'Connell, 2005) and well-being therapy (Fava, 1999; Fava et al., 1998), although used as therapy, have many elements that suggests they may have value for enhancement. Modern CBT has proven to be an extraordinarily flexible therapy able to absorb and assimilate new ideas and techniques notably of mindfulness, acceptance, and compassion. There seems every likelihood that CBT can be developed to incorporate the ideas and findings from positive psychology and used as a basis for programs that can contribute to human mood enhancement.

What is Happiness?

Central to the field of positive psychology is the meaning and measurement of happiness. While some philosophers tell us that "happiness" is far too vague a concept to be meaningful (White, 2006), let alone measurable, there are whole departments of psychologists able to measure it to three decimal places.

I am reminded of Majikthise, a representative of the Amalgamated Union of Philosophers, Sages, Luminaries and Other Thinking Persons, who fears for his job as the computer, Deep Thought, begins calculating the answer to the Ultimate Question of Life, the Universe, and Everything. "I mean" Majikthise say, "what's the use of our sitting up half the night arguing that there may or may not be a God if this machine . . . gives you his bleeding phone number the next morning?" (Adams, 1979).

There are three fundamentally different concepts that psychologists measure (Nettle, 2005):

1. Happiness as a subjective experience. On this view at any moment each of us is experiencing a particular level of happiness or unhappiness. This is the approach of "quantitative hedonism."
2. Happiness as a judgment that each of us can make about our feelings and life experiences. This might be called the "life-satisfaction approach."
3. Happiness as a multidimensional concept covering many aspects of what we might judge to be the various components of a happy and fulfilled life. This might be called the "flourishing approach."

Each approach is associated with a different approach to measurement.

Quantitative hedonism (Kahneman & Riis, 2005) is most clearly measured by asking people to give a quantitative measure as to how happy they feel at this moment on some suitably defined scale. Total happiness over any particular period of time is simply the integral of these *moment utilities*. Kahneman calls this integral *experienced well-being*. Alternatively one can ask people to give a single average measure over a period of time (e.g. over the previous 24 hours). In practice, however, when people are asked to give a single measure of happiness over time they don't so much remember (and integrate) the *moment utilities* as evaluate their overall well-being – what Kahneman calls *evaluated well-being*. There are pros and cons of each of these approaches, but they are not measuring the same thing and they give different, and often contradictory, results.

For both practical and theoretical reasons, therefore, many measures of well-being are essentially evaluations of people's own satisfaction with life over longer or shorter periods of time (Diener *et al.*, 2004). A problem for all self-evaluated measures is the question of whether, for example, my report of, say, seven on a scale means something quite different from your report of seven (Diener et al. 2005).

There is a long history, going back to Aristotle, of a concept of happiness that is multidimensional and, more importantly, where the dimensions are determined not by each individual but are seen as intrinsic to the concept. The term in English usually used for this concept of happiness is "flourishing."

Much of modern positive psychology seeks to investigate the conditions for what one might call a "flourishing" life. The crucial difference between this concept, and the two that I have outlined above, is that a flourishing life includes marked value judgments that are imposed by the experimenter on the participant. Csikszentmihalyi 's concept of "flow" is one example (see discussion below; Csikszentmihalyi, 1992; Nakamura & Csikszentmihalyi, 2005). Another is Seligman and Petersen's 24 human strengths (see Seligman, 2003, page 13). Leadership, for example, is on the list of strengths, but not (as Haidt, 2006, has pointed out) some characteristics of "followers" such as duty, respect, and obedience; neither is independence listed as a strength. This concept of strengths is not whatever an individual client sees as strengths but it is an objective list culled from many sources and endorsed by Seligman and Petersen.

One implication of the different approaches to the concept of happiness is that in developing ways of enhancing mood, and increasing individual happiness, we will need to make some decisions about precisely what we mean by happiness. Which of the concepts outlined above is the one we want to enhance? One of the lessons to be learned from CBT is the value of the scientific approach – to carrying out empirical studies in order to find out what works and develop increasingly effective interventions. Such scientific studies require outcome measures. A position of philosophical paralysis over what is meant by happiness will lead only to stagnation.

Evolution and the Emotions

There is no single theory that provides a unifying structure to the diffuse area of positive psychology. In the absence of such a theory I believe that the best single perspective from which to gain an understanding of positive psychology is that of evolutionary psychology, even though it is underdeveloped and contentious. Evolutionary psychology bridges the gap between individual history and the general features of the human condition that helps to explain both our capacity for happiness and some of the barriers to achieving it. It provides, if not causal theories, at least useful metaphors that can assist both therapists and clients. Of central importance to the issue of the enhancement of human happiness is the idea, which I discuss below, that there may be good evolutionary reasons why we are not in general as happy as we (rationally) should be – at least those of us who have been relatively lucky in the environment in which we live. Such evolutionary reasons are a barrier to happiness, but there are no overwhelming grounds for believing that they are an insuperable barrier.

The modern general evolutionary view of emotions is that they help animals in regulating their effort: how they behave at any one time and how they apportion their time and energy between different types of behavior. Different emotions are connected with different situations and "decisions," and are directed towards different behavior. A broad division can be made between negative emotions, connected with avoidant behavior and precipitated by loss or threat of loss, and positive emotions connected with approach and sustaining behavior.

Why do we have negative emotions?

Consider the gazelle feeding in the savannah, on the look out for predators. Its (perhaps rudimentary) emotion is anxiety, turning to fear when it sees the cheetah. It runs for its life. Could the fear – the emotion that drives the behavior to run away – have been pleasant rather than unpleasant?

If the sensation of fear were pleasant then the gazelle would be rewarded for grazing where cheetahs are common and able to approach. The gazelle would tend to seek out dangerous places. Such gazelles would be prone to an early grave. Their cousins, those gazelles that found the sensation of fear aversive, would be fitter, in the evolutionary sense.

There are therefore good reasons why, once there is the possibility of emotions, the emotions associated with loss or threat of loss are negative.

The dominance of negative emotions: the life/dinner question (Nettle, 2005)

Our poor gazelle is being chased by a cheetah. Which animal should run for longer? The answer is the gazelle. If it is caught it will die. It should keep running until it is about to drop dead from exhaustion. The cheetah, if it gives up too soon, will get no dinner today, but there is a good chance that it will find a dinner in time to prevent starvation. Indeed it will need to be sufficiently healthy to have a good chance of killing the next prospective dinner that happens to wander by. The cheetah should give up running before it suffers significant ill-health from exhaustion.

The fear program therefore should consume almost all of the gazelle's attention and should run until the gazelle is at the point of death. The cheetah's desire program on the other hand should run for some time but should be overridden by other considerations: pain from a stiffening joint, the sight of an easier dinner, or excessive tiredness.

There are therefore good evolutionary reasons for an asymmetry between the fear system and the desire system – and more generally between negative and positive emotions. Negative emotions (some at least) are very powerful at gaining our full attention and at persisting. Evolutionary psychologists argue (Buss, 2000; Nesse, 2005; Nettle, 2005) that we feel the evolutionary legacy of this asymmetry, even though it no longer serves us well, for example when we lie awake all night worrying.

The smoke detector analogy

A second reason why we may suffer negative emotions more than seems useful, at least at first sight, is the smoke detector principle. If the cost of not detecting the danger is very grave and much worse than the cost of falsely detecting a danger then it will be best to set the alarm system such that it gives warning very easily – i.e. that the number of false positives is relatively high. No wonder that our alarm systems, such as anxiety, are easily triggered. This was useful in the savannah. In many modern settings where the real physical dangers are very low indeed, this sensitivity of the anxiety system causes unnecessary distress.

Why negative emotions are often inappropriate

The greater physical dangers that threatened us back in the mists of our evolutionary past is one reason why we are prone to negative emotions that no longer serve us well. Buss (2000) argues that the single most important evolutionarily determined barrier to human happiness is the vastly different size of human groups between the time when many of our emotions were being developed and now. Competition between individuals – for status, or sexual partners – and the emotions associated with comparing ourselves with others (such as envy) probably developed within small groups (of 20–150 individuals). In many domains we can now compare ourselves with some of the best people in the world. An emotion that effectively spurs us on within the small group setting and causes only limited unpleasant sensations becomes a constant source of negativity as we strive for what is completely out of our reach.

A further evolutionary reason for the power of negative emotions is that evolutionary adaptation is designed for competition. Much of evolutionary pressure is about differences between individuals: differential reproductive success, for example, rather than the absolute success. Thus: "humans have evolved psychological mechanisms designed to inflict costs on others, to gain advantage at the expense of others" (Buss, 2000). Since one person's happiness depends partly on another's misery there are evolutionary problems with increasing the happiness of all.

The purpose of positive emotions

Positive emotions are generally those that lead to approach behavior. Modern evolutionary psychologists see positive emotions as valuable in two general situations:

1. in situations that offer a range of opportunities; and
2. in situations where progress is swifter than expected.

Positive emotions, it is thought, are directed at enabling the animal to be open to and curious about the environment. This is valuable in helping to build resources, whether social or physical resources. It is appropriate when physical danger is low. A high-ranking female primate, for example, will in general be able to occupy a safer position (e.g. in a tree) than one lower in rank; and will be positioned in a more secure position within the troupe. Such an animal will be able to devote most of its attention to searching out and eating fruit and in creating social ties, say with a high-ranking male. A higher ratio of positive to negative emotion would be appropriate in such a female compared with a lower ranking individual who will be in greater danger from predators.

The elephant and the rider

The psychologist Jonathan Haidt uses the metaphor of a rider on an elephant to summarize the picture that is developing from both evolutionary psychology and the neuroscience of emotions. The rider is that part of us that can reason consciously. The "elephant" represents our usually barely conscious emotions and judgments. "Reason and emotion," he writes (2006), "must work together to create intelligent behaviour, but emotion (a major part of the elephant) does most of the work. When the neocortex came along, it made the rider possible, but it made the elephant much smarter too." The analogy is not fully worked through but it provides, I believe, a picture that might be useful in considering approaches to mood enhancement. The "elephant" represents our emotions and automatic responses (and for Haidt also our moral "gut feelings"). These can be triggered, without our having much conscious control, by a variety of situations and include both negative and positive emotions. They are determined principally by our evolutionary past and for this reason the "elephant's" reactions are often no longer appropriate to our current situation and often dominated by negative emotions that keep us on the alert for danger, or striving to better ourselves within our social group. Part of Haidt's purpose in the image of the elephant (rather than choosing a lower, or less intelligent animal) is to suggest that the elephant can, under guidance from the rider, come to respond differently and more appropriately, but this will need the rider to understand the nature of the elephant's behavior and it is likely to take time: the elephant is unlikely to respond to a single flash of cognitive insight.

Some Key Ideas and Findings from Positive Psychology Relevant to Developing Methods for Mood Enhancement

(1) There is a significant genetic component to happiness[4]

There are three reasons to be pessimistic about the possibility of increasing personal happiness, but none is convincing.

1. Twin studies suggest that 50–70% of variance in happiness is genetically determined.
2. Happiness is strongly correlated with personality type.
3. The average happiness of most people is remarkably constant over time.

These three facts have led to the idea that we each have a "happiness set point" and that there is very little that we can do to significantly alter our average happiness: that we may have ups and downs but we will always in general revert to the same level of happiness.

Such pessimism is not justified. The genetic data can be reframed as showing that 30–50% of the variance in happiness is not accounted for by genetic factors and may be the result of factors that can be changed. More importantly from the fact that a large proportion of the variance is genetically determined it does not follow that the only way to alter happiness is through altering one's genetic make-up. The variance in the number of life events that a person experiences over a year is largely accounted for by genetic differences. But life events are not generally the direct result of people's genes. There are intermediate causes, such as risk-taking behavior, and many of these intermediate causes can be altered once one knows what they are. The same is likely to be true with happiness.

The three factors cited above are not grounds for pessimism. They show us that at the moment few of us take effective steps to increase happiness. Learning what these steps are and how they can be taken is a major task for positive psychology and the practice of enhancement.

(2) Happiness is relatively independent of circumstances

Despite large increases in wealth over the last 40 years in many Western countries there has been no increase in happiness. The variation in happiness between countries is not strongly correlated with wealth. There is remarkably little difference in happiness between healthy people and those with quite significant disability. Happiness appears surprisingly immune from many external circumstances, as the Café Dôme anecdote (above) suggests.

Perhaps then it is the way that people think that is important. "We must understand the cognitive and motivational processes that serve to maintain or enhance both enduring happiness and transient mood" (Lyubomirsky, 2001). The time seems ripe for developing a cognitive therapy for happiness.

(3) Wanting, liking and the increase in happiness

Common-sense psychology tells us that the reason we want something is because we like it; but modern neuroscience distinguishes wanting from liking. If an electrode placed in a rat's lateral hypothalamus is stimulated the rat will eat more; but its facial expression shows that it does not enjoy the food. It wants food but does not like it. Conversely when given drugs blocking the dopamine system the rat will starve in the midst of plenty. If the food is placed on the rat's tongue its facial expression shows that it likes it (Nettle, 2005).

Wanting and liking are logically, and neurologically, distinct. Just because we want something it doesn't necessarily give us pleasure or an increase our happiness. In developing ways to enhance happiness it will be important to shift people's motivation from following those desires (addictions are an extreme case) that do not lead to happiness.

(4) Adaptation

One of the most startling early findings of positive psychology – startling that is if you are not steeped in the writings of the ancient stoics – is how short-lived the boost in happiness is for those who win large amounts of money on the lottery.[5] This phenomenon is called *adaptation*: the tendency to re-center ourselves, or return to our previous level of happiness, when circumstances change. Adaptation occurs not only to most material gains, once we can comfortably cover the basics in life, but also, to a considerable extent, to disability.

There are good evolutionary reasons for adaptation. In situations where resources are relatively scarce there is a great deal of survival value to the pursuit of material goods and to increasing one's social status. But once a new level has been reached evolution favors those who continue striving; it has little interest in our happiness. Evolution shapes us to be caught on a "hedonic treadmill."[6]

The pursuit of financial success not only fails to bring the happiness that people often expect. Evidence from studies of U.S. college students suggest that those for whom money-related values are central have lower levels of well-being than those whose values are less materialistic (Kasser & Ryan, 1993).

We do not adapt to all changes. People adapt poorly to constant noise and to commuting by car. On the positive side we do not adapt to the happiness that close relationships bring nor to the increases in happiness that come with experiences such as holidays.

The implications of this for enhancement are that if people wish to increase their well-being then pursuing some goals are more likely to be effective than pursuing other goals, such as money and material goods, and that the immediate gain in happiness in achieving a goal is not a good guide to its effect on longer-term happiness.

(5) Comparison – the tiptoe effect

There are evolutionary reasons why we are "programmed" to compare ourselves and to feel bad if we feel we come out poorly from such comparison: those higher in social hierarchy had better chances of survival.

Economists make a useful distinction between positional and non-positional goods. Positional goods are those we value principally because they are markers of our success compared to others. They are the goods we want others to know about. Non-positional goods are valued for themselves – and consumed more privately. "If everyone stands on tiptoe no-one sees any further" and so it is with positional goods. The two reasons why there has been no increase in general happiness in the United Kingdom or United States over the last 40y years is probably a combination of adaptation to increased wealth, and the "tiptoe" effect: that much of wealth is about comparison with others.

Positional goods are a "zero-sum" game. If I buy a smart new Mercedes I might be a little happier (though that won't last for long), but my neighbor is sadder. Overall there is no gain in human happiness.

(6) We are poor at predicting what will make us happy

The previous three findings add up to making us poor at predicting what will make us happy. Our desires are not a reliable guide; we will adapt to many of the things that bring us temporary happiness; and striving to get ahead of others is likely to end in a treadmill of endless striving. It seems that we are very bad at allowing for all these effects. Indeed, Gilbert (2006) argues that we are better predictors of the effects of our choices on our happiness if we leave our own imaginations aside and rely on the reports of people who have made the change we are contemplating. This is why a science of happiness should be able to help enhancement: it will clarify what does make us happy, so that we can rely on proper evidence and not the set of psychological drivers that evolution has rather unhelpfully left us with.

"If money doesn't buy you happiness, you don't know where to shop." The economist Robert Frank (2006) has taken this old joke seriously and used the findings of positive psychology to propose a shopping list for those who do wish to buy happiness. His list looks like this (assuming the basics of food and decent shelter):

1. Time with family and friends
2. Decreasing commuting even if this means living in a smaller house
3. Longer holidays
4. Investing money for future consumption
5. Spend on "inconspicuous" not "conspicuous" consumption – i.e. on goods and activities that are valued for themselves and consumed privately rather than on goods visible to others that have their value (and their price) because of how you think others will see you (designer labels).

I showed this to my 17-year-old daughter but her answer to buying happiness was more shoes: stylish footwear for the hedonic treadmill.

(7) Relationships and some other things that make us happy

If so little of what we strive for will make us happier, what can we do that will be of help? The overwhelming finding from positive psychology is the importance of relationships, and particularly deep relationships.[7] There is also evidence that altruism makes people happier (Haidt, 2006; Piliavin 2003). Control over our lives both in large and small matters is another important and sustained source of happiness (Schulz, 1976),[8] as is doing things that give us a sense of value. This sense of value can come not only from relationships but from gaining knowledge, doing one's job well, or being good at a skill such as sport.

Underlying rational choice theory is the idea that people are best off if they make choices to maximize their preferences or values. The more choices they have, the better. Rational choice theory, however, makes many assumptions about the psychology of how people make decisions that turn out to be wrong (Kahneman & Tversky, 2000). Those who tend to try to maximize good outcomes ("maximisers") are generally less happy, are less satisfied with consumer decisions, are affected more negatively by social comparison, and more sensitive to regret than "satisficers" (those who tend to be concerned only to make decisions that are good enough) (Schwartz *et al.*, 2002).

Some further general rules that seem to enhance happiness are: if you must compare yourself to others do so only to your advantage (Lyubomirsky & Ross, 1997); count your blessings (what your grandmother always told you) (Emmons & McCullough, 2003; Emmons & Shelton, 2005; Lyubomirsky *et al.*, 2006; Tennen & Affleck, 2005); and, savor your pleasures (Lyubomirsky *et al.*, 2006; Wrzesniewski *et al.*, 2003).

(8) The concept of "flow"

The concept of "flow experiences" has received a great deal of attention in the positive psychology literature. The idea originated from studying creativity. Csikszentmihalyi was struck by the fact that creative people, for example artists, persisted with their work, when it was going well, disregarding hunger, fatigue, and discomfort (Nakamura & Csikszentmihalyi, 2005). Across a wide range of activities and people, sport, the arts, science, surgery, and leisure activities, people described a similar experience that they valued greatly: a sense of intense concentration on what one is doing in the present; a loss of self-awareness; forgetting the passing of time; a sense that one can "in principle deal with the situation because one knows how to respond to whatever happens next" (Nakamura & Csikszentmihalyi, 2005). This experience is intrinsically rewarding and arises from activities that are intrinsically and immediately rewarding.

Flow experience occurs during those activities that people find challenging and that use their skills. If the task is too challenging the experience turns to frustration, if insufficiently challenging it turns to boredom. Tasks leading to "flow" have clear goals (most sports are a good example) and immediate and accurate feedback about the person's movement towards those goals. Carr (2004) summarizes how one might create flow within an activity:

1. Set an overall goal and break this down into a number of sub-goals.
2. Decide on a way of measuring progress towards the chosen goals.
3. Concentrate on doing the activity as well as you can while doing it.
4. Gradually increase the complexity of the sub-goals you are aiming for.

Flow is not the same as happiness; there is something of the work ethic about it. "Flow" activities (high challenge, high skill) are associated (at least among American adolescents) with high concentration; high importance to future goals; and high self-esteem. But the category that rates highest for enjoyment and "wish to be doing activity" are those activities in the category of low challenge, high skill. So if it is current enjoyment you are after then flow activities are more of a challenge than is ideal.

Positive Psychology and CBT: Theoretical Links

If the findings of positive psychology are to be transformed into a program of mood enhancement then there will be two broad aspects to such a program: creating a better environment; and helping individuals. It is the second of these that is the concern of this chapter. I believe that CBT provides a good basis for the development of individualized programs for mood enhancement not only because it has demonstrated its ability to improve mood in those who are depressed but also because of theoretical links between positive psychology and CBT.

One of the few underlying theories of positive emotions, Fredrickson's (2005) broaden-and-build model, is essentially cognitive in nature. If this theory is at least in part correct then it suggests that the well-tried methods of CBT will be effective in building positive emotions. The "build" part of this theory is an example of a positive, virtuous cycle. She writes: "positive emotions not only make people feel good in the present, but also – by broadening thinking and building resources – positive emotions increase the likelihood that people will feel good in the future" (Fredrickson, 2005). This third part of the theory "casts positive emotions in a far more consequential role in the story of human welfare" (Fredrickson, 2005). Positive emotions are not simply markers or constituents of well-being: they help to produce well-being and physical health. "Positive emotions fuel human flourishing" (Fredrickson, 2005).

Furthermore some new theoretical ideas in CBT are particularly pertinent to enhancement. Teasdale (1997) has borrowed and developed the idea of a "mind in place" from Ornstein. Teasdale suggests that it is useful to think of ourselves as having many minds although one may be dominant at any one time and could be considered as the current "mind in place." We are, psychologically speaking, like a suite of minds, one of which is dominant, at least from the point of view of consciousness, at any one time. Mood disorders (depression is the example that Teasdale uses) can be thought of as minds in this sense, and minds that tend to be particularly persistent at being "in place." The point of therapy is not so much to chip away at the thoughts that maintain the mood disorder (as the classical cognitive model might have it) but to help clients to bring another, more pleasant and effective, mind into place – shifting the mind that is the mood disorder out of the way. Therapy, and indeed a program for individual mood enhancement, might usefully be directed at building up minds associated with positive emotions helping them to gain strength and to become elaborated.

Conclusion

Cognitive behavior therapy has shown itself to be remarkably flexible in being able to incorporate both theoretical and practical ideas from a range of sources. The rapidly growing field of positive psychology is providing information on, among other things, the psychology of individual happiness. Mood enhancement, I have suggested, might fruitfully be tackled at the individual level, through a combination of these two areas of psychology.

What both CBT and much of positive psychology share is the idea that cognitions are central to our functioning. Sartre went further. In his novel *Nausea* (*La Nausée*) which he published in 1937, and which he may well have partly written while smoking at the Dôme: "My thought is *me*:. . .I exist by what I think."

Notes

1. From Geoffrey Fraser in *Paris Tribune* (quoting p.3 of Graf, 1996).
2. Self-help books on happiness include: Baker and Stauth, 2003 and Hoggard, 2005.
3. One involving group discussions of the practical implications of "pro-happy" and "anti-happy" beliefs; the other involving reading 18 positive statements each morning.
4. Well reviewed in Nettle, 2005 and Layard, 2006.
5. Discussed widely, e.g. in Nettle, 2005, Layard, 2006, and Frank, 2005.
6. The term "hedonic treadmill" was first coined by Brickman and Campbell – see Nettle, 2005, p. 76.
7. For reviews see Reis and Gable, 2003, and Layard, 2006.
8. See Bandura, 1997, for a comprehensive review of self-efficacy, control, and well-being.

References

Adams, D. (1979). *The Hitch-Hiker's Guide to the Galaxy*. London: Pan Books.

Baker, D. & Stauth, C. (2003). *What Happy People Know*. Element (HarperCollins).

Bandura, A. (1997). *Self-efficacy: The Exercise of Control*. New York: Freeman.

Buss, D. (2000). The evolution of happiness. *American Psychologist*, **55**, 15–23.

Carr, A. (2004). *Positive Psychology: The Science of Happiness and Human Strengths*. Hove: Brunner-Routledge.

Csikszentmihalyi, M. (1992). *Flow*. New York: Harper & Row.

Diener, E. *et al.* (2004). Satisfaction with life scale. In A. Carr. (ed.), *Positive Psychology: The Science of Happiness and Human Strengths*. Hove: Brunner-Routledge.

Diener, E., Lucas, R. & Oishi, S. (2005). Subjective well-being: The science of happiness and life satisfaction. In C.R. Snyder & S. Lopez (eds.), *Handbook of Positive Psychology* (pp. 63–73). Oxford: Oxford University Press.

Emmons, R. & McCullough, M. (2003). Counting blessings versus burdens: An experimental investigation of gratitude and subjective well-being in daily life. *Journal of Personality and Social Psychology*, **84**, 377–89.

Fava, G. (1999). Well-being therapy: Conceptual and technical issues. *Psychotherapy and Psychodynamics*, **68**, 171–9.

Fava, G., Rafanelli, C., Cazzaro, M., Conti, S. & Grandi, S. (1998). Well-being therapy. A novel psychotherapeutic approach for residual symptoms of affective disorders. *Psychological Medicine*, **28**, 475–80.

Fordyce, M. (1977). Development of a programme to increase personal happiness. *Journal of Counselling Psychology*, **24**, 511–20.

Fordyce, M. (1983). A programme to increase personal happiness: Further studies. *Journal of Counselling Psychology*, **30**, 483–8.

Frank, R. (2005). Does money buy happiness? In F.A. Huppert, N. Baylis & B. Keverne (eds.), *The Science of Well-being* (pp. 461–73). Oxford: Oxford. University Press.

Frank, R. (2006). Luxury Fever. In J. Haidt (ed.), *The Happiness Hypothesis: Putting Ancient Wisdom and Philosophy to the Test of Modern Science*. London: Heinemann.

Fredrickson, B. (2005a). Positive emotions. In C.R. Snyder & S. Lopez (eds.), *Handbook of Positive Psychology* (pp. 120–35). Oxford: Oxford University Press.

Fredrickson, B. (2005b). The broaden-and-build theory of positive emotions. In F.A. Huppert, N. Baylis & B. Keverne (eds.), *The Science of Well-being* (pp. 217–38). Oxford: Oxford. University Press.

Gilbert, D. (2006), *Stumbling on Happiness*. London: HarperCollins.

Graf, C. (1996). *The Cafés of Paris: A Guide*. London: Constable.

Haidt, J. (2006). *The Happiness Hypothesis: Putting Ancient Wisdom and Philosophy to the Test of Modern Science*. London: Heinemann.

Hoggard, L. (2005). *How to be Happy*. London: BBC Books.

Kahneman, D. & Riis, J. (2005). Living, and thinking about it: Two perspectives on life. In F.A. Huppert, N. Baylis & B. Keverne (eds.), *The Science of Well-being* (pp. 285–304). Oxford: Oxford. University Press.

Kahneman, D. & Tversky, A. (eds.) (2000). *Choices, Values and Frames*. New York: Cambridge University Press.

Kasser, T. & Ryan, R. (1993). A dark side of the American dream. Correlates of financial success as a central life aspiration. *Journal of Personality and Social Psychology*, **65**, 410–22.

Layard, R. (2006). *Happiness: Lessons from a New Science*. London: Penguin.

Lichter, S., Haye, K. & Kamman, R. (1980). Increasing happiness through cognitive training. *New Zealand Psychologist*, **9**, 57–64.

Lyubomirsky, S. & Ross, L. (1997). Hedonic consequences of social comparison: A contrast of happy and unhappy people. *Journal of Personality and Social Psychology*, **73**, 1141–57.

Lyubomirsky, S. (2001). Why are some people happier than others? The role of cognitive and motivational processes in well-being. *American Psychologist*, **56**, 239–49.

Lyubomirsky, S., Sousa, L. & Dickerhoof, R. (2006). The costs and benefits of writing, talking, and thinking about life's triumphs and defeats. *Journal of Personality and Social Psychology*, **90**, 692–708.

Emmons, R. & Shelton, C. (2005). Gratitude and the science of positive psychology. In C.R. Snyder & S. Lopez (eds.), *Handbook of Positive Psychology* (pp. 459–71). Oxford: Oxford University Press.

Nakamura, J. & Csikszentmihalyi, M. (2005). The concept of flow. In C.R. Snyder & S. Lopez (eds.), *Handbook of Positive Psychology* (pp. 89–105). Oxford: Oxford University Press.

Nesse, R. (2005). Natural selection and the elusiveness of happiness. In F.A. Huppert, N. Baylis & B. Keverne (eds.), *The Science of Well-being* (pp. 3–32). Oxford: Oxford. University Press.

Nettle, D. (2005). *Happiness: The Science Behind Your Smile*. Oxford: Oxford University Press.

O'Connell, B. (2005). *Solution-Focused Therapy*, second edition. London: Sage.

Piliavin, J. (2003). Doing well by doing good: Benefits for the benefactor. In C.L.M. Keyes & J. Haidt (eds.), *Flourishing: Positive Psychology and the Life Well Lived* (pp. 227–47). Washington, DC: American Psychological Association.

Reis, H. & Gable, S. (2003). Towards a positive psychology of relationships. In C.L.M. Keyes & J. Haidt (eds.), *Flourishing: Positive Psychology and the Life Well Lived* (pp. 129–59). Washington, DC: American Psychological Association.

Schulz, R. (1976). Effects of control and predictability on the physical and psychological well-being of the institutionalized aged. *Journal of Personality and Social Psychology*, **33**, 563–73.

Schwartz, B., Ward, A., Lyubomirsky, S., Monterosso, J., White, K. & Lehman, D. (2002). Maximizing versus satisficing: Happiness is a matter of choice. *Journal of Personality and Social Psychology*, **83**, 1178–197.

Seligman, M. (2003). *Authentic Happiness: Using the New Positive Psychology to Realize Your Potential for Lasting Fulfilment*. London: Nicholas Brearley.

Seligman, M. (2005). Positive psychology, positive prevention, and positive therapy. In C.R. Snyder & S. Lopez (eds.), *Handbook of Positive Psychology* (pp. 3–9). Oxford: Oxford University Press.

Teasdale, J. (1997). The relationship between cognition and emotion: The mind-in-place in mood disorders. In D. Clark & C. Fairburn (eds.), *Science and Practice of Cognitive Behaviour Therapy*. Oxford: Oxford University Press.

Tennen, H. & Affleck, G. (2005). Benefit-finding and benefit-reminding. In C.R. Snyder & S. Lopez (eds.), *Handbook of Positive Psychology* (pp. 584–97). Oxford: Oxford University Press.

White, N. (2006). *A Brief History of Happiness*. Oxford: Blackwell Publishing.

Wrzesniewski, A., Rozin, P. & Bennett, G. (2003). Working, playing, and eating: Making the most of most moments. In C.L.M. Keyes & J. Haidt (eds.), *Flourishing: Positive Psychology and the Life Well Lived* (pp. 185–204). Washington, DC: American Psychological Association.

17

After Prozac

S. Matthew Liao and Rebecca Roache

Introduction

In *Listening to Prozac*, the psychiatrist Peter Kramer (1993) describes the dilemma he faced when patients cured of their depression by Prozac asked him to continue prescribing the drug in order to help them feel "better than well":

> After about eight months off medication, Tess told me she was slipping. "I'm not myself," she said. New union negotiations were under way, and she felt she could use the sense of stability, the invulnerability to attack, that Prozac gave her. Here was a dilemma for me. Ought I to provide medication to someone who was not depressed?

Kramer's account illustrates both the striking transformative possibilities of pharmacological mood enhancers, and that there is a demand for such enhancers among those who know of these possibilities.

Despite the furor that followed Prozac's introduction in the late 1980s, which focused debate on the acceptability of a drug that could do more than merely cure illness, pharmacological mood enhancement – that is, the use of drugs to improve mood beyond a level that is merely normal or healthy – is much older. Individuals have long been able to take caffeine, amphetamines, barbiturates, benzodiazepines, and other psychopharmaceuticals to affect their moods and emotions. Looking to the future, advances in neurotechnologies and genetic engineering may lead to the development of "neuroceuticals" (neuromodulators that target multiple subreceptors in specific brain neural circuits) and "geneceuticals" that modify the genetic basis of our emotional capacities. With these advances, we may able to produce effects similar to those of current pharmaceuticals with greater efficiency and fewer side effects. As the possibilities and demand for mood enhancement increase, existing legislation will prove inadequate, designed as it is to regulate pharmaceuticals mainly for therapeutic use. In this chapter, we consider why mood enhancement might be desirable, explore some key ethical issues associated with it, and suggest how policy makers can respond to ensure that people use mood enhancement safely and responsibly.[1]

Enhancing Human Capacities, edited by Julian Savulescu, Ruud ter Meulen and Guy Kahane.
© 2011 Blackwell Publishing Ltd

Why Mood Enhancement Might Be Desirable

There are many reasons why we might seek to induce feelings we lack in order to experience a particular emotion or to experience it more fully. Emotions can be a source of insight into or appreciation of what we value in an object, situation, or person. For example, if someone with whom you thought you had a close relationship passed away but it turns out that you do not feel any grief, this may provide some insight into the nature of your relationship with this person. And we may be expected or required by our social roles and relationships to have certain feelings (Liao, 2006a). There are occasions when emotions that seem appropriate for certain circumstances are not forthcoming, for a variety of psychological or physiological reasons. For example, we may want to be happy for a friend who is getting married, but we may be too stressed to enjoy the friend's wedding celebration. Or we may have neurological incapacities that prevent us from feeling a range of affective states. Being able to regulate or induce certain feelings in appropriate circumstances can help us in several ways. We might feel better just by being able to experience emotions that should come naturally. It can be frustrating not to be able to experience joy when one knows one should, and when all those around one seem joyful.

Moreover, we arguably owe the people to whom we stand in close personal relationships certain emotional responses – not because those responses promote their welfare directly or indirectly, but because we cannot relate to them in the way we should unless we have such responses (Liao, 2006b). For example, instead of feeling spontaneous love for their newborn child, it is common for mothers – perhaps owing to postpartum depression – to feel instead estrangement and resentment. Or, step- or adoptive parents might really want to love their step- or adopted children, but find it very difficult to do so. On these occasions, it can be frustrating not to be able to exhibit the kind of love that children need. If pills that could induce the feelings associated with parental love were available, this might enable one to provide the kind of love that children need, thereby relieving this frustration. Indeed, in being able to induce parental love that one does not feel spontaneously, one may also be able at least partially to fulfill a duty to love a child.

Mood enhancement could also benefit the community as a whole. Consider that many societal problems are the result of collective action problems, according to which individuals do not cooperate for the common good. In a number of cases, the impact of any particular individual's attempt to address a particular problem may be negligible, whereas the impact of a large group of individuals working together may be huge. For example, while air travel contributes to climate change, individuals may see little reason to avoid traveling by air, since commercial planes will make their journeys regardless of whether or not any particular individual decides to travel. However, if people were generally more willing to act as a group, and could be confident that others would do the same, we may be able to enjoy the sort of benefits that arise only when large numbers of people act together.

Mood enhancement drugs could potentially help with such collective action problems. While altruism and empathy have large cultural components and are strongly affected by individual moral choices, there is evidence that they also have biological underpinnings. Indeed, test subjects given the prosocial hormone oxytocin were more willing to share money with strangers (Zak *et al.*, 2007), and to behave in a more trustworthy way (Zak *et al.*, 2005). Also, a noradrenaline re-uptake inhibitor increased social engagement and cooperation, and reduced self-focus during a mixed-motive game (Tse & Bond, 2002). And, oxytocin appears to improve the capacity to read other people's emotional state, which is important for empathy (Domes *et al.*, 2007). This suggests that administering these chemicals to individuals could help us act together to solve important problems.

Would Using Mood Enhancements Harm Others?

In modern, liberal societies like the UK and the USA, much concern about novel developments centers on issues about harm and fairness. To what extent is developing these technologies safe, to what extent is using them likely to harm others, and to what extent might it exacerbate existing inequalities?

Harm

That the development of mood enhancement drugs might harm people during clinical trials applies generally to drugs and experimental medical procedures. So the potential harms to people of developing mood enhancement drugs should be minimized using the same methods as those that minimize potential harms arising from medical technology generally.

Once these drugs have been developed, tested, and made available to the public, assessing whether and how mood enhancement technology can be used without significantly harming others requires an assessment of its risks. It is worth remembering that when assessing the risks of novel technology, it can be tempting to focus only on the potential harms, without balancing them against the potential benefits. Many opponents of enhancement fail to take into account its potential benefits, leading to an overly pessimistic view of it (Fukuyama, 2002; Kass, 2003; Sandel, 2004). The enormous market in self-help books alone should give us pause before discounting the potential benefits of mood enhancement: An enormous number of mentally healthy people want to improve their mood, and are willing to pay generously in order to do it.

In assessing how mood enhancement might be harmful, we should take care to distinguish genuine harms from what merely appear to be harms, perhaps because of our cultural viewpoint. In some cases, the circumstances in which using mood enhancement drugs is acceptable might be influenced by cultural considerations. Consider bereavement. In the United States, it is common to prescribe antidepressants for the bereaved if their grief continues for longer than a year. In rural Greece, however, a mother's grief for a lost child, or a wife's grief for her dead husband, is expected to last five years (Schwartz, 1991). Adherents to each of these cultures, then, are likely to disagree about what constitutes an appropriate duration of grief; and consequently views about when it might be appropriate pharmacologically to lift one's mood might vary between these cultures. However, mood enhancement should not just be about helping people conform to cultural expectations. Since it might sometimes be desirable to enhance mood even when doing so does not conform to what is culturally acceptable, it is important to give due consideration to cultural issues and how they might affect one's judgment about the acceptability and harmfulness of mood enhancement.

Keeping these considerations in mind, how might mood enhancement drugs harm others? One way is by inducing emotional and mood states that increase the possibility that the user will harm others. These states could be induced either as intended enhancement effects or as unintended side effects. As an example of an intended effect, guilt is unpleasant to experience, and the anticipation of feeling it can inhibit our behavior, such that we avoid behaving in a way likely to result in guilt. Since guilt, when functioning properly, is felt in response to acting immorally, our avoidance of acting in a way likely to result in guilt helps to prevent us from acting immorally. Except perhaps in cases of people whose guilt may be deemed pathological,[2] altering mood such that our experience of guilt is subdued or diminished may turn out to be disastrous, since it may result in an increase in immoral behavior, which is likely to be harmful to others. As an example of an unintended side effect, someone who believes that he is too shy and unassertive, and who wishes to use mood enhancement drugs to change this, might fail to strike the right balance and render himself overaggressive rather than merely assertive.

Devising policies to guard against this sort of effect demands a multifaceted approach. There is obviously a case for restricting those drugs that are known to induce potentially harmful mood states and for adopting a cautious attitude towards drugs whose effects are not yet fully understood, at least in the absence of known great benefits. But matters are more complicated when we consider the possibility of drugs whose effects are harmless to others when used responsibly but nevertheless induce potentially harmful effects when used recklessly. In such a case, we might adopt similar policies to those governing alcohol use. In other words, we might restrict its use by those deemed incompetent, and respond to other cases of irresponsible use by punishing the resulting antisocial behavior rather than further restricting the drug's use. The latter would introduce an incentive to use mood enhancement drugs in ways that are not harmful to others, and could be combined with educational campaigns designed to inform people about how to enhance responsibly.

Another way in which mood enhancement drugs might harm those who do not choose to use them is through their surreptitious use by unscrupulous governments. Imagine a drug that reduces aggression and renders users more easy-going. When taken by stressed individuals, it may improve well-being by making users more relaxed and contented. However, used on a population-wide scale, it could have the unpalatable effect of making people more accepting of an unjust political regime about which, unmedicated, they would be very angry. That some scientific knowledge and developments can, in the wrong hands, be used to promote unethical ends is a problem that applies to scientific research generally.[3] It is beyond the scope of this chapter to discuss this matter at any length, but we envisage that citizens of liberal and democratic nations would require transparency from their governments and that they would expect to be informed and consulted regarding such possibilities.

Inequality

When they first appear on the market, many novel technologies are expensive and therefore available only to the few who can afford them. If mood enhancement is available only to the rich, the disparity between the quality of life enjoyed by the rich and the poor could become greater as the rich become happier in comparison to the poor, thus adding to the existing advantages that the rich enjoy. Any society that cares about equality should regard it as highly important to minimize this effect. There are a number of ways in which this could be done. One way is to tax those who enhance, and use the proceeds to subsidize enhancement for the disadvantaged. However, such an approach presupposes an infrastructure that recognizes the benefits of using drugs for enhancement as well as for therapy. Such an infrastructure is currently lacking. Drugs are funded, developed, and prescribed for therapeutic use, not for enhancement use. That some drugs turn out to have enhancement effects is a lucky accident, and those healthy individuals wishing to take advantage of a drug's enhancement effects must currently either find an open-minded physician who is willing to prescribe the drug for this purpose, or become diagnosed with some condition that would bring the prescription of the drug under the umbrella of therapy. This infrastructure itself is a potential source of inequality, since those with sympathetic physicians, or with knowledge of how to get themselves diagnosed appropriately, will gain access to enhancement drugs while others go without. Rethinking the way in which we as a society uses prescription drugs therefore seems a necessary step on the way to ensuring that enhancement benefits everyone.[4]

However, even ensuring that the use of mood enhancement drugs does not significantly harm others or exacerbate inequalities is not sufficient for ensuring that they are used responsibly. Consider the users of the fictional soma in Aldous Huxley's *Brave New World*, who exist in a state contented of apathy despite living in a dystopic society. A drug like soma could be used in ways that do not significantly harm others, and could be distributed fairly and equally; but its effects are nevertheless highly disturbing, and few would relish living in a society in which large numbers of people used such a drug. This demonstrates that a society that embraces mood-altering drugs ought not to content itself with addressing concerns about harm to others and equality. We are uneasy about drugs like soma because of their effects on those who use them: users end up living lives that are in some sense impoverished.

We might categorize this worry as one about self-harm. In one sense, the idea of drugs harming those who use them is very familiar: drugs can cause all sorts of harmful side effects that we attempt to minimize by testing them rigorously before making them available to the public. However, there are also varieties of self-harm that are peculiar to mood enhancement, and which should be considered by anyone intending to use mood enhancement drugs, and by any society considering embracing them. We consider some of these issues in the next section.

Would Using Mood Enhancements Harm Users?

Authenticity

One concern about self-harm relates to authenticity; in particular to the question of whether pharmacologically induced emotions would really be "one's own".[5] The notion of ownership here is akin to Harry Frankfurt's (1988) notion of identification.

According to Frankfurt, for a person to be morally responsible for an action, the desire behind it must be one with which that person identifies. For Frankfurt, this means that desire must be endorsed by a higher-order desire: we must desire to act upon that desire. Frankfurt goes so far as to hold that we are not fully responsible for actions that are not "wholehearted", that is, actions that arise from desires opposed by other desires of the same order, or by any higher-order desire. Similarly, some philosophers claim that for an emotion to qualify as one's own, the emotion must be fully consistent with one's beliefs and attitudes (Helm, 2001; Salmela, 2005).

It is certainly true that an emotion unanchored in our beliefs and attitudes would be anomalous. If someone accidentally took a pill that made him feel happy when he thought about his life, but did not believe that he should feel happy, the pill would not have induced the emotions associated with happiness. Also, as Robert Nozick's (1974) "experience machine" and the soma users of Aldous Huxley's (1932) *Brave New World* demonstrate, what matters in life is not simply enjoying pleasant experiences. We also want our experiences to bear the right sort of relation to reality. We want to engage with the world, and we care whether things are going well or badly for us. As a result, we want to be able to recognize when life is going well or badly, and to respond accordingly. This points to the importance of maintaining what we might call a healthy outlook on one's life and the world. Many drugs can induce delusions in users, especially when used recklessly; for example, cannabis can induce psychotic episodes (Thornicroft, 1990).

However, a "wholeheartedness" requirement may be too strong. For one thing, it would deny ownership of emotion whenever we were ambivalent or conflicted. Moreover, we often feel recalcitrant emotions, which seem to conflict with our other attitudes and beliefs, e.g. jealousy at a friend's success or pleasure at a friend's humiliating faux pas. Sometimes, these anomalous emotions may reveal that our real attitudes or beliefs are different than we thought. But that is not always the case. We often have unresolved conflicts among our attitudes and beliefs. If our conflicting emotional responses arise from such conflicting attitudes and beliefs, we regard those responses as fully our own. Wholeheartedness demands too much. In any case, attempts to induce emotions pharmacologically will often be induced by consonant beliefs. It is just because we believe an emotion to be warranted, if not required, that we seek to induce it.

Related to this is the concern that pharmacologically inducing emotions can drastically alter one's temperament and thereby alienate one from one's older, "genuine" self (Elliott, 2003; Kramer, 1993; President's Council on Bioethics, 2003). For example, a person with a morose temperament might develop a cheery one as a result of taking a euphoria-inducing drug to get through a crisis. If he valued and identified with his older, morose self despite his willingness to brighten his mood in exigent circumstances, he would likely find his new temperament profoundly distasteful; the drug would have alienated him from his older self.

It seems quite possible that some emotion-inducing drugs could have such long-term side effects. If it turns out that they do, it is imperative to make people aware of the risk. On the other hand, a person might take such a drug voluntarily, fully aware of its personality-changing effects. If so, concern about alienation becomes less acute; there is no reason why he should be prevented from choosing to fashion himself into a different person and instead be encouraged to preserve his old personality.

Self-knowledge

Another concern is that pharmacologically induced emotions might undermine valuable opportunities to acquire self-knowledge. Our present emotions often give us important insight into ourselves, because they reflect and call attention to our present beliefs, especially those we ignore or suppress. Inducing emotions pharmacologically may obscure beliefs that we are reluctant to acknowledge and confront, by giving affective support to the contrary beliefs we more readily acknowledge. Perhaps we did not value the deceased as much as we think we should have, for reasons it is difficult for us to understand or admit to ourselves. Perhaps we have misgivings about our friend's wedding, out of prudential concerns about the match.

This said, it is worth noting that some people object to the use of SSRIs such as Prozac on similar grounds (Manninen, 2006). The use of SSRIs is based on a belief that depression is caused in part by a serotonin deficit and can be treated by increasing the brain's level of serotonin. Critics of SSRIs argue that serotonin levels (also) change in response to external events and features of oneself. They fear that taking SSRIs can prevent one from having to confront those events and features. Like depression, a limited capacity to experience certain emotions may reveal hidden problems that we are better off knowing. If this is so, we should certainly be cautious about immediately resorting to pills to induce emotions whenever we find ourselves unable to experience them.

However, such caution is fully consistent with the recognition that in other circumstances, our emotional capacities may be incapacitated beyond our power to restore by self-examination. Very few people would argue against the use of SSRIs by an individual with severe, protracted depression (Wolpert, 2001). And severe depression is hardly the only emotion-blocking condition that is beyond our control. If depression can blunt our capacity to feel emotion, trauma can cause us to repress it.

It is also possible that individuals can know the roots causes of their problems without being able to resolve them on their own. For example, a person with severe depression may already know why she is depressed, but simply be unable to get out of it by her own efforts.

Furthermore, whether it is appropriate to enhance one's mood might also depend on the manner in which the mood is experienced. For example, while the ability to experience acute pain can be beneficial since it can alert us to problems with the body, there is less to be gained from being able to tolerate chronic, pathological pain, such as the pain that amputees sometimes feel in their phantom limbs. In the case of the latter, it seems better where possible to alleviate the pain rather than to attempt to remove the source. The acute-chronic model is instructive in thinking about emotional and mood states. While some unpleasant states like anxiety and depression may be appropriate and valuable in some cases, they can be disruptive and disabling if they continue indefinitely and bear no relation to the state of the subject or the world around her. There may be a case for enduring some of the former, "acute", types of state; but the latter, "chronic", types of state serve no useful function and are better alleviated.

However, even if inducing emotions with a pill denies self-knowledge or self-protective insight, it is worth asking why we should object if someone with mild incapacities does so. Safety issues aside, why should we discourage him from trying to treat his emotional incapacities pharmacologically when we do not discourage people from taking medicine for mild colds and mild depression, even when it may be better in the long run for them to acquire natural resistance or work out their problems? Without conveying disapproval, though, we may remind the individual that that his mild incapacities can become more severe unless he takes the time to examine their root causes.

In this regard, it is worth noting that there is evidence to suggest that mentally healthy individuals hold a variety of overly positive illusions about themselves, and that their mental health is tied to their holding such illusions; whereas mentally unhealthy people perceive themselves, the world, and their future more accurately (Taylor & Brown, 1988). This research has been disputed (Colvin & Block, 1994), but if there is any truth in the claim that illusions about oneself and the world can promote mental health, there are implications for our assessment of mood enhancement drugs. Specifically, focusing too heavily on the desirability of developing self-knowledge may be counter-productive for our attempts to enhance mood. We may ultimately be forced to choose between two highly valuable mental capacities: happiness and accurately perceiving reality.[6]

Narcissism

Emotions could become narcissistic, that is, overly self-absorbed, when the focus shifts from their object to their subjective experience (Pugmire, 2005). One would certainly feel that the experience of mourning had become debased if the conversation at a funeral was almost exclusively about the survivors' feelings rather than the deceased's life.

At the same time, the claim can be overstated. It is surely not narcissistic for a parent to take notice of her lack of emotional sensitivity to her children's tribulations and triumphs, especially if that notice leads her to take a greater interest in her children's lives. Of course, if she took a pill to increase her emotional sensitivity without attempting to increase her involvement in her children's lives, her effort might well seem cosmetic. But if she took the drug to deepen her emotional and social involvement in her children's lives, it would appear to be an acceptable means to achieving a stronger relationship with them.

Instrumentalization

A further worry about the pharmacological induction of emotions is that it may involve treating ourselves as mere means, or instrumentalizing ourselves, rather than treating ourselves as ends (Freedman, 1998). According to this line of thought, we are ends because we are rational agents capable of moral deliberation. We treat ourselves as ends when we try to modify our emotions by engaging with our beliefs, but we treat ourselves as mere means when we fail to engage with our beliefs. Using pills to induce emotions means that we fail to engage with our beliefs. Therefore, in doing so, we treat ourselves as mere means.

This objection certainly has some force in third-person contexts, for example, where one person is advising another regarding whether to take this kind of pill. If a counselor advised someone to take a grief pill without finding out whether he really believed that he should grieve relative's death, it could be argued that the counselor was not treating the patient as an end. However, suppose that advice concluded a thoughtful, probing discussion with the patient, which revealed the strength of his attachment to his relative and his recognition of a duty to mourn the relative. Arguably, the counselor would have respected the individual as an end in advising him to take the pill.

This contrast is equally relevant in first-person contexts. If I took such a pill without even thinking about whether it was the right course of action for me, then I may indeed be instrumentalizing myself by failing to engage with my beliefs and values. However, if I take the pill after careful self-examination, I arguably have treated myself as an end. I hardly fail to engage with my beliefs if I seek to deepen or intensify them by inducing appropriate feelings. It is only if I ignore my beliefs or the conflicts among them that I treat myself with disrespect.

Duty

One way in which the capacity to regulate emotions pharmacologically may affect our responsibility for our emotions is in limiting our excuses for failing to have the appropriate ones. Even if we have a duty to have certain emotions, we are excused from fulfilling it if our best efforts are unavailing. Alternatively, our duty may be only to make our best efforts. The availability of a pill may limit our excuses by making our efforts more likely to succeed.

This hardly means that someone who is initially deficient in a required emotional response must immediately take a pill. It is important to remember that when natural emotions are not forthcoming, there are various other means of coaxing or evoking them. Those other means may be at least as effective as a pill, and have fewer of the moral risks outlined above. That said, we might sometimes find a pill more efficient than, or simply preferable to, other means. If so, then assuming that the conditions of authenticity are all met, and that we are aware of the problems of self-knowledge, narcissism, and self-instrumentalization, it may well be acceptable to take a pill as means to discharge one's duty. It may even be morally incumbent on us to do so if no other means of inducing the emotion are effective.

The government's role in preventing self-harm

How can a government act to ensure that its citizens use such drugs in ways that do not cause the sort of self-harm described above?

We can begin by noting that, in most liberal societies, people expect the state to intervene and prevent mentally sound citizens from pursuing a given activity only when it has compelling reasons to do so. Such reasons usually involve the possibility of significant harm to others. For example, it is impermissible to drive while drunk because of the increased possibility of harming others in a collision. Legislation to prevent mentally sound people from pursuing activities unlikely significantly to harm anyone – such as legislation restricting the practice of homosexuality – is increasingly viewed as an unacceptable infringement on liberty, as attested by the increasing number of Western countries that legally recognize same-sex civil partnerships. Restricting the use of mood enhancement drugs because of concerns about the sorts of self-harm just described would, therefore, go against the grain of liberalism.

However, there are ways in which policy makers can help to ensure that people do not harm themselves that do not involve restricting resources or activities that could potentially harm users. People can harm themselves by eating an unhealthy diet, having sex without using a condom, crossing the road without first checking for oncoming traffic, and getting insufficient sleep; yet the government does not respond by legally requiring that people eat healthily, have safe sex, cross the road responsibly, and sleep well. Instead, the government funds educational campaigns designed both to inform people about the importance of eating healthily, having safe sex, and so on, and to provide guidelines on what sort of behavior qualifies as eating healthily and having safe sex. Consider, for example, the UK government's "five-a-day" campaign, which encourages people to eat at least five portions of fruit and vegetables per day.[7] The campaign website explains why healthy eating is important and how to eat healthily, as well as providing resources to make the message easy to understand. As such, the government sets out to achieve its aim of having people eat healthy food by providing information, education, and encouragement, rather than by legislation that restricts consumption of less healthy food. A similar approach might be appropriate in the case of mood enhancement drugs: those drugs that pose a serious risk of harm to users and others could be restricted or made available only on prescription from qualified professionals, while other drugs could be made more freely available, and accompanied by a high-profile awareness campaign to help ensure that people use enhancement in ways that do not cause more subtle forms of self-harm.

Policy Implications

To summarize, the benefits of using mood enhancement drugs, both for the individual and for the community, are potentially great. In order to make the most of these benefits while still taking a responsible stance towards enhancement, policy makers in liberal societies would be advised to guard against being overly risk-averse when evaluating this technology. It is easy to fall into the trap of supposing that the current status quo represents an acceptable state of affairs, from which point of view losses loom larger than gains. However, doing so could squander many beneficial opportunities.

Harm to others and inequality are of great importance when formulating mood enhancement policy. In assessing harms, policy makers should take care to consider only genuine harms that are not overly influenced by cultural considerations. We have suggested that their aim should be to protect citizens, not to ensure that they conform to a culturally desirable model.

Guarding against inequality may require some fundamental changes to the way in which medicines are developed and licensed. While subsidizing enhancement for the poor is worth considering, turning this into a workable solution requires viewing enhancement as a worthwhile use of medicines.

Considerations of harm to others and inequality take us only part of the way towards an acceptable mood enhancement policy, however. We have seen that the dangers of self-harm should not be underestimated. Minimizing the risks of these dangers may best be achieved through educational and awareness campaigns rather than by legis-lation to restrict the use of mood enhancement drugs. Such an approach would be commensurate with the way in which liberal governments attempt to deal with issues of self-harm more generally.[8]

Notes

1. We assume throughout this chapter that it is possible to regulate or induce pharmacologically certain emotions in appropriate circumstances (Liao, 2006b; Wasserman & Liao, 2008).
2. For example, some people feel guilt in response to eating (Frank, 1991).
3. For a discussion of the problem see Selgelid, 2007.
4. For a more detailed discussion of the problems created by the view that the proper use of drugs is exhausted by their therapeutic use, see Bostrom and Roache, chapter 9, this volume.
5. This section draws on Wasserman and Liao, 2008.
6. For an account of how we might use enhancement to realize both increased happiness and an accurate perception of oneself and the world see Roache, 2007.
7. www.5aday.nhs.uk.
8. We would like to thank Steve Clarke for his very helpful comments on an earlier version of this chapter.

References

Colvin, C.R. & Block, J. (1994). Do positive illusions foster mental health? An examination of the Taylor and Brown formulation. *Psychological Bulletin*, **116**, 3–20.

Domes, G., Heinrichs, M., Michel, A., Berger, C. & Herpertz, S.C. (2007). Oxytocin improves "mind-reading" in humans. *Biological Psychiatry*, **61**(6), 731–3.

Elliott, C. (2003). *Better Than Well: American Medicine Meets the American Dream*. New York: W.W. Norton.

Frank, E.S. (1991). Shame and guilt in eating disorders. *American Journal of Orthopsychiatry*, **61**, 303–6.

Frankfurt, H. (1988). *The Importance of What We Care About: Philosophical Essays*. Cambridge: Cambridge University Press.

Freedman, C. (1998). Aspirin for the mind? Some ethical worries about psychopharmacology. In E. Parens (ed.), *Enhancing Human Traits: Ethical and Social Implications* (pp. 135–50). Washington, DC: Georgetown University Press.

Fukuyama, F. (2002) *Our Posthuman Future*. New York: Farrar, Straus and Giroux.

Helm, B. (2001). *Emotional Reason: Deliberation, Motivation, and the Nature of Value*. Cambridge: Cambridge University Press.

Huxley, A. (1932). *Brave New World*. New York: Harper Perennial.

Kass, L. (2003). Ageless bodies, happy souls: Biotechnology and the pursuit of perfection. *The New Atlantis*, Spring, 9–28.

Kramer, P.D. (1993), *Listening to Prozac*, 2nd edition. London: Penguin.

Liao, S.M. (2006a). The right of children to be loved. *Journal of Political Philosophy*, **14**(4), 420–40.

Liao, S.M. (2006b). The idea of a duty to love. *Journal of Value Inquiry*, **40**(1), 1–22.

Manninen, B.A. (2006). Medicating the mind: A Kantian analysis of overprescribing psycho-active drugs. *Journal of Medical Ethics*, **32**, 100–5.

Nozick, R. (1974). *Anarchy, State and Utopia*. New York: Blackwell.

President's Council on Bioethics (2003). *Beyond Therapy. Biotechnology and the Pursuit of Happiness*. New York: Regan Books.

Pugmire, D. (2005). *Sound Sentiments: Integrity in the Emotions*. Oxford: Oxford University Press.

Roache, R. (2007). Should we enhance self-esteem? *Philosophica*, **79**, 71–91.

Salmela, M. (2005). What is emotional authenticity? *Journal for the Theory of Social Behaviour*, **35**(3), 209–30.

Sandel, M. (2004). The case against perfection. *The Atlantic*, April, 1–11.

Schwartz, R.S. (1991). Mood brighteners, affect tolerance, and the blues. *Psychiatry*, **54**, 397–403.

Selgelid, M. (2007). A tale of two studies: Ethics, bioterrorism, and the censorship of science. *Hastings Center Report*, **37**(3), 35–43.

Taylor, S.E. & Brown, J.D. (1988). Illusion and well-being: A social-psychological perspective on mental health. *Psychological Bulletin*, **103**, 193–210.

Thornicroft, G. (1990). Cannabis and psychosis. Is there epidemiological evidence for an association? *British Journal of Psychiatry*, **157**, 25–33.

Tse, W.S. & Bond, A.J. (2002). Difference in serotonergic and noradrenergic regulation of human social behaviours. *Psychopharmacology*, **159**(2), 216–21.

Wasserman, D. & Liao, S.M. (2008). Issues in the pharmacological induction of emotions. *Journal of Applied Philosophy*, **25**(3), 178–92.

Wolpert, L. (2001). *Malignant Sadness: The Anatomy of Depression*. London: Faber & Faber.

Zak, P.J., Kurzban, R. & Matzner, W.T. (2005). Oxytocin is associated with human trustworthiness. *Hormones and Behavior*, **48**(5), 522–7.

Zak, P.J., Stanton, A.A. & Ahmadi, S. (2007). Oxytocin increases generosity in humans. *Public Library of Science*, **2**(11), 1–5.

Part IV
Physical Enhancement

18

Physical Enhancement

Hidde J. Haisma

Doping

Doping is of all times. In the Greece of the Antique, athletes were trying to increase their physical strength by eating different kinds of herbs and funguses prior to the games (Papagelopoulos *et al.*, 2004). Currently athletic performance may be increased in many ways, some of which are permitted and some of which are prohibited by the governing sports bodies. An example of the latter is the use of performance-enhancing drugs, or doping.

The first International Olympic Committee (IOC) banned substances list was produced in 1963, just before the doping-related death of cyclist Tom Simpson in 1967. Testing of athletes for performance-enhancing drugs did not begin until 1964, at the Tokyo Olympic Games. Subsequently the World Anti-Doping Agency (WADA) was created in 1999 through a collective initiative of sporting organizations and governments led by the IOC. In 2003, all major sporting federations and 73 governments approved a resolution accepting the WADA Code as the basis for the fight against doping (Striegel *et al.*, 2005).

Doping can be both of chemical and protein nature or may involve prohibited methods, such as illegal blood transfusions. The percentage of athletes that test positive in doping tests has fluctuated between 1.5% and 2.5% over the last few years (World Anti-Doping Agency, 2009).

The past has shown that some athletes (and their staff) go to great lengths to gain a competitive advantage. Athletes have access to the latest drugs, as exemplified by the finding in athletes' urine of a third-generation form of erythropoietin, CERA (continuous erythropoiesis receptor activator) which was developed for patients with kidney disease and is a form of erythropoietin (EPO) that has a longer lasting effect without repeated dosing (Schoffel *et al.*, 2008). Pharmaceutical products have been found that had not yet been sufficiently tested for side effects as was the case with efaproxiral, an allosteric modifier of hemoglobin (Jimenez *et al.*, 2004). This shows that even when it can be expected that the use of certain products will have serious health consequences, some athletes are willing to serve as subjects in an uncontrolled trial.

Enhancing Human Capacities, edited by Julian Savulescu, Ruud ter Meulen and Guy Kahane.

Gene Doping

The elucidation of the complete human genome with approximately 30,000 different genes will lead to new possibilities for diagnosis and prevention of a wide variety of diseases. In addition, this knowledge may be used for the design of new therapeutics, based on the DNA sequence information. The rapidly increasing number of genetic therapies as a promising new branch of regular medicine, has raised the issue whether these techniques might be abused in the field of sports (Haisma & de Hon, 2006). Both WADA and the IOC have expressed concerns about this possibility. As a result, the method of gene doping has been included in the list of prohibited classes of substances and prohibited methods.

At this time, almost 200 genes have been identified that are associated with health and fitness (Bray *et al.*, 2009). For example, some specific alleles of the *ACE* gene are associated with improved endurance. This ultimately allows for the selection of athletes ideally suited for a particular sport. Genetic screening at an early age may indicate the greatest potential for a specific child to develop into a top athlete and a specific training program may be designed. On the other hand, genetic screening of athletes may be used to select specific training methods to enhance or improve his or her genetic predisposition.

Many genes are readily available and evaluated for their treatment potential in animal disease models and patients. Genes encoding growth factors may be used to improve regeneration of sports-related injuries, including muscle injuries, ligament and tendon ruptures, meniscal tears, cartilage lesions, and bone fractures (Huard *et al.*, 2003). Other genes may possibly have an effect on athletic performance such as erythropoietin for increasing endurance or insulin-like growth factor for improving muscle strength. In addition, gene-modulating small molecules are being developed to indirectly increase gene expression. These include orally active small molecules in clinical development for the treatment of anemia (Hsieh *et al.*, 2007; Jelkmann, 2009) and Id2 which is a small molecule-inducible modulator of PPARγ expression which affects endurance (Park *et al.*, 2008).

Risks of Gene Doping

Gene therapy is currently an experimental therapy delivered to patients in a well-controlled setting. Recent clinical data show encouraging gene therapy results in major diseases: patients with x-linked severe combined immunodeficiency disease (Fischer *et al.*, 2005), adenosine deaminase deficiency (Aiuti *et al.*, 2009; Podsakoff *et al.*, 2008), chronic granulomatous disease (Kim *et al.*, 2008), or patients with hemophilia B (Viaala *et al.*, 2009). In addition, angiogenic gene therapy with vectors expressing the human vascular endothelial growth factor for the treatment of coronary artery disease, showed improvement in angina complaints (Hedman *et al.*, 2009). The gene transfer vectors used have been produced in certified laboratories and have been extensively tested for toxicity and safety. If gene therapy was be used to improve athletes' performance it is very likely that such a setting will be absent. The risks involved with gene therapy would then increase tremendously. The use of medicines by healthy people, gene therapeutics or others, always involves a certain risk. The drugs are developed to treat ill people – improving the performance of healthy people is a different indication which may result in specific side effects.

General Health Risks

The risks involved in gene doping are several, and are related both to the vector used (DNA, chemical, viral) and to the encoded transgene. So far, clinical gene therapy studies have been relatively safe (Kimmelman, 2005). Over 3,000 patients have been treated and only one patient died due to a chronic liver disease and an overdosing of vector (Raper *et al.*, 2003). In three other patients, who were cured for their life-threatening immune deficiency disease, leukemia-like symptoms developed (Hacein-Bey-Abina *et al.*, 2002). One of these patients died from this malignancy. Since then, other groups have treated similar patients with comparable therapeutic results, without any side effects (Aiuti *et al.*, 2009; Gao *et al.*, 2004). These studies were aimed at lifelong cure of the patients with integrating vectors that will not be used for performance enhancement. Therefore, these side effects will not occur in athletes taking gene doping.

Recently an autoimmune response to endogenous and transgene derived protein was reported in monkeys. Adeno-associated virus was used for EPO gene delivery and some animals developed severe anemia due to an autoimmune response (Gao *et al.*, 2004). So far, this inadvertent autoimmunity has not been observed in other studies, but may pose a serious problem if it were to develop likewise in humans.

Other side effects from gene therapy that have been reported are mostly flu-like symptoms. There have been no reports on transfer of gene therapy vectors from treated patients to next of kin or to germ cells (Arruda *et al.*, 2001; Griscelli *et al.*, 2003). However, if gene transfer vectors were produced in non-controlled laboratories, the preparations may be contaminated with chemicals and other impurities from the production and purification process, including pyrogens and virulent viruses. The potential for generating new viruses, known as replication-competent viruses (RCV) is a major safety concern. There is no way to predict the virulence or disease potential of recombinant viral vectors. These impose great safety risks for the people who would receive these agents.

Specific Health Risks

Health risks related to the specific proteins expressed in gene doping are similar to those of other doping forms. Healthy people who unnaturally boost their EPO levels increase their chances of stroke and heart attack because adding red blood cells makes the blood thicker. As the blood gets thicker, it becomes more difficult for the body to pump it successfully to all tissues of the body, causing clots wherever vessels cannot compensate for this increased density. Whereas the athletes using synthetic EPO today face similar risks (Lage *et al.*, 2002), after a few weeks the risk subsides as EPO is cleared from the body and red blood cell production returns to normal levels. But if EPO were delivered by gene therapy, the level and duration of EPO production is less controllable. The hematocrit would be less manageable and could continue almost indefinitely, giving rise to pathological EPO levels.

Other genes may give different health risks if the expression is not controlled. It may be envisioned that genetic growth hormone treatment with IGF-1 or VEGF may give rise to tumor development. Therefore, it is crucial that selected pharmaceutical grade gene delivery vectors are used, which will have a known and controlled gene expression pattern.

Environment Risks

Athletes that would have received gene therapy may have genetically modified cells or excreta that contain the gene transfer vector. This may potentially pose a risk for people in close contact with the athlete, because they may be exposed to the gene. In current gene therapy trials, patients treated with viral gene therapy vectors are closely monitored for shedding of the gene therapy vectors and in most instances should have no detectable gene therapy vector in blood, stool, urine, semen, or saliva before they are allowed to leave the hospital. Although there have been no reports of unwanted gene transfer from shed gene therapy vectors in clinical studies, this cannot be excluded when athletes are treated with these vectors in a less controlled environment.

Detection of Gene Doping

A concern in the athletic community, especially among doping control agencies, is that no one knows how easily gene doping can be detected, if at all. The DNA which is used for gene transfer of the gene is of human origin, and therefore not different from that of the person applying gene doping. Labeling of gene transfer products with genetic "bar codes," as has been suggested with genetically modified agricultural produce, may be an option, however, this would require the complete cooperation of scientists, ethicists, athletes, sports authorities, medical practitioners, professional societies, pharmaceutical and biotech industries, and the public to avert misuse. Gene doping will be delivered by a vector-containing DNA, with or without chemicals to enhance gene transfer or by a viral vector. Muscle-based therapies will be confined to the injection site or tissue in the direct vicinity. Therefore, many of the muscle-based gene technologies are unlikely to be detected by urine or blood testing as is currently done in elite athletes. The detection of associated chemicals or viral particles may be of use but this would involve tissue sampling. It will be unlikely that athletes can be forced to give consent to this procedure given the invasive nature of the biopsies.

Detection of Gene Doping: DNA, Vector Protein, Effect, Proteomics

Many forms of genetic doping do not require the direct injection of genes in the desired target organ, i.e. the *EPO* gene may be injected into almost any site of the body to locally produce the EPO protein which will then enter the blood stream and stimulate the bone marrow. Finding the site of injection will be like looking for a needle in a hay stack. With injectable EPO use, close medical monitoring ensures that red blood cell parameters can be contained within set levels, making it difficult to even be suspicious that illicit gene doping may have occurred. According to Larry Bowers, the lead toxicology and testing expert with the U.S. Anti-Doping Agency, there would be no way to test for gene doping with current technologies (www.msnbc.msn.com/id/10628586/). The authors of a *Scientific American* article (Andersen *et al.*, 2000) conclude their assessment by saying, "[F]or all intents and purposes, gene doping will be undetectable." It may be impossible to detect the agents used in gene doping, but the effects can be measured.

The gene doping will in most instances result in the production of a human protein, which by itself is identical to the person's own proteins. A recent publication indicates that even in these cases a difference between the native protein and the gene therapy product may be detected, on the basis of different glycosylation patterns in different cell types. It remains to be seen if this will be the case for all types of gene doping (Lasne *et al.*, 2004).

Only the (blood) level of the protein may be indicative for doping abuse. In the case of EPO-type treatment, this might be detectable, because of the resulting increase in hemoglobin and hematocrit. However, genes may be turned on and off by taking specific medicines. Studies in monkeys have shown that EPO levels can be controlled in this way, resulting in desirable hematocrit levels (Ye *et al.*, 1999).

A possible solution is the use of RNA or protein markers as indicators for disruption of normal physiology. In a recent study microarrays were used to identify the effects of tetrahydrogestrinone (THG) on the expression of the genes of the mouse genome in muscle (Labrie *et al.*, 2005). An anabolic steroid-specific signature was identified, describing a proteomics technique for the detection of human growth hormone (hGH) in blood. Plasma proteins were reduced, alkylated, and digested with trypsin, and the resulting peptides were separated on a capillary C-18 column and then detected by ion-trap mass spectrometry (1D LC/MS). This study provided a global view of the serum proteome with over 200 plasma proteins being preliminarily identified. In the MS/MS analysis, hGH was detected by characterization of the first tryptic peptide. The detectable amount of growth hormone was 10-fold above normal *in vivo* levels, representing concentrations that may be present in doping measurements. These studies have demonstrated that shotgun sequencing approaches (LC/MS/MS) can not only profile high-abundance proteins in complex biological fluids but also have the potential to identify and quantitate low-level proteins. These techniques may be used to identify gene doping in the future. It will require the sampling and analysis of sets of RNA or proteins at the level of the individual athletes' physiology over time. It is conceivable that testing will be limited to urine and blood samples, as athletes are unlikely to accept tissue sampling. These techniques will require storage of samples at low temperatures and thus demands either onsite testing or new handling regiments. With progress in RNA array and proteomic techniques, which allow the simultaneous screening of the expression of hundreds of proteins, this technique may become valuable for anti-doping testing.

In conclusion, the sporting world will eventually be faced with the phenomenon of gene doping to improve athletic performance. A combination of developing detection methods based on gene arrays or proteomics and a clear education program on the associated risks seems to be the most promising preventive method to counteract the possible application of gene doping.

References

Aiuti, A., Cattaneo, F., Galimberti, S., Benninghoff, U., Cassani, B., Callegaro, L. *et al.* (2009). Gene therapy for immunodeficiency due to adenosine deaminase deficiency. *New England Journal of Medicine*, **360**(5), 447–58.

Andersen, J.L., Schjerling, P. & Saltin, B. (2000). Muscle, genes and athletic performance. *Scientific American*, **283**(3), 48–55.

Arruda, V.R., Fields, P.A., Milner, R., Wainwright, L., De Miguel, M.P., Donovan, P.J. *et al.* (2001). Lack of germline transmission of vector sequences following systemic administration of recombinant AAV-2 vector in males. *Molecular Therapy*, **4**(6), 586–92.

Bray, M.S., Hagberg, J.M., Perusse, L., Rankinen, T., Roth, S.M., Wolfarth, B. *et al.* (2009). The human gene map for performance and health-related fitness phenotypes: The 2006-2007 update. *Medicine & Science in Sports and Exercise*, **41**(1), 35–73.

Fischer, A., Hacein-Bey-Abina, S., Lagresle, C., Garrigue, A. & Cavazana-Calvo, M. (2005). Gene therapy of severe combined immunodeficiency disease: Proof of principle of efficiency and safety issues. Gene therapy, primary immunodeficiencies, retrovirus, lentivirus, genome. *Bulletin de l'Academie Nationale de Medecine*, **189**(5), 779–85.

Gao, G.P., Lebherz, C., Weiner, D.J., Grant, R.L., Calcedo, R., Bagg, A. *et al.* (2004). Autoimmune anemia in macaques following erythropoietin gene therapy. *Molecular Therapy*, **9**, S130.

Griscelli, F., Opolon, P., Saulnier, P., Mami-Chouaib, F., Gautier, E., Echchakir, H. *et al.* (2003). Recombinant adenovirus shedding after intratumoral gene transfer in lung cancer patients. *Gene Therapy*, **10**(5), 386–95.

Hacein-Bey-Abina, S., le Deist, F., Carlier, F., Bouneaud, C., Hue, C., De Villartay, J. *et al.* (2002). Sustained correction of X-linked severe combined immunodeficiency by ex vivo gene therapy. *New England Journal of Medicine*, **346**(16), 1185–93.

Haisma, H.J. & de Hon, O. (2006). Gene doping. *International Journal of Sports Medicine*, **27** (4), 257–66.

Hedman, M., Muona, K., Hedman, A., Kivela, A., Syvanne, M., Eranen, J. *et al.* (2009). Eight-year safety follow-up of coronary artery disease patients after local intracoronary VEGF gene transfer. *Gene Therapy*, **16**(5), 629–34.

Hsieh, M.M., Linde, N.S., Wynter, A., Metzger, M., Wong, C., Langsetmo, I. *et al.* (2007). HIF-prolyl hydroxylase inhibition results in endogenous erythropoietin induction, erythrocytosis, and modest fetal hemoglobin expression in rhesus macaques. *Blood*, **110**(6), 2140–7.

Huard, J., Li, Y., Peng, H.R. & Fu, F.H. (2003). Gene therapy and tissue engineering for sports medicine. *Journal of Gene Medicine*, **5**(2), 93–108.

Jelkmann, W. (2009). Erythropoiesis stimulating agents and techniques: A challenge for doping analysts. *Current Medicinal Chemistry*, **16**(10), 1236–47.

Jimenez, C., Ventura, R. & Segura, J. (2004). Detection in urine of efaproxiral (RSR13), a potential doping agent, by a routine screening procedure based on methylation followed by gas chromatography/mass spectrometry. *Analytica Chimica Acta*, **505**(2), 227–9.

Kim, J.G., Ahn, H.S., Kang, H.J., Kim, S., Hong, Y.T., Joo, C.W. *et al.* (2008). Retroviral gene therapy for x-linked chronic granulomatous disease: Results from Phase I/II trial. *Blood*, **112**(11), 818.

Kimmelman, J. (2005). Recent developments in gene transfer: Risk and ethics. *British Medical Journal*, **330**(7482), 79–82.

Labrie, F., Luu-The, V., Calvo, E., Martel, C., Cloutier, J., Gauthier, S. *et al.* (2005). Tetrahydrogestrinone induces a genomic signature typical of a potent anabolic steroid. *Journal of Endocrinology*, **184**(2), 427–33.

Lage, J.M.M., Panizo, C., Masdeu, J. & Rocha, E. (2002). Cyclist's doping associated with cerebral sinus thrombosis. *Neurology*, **58**(4), 665.

Lasne, F., Martin, L., de Ceaurriz, J., Larcher, T., Moullier, P. & Chenuaud, P. (2004). Genetic doping with erythropoietin cDNA in primate muscle is detectable. *Molecular Therapy*, **10**(3), 409–10.

Papagelopoulos, P.J., Mavrogenis, A.F. & Soucacos, P.N. (2004). Doping in ancient and modern Olympic Games. *Orthopedics*, **27**(12), 1226–31.

Park, K.W., Waki, H., Villanueva, C.J., Monticelli, L.A., Hong, C., Kang, S. *et al.* (2008). Inhibitor of DNA binding 2 is a small molecule-inducible modulator of peroxisome proliferator-activated receptor-gamma expression and adipocyte differentiation. *Molecular Endocrinology*, **22**(9), 2038–48.

Podsakoff, G., Engel, B.C., Sokolic, R., Carbonaro, D.A., Muul, L., Garabedian, E. *et al.* (2008). Gene therapy for adenosine deaminase (Ada)-deficient severe combined immune deficiency (Scid): Comparative results with or without Peg-Ada withdrawal and myelosuppressive chemotherapy. *Biology of Blood and Marrow Transplantation*, **14**(2), 27–8.

Raper, S.E., Chirmule, N., Lee, F.S., Wivel, N.A., Bagg, A., Gao, G.P. *et al.* (2003). Fatal systemic inflammatory response syndrome in a ornithine transcarbamylase deficient patient following adenoviral gene transfer. *Molecular Genetics and Metabolism*, **80**(1–2), 148–58.

Schoffel, N., Borger, J.A., Quarcoo, D., Scutaru, C. & Groneberg, D.A. (2008). Erythropoietin – State of science. *Sportverletzung-Sportschaden*, **22**(4), 201–6.

Striegel, H., Rossner, D., Simon, P. & Niess, A.M. (2005). The World Anti-Doping Code 2003 – Consequences for physicians associated with elite athletes. *International Journal of Sports Medicine*, **26**(3), 238–43.

Viaala, N.O., Larsen, S.R. & Rasko, J.E.J. (2009). Gene therapy for hemophilia: Clinical trials and technical tribulations. *Seminars in Thrombosis and Hemostasis*, **35**(1), 81–92.

World Anti-Doping Agency (2009). The World Anti-Doping Code, the 2009 Prohibited List, www.wada-ama.org/rtecontent/document/2010_Prohibited_List_FINAL_EN_-Web.pdf.

Ye, X.H., Rivera, V.M., Zoltick, P., Cerasoli, F., Schnell, M.A., Gao, G.P. *et al.* (1999). Regulated delivery of therapeutic proteins after in vivo somatic cell gene transfer. *Science*, **283**(5398), 88–91.

19

Physical Enhancement: The State of the Art

Andy Miah

In June 1969, *Sports Illustrated* outlined the state of the art in doping technology. At the time, global concern about sports doping was just beginning, but what has changed in the 40 + years since then? There is still considerable uncertainty about whether many substances actually enhance performance and there is still little known about the health risks posed by doping methods, as there is nearly no evidence base detailing the utilization of medical products by healthy, trained athletes. There is also an absence of evidence about how the medical supervision of doping methods might affect this risk, both by allowing more insight into its management and by ensuring that the products themselves are from reliable distributors, rather than illegal markets.

Similarities between then and now are also apparent in the moral equivocation about lifestyle modifications. While the sports movement generally focuses on doping methods that affect fair competition, cases such as that of American swimmer Michael Phelps in 2008 who was photographed smoking marijuana raises further questions about whether the role of sports organizations also extends to regulating moral behavior outside of sports' primary concern. In such cases the common ground is also to do with whether lifestyle drugs have an effect on performance, and discussions about alcohol today.

Gilbert (1969) also inquires into whether the concern about physical enhancement in sport should be seen as a matter of public interest, rather than private sport concern. To support this case, the American Academy of Pediatrics (2005) outlined that enhancement was a broader cultural phenomenon where body boosting for *performance* or *appearance* were both major factors in what led young people in particular to enter into off-prescription substance use.

Today, the World Anti-Doping Code (2009) encompasses a wide range of methods that reflect the expansion of doping techniques. These include anabolic agents, hormones, beta-2 agonists, agents with anti-estrogenic activity, diuretics and other masking agents, oxygen transfer enhancers, chemical and gene doping, stimulants, narcotics, cannabinoids, glucocorticosteroids, alcohol, and beta blockers. However, there remain numerous enhancement practices that extend beyond what the Code covers, and understanding how these technologies are integrated with elite sports

Enhancing Human Capacities, edited by Julian Savulescu, Ruud ter Meulen and Guy Kahane.
© 2011 Blackwell Publishing Ltd

practices is essential to coming to terms with how risk is negotiated by athletes around physical excellence.

This chapter examines the state of the art of physical enhancement, demonstrating how the problem of regulating excellence is becoming more difficult as technology advances. Modifications are grouped into the following categories, building on Ellul's (1964) seminal discussions on philosophy and technology: *technique, equipment*, and *biology*.

Technique

Technical enhancements are those that involve knowledge-based innovations, which lead to improved performance. Such examples encompass modifications arising from scientific insights, such as better understanding about the effect of nutrition. However, they also include the way that knowledge affects our understanding of technique. For example, in the 1960s, the Fosbury flop transformed high-jumping in such a way as to alter what we now understand by this athletic endeavor. These insights can sometimes arise from spontaneous discoveries, though the expansion of sports science has led to the careful design of such transformations (Busch, 1998).

Modifications of this kind do not tend to attract the interest of doping authorities, though often this is because their use does not imply any misuse of medical technology, which is a primary concern of the anti-doping authorities. Yet, they are forms of enhancement and their development dramatically affects fair competition. An example that occupies the mid-point between such innovations in technique and medical intervention is the hypoxic chambers (Levine, 2006; Loland & Murray, 2007). Hypoxic training is a long-established tradition of athletic competition and involves athletes moving from one altitude to another to optimize performance. However, hypoxic *chambers* are a relatively new technology that simulates this effect, while remaining in one location. In 2006, the world of sport debated their ethical status where concerns arose about the reliance on "expert systems" to bring about performance advantage, but it is important to note that such expertise is contested. Scientists differ on how best to utilize hypoxic chambers to promote enhancement and so it remains a strategic choice to use, rather than a sure way of gaining an advantage. The risks posed by such chambers are also unclear and, in 2006, after extensive review, the World Anti-Doping Agency concluded that there was no evidence to suggest they are especially dangerous and they remain a permissible means of enhancement.

Another emerging technology is the "Glove," developed by Heller and Grahn. This innovative cooling device has been utilized by the San Francisco 49ers and it demonstrates the blurred boundary between therapeutic use and enhancement. The problem addressed by this technology is overheating during exercise, which significantly diminishes performance. The glove device "is used to apply a 35- to 45-mmHg subatmospheric pressure to an entire hand to draw blood into the hand and increase the filling of the venous plexus underlying the palmar surface. A heat sink applied to that palm extracts heat and cools the venous blood" (Grahn *et al.*, 2005, p.972). Research on trained persons – military, sportspersons, emergency services – demonstrates between 30% and 60% enhancement of endurance capacity after use. This means that the subject can work for an additional 30–60% before exhaustion through overheating when working at maximal load. Presently, such a device is not of immediate concern to the World Anti-Doping Agency – and there are many devices that attempt to address overheating – though it remains to be seen whether similar such devices will soon be part of the anti-doping list. Guthrie (2008) describes one of the tests undertaken by the scientists on a trained athlete:

> His routine included 100 pull-ups. One day, Grahn and Heller started using an early version of the Glove to cool him for 3 minutes between rounds of pull-ups. They saw that with the cooling, his 11th round of pull-ups was as strong as his first. Within 6 weeks of training with the cooling breaks, Cao did 180 pull-ups a session. Six weeks later, he went from 180 to 616.

Equipment

The "glove" leads us to forms of enhancement that arise from innovations in equipment design, though even this concept has expanded in remarkable ways recently. While sports have always evolved alongside technological developments, equipment has sometimes been controversial and this often has to do with its transformative effect. For example, in the 1980s, javelins were redesigned due to the fact that athletes were becoming so capable that their distances posed a risk to spectators in the far side of the stadium. Thus, rather than change the size of the arena, the javelin was adapted. The result was an alteration of the skills needed to be a competent javelin thrower and this meant a change in the kinds of athletes who were successful. Alternatively, there are *unintended consequences* arising from technological change. For example, the development of the plastic helmet in American football was designed to protect athletes from head injuries, but was widely reported to have led to more risky behavior (Gelberg, 1995). Examples like this emphasize how difficult it is to preview how an innovation affects performance. As technology improves, equipment finds itself in close proximity to doping discussions. For example, swimming costumes have attracted such alarm in recent times and were, until very recently, a recurrent technological story around major competitions. The evidence base to support their enhancing properties is dubious, though the psychological edge athletes may achieve by such campaigns could be considerable. In any case, during 2009, FINA was under pressure to react to a latest costume design, the use of which a number of high-profile athletes protested. Among the protestors was Michael Phelps, the most successful Olympic swimmer of all time, who threatened withdrawal from the sport unless a ban was enforced. The outcome was a complete ban on swimsuit technology, marking the end of an era of alleged technological enhancement. Again, what interests us here is less the final decision and more the process through which the decision took place, which did not involve the arena of anti-doping concern at all. Instead, judgments arose from within the swimming federation's technical rules commission. Historically, equipment and biological enhancements have often been completely separate debates, yet they raise similar philosophical issues (Miah, 2005).

Prosthetic devices

The expansion of equipment to prosthetic devices is also provoking new philosophical questions about what constitutes athletic performance. In 2008, the world-record breaking South African sprinter Oscar Pistorius campaigned to take part in the Beijing Olympic Games as well as the Paralympic Games. A double below-the-knee amputee, Pistorius is able to attain sprint times that approximate athletes competing in the Olympic Games. His achievements reflect the convergence between Olympic and Paralympic athletes that is brought about by prosthetic devices. While Pistorius did not succeed in 2008, it is likely that he will be the first of many athletes who are able to compete at Olympic level. The reason for this is relatively simple: as prosthetic technology improves, it reduces the performance inhibition arising from the technology, slowly creating a device that seamlessly approximates the capacities of a human leg. When this reduction is optimized, Paralympians will be competing on the same biomechanical basis as Olympians and it is likely that we will see even greater challenges to biology as the exemplar of human excellence. However, the major problem for sports is what may happen when the devices *exceed* the capacities of their biological counterpart. In such an era, it may signal the end of biologically governed sports performance.

Biology

Prosthetic devices articulate how biology and artifice intersect and, while all of the previous examples affect an athlete's biology in some way, perhaps the most controversial physical enhancements arise from interventions that alter an athlete's biology from the inside. The methods by which this is achieved vary considerably, as do the risks. My final section offers insight into some of the major, emerging biotechnological enhancements that affect physical capabilities. Together, they articulate the challenge faced by regulatory authorities – both sports and medical – as greater demands are placed on the medical industries.

Designer steroids

In 2003, a phial filled with an unknown substance was left by an unknown individual at the U.S. Anti-Doping Authority laboratory. Upon analysis, it became characterized as a designer steroid called tetrahydrogestrinone (THG) and its discovery led to the BALCO scandal, which saw the demise of high-profile U.S. athletes Marion Jones and Tim Montgomery among others. THG demonstrated that so-called designer steroids pose one of the major challenges to the world of sport (Sekera *et al.*, 2005). While in many ways similar to traditional steroids, what distinguished THG – and other designer steroids – was the fact that it was not a substance available commercially and, as such, very little could have been known about it in advance of its discovery. No authorities were testing for it in sports, as they did not know it existed. This shift from steroid use that arises from the nonmedical use of medically available products to a situation where doping communities are developing their own products on the basis of pre-clinical data, changes what anti-doping authorities must do to keep up with dopers. Now, there is more need than ever to ensure that anti-doping authorities are not just studying what is available, but that they have access to research at the developmental stage.

Additional scientific advancements in steroid-like enhancements arise through SARMs (selective androgen receptor modulators), another emerging enhancement. Through the use of SARMs, athletes may be able to target specific tissue more effectively, avoid having to use injections, and can minimize some of the side effects common to steroids, such as conversion to estrogen or the inhibition of naturally produced testosterone.

Nutritional supplements, customized vitamins, and functional foods

While various forms of drugs clearly engage various authorities, the use of nutritional supplements by athletes is much more ambiguous. However, they have been a matter of concern for to the sports world for over 10 years and, in the 1990s, it was commonplace for athletes to attribute positive tests to poorly labeled nutritional supplements or food products (Hon & Coumans, 2007). Supplements are not prohibited methods of performance enhancement, though their use is discouraged due to the quality control problem. Labeling issues continue to arise in the context of standard sports products, as in the recent cases of *Vitaminwater*, which contains caffeine, a controlled substance in some anti-doping codes, or *6-OXO Extreme*, an anti-estrogenic substance used to build muscle mass.

Additionally, *nutrigenomics* is creating a new generation of functional foods, whether through enhancing crop properties or by feeding animals with enhanced diets that will, in turn, enhance humans through their consumption (Twine, 2007). Again, the overlap between sport and society at large is central to understanding the challenge arising from the regulation of such products in competitive situations.

Elective surgery

A further means by which physical enhancements are achieved is through elective surgical procedures. For instance, leg extensions using reconstructive surgery, or reparative surgical procedures that translate into improved performance capabilities, are examples that beckon an age of enhancement. One example of this is laser eye surgery, which was famously utilized by world champion golfer Tiger Woods. Alternatively, injured athletes may enter into surgery in order to have a chance of returning to competition. One such treatment is Tommy John's surgery, utilized by baseball pitchers who tear their ulnar collateral ligament. Such athletes face the hard choice of never competing again, or undergoing invasive surgery and strenuous rehabilitation. While in its early years, this procedure had a very poor likelihood of success, recent anecdotal evidence suggest the additional complication that post-surgery athletes are returning to the field pitching harder and faster than before they were injured. This raises questions over whether athletes may even elect for such surgery prior to injury, just to reinforce their biological capabilities. A similar proposition arises in the context of the earlier discussion about prosthetic devices. While athletes might not choose to replace a limb with a prosthetic, the strengthening of tendons and other connecting tissue may appeal.

Growth factors

The utilization of growth factors and hormones has been commonplace in sports for many years particularly through human growth hormone (HGH), which is used to promote the secretion of insulin-like growth factor 1 (IGF-1), which can play a role in muscle and organ growth. Side effects of HGH can include diabetes, "worsening of cardiovascular disease, muscle, joint and bone pain; hypertension and cardiac deficiency; abnormal growth of organs; accelerated osteoarthritis" (World Anti-Doping Agency, 2009). While developing a test for HGH has taken some years, recent science proposes utilizing nanotechnology to identify the substance (Shipley, 2008). Moreover, a "marker method" (Stow *et al.*, 2009) is becoming a preferred anti-doping method for the indirect detection of a number of new substances. Other growth factors, such as vascular endothelial growth factor (VEGF), can be used to enhance blood vessels, allowing more oxygen to muscles.

Pain modulation

Enhancements often provide their advantage by addressing the debilitating physiological effects of extreme exercise, as for the glove. However, there are also biochemical mechanisms through which pain may be managed to enhance physical performance. One candidate is Downstream Regulatory Element Antagonistic Modulator (DREAM), which is a "critical repressor for pain modulation" (Cheng *et al.*, 2002). Recent research suggests that DREAM could provide useful information about the function of pain and how it might be managed, which could revolutionize how pain is addressed by medicine (Cheng *et al.*, 2002; Cheng & Penninger, 2003). The DREAM protein functions by blocking the production of prodynorphin (the precursor to dynorphin, an endogenous analgesic), which is a chemical produced in response to pain or stress. Research with mice suggests that the absence of DREAM (the gene) leads to increased levels of dynorphin and a decreased sensitivity to inflammatory, acute, and neuropathic pain.

Blood boosting

A range of methods of performance enhancement involve the manipulation of blood, particularly the boosting of red blood cells to improve oxygen delivery, which promotes endurance. Early forms of blood modification include the practice of blood transfusions, which, in the 1960s, was not a banned method, due to a clause in anti-doping law that required a test to be available in order for a method to be banned. Since the removal of this clause, blood doping has gone through various histories of use. Most recently, autologous blood transfusion has become prominent, often using *dry blood* that is extracted, frozen, stored, and then reintroduced to the athlete's blood stream.

Since its emergence in 1989, recombinant human EPO (rHuEPO) has become a popular drug through which to boost endurance, though a test for its detection has led to the creation of various forms, such as CERA (continuous erythropoiesis receptor activator), which does not require as frequent injections as rHuEPO. The risks of such use include the thickening of blood to such a degree that clots can form, increasing the chances of heart disease, stroke, and cerebral or pulmonary embolism.

Alternatively, the practice of *blood spinning* (platelet-rich plasma therapy) has become a common therapeutic device, which enhances recovery. The method involves drawing blood from an athlete, spinning it to isolate the platelets, which clot and promote healing. The platelets are then injected into the injured part of the body to repair tendons. Its status is unclear as a method of doping, but the case emphasizes how the problem of sports arises when therapeutic interventions become extraordinarily effective – arguably transforming natural healing processes.

More modest means of boosting the oxygen content are also available on the market. For example, *canned oxygen* has become prominent in some sports and is available as a recreational sports product. However, WADA has recently given notice of its prohibition as an illegal method of oxygen transfer, raising further questions about how sports regulate practices outside of elite competition. While the use of bottled medical oxygen itself is classified as a drug in some countries, recreational canned oxygen is not. Yet, there is no proven enhancement to athletes, despite its widespread use in high profile sports such as the National Football League (NFL). Similar questions arise from the present discussions about Viagra (sildenafil citrate), which is currently not a banned substance, but which may find itself on the prohibited list, due to its potential to boost oxygen levels and affect performance at modest altitudes (Hsu *et al.*, 2006). By delivering such substances via "Viagra tattoos" (Magnay, 2008) located under the skin, doping can be even harder to detect due to its slow release and low quantities.

Conclusion

What unifies these examples of physical enhancements is their utility for activities beyond sport. One can imagine numerous forms of labor that would benefit from greater endurance, strength, or ability. Elite sports have always been a test space for enhancements and their rule-governed nature offers a useful structure through which to address how questions of justice would be played out within an enhancement-led society. Yet, is also apparent that enhancement is not just a functional quality, as many such modifications are utilized to improve appearance as much as performance.

The key challenge for enhancement advocates is to bridge the ethical gap between therapy and enhancement, to reach a point where new medical products can be developed and characterized for use by healthy subjects. While it is apparent that the medicalization of various conditions may be leading to this situation, an explicit shift in how medicine progresses will be necessary before a strong enhancement culture can emerge. Many forms of enhancement rely on the use of therapeutic technologies, which bring about transformations in the concept – such as the use of stem cells to promote tissue repair (Templeton, 2006). As these technologies begin to arise, an increasing number of questions will emerge about whether sports can stem the tide of enhancements alone, or whether broad social structures will intervene.

References

American Academy of Pediatrics (2005). Policy statement: Use of performance-enhancing substances. *Pediatrics*, **115**, 1103–106.

Busch, A. (1998). *Design in Sport: The Cult of Performance*. London: Thames & Hudson.

Cheng, H.-Y.M. & Penninger, J.M. (2003). When the DREAM is gone: From basic science to future prospectives in pain management and beyond. *Expert Opinion on Therapeutic Targets*, 7(2), 249–63.

Cheng, H.-Y.M., Pitcher, G.M. *et al.* (2002). DREAM is a critical transcriptional repressor for pain modulation. *Cell*, **108**, 31–43.

Ellul, J. (1964). *The Technological Society*. New York: Vintage Books.

Gelberg, J.N. (1995). The lethal weapon: How the plastic football helmet transformed the game of football, 1939-1994. *Bulletin of Science, Technology, and Society*, **15**(5–6), 302–9.

Gilbert, B. (1969). Problems in a turned-on world. *Sports Illustrated*. June 23.

Grahn, D.A., Cao, V.H. *et al.* (2005). Heat extraction through the palm of one hand improves aerobic exercise endurance in a hot environment. *Journal of Applied Physiology*, **99**, 972–8.

Guthrie, J. (2008). Cool invention helps tired players bounce back. *San Francisco Chronicle*. September 22.

Hon, O. & Coumans, B. (2007). The continuing story of nutritional supplements and doping infractions. *British Journal of Sports Medicine*, **41**, 800–5.

Hsu, A.R., Barnholt, K.E. *et al.* (2006). Sildenafil improves cardiac output and exercise performance during acute hypoxia but not normoxia. *Journal of Applied Physiology*, **100**(6), 2031–40.

Levine, B.D. (2006). Editorial: Should "artificial" high altitude environments be considered doping? *Scandinavian Journal of Medicine and Science in Sports*, **16**, 297–301.

Loland, S. & Murray, T.H. (2007). Editorial: The ethics of the use of technologically constructed high-altitude environments to enhance performance in sport. *Scandinavian Journal of Medicine and Science in Sports*, **17**, 193–5.

Magnay, J. (2008). Tattoo your way to tarnished gold. *The Age*. August 5.

Miah, A. (2005). From anti-doping to a "performance policy': Sport technology, being human, and doing ethics. *European Journal of Sport Science*, **5**(1), 51–7.

Sekera, M.H., Ahrens, B.D. *et al.* (2005). Another designer steroid: Discovery, synthesis, and detection of "madol" in urine. *Rapid Communications in Mass Spectometry*, **19**, 781–4.

Shipley, A. (2008). Local company says it has developed urine test for HGH. *The Washington Post*. July 24. www.washingtonpost.com/wp-dyn/content/article/2008/07/23/AR2008072303639_pf.html.

Stow, M.R., Wojek, N. & Marshall, J. (2009). The UK Sport perspective on detecting growth hormone abuse. *Growth Hormone and IGF Research*, **19**, 375–7.

Templeton, S.-K. (2006). Footballers use babies for "repair kits." *The Sunday Times*.

Twine, R. (2007). Thinking across species – A critical bioethics approach to enhancement. *Theoretical Medicine and Bioethics*, **28**, 509–23.

World Anti-Doping Agency (2009). The World Anti-Doping Code, the 2009 Prohibited List, www.wada-ama.org/rtecontent/document/2010_Prohibited_List_FINAL_EN_Web.pdf.

20

Enhanced Bodies

Claudio Tamburrini and Torbjörn Tännsjö

Introduction

Recent developments within genetics are encouraging. Many ill people have already been treated with genetic therapy with positive results and virtually no negative side effects (Haisma & de Hon, 2006). Parallel to this positive prospect, worries have been expressed about the possible application of the new medical techniques for enhancement purposes. The use of genetic technology in the world of sports has been conceived of as especially problematic, since in some cases it might violate the present ban on gene doping.

In this chapter we will present a brief account of current discussion on the enhancement of human physical capacities, particularly in (elite) sports. First the natural scientific picture will be sketched, followed by a discussion of the ethical implications of enhancement technologies.

Scientific Questions

Enhancement as distinct from therapy?

A clear-cut demarcation line between therapeutic and enhancement intervention is difficult to draw. Usually, this distinction is advanced with the purpose of distinguishing between legitimate and illegitimate health care, or between health care that should be publicly funded and health care that should be paid for privately.

However, a tentative distinction might be made between *negative* medical interventions, performed with the aim of curing a disease or eliminating a handicap or disability, *positive* interventions aimed at improving the functioning of a human organism within a natural variation, and *enhancement proper* that takes an individual beyond normal functioning. To provide antibiotics to someone affected by pneumonia is a typically negative intervention. To give human growth hormone to an unusually small child in order to increase the child's length would be a positive intervention. To radically reduce the need of sleep of a person to, say, three hours per night would be a typical case of enhancement.

Enhancing Human Capacities, edited by Julian Savulescu, Ruud ter Meulen and Guy Kahane.
© 2011 Blackwell Publishing Ltd

"Old-fashioned" doping

There is no clear definition of what constitutes doping. In practice, doping is everything (substances as well as training methods) that is included in the doping lists. According to the World Anti-Doping Agency (WADA), a substance or training method is a proper candidate to be banned when it satisfies at least two of the following three characteristics: it is (i) *contrary to the spirit of sport*; (ii) *unfair*; and (iii) *dangerous* for the athlete's health.

The new genetics

The new genetic technologies might be applied in several areas of general medicine. In sports they might instead be used to help athletes to perform better ("gene doping"). Gene therapy may be applied to re-engineer a sportsperson's body thereby enhancing athletic performance. The most relevant genes available with a potential to enhance athletic performance are erythropoietin (EPO), insulin-like growth factor-1 (IGF-1), vascular endothelial growth factor (VEGF), myostatin, and endorphins.

In recent years, gene doping was taken up in the doping list where it is defined as "... the non-therapeutic use of genes, genetic elements and/or cells that have the capacity to enhance athletic performance" (WADA, 2005, www.wada-ama.org/en/prohibitedlist.ch2).

The application of the new genetics in sports

Erythropoietin (EPO) is a potent hormone produced in the kidneys that regulates the amount of the oxygen-carrying red blood cells.
Uses in sports: Increasing hematocrit levels from 40 to 50 % might increase endurance by perhaps 10%.

Insulin-like growth factor-1 (IGF-1) is produced in the liver as well as in the muscles and has anabolic effects.
Uses in sports: This treatment might be used to strengthen a tennis player's shoulder muscles, a sprinter's calves or a boxer's biceps. Such gene therapy is probably relatively safe as the effects seem to be localized to the targeted muscle. Human trials might be expected to start in the coming years.

Vascular endothelial growth factor (VEGF) is a vascular endothelial growth factor for blood vessels. It is among the front runners in gene therapy trials and has already been tested in humans.
Uses in sports: Possibly a hyper supply of oxygen and other nutrients to the tissues by improving blood vessel production.

Myostatin is a negative regulator of muscle growth. Administration of myostatin blockers such as follistatin, mutant activin type 2 receptors, and myostatin propeptide results in increased skeletal muscle mass due to increased number of muscle fibres (hyperplasia) and thickness of fibers (hypertrophy) and less fat and connective tissue.
Uses in sports: Athletes could use these inhibitors as anabolics in the near future.

Endorphins act upon muscular exhaustion that causes hyperacidity, which prevents the detoxication of the lactic acid and waste products of matrix and causes pain.
Uses in sports. Pain relief could potentially help athletes to perform better or for a longer period of time.

Can gene doping be detected?

The DNA of the artificial gene itself can be detected but this requires (i) that the sequence is known and (ii) that a sample of the tissue containing the DNA can be acquired. If a virus carrier is used then some of the blood cells might also contain the artificial DNA and a blood test could be used for detection. However, if a direct injection of DNA into the muscle or modified muscle cells is used, the DNA would only be present in the injected muscle. Thus, a doping test would require a biopsy from the specific muscle.

Regarding blood boosting, the use of EPO gene therapy might go undetected since the EPO would be similar to the endogenous EPO and only slightly above the normal level. A possibility, however, that has been discussed during the last years is to map the blood profile of an athlete and try to detect abnormal variations in her/his historical hematocrit level.

When could gene doping be in use?

Given current knowledge, the risk of serious health damage would still be very high. Therefore we might expect that the main breakthrough for gene doping will have to wait until gene therapy becomes an established procedure, probably within the next 10–15 years.

Is gene doping different?

There are some aspects that suggest that gene doping might be worse than traditional performance enhancers. Shortly, it might be said that:

- Particularly regarding germline alterations, modifications performed in the genome of an individual through gene therapy will be transmitted to her offspring. This notwithstanding, there have been no reports on transfer of gene therapy vectors from treated patients to next of kin or to germ cells (Arruda *et al.*, 2001; Griscelli *et al.*, 2003; Tenenbaum *et al.*, 2003).
- Gene doping implies environmental risks as genetically modified athletes may have genetically modified cells or excreta that contain the gene transfer vector. People in close contact with the athlete might be exposed to the gene.

Ethical Questions

Genetic enhancement, particularly of the third kind above, which goes beyond species normalcy standards, is seen by many critics as a serious threat to sports and wider society. In the second part of this chapter we will try to ascertain some ethical aspects of the foreseeable impact of the new genetic technology on society and (elite) sports.

Coercion

Due to the situation of hard competition that characterizes professional sports, it has been argued that allowing doping (either traditional or of the genetic kind) implies coercing sportspersons to dope themselves. Otherwise they will be left behind by their more risk-inclined competitors.

However, speaking of coercion in this context would be an overstatement. Athletes reluctant to dope will no doubt be put under pressure to emulate their less prudent colleagues. But nothing hinders them from still refusing to dope. They will not then be part of the reduced group of habitual winners. In competitive activities, however, not everyone can win. It is a well-established principle of professional ethics that benefits and rewards should be distributed according to efforts and risks undertaken. Athletes should not be treated differently. If an athlete risks her health to attain victory, while others are more prudent, it is only fair that the victory goes to the former. Or so it has been argued.[1] Seen from this perspective, doping would then not be morally problematic.

Furthermore, all kinds of enhancements that go well put a pressure on others to emulate the positive intervention that has been performed on the patient/client. Shall we for instance oppose to efficient educational programs on grounds that, due to their success, they will push others to go through them and get "culturally enhanced"?[2] Or should literacy be opposed to an illiterate society on the grounds that this puts a pressure on future generations to learn to read and write as well?

Autonomy

Some authors fear the adoption of the new genetics might jeopardize individuals' autonomy. According to one ideal of autonomy, a person is (more or less) autonomous in relation to the degree to which she can decide upon and carry on her own life projects, goals, and plans. Embryos, however, cannot choose for themselves. So, if parents or tutors were to design their physical traits and capacities in advance (for instance, to secure a successful sporting career for their offspring), wouldn't they be manipulating those future lives in an ethically improper way?[3] Some critics affirm that germline modifications (that is, genetic interventions at the embryonic level) violate individuals' autonomy, as prospective persons are designed to fit certain activities before they are even born. To be pre-programmed to develop a certain repertoire of skills, traits, interests, etc., would thus be tantamount *to be deprived of one's right to an open future*.

This objection rests on the predominant view of autonomy according to which individuals possess certain negative rights. In this view, autonomy sets up restrictions or side-constraints on how other agents should treat an autonomous person. Many people feel that this negative right would not be properly honored if we adopted a medical practice that consisted in shaping next generations according to the traits (physical, cognitive, mood, etc.) that we now happen to value.

However, even if genetic engineering might predispose an individual to develop certain traits and skills, she might still retain the capacity of making her own choices. The deterministic picture presupposed in the present objection is simply not true. Whether or not a child develops certain (genetically conditioned) traits depends to a great degree on environmental and social factors as well. And even if the new techniques introduced a (further) manipulative factor in the pedagogical process, gene technology would not then be essentially different from traditional education. Also a bad educator may reduce the educand's control over her life options.[4] Thus, the decisive question is not whether the improvement is made with the individual's consent but whether the individual retains her/his capacity to freely choose what path of life to pursue. Provided genetic enhancement *adds* to the capacities and aptitudes possessed by the individual without neutralizing or annulling others, there would be no problem in widening the individual capacity repertoire in this way. Of course, we know very little, if anything, at present on those matters. But that question is for natural scientists and the medical profession to answer. Provided it was satisfactorily solved in the future, no objection to genetic enhancement could be raised from an autonomy point of view.

Self-realization

Recently a different, positive notion of autonomy has taken form in the bioethical debate which emphasizes *self-realization* instead of side-constraints. This ideal underlines the value of living one's life in accordance with one's own basic authentic desires, actualized by one's own decisions and actions. If a person knows in advance about her future genetic predispositions (included the propensity to develop certain diseases), she is simply in a better position to plan her life in accordance with her own basic wishes. This line of reasoning is often used to justify offering assisted reproductive technologies and prenatal diagnosis, as it is considered that these medical procedures promote reproductive autonomy by helping couples to realize their family plans (Chadwick *et al.*, 1999). The same argument might be used regarding the modification of our offspring through genetic means.

However, although this newly developed autonomy ideal apparently promises to settle the question of genetic enhancements, it also raises further complications. The most disturbing one is concerned with the *pre-selection* of individuals for certain activities on grounds of genetic testing. Through genetic testing, children might be selected to participate – or not be allowed to be a part of – in a particular sport discipline on the grounds of their genetic predisposition to be successful. Thus, even if knowledge about what kind of (sporting) activity a person is most fitted to perform is in itself no threat to that person's autonomy, the way in which that information is used by others (for instance, sport managers, sport officials, and coaches) might constitute a serious threat to the individual's possibility of making an own choice.

Another concern that has been expressed regarding the ideal of self-realization is related to *authenticity*. On a reasonable interpretation of the autonomy ideal, it is not enough that the individual be capable of doing what she desires: these desires must also be her own in the sense of not being originated by deception, manipulation, indoctrination, etc. (Tännsjö, 1998, chapter 4). Genetically pre-implanted traits, critics would say, can hardly satisfy this requirement. Is that really so?

Authenticity

It might be argued that enacting desires and preferences that rest on traits and skills that have been instilled in us through genetic engineering cannot possibly be seen as acting on our own, authentic reasons. Thus, even if the decision itself to carry on with our life plans would be a free one (nobody would be coercing us), and in a certain sense autonomous (we would be able to act as we desire), it would nonetheless be an inauthentic decision due to the character of the desires and preferences we would be acting upon.[5]

Niklas Juth (chapter 3, this volume) asks what it means to govern the forming of a desire. Are not all desires formed by factors the subject does not control if the story of the forming is told from the start? This seems to suggest that the authenticity of desires should not be understood in terms of self-governance regarding the creation of desires. According to this alternative account, the conditions of authenticity should be understood as a pro-attitude towards the desires one happens to have, given knowledge about why one has these desires. The more it is approved of, given a certain level of knowledge, the more authentic it is. In this view, authenticity is a matter of degree depending on two factors: level of knowledge and level of approval. It is thus not the approval, or liking, or acceptance of the *explanation* that is of relevance in itself but rather the approval (or liking, or acceptance) of the *desire itself, given knowledge about why one has it.*[6] It is not difficult to grasp that, provided she approved of the desires, life plans, goals, etc., the traits genetically designed before her birth have given rise to, an individual who was submitted to germline genetic transformations (say, to be able to become a talented athlete) might not only fulfill the condition of acting autonomously (authentically), but even of getting her autonomy enhanced as a result of a broader dominion of life options in the future.

Reinforcing suspect cultural values

What about the charge that genetic enhancements might reinforce elitist cultural values? Confronted with the prospect of genetically modifying our genome, some authors would like to remind us of the eugenic experiments of the Nazi regime. Others argue instead that this parallel is not justified as these genetic modifications would now be voluntarily chosen by individuals themselves rather than imposed by totalitarian authorities, as in the Nazi state.

There is, however, another critical aspect related to the present objection that is independent of the kind of political system we live in. It runs as follows: allowing lower-performing individuals to modify themselves in order to get characteristics (physical, cognitive, or of other sort) that belong to the best-situated part of a population implies disrespecting the idiosyncrasy of those who are considered as different and amounts to indirectly reinforcing "the tyranny of the normal." Instead of showing respect for what individuals – all individuals – do, by letting low performers become genetically modified we would be indirectly encouraging them to adopt the standards of the genetically best fitted as a condition for social recognition. This phenomenon is particularly evident in the disability debate. As it has been explicitly stated in the discussion on deafness culture, many disabled people refuse to emulate, sometimes even to adapt to, "normal" standards and demand instead to be recognized for what they are.

This objection, however, has not gone unanswered. Encouraging low performers or disabled people to reach the levels of performance that hitherto have been achieved by physically able individuals (or athletes) would not necessarily imply any form of disrespect for the lower performers. First, both low performers and disabled athletes already emulate the performance standards of fully physically able individuals/athletes. Should they then be blamed for lack of respect for their companions? Second, it is not a question of respect, but rather of granting everyone the right of improving herself as she sees most suited. In that regard, what is at stake is the eventual aggregate effect of a collective's actions (that is, the reinforcement of majority's standards that might occur when many individuals choose to get enhanced) versus the tangible welfare (happiness, hedonistic, etc.) gain for each individual that follows from getting rid of a trait that she experiences as burdensome. Take for instance stammer. Suppose it were possible to get rid of that troublesome speech dysfunction by means of genetic engineering. In so doing, a stammerer would according to the present objection be reinforcing the speech standards of the majority. Why not accept that there are stammerers and simply see it as a different way of talking? Well, one could also say: why not asking stammerers what they want? After all, they are the ones who experience the feeling of not being able to communicate in a fluent way with others. Why should these individuals bear the burden of not reinforcing majority standards by not getting rid of a trait they experience as burdensome? As a matter of fact, the same reasoning might be advanced concerning every other physical or psychological shortcoming. Some of them will clearly fall within the category of illness. In that case, opponents of gene technology might argue that we are not reinforcing dubious majority standards, but instead curing an individual from a scientifically provable pathological condition. Other people will instead argue that what really matters is how the condition is experienced by the subject, rather than whether it falls into a well-established and recognized illness diagnosis. In other words, here we meet again all the difficulties related to the distinction between therapy and enhancement we accounted for before. It is to put it mildly not easy to see how this issue could be settled, other than simply by leaving those decisions to the individuals affected. This does not mean that all these interventions should be financed by taxpayers. Perhaps it might be possible to pinpoint a criterion to draw a line between publicly financed genetic interventions and those which should reasonably be paid by the patient. But at least one thing emerges as crystal-clear in this discussion: the state should not be involved in telling people how they should feel regarding certain physical or psychological conditions.

More directly relevant for (elite) sports, a related objection says that enhancing *elite athletes* would be particularly problematic, due to the importance they have as role models for the young. In a world in which athletes become transhumans (or, rather, super-humans), this might be interpreted by the younger generation as a signal that the weak, the ugly, or the less intelligent should be despised.

On the opposite side of this controversy, we find authors affirming that we should not exaggerate the impact on the young that a genetically enhanced sports world might have. Rather than cementing fascistoid attitudes among them, what these authors at worst foresee is the definitive discredit of *commercialized* elite sports. Even more than today, it will then become a freak show. But rather than being a problem, this might lead people to choose to spend their time practicing recreational sports instead of expressing their ethically dubious admiration for the winner in commercialized sport arenas. Is it really so evident that such a development would be noxious for society?

Finally, it has also been argued that, in spite of the objections to genetic improvements, the context is already settled by current scientific developments. Perhaps there is something wrong with this development. It might lead, for instance, to the creation of a new, superior species endowed with better tools to cope with the circumstances of life than we have at present. This, however, is not necessarily to the detriment of others. Depending on how it is implemented, such a development might even turn out to be beneficial for other people than the enhanced individuals themselves.[7] It is true that inequality will probably be increased in an enhanced new world. But, even then, everyone who can be benefited by it will probably in fact be benefited.

Self-defeatingness

A further observation to be made is related to the fact that, if everyone gets enhanced, then the competitive advantage an enhanced person might get at the beginning will soon be erased, with the result that everyone will be performing at a higher level but now with the initial equality (or inequality) in performance restored. This phenomenon is usually discussed as "the looping effect."

Against this two arguments might be raised. First, even if some enhancements only have competitive value, we should not forget that others are positive in a non-relative manner, in the sense of benefiting the person enhanced independently of what others do. If I get enhanced in order to diminish my sleep need and work harder, other people might soon erase this competitive advantage by doing the same. No one is better off, neither in competitive terms (we all work longer now) nor in well-being terms (probably most people will feel worse due to increased labor burden). But if I get my taste sense enhanced (thus being able to experience different and richer flavors than before), or if I improve my reading abilities so that I now am able to get acquainted with much more of the world literature than before (I simply read faster and understand better!), then that will most probably allow me to enjoy more of the goods things in life no matter what others do.

Secondly, the objection from the looping effect presupposes that all people will have equal and direct access to genetic improvements. Otherwise, how could it be argued that, as soon as some person or group gets enhanced, others will follow the example and do the same? However, as it will be stressed in the following section, it is far from obvious that this scenario will obtain. Let us therefore now discuss the distributive aspects of the new genetics.

Distributive justice

A majority of authors fear that, as getting the necessary or desired genes either into somatic or germ cells will be prohibitively expensive for many people, only those who can afford the new genetic technology will be able to benefit from it (Buchanan *et al.*, 2000). Is it not unjust to discriminate against disadvantaged groups in society, making new medical advances available only for the better off?

According to a (modified) Rawlsian approach, the increased gap in genetic fitness between the poor and the rich will have a negative impact on individuals' life projects and plans. Cognitive and emotional skills, for instance, are directly relevant for career opportunities. Thus, the unfair distribution of these (genetically enhanced) traits will affect individuals' chance to realize their career and life plans. A similar reasoning might be advanced regarding at least certain genetic modifications of our physical condition. It is true that career opportunities, at least in our part of the world, are barely related to our capacity to excel physically. With the obvious exception of elite sports, enlarged muscle mass or increased capacity for oxygen intake beyond what is considered as normal levels are seldom decisive for our possibilities of success in today's professional world (although they might be decisive for individuals' survival in other, less economically developed areas of the planet). But a large number of genetic enhancements of our physical condition will aim to enhance our health. And a healthy person has no doubt better chances to success in the professional world, even in a predominantly knowledge-based and nonphysical labor market as ours. So, inequality in the distribution of genetic assets will deprive the poor, and perhaps further social strata in society, from career achievements that are directly related to their well-being.[8] Or so would a sophisticated Rawlsian argue.

On the other hand, it might be asked why society *should grant to the contemporary poor a right to veto a development that will be positive for all at a later stage of society.* Historically, the adoption of new medicines and medical techniques always took place in a socioeconomic situation of inequality. Although antibiotics, for instance, were first unavailable to the poor, they are now used by the majority of the world's population, regional inequalities notwithstanding. By the same reasoning, genetic technology could probably become available to the poor of the future, although not for the *contemporary* poor. I will not extend myself further on this issue.

Gender equity

There are in my view two different issues related to gender equity and variation in gender roles (or lack thereof) that deserves attention. One is the issue of women's reproductive freedom; the other is the supposedly male-biased character of most of the physical enhancements suggested for women in sports.

Although this is far from being a real possibility yet, enhancement technologies might be used to further women's reproductive freedom, for instance by allowing them to freely choose at what moment in life to have children. From time to time we hear of women who become pregnant and give birth at postmenopausal age. Would it be desirable to do this by genetic means? And how would sports governing bodies and the sporting community react to that (Spallone & Steinberg, 1987)? One of the authors of this chapter has argued elsewhere for the possibility that this kind of genetic modifications might end up among the candidates to be included in the list on banned doping substances and training methods, mainly due to the fact that postponed motherhood (i) renders a competitive advantage in elite sports and (ii) might require in the future using gene technology. If this happens, then we might confront a situation in which an application of gene technology probably deemed as socially desirable (it would contribute to increasing gender equity in society) was forbidden for sportswomen.[9]

Another interesting issue when discussing (genetic) enhancements is related with what is traditionally considered as masculine/feminine. Unlike other kinds of (genetically induced) enhancements discussed at present (for instance, improvements of our cognitive skills and mood condition), the sort of physical enhancements hitherto envisioned in the world of sports appear to be clearly male-biased. Mostly, what is hoped the new technologies will achieve in a not so far away future are improvements in strength, length and speed beyond species-normal levels, all of which are univocally understood as male attributes, at least at the present stage of our evolutionary history. So, the question might be posed: are these genetics enhancements male-biased? And, if so, what would be the point in promoting them?

This objection has been indirectly met in Tännsjö and Tamburrini (2005). There we questioned the underlying assumption on which the above objection rests, namely that strength, length and speed are *essentially* male attributes, rather than (to a relevant degree) the result of cultural processes. We therefore do not develop this argument here. However, there is another response to this criticism that, although it was advanced in Tännsjö and Tamburrini (2005), it can nonetheless be underlined once more here. We cannot in advance exclude the possibility that at least some men might also want to change their genetic constitution to acquire physical traits in which women were previously superior. And if this scenario appears as improbable, then we might try to design appropriate social policies in order to encourage men to give up their muscular supremacy. Why not for instance offer tax reductions to those men willing to contribute to a more equal, and more diversified, gender order?

Sport ethos

The notion of "the ethos of sports," in itself very vague, is usually characterized as a tacit agreement, partly based on tradition, on how the game should be played. Central to this notion is the concept of *fairness in competition*. There is a wide agreement among sports philosophers on the importance of this notion as a central ingredient of the sports ethos. Fairness in sports might be characterized in a narrow way (competing in accordance to the regulations)[10] or in a wider way (competing only through the skills and excellences that are relevant for the sports discipline in question).[11] In line with this latter interpretation, many people think artificial enhancing methods are obviously unacceptable, and are inclined to the idea that only natural talent should decide the outcome of a sporting competition.

On the other hand, it has been asked why only congenital, genetically determined traits can justify a sporting victory but not acquired ones. Elsewhere we have argued that such a notion of justice is not only flawed, it is also becoming obsolete, due to the fast medical development that is taking place today. There is no reason to let the genetic lottery decide a sports competition, when the winning odds of the competitors might be leveled out by intentional and goal-oriented efforts to achieve a higher sports performance level.[12]

Furthermore, suppose we some day had the possibility of genetically modifying our offspring before the affected individuals are even born. Should our children then be banned from competition? By resorting to the dubious distinction between "natural" and "artificial" qualities, one could at most ban our children from competition, but not their offspring (it might for instance be argued that our children, unlike their offspring, achieved the relevant physical traits through a genetic intervention and not by birth). If one still wants to prohibit this kind of genetic enhancement, then it will be necessary to proscribe a whole family, included generations yet to come. Otherwise, if our children's offspring were allowed to participate in sports competitions on the grounds that they are not responsible for their physiological characteristics, the ban on genetic enhancements will become toothless.

Privacy

There is another problematic aspect of the ban on genetic enhancements in sports. In order to control that athletes abide by the prohibition, it will be necessary to test them for genetic traits. This constitutes a violation of athletes' right to privacy. To begin with, the tests might reveal information they don't want to have, for instance on their propensity to develop certain serious diseases. Secondly, this information might come to be misused by third parties, for instance insurance companies and employers, against the athletes.

But do private organizations such as the IOC and other sport federations not have the right to define the rules according to which they want their competitions to be carried out? After all it might be argued that if you want to be a part of the game then you have to abide by its rules.

Things, however, are not that easy, Let us recall for instance that the IOC itself abolished sex testing before the Olympic Games at Sydney 2000 with the argument that such testing violated women athletes' privacy. It is true that, at the time it was abolished, sex testing had become discredited among women athletes and the public opinion. But the same could be said about genetic testing. Most of us feel, and rightly so, that revealing our genetic constitution is a threat to our privacy. Besides, even if the World Anti-doping Agency (WADA), the IOC, and other international sport federations could manage to get "acceptance" for the genetic testing from athletes, we should not forget that, by testing the athletes, the genetic constitution of their relatives will also be revealed. So, their families too will be given information on their genetic constitution that they might not wish to have. And they might also be submitted to the risk of being discriminated by employers or insurance companies. So, testing for gene doping violates not only the privacy of those submitted to the testing, it also exposes third parties to harm (Tamburrini, 2005, pp.86–8).

Sports medicine

Two issues related to gene doping have particular relevance for sport medicine: safety and the ethical aspects of testing procedures.

Safety As stated above, potential health risks is one of the criteria that determines which substances and methods are included in the doping list. The vast majority of the traditional doping procedures satisfy that condition, and the same applies to gene doping. As a general conclusion, it can be said that gene therapy, though the trials performed have been relatively safe, is still a potentially very dangerous technique only available in a few experimental laboratories. However, as gene therapy becomes a more established technique comparable to normal treatments, safety and availability might be increased *provided treatment is performed in controlled environments*. In general, the potential risks of gene therapy increase when the procedures are implemented in uncontrolled environments, as the ones cheating athletes will have to resort to in order to (gene) dope. In order to reduce the risk of overproduction of genetic elements it would be required that doctors monitor the production level. But sports medicine doctors are impeded to participate in any genetic procedure classified as doping by sport governing bodies. This poses a challenge to the sport medical profession. Most probably, sport medicine doctors in the future will have to choose between acting as (gene) doping police or contributing to minimize harm by offering their counseling to athletes who wish to dope. It should be recalled that, unlike traditional doping, genetic enhancements will be a part of medicine, legally permitted and socially accepted. Is it really ethically defensible for a sport medical doctor to refuse to reduce harm by supporting the chase against dopers in the name of a supposed "purity of sports"?

On the other hand, although Peter Schjerling (2005) believes that, "Perhaps the danger would be relatively small if used in organised sports teams where physicians are involved as well," he issues a warning: "However, the physicians may also be pressed to allow the use to go too far to achieve the maximal effect."[13] A similar viewpoint has been advanced by Holm (2007). In his chapter "Is doping under medical control possible?" he purports to show "that we have no reason to believe that the legalisation of doping will lead to a situation where open doping under medical control will become the norm." Particularly if the sportsperson is contracted by a specific club or sporting association, Holm argues, the sport doctor might feel loyal to her employer rather than to the sportsperson. A contracted sportsperson's chance of getting impartial advice might therefore be seriously jeopardized by the sport doctor's dependent position to her employer.[14]

No matter how certain the predictions made by Schjerling and Holm might turn out to be, they cannot possibly be a justification of the doping ban. If sport doctors all too often forget to serve their patients (in this case, the sportspersons) due to exaggerated career ambitions, then the answer is reinforcing the code of professional ethics under which they have to act and/or increasing control in order to be sure they act as they are expected to do when exercising their profession. But none of these alternatives seem to presuppose keeping the doping ban.

The ethics of testing Another issue related to (gene) doping that is relevant for the incipient sport medical ethical discussion is how the testing procedures will be carried out. According to current knowledge among natural scientists and geneticists, to discover gene dopers it will be required to analyze a tissue sample. However, a test based on taking pieces of the athlete's muscle is not likely to be ethically accepted. This has a direct bearing on the question of the reliability of the testing methods as well. If doping controllers will be impeded from using the most effective and reliable testing procedures for ethical reasons, then the possibility that gene doping might go undetected increases. A ban that is not appropriately controlled is a poor warrant of fairness in competition: if a sufficient number of cheaters get away with their (gene) doping, rule-complying athletes will be competing in a situation of inferiority. So, a further issue to be discussed is how the sport medical profession will relate to the latent conflict between on the one hand sportspersons' right to (i) privacy and (ii) not to be submitted to too intrusive testing procedures, and on the other hand the need to develop reliable testing procedures to detect gene dopers. To put it briefly: is transparency in sports worth the prize of sacrificing a group of patients,' (namely, sportspersons) rights vis à vis their doctors? And, if transparency is worth that much, would it not be preferable to attain it through lifting the ban rather than through chasing dopers?

The detection difficulties mentioned above are not limited to "muscle doping." Contrary to what was believed until recently, there might also be problems with detecting EPO doping. To begin with, according to some recent studies, we all have rather big daily variations in our hematocrit levels, which are even more accentuated if we train intensively. This being so, it might prove to be meaningless to start mapping blood profiles.

A further difficulty related to EPO testing has to do with the fact that there are many substances that may activate the EPO receptor that are not EPO. This means that it is possible to enhance the endogenous EPO production without taking rHuEPO. These substances might of course also be tested for, but at present it is not worth the trouble: the list will be too long and – therefore – the testing will be very expensive. Another possibility are prolyl hydroxylase inhibitors. They will also increase the endogenous EPO production without the need of taking rHuEPO. Again, it is doubtful whether it would be worth testing for these inhibitors as the list will grow almost indefinitely.

Another conclusion (perhaps the most important for the justification of the doping ban) arrived at in these studies was that EPO increases red-cell mass but also decreases blood plasma volume. This means most probably that EPO is not as dangerous as we thought, as the risk of blood clots is not as high if the total volume of blood is increased (Lundby *et al.*, 2008). In that regard, it seems to be more rational to introduce maximum levels of blood density and not allow athletes to compete when they show levels above the permitted limit. But no endeavors can reasonably be devoted to show how athletes achieve a particular hematocrit level.

Conclusions

The conclusions arrived at in this chapter can be summed as follows:

1. Although gene therapy appears to be a safe medical technique, gene doping might prove to be hazardous for sportspersons' health. This fact, however, would be mainly due to the existence of the prohibition and the difficulty it creates in carrying out research that might lead to the development of harmless doping substances and methods.
2. The prospect of developing effective testing methods in order to disclose doping use seems at present not to be very encouraging. First, invasive methods seem to be required to disclose the use of banned anabolic steroids, as for instance the collection and storage of muscle samples by biopsies. If the testing consists of

controlling certain physiological markers that might indicate the use of forbidden gender transfer technologies, then an obstacle would be that the testing might also disclose a predisposition to develop certain pathological conditions that might be present both in the athlete as well as in her/his family. Finally, regarding blood doping (for instance with EPO), it seems that mapping athletes' previous blood profiles might not be of much use, given the great variation in hematocrit level showed by healthy individuals, particularly when they are submitted to hard training programs. In addition to that, EPO use appears in some recent studies as relatively harmless, as the total density of the blood remains unchanged. This is due to the fact that, although the red cell volume increases using EPO, the plasma volume is decreased to a similar degree.

3. Regarding autonomy and other related ethical notions usually discussed in the (gene) doping debate, it seems as if no serious threat is posed to individual autonomy or, for that matter, to the authenticity we usually desire our choices and decisions be characterized by. Provided the individual has a pro-attitude towards the desires he happens to have, and given knowledge about why he has these desires, there is no reason to consider such desires and choices as inauthentic. If we did, we should as a matter of fact have to accept there are no authentic desires.

4. On the charge that genetic enhancing might reinforce suspected cultural values, it has been argued here that the impact on the young that a genetically enhanced sport world might have should not be exaggerated. Rather than cementing fascistoid attitudes among them, what we might foresee is the discrediting of *commercialized* elite sports.

5. On the supposedly self-defeating effect of enhancements, it was concluded that most improvements of our human capacities allow us to increase our capacity of enjoying certain valuable activities in life, irrespectively of how other people respond to these enhancements.

6. On the issue of distributive justice, it was argued that to object to the implementation of new genetic technologies on the grounds of the unequal distribution of genetic assets that might occur during the first period of implementation, we need to answer the question of *why society should grant to the contemporary poor a right to veto a development that will be positive for all at a later stage of society.* Most probably, genetic technology will become available to the poor of the future.

7. Although this is far from being a real possibility yet, enhancement technologies might be used to further women's reproductive freedom, for instance by allowing them to freely choose at what moment in life to have children. Furthermore, we might come to experience in the future more varied gender roles, with physically stronger females and more rhythmic and agile men, thanks to physiological transformations made possible by the new genetic technologies.

8. On the underlying notion of fairness in competition that seems to animate the sport ethos ideal, it was asked why only congenital, genetically determined traits can justify a sporting victory but not acquired ones. In that sense, such a notion of justice was found not only flawed but also obsolete, due to the fast medical development that is taking place today.

9. Privacy is another problematic aspect of the ban on genetic enhancements in sports. In order to control that athletes abide by the prohibition, it will be necessary to test them for genetic traits. Thus, the tests might reveal information about their propensity to develop certain serious diseases (as well as their relatives'). There is a risk that this information would be misused by third parties, for instance insurance companies and employers.

10. As the potential risks of gene therapy increase when the procedures are implemented in uncontrolled environments, a challenge is posed to the sport medical profession. Is it really defensible to act as (gene) doping police? Or should sport medical doctors instead try to minimize harm by offering their counseling to athletes who wish to dope? This question is particularly relevant in a context in which, unlike traditional doping, genetic enhancements are becoming a part of medical practice.

Furthermore, and related to (2) above, if doping controllers are impeded from using the most effective and reliable testing procedures for ethical reasons, then the possibility that gene doping might go undetected increases. Among other things, a ban that is not appropriately controlled is a poor warrant of fairness in competition.

The final result of the ethical discussion on (genetic) enhancements in elite sports suggests the following reflections. In the first place, there seems to be a need for increased insight about how eventual conflicts between socially desirable goals and the limits imposed by the official sport ethos should be decided. If the arguments above are right, sport officials and sports organizations might be compelled to choose between either proscribing a positive practice for society or allowing a certain genetic technique which enhances sport performance.

Secondly, we need to conduct an open and unprejudiced discussion on how sports governing bodies should handle the fact that in the future most people will, in one way or another, already have undergone genetic enhancement before the age of adulthood. Should all these people be banned from sport competitions? Such cases might be a reality in, say, the next 10–15 years.

Finally, the arguments advanced in this chapter should draw our attention to the rationality of coping with the new challenges posed by medical-technical developments with the old paradigm of prohibition. In that regard, society and the sports community are in an urgent need of developing alternative ways of addressing these issues.

Notes

1. See, for instance, Tamburrini (2000), mainly pp. 50–1.
2. For a more thorough account of this position, see Tamburrini (2000, 2002).
3. See, for instance, Tamburrini (2005) and van Hilvoorde (2005).
4. See, for instance, Tamburrini (2005, pp. 84–5).
5. According to some influential contributors to the autonomy debate, authenticity is the most fundamental component of autonomy. See e.g. Christman (1998).
6. See Juth, chapter 3, this volume. This account of authenticity is more fully explicated in Juth (2005, chapter III).

7. What is usually suggested in that case is the prospect of developing individuals, or a new species, with improved empathy and social engagement.

8. Here it could be retorted by a convinced Rawlsian that to block access to the privileged positions to those who are less genetically endowed would be discriminatory and therefore contrary to the difference principle. However, it should be recalled that Rawls' principle in this regard is not completely egalitarian. Rather, what the difference principle commits us to do is not to block access to positions to individuals *due to irrelevant criteria*. To perform worse at work, even as a consequence of inherited genetic inferiority, is not an irrelevant discriminatory criterion. Thus, the inadequacy of the difference principle to deal with the distributive challenge posed by the new genetics still remains. According to that principle, *any reasonable* improvement in the situation of the worse-off part of the population will do, even when – as the case is with genetic enhancement – this perpetuates the situation of social and economic disadvantage of the poor.

9. See Tamburrini (2009).

10. See Tamburrini (2000), particularly chapter 2.

11. For a thorough discussion of different notions of fairness in competition, see Loland (2002).

12. This argument is advanced in an article – "The genetic design of a new Amazon," which is included in *Genetic Technology and Sport – Ethical Questions,* an anthology co-edited by Torbjörn Tännsjö and Claudio Tamburrini (2005).

13. In "The basics of gene doping", included in Tännsjö and Tamburrini's above quoted anthology from 2005 (quotation on p. 29).

14. Although a sportsperson who lives on her own prize money and publicity earnings, and who also employs her own advisors, apparently would have more possibility of getting impartial advice from a sport doctor, Holm draws our attention to the fact that elite sportspersons might have an interest in using a drug or doping method long before it has been properly tested by the pharmaceutical industry. So, even independent sportspersons will probably be subjected to health risks if the ban on doping were lifted. Having said this, it should be noted that Holm does not advance his arguments in support of the doping ban. He simply states (2007, p.144) that, if he is right, then "one of the alleged positive effects of legalising doping is unlikely to occur. This does not show that doping should not be legalised, but just that we should not expect the world of sports to become a much better place if it is, or doping a much safer practice."

References

Arruda, V.R., Lima, C.S., Grignoli, C.R., Melo, M.B., Lorand-Metze, I., Alberto, F.L. *et al.* (2001). Increased risk for acute myeloid leukaemia in individuals with glutathione S-transferase mu 1 (GSTM1) and theta 1 (GSTT1) gene defects. *European Journal of Haematology,* **66**, 383–8.

Buchanan, A., Brock, D.W., Daniels, N. & Wikler, D. (2000). *From Choice to Chance – Genetics and Justice.* Cambridge: Cambridge University Press.

Chadwick, R. *et al..* (eds.) (1999). *The Ethics of Genetic Screening.* Kluwer.

Christman, J. (1998). Autonomy, independence, and poverty-related welfare policies. *Public Affairs,* **12**(4), 383–405.

Griscelli, F., Opolon, P., Saulnier, P., Mami-Chouaib, F., Gautier, E., Echchakir, H. *et al.* (2003). Recombinant adenovirus shedding after intratumoral gene transfer in lung cancer patients. *Gene Therapy,* **10**, 386–95.

Haisma, H.J. & de Hon, O. (2006). Gene doping. *International Journal of Sports Medicine*, **27**, 257–66.

Holm, S. (2007). Is doping under medical control possible? In C. Tamburrini & T. Tännsjö (eds.), *Sport, Ethics and Philosophy* (Official Journal of the British Philosophy of Sport Association), *Special Issue: The Ethics of Sports Medicine* (pp. 135–45). London: Routledge.

Juth, N. (2005). *Genetic Information: Values and Rights. The Morality of Presymptomatic Genetic Testing.* Göteborg: Acta Philosophica Gothoburgensia.

Loland, S. (2002). *Fair Play in Sport. A Moral Norm System.* London: Routledge.

Lundby, C. *et al.* (2008). Erythropoietin treatment elevates haemoglobin concentration by increasing red cell volume and depressing plasma volume. *Journal of Physiology*, **586**(1), 305–6.

Schjerling, P. (2005). The basics of gene doping. In T. Tännsjö & C. Tamburrini (eds.), *Genetic Technology and Sport – Ethical Questions.* London: Routledge.

Spallone, P. & Steinberg, D.L. (1987). *Made to Order. The Myth of Reproductive and Genetic Progress.* Oxford: Pergamon Press.

Tamburrini, C. (2000). *The "Hand of God"? – Essays in the Philosophy of Sports.* Göteborg, Sweden: Acta Universitatis Gothoburgensis.

Tamburrini, C. (2002). After doping, what? The morality of the genetic engineering of athletes. In S. Eassom & A. Miah (eds.), *Research in Philosophy of Technology – Special Edition on Sport Technology: History, Policy and Philosophy, Vol. 21.* New York: Elsevier Science.

Tamburrini, C. (2005). Educational or genetic blueprints, what's the difference? In T. Tännsjö & C. Tamburrini (eds.), *Genetic Technology and Sport – Ethical Questions.* London: Routledge.

Tamburrini. C. (2009). Genetic technology, postponing motherhood and the doping ban. In V. Möller, M. McNamee & P. Dimeo (eds.), *Elite Sport, Doping and Public Health.* Odense. University Press of Southern Denmark.

Tännsjö, T. (1998). *Vårdetik (Ethics of Care)* Stockholm: Thales.

Tännsjö, T. & Tamburrini, C. (eds.) (2005). *Genetic Technology and Sport – Ethical Questions.* London: Routledge.

Tenenbaum, L., Lehtonen, E. & Monahan, P.E. (2003). Evaluation of risks related to the use of adeno-associated virus-based vectors. *Current Gene Therapy*, **3**(6), 545–65.

21

Physical Enhancement: What Baseline, Whose Judgment?

Søren Holm and Mike McNamee

The purpose of this chapter is to analyze the ethical issues that arise in the context of the use of physical enhancement techniques, i.e. techniques that aim at enhancing one or more physical functions of human beings. Such techniques have been used for millennia since any training aimed at improving strength or skill, for instance, may to some extent count as an enhancement technique. But new biomedical technologies have increased the scope and range of possible enhancements immensely and it is certain that we will see further developments in the future.

In this chapter we will first discuss the many different types of physical enhancement and make the point that one of the most discussed areas of physical enhancement, doping in sports, is only a minor part of the whole enhancement field. Despite this protestation we will, however, also devote considerable attention to enhancement in sports, primarily because of the extensive extant literature. We will then move on to problematize the concept of enhancement and we will show that deciding whether something should count as an enhancement is not a matter for pure personal decision. Having cleared the ground in this way we will then be able to engage with the ethical arguments that have been put forward in the enhancement debate. We will show that the validity of both the pro- and the anti-enhancement arguments is context-dependent and more specifically that some of the arguments against doping in sport are valid.

The Many Types of Physical Enhancement

Let us accept a broad conception of physical enhancement where any development that improves a physical function of a human body, without (net) deleterious side effects, counts as an enhancement. Then it is easy to see that some enhancements are sought for, or are useful for, specific purposes and some for much more general purposes.

It is obvious that some physical enhancements can be classified as other kinds of enhancement as well. Surgical laser correction of myopia which can lead to better than normal sight changes a physical function, i.e. the refraction of light in the eye but it

Enhancing Human Capacities, edited by Julian Savulescu, Ruud ter Meulen and Guy Kahane.
© 2011 Blackwell Publishing Ltd

enhances one of our most important senses. It is, however, not particularly important for our arguments here whether a given intervention is a "pure" physical enhancement or not.

A physical enhancement may be pursued because it is useful in relation to a specific task or set of tasks that the individual in question is engaged in. Athletic enhancements are pursued in order to become a better athlete (in the non-ethical sense of better).[1] But the word "better" is the most general of positive evaluations and does not specify any particular context-free content. Thus what is better for the athlete is that which increases the chance of winning in athletic competitions. Enhancement of specific skills may be sought in work environments or to pursue specific leisure pursuits.

Many of the enhancements pursued or desired are of limited use outside of the specific contexts of their application. The fine motor skills needed to paint tin soldiers (or perhaps more relevant to present adolescents Warhammer 3000™ figures) are of little or no use in general life. And enhancing one function may make it impossible or more difficult to enhance others. Thus the male gymnast who significantly increases the girth of his quadriceps muscles to have greater power for floor work or vaulting, finds that his ability to move his legs around the pommel horse have been made all the more difficult because of the increased musculature which makes it harder to navigate the equipment. Similarly, specialization in one discipline by athletes in the decathlon and heptathlon (and to an even more extreme degree by competitors in the modern pentathlon) typically renders them less competitive in others that comprise the activity.

The likelihood that enhancements might not be compatible was already made by Aristotle in relation to the development of general human potentials (*Metaphysics*, Book 5 Ch 4, Book 7 Ch 4). In discussion of such Scheffler (1991) notes that there are three myths of human potentials: human potentialities are neither fixed, nor harmonious, nor uniformly valuable. In keeping with these thoughts we should not expect enhancements to be equally valuable in the life of all or any particular agents. Nor should we expect that we may combine any or all enhancement that are desired by any particular agent, a point commonly made of the heterogeneity of value as well as desire. Finally, given our developmental nature we ought to expect that certain goods are time dependent (Slote, 1993) and therefore that any enhancements are likely to differ in their desirability according to the role that the capacity plays in the lives of the enhanced at various points during the life course.

A physical enhancement may also, however, be sought because it is of more general use. There are powerful reasons to pursue fitness and improvement (or simply maintenance) of muscle strength, cardiovascular function, and bone density through regular exercise. Such enhancement may ameliorate, prevent, or reduce the risk of a wide range of health problems.

Given a broad conception of enhancement it thus becomes obvious that most activities aimed at achieving physical enhancement are not directed towards athletic goals, and indeed may be completely unrelated to sports. Thus the most commonly used pharmaceutical enhancement is probably Viagra and similar drugs and the enhancement sought through their use is completely non-athletic.[2] Thus the attention being paid to doping in sport as an exemplar of physical enhancement is out of proportion with the magnitude of the problem, especially if doping is seen as a problem primarily of athletic competition, While data is uncertain here, there is regular reporting of between 3–12% of high school uptake of anabolic androgenic steroids (American Academy of Pediatrics[3], 1997; Calfee & Fadale, 2006; Yesalis & Bahrke, 2000) though the figures are typically for males, not females (whose use is more typically between 1–2%). Moreover, the majority of studies are based in North American high schools making generalizations more problematic given its idiosyncratic nature. Finally, the validity of self-report questionnaires, which is the standard method, has also been questioned (Kanayama *et al.*, 2007). Doping in sport is far from being a typical enhancement activity. It occurs in specific contexts that are by definition competitive and whose users aim at the improvement or even perfection of performance in a narrowly circumscribed activity. Most physical enhancements that people pursue are not bounded in this way.

Beyond athletic contexts, a separate and more widespread issue arises in relation to changes in physical appearance like those created by cosmetic surgery, tattooing, scarification, and other body modifications. Most of these modifications do not change any physical function or capacity. Without falling into complete subjectivism about beauty it seems reasonable to hold that beauty is not straightforwardly analyzable as a pure function of the beautiful body and that cosmetic interventions are therefore not straightforwardly functional. Nevertheless, such modifications are at least sometimes sought because they are believed to be enhancing in a broader sense. It may thus make sense to consider them as physical enhancements in a slightly extended sense of that term, also because they fall within the scope of a right to "morphological freedom" advocated by some transhumanists (Sandberg, 2001).

What Counts as an Enhancement?

Until now we have accepted a conception of enhancement that is cashed out in terms of improvement of function. Yet articulating more precisely the concept of improvement is not without problems. There are two intersecting accounts of improvement that are at play: one that makes a distinction between objective (or inter-subjective) and subjective improvements and a second that makes a distinction between improvement in relation to a norm and improvement purely in relation to the *status quo ante*. And it is helpful to keep these apart at least for analytical purposes.

The first distinction is concerned with who is to judge whether a certain change is an improvement. Thus we can ask of any purported enhancement whether it is determined objectively (or inter-subjectively at least) or whether it is exclusively a matter for personal judgment. The second distinction is concerned with what the proper baseline is for judging or measuring improvements. Is it, for instance a species-based norm, or is it the function of one specific individual.[4]

These two intersecting distinctions give rise to four different ways of (mis)understanding improvement and *a fortiori* enhancement. The most restrictive of these is the objective, norm-based account which usually underlies arguments making a distinction between therapy in the sense of bringing a person (or restoring them) to a normal level of functioning and enhancement in the sense of improving function above the normal (Daniels, 2007). The most expansive account is the subjective, status quo account, which essentially entails that any physical change a person deems to be an improvement

Table 21.1   Four different understandings of enhancement

Improvement	Norm based	Status quo based
Objective	Most restrictive Treatment/enhancement distinction	For example the sports "doping" account
Subjective	Rarely held	Least restrictive For example often implied in transhumanist writing

of his function is an improvement (Harris, 2009). The four options can be illustrated as shown in Table 21.1.

Each of the four basic accounts can be further refined. As noted above improvements can be specific or general in relation to function, but it is also possible to conceive of physical improvements which do not strictly improve any particular function yet still improve the welfare of the person.

Within the subjective accounts further distinctions can be made in relation to whether the subjective judgment is personal or social and whether it can be fallible or not. A personal subjective account holding that a person's judgment concerning improvement is infallible is clearly implausible. I may think that an increase in manual dexterity improving my game of tiddly-winks is an improvement, but I may clearly be wrong. Similarly I may be wrong in my belief concerning whether or not a having a specific tattoo is likely to be an enhancement or not.[5] That such judgment can be wrong and that this is not an infrequent occurrence is sometimes overlooked because there are possible liberal ethical arguments for allowing people to act on erroneous judgments (see the discussion below of Mill's so-called harm principle). My choosing a harmful act, wrongly thinking it to enhance my welfare, may be permissible but it is not thereby an accurate estimation of enhancement. Liberal ethical arguments cannot, however, make erroneous arguments correct. The personal subjective account furthermore suffers from the problem that whether something counts as an enhancement is likely to fluctuate markedly over time. I may think my prominent tattoo an enhancement now, but not when I appear before a sober panel in a crucial job interview in five years' time. This is clearly a problem if the concept of enhancement is to bear any positive ethical weight. That is to say, if the fact that something counts as an enhancement is to give people (other than the allegedly enhanced person) a reason to help him or her in pursuing it or even a reason to remove obstacles to its pursuit, the estimation of its status as a potential enhancement must in principle be made or endorsed by an external source.

A slightly more technical reason to be mindful of the many different ways in which an improvement might be defined is that the transitivity of "better than" is only secured if all instances are evaluated according to the same standard. That "A is better than C" only follows with certainty from the two premises that "A is better than B" and "B is better than C" if "better than" is used in the same sense in the two premises. If insufficient attention is given to the different possible senses of "better than" the possibility for equivocation is great.

The Ethics of Physical Enhancement

There is one anti-enhancement argument and one pro-enhancement argument that are often used as if they can work as "hole in one" arguments that are able to solve once and for all whether physical enhancement is ethically acceptable or not.

The anti-enhancement argument relies on the treatment/enhancement distinction whereas the pro-enhancement argument relies on an application of Mill's harm principle. Both arguments are problematic and their scope much narrower than is typically assumed by their proponents. Both arguments are also discussed extensively in other chapters in this book, so our exposition and critique here will be brief.

Let us first look at the general anti-enhancement arguments. The argument relying on making a distinction between treatment and enhancement posits that there is a difference between treating persons who are deficient in some function and bringing them up to normal functioning and enhancing people above the normal functioning range (Daniels, 2007). Restoring or normalizing function is consistent with dominant understandings of medical treatment and therefore morally unproblematic, whereas enhancing someone is thought to be morally problematic.

There are two main problems with this line of argument. The first is that the treatment/enhancement distinction is not clear and therefore inoperable (Harris, 2007) and the second is that even if it was clear it is unclear whether the moral value that is put on it can be justified (Murray, 2006).

In order to draw the line between treatments and enhancements reference is most often made either to what is normal, for instance species-typical functioning on Boorsean lines or to a notion of what is natural. Both the concepts of normality and the natural are problematic in themselves (Holm, 2006, 2007).

Moreover, the distinction is afflicted with other problems because there are many examples of interventions where it is unclear whether they bring about treatments or enhancements and where the same intervention can be both. Improving muscle function can be a treatment in some people and an enhancement in others. Everything then hangs on what is regarded as the baseline for comparison. A standard example from the literature is that of immunization. In preventing a virus developing into a deleterious condition the immune system is boosted above normal levels – that is to say it is enhanced. Yet, objectors reply, it is widely agreed to be an accepted medical intervention. It can be argued that this example does not quite have the power that it seems. It may be that the act is in its nature preventative, and that the enhancement of functioning is merely a consequence rather than the aim of the intervention or that immunization merely activates an inherent potential of the immune system (i.e. that although the measles vaccine is artificial it activates a natural response, because a similar response is activated by measles infection).

A more problematic example is where the standard treatment for a condition takes the individual beyond their normal functioning. This type of example has occurred frequently in elite sports. There are many examples of baseball pitchers whose elbow surgery has increased their pitching capacity. And Floyd Landis, the winner of the 2006 Tour de France, underwent a hip replacement operation that increased his functional capacity.

A more general response may be made from informal logic. It pertains to the matter of conceptual vagueness. Color predicates are a paradigmatic example of conceptual vagueness. Yet their uncertainty (when precisely is something yellow and not orange, orange but not red etc.) does not make them meaningless, useless, or even less useful. It does not follow that the existence of borderline cases necessarily renders us unable to use the distinction between those predicates. Thus, merely from the fact that there are fuzzy borders between treatment and enhancement, and that there may be interventions that count as both at the same time, does not imply that there are no clear cases. To use an analogy the monotremes (i.e. the platypus and the echidna) are borderline mammals but the fact that they exist does not show that no animals can definitely be identified as mammals.

With regard to the second problem the issue is simply that it does not even *prima facie* seem to be the case that all improvements moving someone from normality or from what is natural to a state of even better functioning are necessarily morally problematic.

The overarching pro-enhancement argument relies on Mill's harm principle as expressed in *On Liberty*:

> The object of this Essay is to assert one very simple principle, as entitled to govern absolutely the dealings of society with the individual in the way of compulsion and control, whether the means used be physical force in the form of legal penalties, or the moral coercion of public opinion. That principle is that the sole end for which mankind are warranted, individually or collectively, in interfering with the liberty of action of any of their number, is self-protection. That the only purpose for which power can be rightfully exercised over any member of a civilized community, against his will, is to prevent harm to others. His own good, either physical or moral, is not a sufficient warrant. He cannot rightfully be compelled to do or forbear because it will be better for him to do so, because it will make him happier, because, in the opinions of others, to do so would be wise, or even right. These are good reasons for remonstrating with him, or reasoning with him, or persuading him, or entreating him, but not for compelling him, or visiting him with any evil, in case he do otherwise. To justify that, the conduct from which it is desired to deter him must be calculated to produce evil to some one else. The only part of the conduct of any one, for which he is amenable to society, is that which concerns others. In the part which merely concerns himself, his independence is, of right, absolute. Over himself, over his own body and mind, the individual is sovereign (Mill, 1978)

When this argument is applied to enhancement one can reach the conclusion that enhancements can only be prohibited by society if their pursuit causes harm to other people. And harm is most often explicated in terms of direct, significant harm thereby excluding for instance symbolic or positional harm.

But the Millian pro-enhancement position also suffers from significant problems. There is a pragmatic problem in the sense that we have not generally organized our societies on Millian lines. Modern welfare states already intervene regularly in a very wide range of human activities that are only indirectly harmful to other people or where the harm in question is primarily symbolic (e.g. restrictions of sexually explicit advertising). In some sports within liberal societies, as we shall discus below, there are prohibitions on the individual that mitigate autonomously chosen self-harming activities too. At a more theoretical level problems arise because the justification for the harm principle is not sufficiently robust. It cannot be based in the idea that people are never wrong about what is in their own interest, because we know that that idea is false. We know that people can be very and even sometimes disastrously wrong in such assessments. It can furthermore not be justified by the idea that outsiders are never in a better position than the person himself to judge these matters, because we also know that that idea is false. Outsiders are sometimes in a much better position to judge where a person's best interest lies. Thus, at its strongest, the harm principle can only be used to justify a rebuttable presumption against societal intervention or prohibition.

We shall now proceed to discuss some ethical issues related to specific enhancement contexts.

Doping and Performance Enhancement in Sports

Some activities discussed in the context of enhancement are defined purely or predominantly in terms of conventional rules. This class of activities includes all organized sports and a variety of other social activities (e.g. the Muslim *Haj*). This has implications for an analysis of physical enhancements within the context of such activities. The first and obvious implication is that given that the rules are conventional there can be nothing ethically wrong in having a rule against specific forms of enhancement as long as that rule is not discriminatory or harm-producing. This does not mean that rules prohibiting (or for that matter requiring) specific enhancements cannot be discussed, promoted or criticized, just that the arguments in that discussion have to relate themselves to the purpose and meaning of the specific rule-bound activity.

But from the conventional nature of the rules follows little about what their content should be. All sets of conventional rules restrict the freedoms of those who participate in the activity and this fact restricts the possibility to appeal directly to ideas concerning liberty to challenge them. It may be true that doping rules restrict the liberty of athletes, but so do rules concerning the number of players on the field or the ways in which players may legitimately move the ball.

A distinction originally found in the writing of Kant between constitutive and regulative rules is commonly drawn in the literature of the philosophy of language (Searle, 1969) and the philosophy of sport (e.g. Loland & McNamee, 2002). While Searle is often referred to as the modern *locus classicus*, it is notable that an earlier essay by Geoffrey Midgley had in fact employed the Kantian distinction to the same effect. He writes "...I shall describe rules of this kind as constitutive rules, and suggest that a system of abstract objects is constituted by such rules. Constitutive rules are not prescriptive of actions, though they are intimately related to rules which are; they cannot be kept or broken, though they are reflected in rules which can be, which are concerned with whether an abstract system so constituted is correctly or incorrectly realised in some concrete manifestation" (Midgley, 1959, p.281).[6] So examples of constitutive rules[7] include those that demarcate the playing dimensions, the numbers of participants, the size or weight of relevant objects such as balls or bats, the time of the event, and so on. It could be argued that even these rules have ethical import since they function *inter alia* to preserve the equality and/or fairness or integrity of the contest. Literally, they are designed so that contestants share the same, or relatively similar, test conditions.[8] These typically, though not exclusively, function to preserve important notions such as respect. Regulative rules, however, refer to the quality of the action therein. They are logically dependent upon the constitutive rules (McFee, 2004). They both prescribe – but more typically – proscribe, actions within the activity. Consider the hand ball rule in football (soccer). No outfield player is permitted to use their hand/arm to control the ball. But some rules have greater ethical import. Thus in rugby, a very effective way of preventing the opposing team ball carrier from making progress is to tackle head-high. This usually stops the ball carrier in their tracks. One is not at liberty to do so, however, since it often occasions serious harm and potential quadriplegia. So the high-tackle law in rugby serves to prohibit otherwise efficacious actions to prevent the opposition gaining strategic advantage. Clearly, the law serves to instantiate the basic moral notion of respect for persons and their physical integrity. Examples abound in all sports and the more serious the potential harm the greater the prohibition which attaches to the restricted action.

While the standard case is designed to respect competitors *qua* persons, and to prevent or limit harm to them, there are also rules that act so as to prevent or reduce self-harm. Professional boxers must undergo strict medical examinations including brain scans at appropriate intervals before being passed fit to compete. Equally, professional cyclists are also open to paternalistic intervention. Erythropoietin is a glycoprotein that governs red cell production in the human body. It is critical for transporting oxygen around the body to supply human effort. If there is too great a concentration of it, however (whether as naturally occurring abnormality or by exogenous use), the athlete may have excessive blood viscosity and become susceptible to myocardial infarctions. Thus, professional cyclists whose erythropoietin levels exceed 50 are not permitted to start races such as the Tour de France by their governing body, the Union Cycliste Internationale (UCI).

In addition to the constitutive and regulative rules of sports, there is a subset of rules which "specify and regulate eligibility, admission, training" and other activities outside the realm of the competition itself. These are by Meier (1985 p. 10) called "auxiliary rules" and do not fall neatly into either category, and which appear to characterize anti-doping rules. These may refer either to the rules of particular sports, or to the rules of the global anti-doping body, the World Anti Doping Agency as set out in the World Anti Doping Code (2009).

Thus, rules define and regulate conventional activities such as sports. Just as they enable game playing they constrain actions therein. So the mere fact that a conventional rule in a specific sport is liberty-restricting is an insufficient and very weak criticism against enhancement-restricting rules. In some cases it may even be irrelevant in determining whether it is a good rule, or a rule that should be upheld, or a bad one that ought to be rejected or withdrawn.

It is also important to note that not all sports would be enhanced by the physical enhancement of the athletes. The most obvious example of this is the various throwing competitions in athletics. One of the purely conventional limitations on javelin and hammer throwing is that athletic stadia have a fairly fixed layout caused by the 400 meter running track with 100 metre straights encircling the centre of the stadium.[9] This layout has as an (unintended?) consequence that throws approaching 100 meters become dangerous to other athletes, officials, or spectators. Better is not always good as

Erik Parens (1998) has observed. At least not for the runners at the top of the bend if the throw exceeds the limitations of the allocated space! So when athletes began, by better technique and greater power, to throw such distances as endangered others, biomechanical modifications were made to the javelin in order to alter its center of gravity and bring the point of the javelin down more steeply and thus reducing the length of the throw. Of course the limitations placed on javelin throwers in this example are predicated on a prevention of harm to others, but we could have decided instead to clear that end of the stadium. But there exist also cases where an enhancement disables, or at least diminishes the functional capacity of, the athlete in performance terms.

Consider for example a wrestler whose increases in muscularity take him into a higher weight class. Thus before the additional muscle bulk was built up – with or without the use of androgenic anabolic steroids – they may have been among the strongest in their weight class but following weight gain they may be forced into a heavier class of contestants where they become the weakest in virtue of their enhanced muscularity. Equally, an athlete who uses such steroids not merely to increase muscle bulk but also to heighten their aggression, may find their performances diminish because of their inability to control the expression of their new-found force. Examples such as these are commonplace because sports, while they are often referred to as physical activities or thought of as paradigmatic examples of physical excellence, are in reality always tests of a complex of embodied and psychological powers.

A slightly more complicated example can be found in golf. Although golf courses do not have a fixed layout they have been designed based on extant evaluations of the lengths to which players can "drive" the ball from the tee. Yet it is not obvious that significantly increased drive lengths would actually enhance the game. As the well-known phrase among golfers has it: you drive for show, but you putt for dough! It is little good if the golfer, having driven 500 yards to the green, then takes four putting strokes on the green before sinking the ball into the hole.

More generally many sports have restrictions on the equipment that can be used legitimately even though it is known that improved equipment is available that could "improve" specific aspects of the game For example, one of the cardinal sins of cricket occurs when a player "tampers with the ball." Anyone who tampers with the ball cannot be an ethically admirable player (or a "true gentleman" in older parlance: see Fraser, 2005), as was evidenced by a high-profile libel case centering on allegations of ball tampering and some years later a refusal by the Pakistan team to continue play in a test match against England after one of their players was adjudged to have tampered with the ball. But tampering with the ball is, from one perspective, merely a case of adapting or changing the equipment to improve certain aspects of bowling perfor-mance. While this example depicts enhanced performance by an action defined by the rules as cheating, there are enhancing technologies or strategies that have been restricted because they usurp the delicate balance of the contest between participants. Fraleigh (1984) has aptly called this the "sweet tension" of outcome uncertainty. Thus in limited-overs cricket, for example, the bowler (pitcher) may only bowl one dan-gerous delivery (a short-pitched "bouncer") per over (six balls). Equally, tennis balls were recently modified to make them travel more slowly through the air (NASA, 2000). This change was effected so that the game was not dominated by a single stroke (i.e. the serve) to the detriment of the complex of strategy, skill, and embodied capacities that tennis at its best represented. These then represent a few perfectly acceptable performance-enhancing restrictions on the athlete.

In so far as similar judgments can be made concerning a specific level of physical enhancement within the context of a specific sport there seems to be nothing wrong in principle with prohibiting that enhancement.

Justice in Enhancement

A further class of arguments in the enhancement debate focuses on issues of justice either in general or specifically within the context of the allocation of resources within the health care system.

General issues of justice arise if the physical enhancement in question (i) either provides competitive advantage and therefore counts as a positional good or provides significant welfare improvements and (ii) the enhancement will not be available to all who need or want it. It is predictable that enhancements that share these two characteristics will primarily be available to the rich and that their distribution across society will be unequal. It will then be a matter of argument from case to case to decide whether the enhancement is so important and the resulting inequality so great that it breaches standards of justice. We live in societies that accept varying degrees of inequality in the distribution of common goods, but every society has its limits as to what is deemed (un)acceptable.

The more specific issue about resource allocation in health care arises in health care systems that are tax-based or based on compulsory, non-risk assessed insurance. In such health care systems there is a common pool of resources and the validity of claims on this pool is independent on the amount a person has contributed to the pool. This gives rise to the question how interventions that are enhancing should be treated in resource allocation. How do we decide how important the claims they give rise to are? There are in general at least two factors that can influence the strength of a health care claim: (i) the initial position of the claimant; and (ii) the consequences of the claim being fulfilled.[10] If we are choosing between two claimants who can achieve the same amount of welfare gain, but where one of them has low welfare and the other already has average welfare most people will allocate the resources to the person who has the lowest initial position on the welfare scale, and this judgment does not change much even if the welfare gain that can be achieved is slightly lower than in the healthy person. Such choices are incompatible with welfare maximization and with the standard approaches of health care economics, e.g. quality adjusted life year maximization. One case of potential enhancement that has been extensively discussed is the use of growth hormone as a height enhancer in children with no known growth hormone deficiency. This case illustrates the complexity of the judgments that have to be made. Let us first note that Peter Singer has argued that we might have good reasons not to enhance the height of people because taller people use more resources, they need to eat more, they are heavier, and transporting them takes up more energy etc. It is therefore better from an environmental point of view not to enhance (Singer 2003). Second, the example simultaneously shows the problems with and the relevance of the treatment/enhancement distinction. If we have two children who are both expected to attain an adult height significantly below the average for the population, then it does not seem to matter much for their claim to growth hormone intervention that one of them has growth hormone deficiency and can be *treated* and the other has no deficiency and needs to be *enhanced*. But if we are talking about someone who has an expected height significantly above the normal then his or her claim on the intervention is much weaker, precisely because it is an enhancement and not a treatment. Third, the example illustrates (along with others discussed above) that mere physical improvement may not be enhancing. Hormone injections are also sometimes used to achieve fusion of the growth discs in the long bones to prevent excessive height, precisely because being very tall may well be a positional good, but it also imposes social disabilities in relation to furniture, airline seats, clothes, and even conversations.

All of these considerations add up to the conclusion that growth hormone treatment in a public health care system can only be justifiably claimed if it aims at giving someone a height in the normal range.

Conclusion

In this chapter we have argued for five main conclusions:

1. That in discussion of enhancement one must first clarify the baseline against which enhancements must be judged.
2. That the existence of conceptual vagueness regarding therapy and enhancement does not render the distinction inoperable.
3. That the concepts of physical improvement and enhancement are not simple and that some confusion may occur if the concept that is being used is not specified.
4. That the area of physical enhancement extends beyond sports contexts which are themselves unhelpfully dominated by the issue of performance enhancement in competitive sport, i.e. doping.
5. That there are no knockdown ethical arguments for or against physical enhancement but that some arguments are persuasive against some enhancements in some contexts.

If we are right the debate about physical enhancement has to become considerably more nuanced than it is at present. It has to take more account of the concrete contexts in which a specific enhancement is being sought. It has to be wearier of using analogies without proper investigation of their scope and applicability. And, most importantly, it has to be less ambitious. There are no "hole in one" arguments that score against the whole enhancement field. It must be unpicked, enhancement by enhancement.

Notes

1. Since we do not subscribe to simple perfectionism where the faster athlete is also, by that very fact the morally superior athlete. It is notable, too, that in John Harris' (2007) book on enhancement there is very little discussion of the ethical sense of being "better" despite the

subtitle being "the ethical case for making better people". Rather he discusses a range of genetic, pharmaceutical, and other cognitive and physical enhancements which, by analogy, he argues ought to be accepted given the relevantly similar enhancements that are already accepted in society.

2. Although one of the Danish slang terms for the activity in which Viagra plays a role is best translated as "bed sheet gymnastics."

3. This is a revised position statement by the American Academy of Pediatrics Committee on Sports Medicine and Fitness providing information on adolescent use of anabolic steroids.

4. We might even subdivide the latter category according to a particular time slice in the life of an individual. Many of us unreasonably (foolishly?) compare our current levels of fitness with those of decades long gone. Enhancement under such a conception might be seen as an act of recovery.

5. And wrong in my assessment of whether the tattoo will make me more or less attractive as a sexual partner.

6. See also Reddiford (1989, p. 41ff), for a discussion of how rule systems in sport include definitions, constitutive rules, and regulative rules.

7. Notably cricket and rugby call them not rules but "laws." Though the semantic difference has an interesting social history it is not relevant for our purposes. See Fraser (2005).

8. Some deviations in test conditions may be inevitable and not inequitable. Consider a tennis match where the sun is in the eyes of the server only when one of them is serving from one end. When the clouds block the sun out for his/her competitor we complain of bad luck not unfairness or inequality. One might consider downhill skiing conditions that vary on a minute by minute basis. Examples abound. See Loland (2002).

9. This limitation is conventional because the layout of the running track could have been otherwise or throwing competitions could have taken place elsewhere.

10. Other factors discussed in the very large literature on resource allocation in health care include merit, past contribution to society, future contribution to society, and whether or not the person is personally responsible for bringing about the condition that requires health care.

References

American Academy of Pediatrics (1997). Adolescents and anabolic steroids: A subject review. *Pediatrics*, **99**, 904–8.

Calfee, R. & Fadale, P. (2006). Popular ergogenic drugs and supplements in young athletes. *Pediatrics*, **117**(3), 577–89.

Daniels, N. (2007). Can anyone really be talking about ethically modifying human nature? In J. Savulescu & N. Bostrom (eds.), *Human Enhancement*. Oxford: Oxford University Press.

Fraleigh, W.P. (1984). *Right Actions in Sport*. Champaign, IL: Human Kinetics.

Fraser, D. (2005). *Cricket and the Law: The Man in White is Always Right*. London: Routledge.

Harris, J. (2007). *Enhancing Evolution*. Princeton: Princeton University Press.

Harris, J. (2009). Enhancements are a moral obligation. In J. Savulescu & N. Bostrom (eds.), *Human Enhancement* (pp. 131–54). Oxford: Oxford University Press.

Holm, S. (2006). The nature of human welfare. In C. Deane-Drummond & P. Manley Scott (eds.), *Future Perfect?* (pp. 45–55). London: T & T Clark.

Holm, S. (2007). Naturalness and anthropology in modern bioethics, with a special view to trans- and post-humanism. In H. Kragh (ed.), *Theology and Science - Issues for Future Dialogue* (pp. 17–29). Aarhus: University of Aarhus.

Loland, S. (2002). *Fair Play*. London: Routledge.

Loland, S. & McNamee, M.J. (2000). Fair play in sport: An eclectic philosophical framework. *Journal of the Philosophy of Sport*, **27**, 63–80.

Kanayama, G., Boynes, M., Hudson, J.I., Field, A.E. & Pope Jr., H.G. (2007). Anabolic steroid abuse among teenage girls: An illusory problem? *Drug and Alcohol Dependence*, **88**, 156–62.

McFee, G. (2004). *Sports, Rules and Values*. London: Routledge.

Meier, K.V. (1985). Restless sport. *Journal of the Philosophy of Sport*, **12**, 64–77.

Midgley, G.C.J. (1959). Linguistic rules. *Proceedings of the Aristotelian Society*, 271–90.

Mill, J. (1978). *On Liberty*. Indiana: Hackett.

Murray, T.H. (2006). Enhancement. In B. Steinbock (ed.), *The Oxford Handbook of Bioethics* (pp. 491–515). Oxford: Oxford University Press.

NASA (2000). NASA tests tennis balls, expands student minds. www.nasa.gov/centers/ames/news/releases/2000/00_58AR.html (accessed March 13, 2009).

Parens, E. (1998). Is better always good? The enhancement project. In E. Parens (ed.), *Enhancing Human Traits* (pp. 1–29). Washington, DC: Georgetown University Press.

Reddiford, G. (1989). Institutions, constitutions and games. *Journal of the Philosophy of Sport*, **12**, 41–51.

Sandberg, A. (2001). Morphological freedom – Why we not just want it, but *need* it. www.nada.kth.se/~asa/Texts/MorphologicalFreedom.htm (accessed March 13, 2009).

Scheffler, I. (1991). *In Praise of the Cognitive Emotions*. London: Routledge.

Singer, P. (2003). Shopping at the genetic supermarket. In S.Y. Song, Y.M. Koo & D.R.J. Macer (eds.), *Asian Bioethics in the 21st Century*. (pp. 143–56). Tsukuba: Eubios.

Searle, J. (1969). *Speech Acts*. Cambridge: Cambridge University Press.

Slote, M. (1993). *Goods and Virtues*. Oxford: Clarendon Press.

World Anti Doping Code (2009). www.wada-ama.org/rtecontent/document/code_-v2009_En.pdf (accessed March 18, 2009).

Yesalis, C.E. & Bahrke, M.S. (2000). Doping among adolescent athletes. *Best Practice & Research Clinical Endocrinology & Metabolism*, **14**, 25–35.

22

Le Tour and Failure of Zero Tolerance: Time to Relax Doping Controls

Julian Savulescu and Bennett Foddy

2007 will be remembered as the year in which the Tour de France died. Race leader and likely eventual winner, Michael Rasmussen, was eliminated near the end on an allegation of doping (without evidence). Pre-race favourite Vinokourov was expelled after blood doping and his team Astana withdrew and fired its management. The Cofidis team withdrew from the Tour de France following the news that their Italian rider Cristian Moreni tested positive for testosterone. Even the eventual winner had to fend off questions about the legality of his victory. The winner's team, which once was home to the Tour legend Lance Armstrong, disbanded because it could not secure sponsorship (Austen, 2007). By all accounts, drug scandals have ripped the sport of professional cycling to shreds. The Tour moved from being the greatest test of human endurance to a petty media-fest of allegations, recriminations and scandals, with the world's best athletes being expelled like shabby contestants in a reality TV show.

For the competitors, doping is a part of the spirit of Le Tour. Since it began in 1903, riders have invariably used performance-enhancing substances in an attempt to get through the grueling 21-day test of human endurance. They have taken alcohol, caffeine, cocaine, amphetamines, steroids, growth hormone, erythropoietin (EPO), and undergone blood doping. Fausto Coppi, who won the golden jersey in 1949 and 1952, summed it up when he was asked whether he ever used amphetamines, or "La Bomba," and replied, "Only when absolutely necessary." When asked how often that was, he said, "Most of the time." The 1967 Tour saw a rider collapse and die during the competition with amphetamines in his pocket (Wheatcroft, 2007).

The Tour requires a superhuman effort, and it seems there have been few winners who won within their human limits. Bjarne Riis, 1996 Tour winner, admitted taking EPO (Associated Press, 2007). The 1997 winner, Jan Ulrich, was later alleged to be taking drugs. Floyd Landis, 2006 winner, was disqualified testing positive for testosterone, and he has since accused seven-time winner Lance Armstrong of doping in 2002

Enhancing Human Capacities, edited by Julian Savulescu, Ruud ter Meulen and Guy Kahane.
© 2011 Blackwell Publishing Ltd

and 2003 (Hart, 2010). The only recent winner of the Tour not to be found taking drugs is Carlos Sastre, who won in 2008.

Since the 1960s, the idealistic drug crusaders have been on a mission to reverse the course of history, and eliminate drugs from the sport. But this "zero tolerance" strategy to drugs has failed, as 2007's Tour spectacularly showed. And it is bound to fail. Only around 10–15% of professional athletes are drug tested. There are enormous pressures to win. And the development of new drugs is clearly outstripping our capacity to develop effective tests.

Many modern doping agents like EPO and growth hormone mimic natural hormones and are extremely difficult to detect. If these agents are developed in secret, either by underground labs or by government-funded researchers, there is no way to detect them until samples are discovered by the authorities. The Bay Area Laboratory Cooperative (BALCO) secretly developed the "designer" steroid THG, and marketed it to elite sportspeople like baseball legend Barry Bonds and athletics superstar Marion Jones. The drug was a well-kept secret, and a test was only developed after a sample was anonymously mailed to the authorities by Jones' coach, Trevor Graham (Hersh, 2006).

As gene doping becomes more efficient, it is likely to offer great opportunities for doping in sport and is likely to be very difficult to detect, whether samples are discovered or not. For example, insulin-like growth factor injected into the muscles of mice increases strength. Direct injection into the muscles of athletes would be simple and very difficult to detect as DNA would be taken into muscle DNA, requiring muscle biopsy (which is dangerous and difficult) to detect it. Vascular endothelial growth factor stimulates the development of new blood vessels and could also be of use to athletes in the future. EPO genes could be directly integrated into host DNA. Since such gene therapy works in animals, there is no reason why it could not be attempted by athletes now.

Some people claim that these recent positive tests show that we are winning the war on drugs. All prohibitionist policies – on alcohol, prostitution, recreational drugs – will fail because they involve "victimless crimes" and because the financial incentives to engage in these activities are so strong. And there is no evidence that the current policy is picking up competent cheaters. Riis was never detected – he confessed. Alexander Vinokourov was ejected from Le Tour in 2007 for blood doping, causing his entire team to withdraw. But it is alleged that he was only picked up because he was using someone else's blood (Wyatt, 2007). He would not have been caught if he had used his own blood. Landis is alleged to have used testosterone to win a stage after an appalling performance the day before. But testosterone takes weeks to increase a rider's muscle mass – it does not confer any instantaneous performance enhancement. If it is true that he was using testosterone, a much plausible explanation was that he donated some of his own blood months before, while training but on testosterone, and that testosterone remained in the blood that was given back during the Tour. He was caught because of incompetence on his part, not because of the success of the testing program. It is likely that many riders in the Tour are doping in one way or another, but they remain undetected simply because they are more careful than Landis.

There are only two options. We can vainly try to ratchet up our war on doping. Or we can take a rational approach to the use of performance enhancers: allow drugs which are safe and do not corrupt the spirit of a sport, as a display of human physical excellence. How would such a policy have helped the Tour?

Le Tour, Blood Doping, and EPO

The ability to perform well in endurance-based sporting events is determined by the ability to deliver oxygen to muscles. The more red blood cells you have, the more oxygen you can carry. EPO is a natural hormone that stimulates red blood cell production, raising the hematocrit (HCT) – the percentage of the blood made up by red blood cells. EPO is produced in response to anaemia, haemorrhage, pregnancy, or living at high altitude. At sea level, the average person has an HCT of 40–50%. HCT naturally varies – 2.5% of all men have a HCT above 50% (Lichtman, 2006).

Raising the HCT too high can cause health problems. Your risk of harm rapidly rises as HCT gets above 50%, especially if you also have high blood pressure (O'Toole *et al.*, 1999). When your HCT is over 56%, you are at high risk of stroke, heart, and lung failure. In the four years after EPO became available in Europe, twenty cyclists died of sudden and unexpected cardiac problems (Eichner, 2007). Use of EPO is endemic in cycling and many other sports. EPO is extremely hard to detect and its use has continued despite the emergence of sophisticated testing methods.

Athletes have also moved back to blood doping, where they donate a unit of their own blood months before and have it retransfused during the race, after their own levels have been replenished. This increases the concentration of red blood cells in the body without leaving any chemical trace, and no physical trace other than, perhaps, a puncture mark, which provides no evidence of wrongdoing since riders are routinely put on intravenous nutrition and hydration because they cannot eat or drink enough naturally to cope with the demands of today's Tour.

Partly due to the existence of undetectable blood doping, the International Cycling Union requires athletes to have an HCT no higher than 50%. This criterion casts a net which ensnares those who inject too much EPO, perform too much blood doping, and those who are born with a naturally elevated hematocrit. Athletes with a naturally elevated level of HCT cannot race unless doctors can prove they have not elevated their HCT artificially. Charles Wegelius was a British rider who was banned and then cleared in 2003. He had had his spleen removed in 1998 following an accident – since the spleen removes red blood cells, this increased his HCT (Anonymous, 2003). Finnish cross country skier Eero Maentyranta won two Olympic gold medals in 1964. Subsequently, it was found he had a genetic mutation that meant that he "naturally" had 40–50% more red blood cells than the average competitor (Roush, 1995).

There are other ways to increase the number of red blood cells which are legal. Altitude training can push the HCT to dangerous, even fatal, levels. More recently, hypoxic air machines have allowed athletes to simulate altitude training at sea level. The body responds to an oxygen-poor environment by releasing natural EPO and growing more blood cells, so that the body may absorb more oxygen with every breath. The results of a haematocrit test show no difference whether you elevate your blood count by altitude training, by using a hypoxic air machine, by having an elective splenectomy, or by taking EPO.

At present, the authorities use haematocrit tests to identify people who are cheating, and make special allowances for those who are born different, or who like Wegelius have become different through some medical procedure. In practice, these tests are only capable of catching those who are incompetent at cheating, and even then there is only a small chance that each incompetent cheater will be caught. The present situation is inherently unfair. It is unfair to those riders who have not had their spleen removed. It is unfair to those riders who cheated like all the others, but who were unlucky enough to be tested at the wrong time. And it is unfair to those who cannot afford hypoxic training facilities. The current system rewards the competent cheaters, the fortunate, and the rich.

A fairer, more effective option would be to forget about finding the cheaters, to forget about making special allowances, and simply measure every cyclist's haematocrit. This would not catch many cheaters, but it would entirely solve the cheating problem. The test is simple, cheap and reliable, and could be done at the beginning of a race. We could pick a safe level for competition. The International Cycling Union currently sets this at 50% but we could revise that. If that is the safe limit, we should let people dope to that limit.

Currently, it is illegal to use EPO or blood doping to move your haematocrit from 48 to 49% (though it is legal to do it by using a hypoxic air machine or altitude training) even though some people will have a normal level of 49%. But if 50% is the safe limit, anyone should be allowed to raise their red cell count to that level and all those above should be excluded for health reasons, even if their HCT is naturally elevated. Alternatively, these people's red cell count could be lowered to safe levels by diluting their blood.

Athletes do not cheat when they take legal performance enhancers like caffeine or creatine. Under blanket haematocrit limits, every blood-based performance enhancer would be like these legal drugs.

A similar strategy could be adopted for anabolic steroids. While we test athletes for unsafe levels of haematocrit, we could test every athlete for the *symptoms* of dangerous steroid overuse. This would mean regularly testing each athlete for liver damage, cholesterol, blood pressure and left-ventricle hypertrophy, which increases the risk of heart attack and sudden cardiac death (Mottram, 1996).

It makes no moral difference whether an athlete has liver damage or high cholesterol from steroids or from poor diet. If their cholesterol level puts them at risk of death during intense athletic competition, they should be excluded for safety reasons. Conversely, if their use of steroids has not produced symptoms of harm, they ought to be allowed to compete, regardless of whether or not they are clean.

A regulated permissive policy would paradoxically reduce risk to athletes. The present system creates an environment of risk to the athlete. Since nearly all doping is illegal, the pressure is to develop undetectable performance enhancers with no mind to safety. Furthermore, the penalties are the same no matter what dosage an athlete takes, and no matter how effective the drug is, so athletes are forced to take massive doses of the most effective drugs. Performance enhancers are produced on the black market and administered in a clandestine, uncontrolled way with no monitoring of the athlete's health. Allowing the use of safe performance enhancers would make sport safer as there would be less pressure on athletes to take unsafe enhancers. Blanket safety testing of every athlete would create a powerful incentive to limit the use of existing enhancements to safe doses. If the safe doses were ineffective at producing a performance benefit, it would create a powerful pressure to develop new performance enhancers which are effective at a safe dose.

Allowing the safe use of performance enhancers would not eliminate risk to athletes' health but it could reduce it to an arbitrarily low level. If we make sure to test *every* athlete for medical indications of risk, it will become more difficult for cheaters to endanger their health by using unsafe dosages or toxic enhancements. Such a system would be effective against most clandestine undetectable drugs, and it would improve the health of the athletes.

Enhanced Recovery and Athlete Health

Sporting bodies, pundits, and players often talk about what's good for their sport. Drugs are often said to be bad for a sport. But this is an oversimplification. Any change – whether technological, regulatory, or pharmaceutical – can be good for players and bad for fans, or vice versa. Whether a drug is good for the fans or for the players depends on what kind of drug it is.

Sometimes, a technology or method of training appears which is good for both the players *and* the spectators. Ironically, the two best examples of such a win-win technology are the most infamous performance enhancements available – anabolic steroids and EPO.

One of the effects of steroid use is that it aids players in recovering from injury and training. Accelerated recovery is an artificial enhancement, but it is not the type of enhancement that makes anybody worse off. To the contrary, when an athlete takes a long time to recover from injury, it is bad for everyone – his fans, his teammates, and the athlete himself.

Players have often used steroids with this recuperative purpose in mind. The American baseball player Chad Fox said this in 2003, in the midst of Major League Baseball's recent doping scandals:

> With all the injuries I've had, I could have taken steroids. But my family is too important (Bloom, 2003).

When he made this statement, Fox was referring to the period before testing began, so he could not have meant that his family would suffer if he was banned for doping. He meant that his family would be put at grave risk by the side effects steroids would have on his body. But this reflects a gross exaggeration of the dangers of steroid use. Doctors regularly prescribe anabolic steroids to "civilians" who are recovering from injuries or surgery. Taken in clinical doses, anabolic steroids are extremely safe and effective at reducing recuperation time (Evans, 2004). In order to elicit both the muscle-building effects of steroids and its famous health-endangering side effects, an athlete must take very large quantities of the drug or take it for a very long time.

In other words, if Fox had taken the steroids in modest doses, it would have only lengthened his career and helped him to recover from injuries, which would have been good for the spectators, for Fox, and certainly for his family.

EPO is medically beneficial in a similar way. To train in any professional athletic sport is very demanding – in fact, it could be compared to a medical pathology. Female athletes training in intense sports like cycling are at high risk of developing a dangerously low haematocrit, also known as anaemia (Ireland & Ott, 2004). Various unrelated complaints can also cause anaemia in male athletes. These athletes would be healthier and safer if their haematocrit was artificially buoyed with EPO. In both men and women, EPO would also be beneficial if their haematocrit were genetically or medically depressed. EPO also has a number of beneficial effects which are not related to its ability to increase HCT. For example, EPO has been shown to stimulate wound healing in mice (Sayan *et al.*, 2006).

More importantly, athletes who increase their fitness by taking EPO do not need to train as hard. We need to acknowledge that training is very hard on the human body. Intense training for a sport like cycling causes traumatic injuries, stress injuries, inflammation, and immunosuppression (O'Kennedy, 2000). It is similar to a medical pathology. If we are serious about protecting the health of athletes, we need to make available the treatments which doctors would prescribe for a pathology of this nature. Like steroids and EPO.

The Spirit of Sport

Sport is the pursuit of human physical excellence (skill or strength) in a rule-governed activity. The rules of any sport aim to define some activity which will bring out the display of certain skills or strengths, and allow the players to compete meaningfully in the expression of those skills. But the rules are essentially arbitrary. Why then do we have rules prohibiting beneficial substances?

One explanation that is often given is that taking performance enhancers is inherently contrary to the spirit of sporting competition. But this objection cannot be what drives current anti-doping policy, since we allow many technologies and practices which significantly enhance performance. Caffeine is not illegal, even though it can strongly increase performance. In endurance sports, caffeine helps to mobilize the fat stores of an athlete (Costill *et al.*, 1978). It can make as much as a 20% difference in the time to exhaustion among competitive athletes, depending on how the trial is performed (Passman *et al.*, 1995). In the context of elite sport, that can be a massive difference. The legal dietary supplement creatine is similar to the banned drugs EPO, growth hormone and testosterone, in that it supplements an endogenous substance. Creatine's other similarity to the banned drugs is that it is effective – it can increase an athlete's time to exhaustion in anaerobic exercise by over 10% (Bosco *et al.*, 1997; Prevost *et al.*, 1997). The reason that these performance enhancers are permitted is because they are safe. It is inconsistent not to allow other performance enhancers if they are safe enough.

Of course we do not wish to argue that athletes should employ any and every safe technology in order to gain a competitive advantage. If we allowed cyclists to ride the Tour on motorcycles, they could win even if they were fat, old, and unfit. This kind of enhancement clearly is contrary to the spirit of competitive cycling, and it would clearly diminish meaningful competition and prevent cyclists from displaying their athleticism.

If the point of sport is to display athletic ability and allow meaningful comparisons between athletes, then it is reasonable to impose rules which prevent athletes from subverting these goals. But enhancements like steroids and EPO are not like motor-cycles in cycling or flippers in swimming. If we allow cyclists to ride the Tour on steroids or EPO, they will only win if they are strong, fit, and fast. These drugs do not subvert the nature of the sport; indeed, they encourage athletes to become paragons of the sporting ideal: supermen.

Cycling better than any other sport shows that drugs can be a part of the culture of that sport and not prevent the display of human physical excellence – doping is as old as human competition and the Tour, because of the superhuman demands it makes, is just a very vivid example of that.

A Rational Doping Policy

A rational policy on doping would allow safe performance-enhancing interventions which are consistent with the spirit of a particular sport. Firstly, we should develop safer performance-enhancing drugs or interventions. These need to be as effective as riskier options. Ideally, they need to be no more effective when taken in harmful megadose quantities. They need to be provided at a price which makes them available to poorer athletes.

Secondly, we should focus detective efforts on those drugs and practices which detract from the athlete's project – enhancing his body's performance. Some changes, like allowing swimmers to use flippers, would reduce the importance of athleticism in a sport. But blood doping in cycling does not.

Thirdly, we should test *every* athlete to make sure they are fit to compete – regardless of whether or not they are using drugs. It is far easier to test haematocrit (the amount of red blood cells in the blood), and set a safe level (such as 50%) and to ban anyone who is above that level and at risk, than it is to detect the cause of that elevation, which could be natural, autotransfusion, use of hypoxic air tent, gene doping, or exogenous EPO. It is also relatively easy to test for liver damage, blood pressure, and cholesterol. We should test heart structure and function, not to see if athletes are guilty of taking steroids, but to make sure they aren't at risk of heart attack. We could also test immunocompetence, testosterone levels and joint structure and function – all of which can be influenced by steroid overuse or simply by training too hard.

In Australia, boxers are excluded from competition if they are shown to have suffered brain damage on a magnetic resonance imaging scan. But recent results suggest that their brains could also be protected by prescribing EPO, which provides protection against traumatic brain injury (Verdonck *et al.*, 2007).

The question is: What risks should athletes be exposed to? It is not: What is the origin of that risk? Setting the acceptable risk level for performance-enhancing drugs should be consistent with the magnitude of risk which athletes are allowed to entertain in elite sport. Elite sport can be extremely harmful. More riders die in crashes than from drugs. Even clean elite athletes have to accept serious harms to be competitive. There is nothing special about a drug-related risk which demands that we intervene, when we permit these unnecessary non-drug risks to exist.

The limits to the use of drugs and other performance enhancers in sport should be on safety grounds, based on a consistent comparison with other risks taken in elite sport, and their use should not diminish the need for athleticism in the athlete (e.g. using flippers in swimming or motorcycles in cycling) and the spirit of a particular sport as a display of a human physical excellence.

We should redirect resources away from the war on performance-enhancing drugs, and use them to protect athletes' health. We should be less concerned with whether some biological substance or intervention improves performance *per se*. Zero tolerance to performance enhancement has failed. It is unfair, unsafe, and ruining the sport.

Jacques Anquetil during a TV debate, asked a French politician if "they expect us to ride the Tour on mineral water" (Wheatcroft, 2005). But today we demonize the men who courageously push themselves to the human limit and beyond. We should admire them, rather than denigrate them. They give us the spectacle we want, and we complain when they push themselves to the limits we expect.

Cheating occurs when the rules are broken. But we set the rules. The rules should define the nature and spirit of a sport, protect athletes' health, provide a reasonable spectacle and be enforceable in a fair and reasonable way. The rules should allow athletes to access medicines which protect their livelihood and help them to recuperate. The current rules are not enforceable. They are ruining the spectacle of cycling and they are ruining the sport for the cyclists as well. We can achieve these goals better with a more regulated permissive approach to doping.

We have two choices: to vainly try to turn the clock back, or to rethink who we are and what sport is. Our crusade against drugs in sport has failed. Rather than fearing drugs in sport, we should embrace them. Performance enhancement is not against the spirit of sport; it is the spirit of sport. To choose to be better is to be human.

References

Anonymous (2003). British rider Wegelius cleared of doping', *Agence France Presse – English*. December 2, Tuesday, Sports.

Associated Press (2007). German team doctor admits he gave cyclists testosterone. *New York Times*. May 27, p. 8.5.

Austen, I. (2007) Tour de France Winner's Team Will Disband. *The New York Times*. August 10, Friday, Sports.

Bloom, B.M. (2003). Many players applaud testing. MLB.com Retrieved August 13, 2007, from www.mlb.com/news/article.jsp?ymd=20031114&content_id=604197&vkey=news_mlb&fext=.jsp&c_id=mlb.

Bosco, C. *et al.* (1997). Effect of oral creatine supplementation on jumping and running performance. *International Journal of Sports Medicine*, **18**, 369–72.

Costill, D., Dalsky, G. & Fink, W. (1978). Effects of caffeine ingestion on metabolism and exercise performance. *Medicine and Science in Sports and Exercise*, **10**, 155–8.

Eichner, E.R. (2007). Blood doping: Infusions, erythropoietin and artificial blood. *Sports Medicine*, **37**(4–5), 389–91.

Evans, N.A. (2004). Current concepts in anabolic-androgenic steroids. *American Journal of Sports Medicine*, **32**(2), 534–42.

Hart, S. (2010). Floyd Landis puts Lance Armstrong at the centre of new drug allegations. *The Telegraph*. 20 May 2010. Thursday. Sport.

Hersh, P. (2006). Graham indicted in BALCO scandal: Track coach who turned in the syringe that led to the doping case is accused of lying to federal agents, becoming the sixth indictment. *Los Angeles Times*. November 3, p. D.7.

Ireland, M.L. & Ott, S.M. (2004). Special concerns of the female athlete. *Clinics in Sports Medicine*, **23**(2), 281–98.

Lichtman, M.A. (2006). *Williams Hematology*. New York: McGraw-Hill.

Mottram, D.R. (1996). *Drugs in Sport*, 2nd edition. London: Taylor and Francis.

O'Kennedy, R. (2000). The immune system in sport: Getting the balance right. *British Journal of Sports Medicine*, **34**, 161.

O'Toole, M.L., Douglas, P.S., Hiller, D.B. & Laird, R.H. (1999). Hematocrits of triathletes: Is monitoring useful? *Medicine and Science in Sports and Exercise*, **31**(3), 372–7.

Passman, W.J., van Baak, M.A., Jeukendrup, A.E. & de Haan, A. (1995). The effect of different dosages of caffeine on endurance performance time. *International Journal of Sports Medicine*, **16**, 225–30.

Prevost, M.C., Nelson, A.G. & Morris, G.S. (1997). Creatine supplementation enhances intermittent work performance. *Research Quarterly for Exercise and Sport*, **68**, 233–40.

Roush, W. (1995). An "off switch" for red blood cells. *Science*, **268**, 27–8.

Sayan, H., Ozacmak, V.H., Guven, A., Aktas, R.G. & Ozamak, I.D. (2006). Erythropoietin stimulates wound healing and angiogenesis in mice. *Journal of Investigative Surgery*, **19**(3), 163–73.

Verdonck, O., Lahrech, H., Francony, G., Carle, O., Farion, R. *et al.* (2007). Erythroprotein protects from post-traumatic edema in the rat brain. *Journal of Cerebral Blood Flow and Metabolism*, **27**, 1369–76.

Wheatcroft, G. (2005). Lance boiled. *Wall Street Journal*. August 26, p. A.12.

Wheatcroft, G. (2007). *Le Tour: A History of the Tour de France*. London: Simon & Schuster.

Wyatt, E. (2007). Tour is hit with another blow as a favorite fails a drug test. *New York Times*. July 25, p. D.1.

23

Enhancing Skill

Bennett Foddy

There is a wide range of physical actions which we can perform with our bodies. For a certain subset of these actions, it can be said that the action is done well or done poorly. All such variations in performance are mediated, at least in part, by the actor's brain, spinal cord, and peripheral nervous system. Neurological systems determine how quickly we react to catch an incoming ball, how accurately we can throw a dart, and how well we can time a dance-step.

But the capacities which we normally conceive of as purely physical or "somatic" capacities are also governed by neural processes. Neurological systems play a role in determining how far we throw a javelin, how deeply we breathe while swimming, how many hot dogs we can eat in a row, and how long we can withstand the pain of endurance cycling.

The most famous enhancement technologies in use are those which enhance purely physical systems like muscle strength or hematocrit, like steroids and erythropoietin do. These enhancements do not involve neural processes at all. Increasingly, we are also familiar with pure cognitive enhancements, which aim to improve pure cognitive capacities such as memory or attention for use in academic pursuits, like pregnenolone and methylphenidate (Ritalin). Cognitive enhancements improve neurological performance only.

There is a third category of enhancement technologies which target neural systems – particularly systems in the peripheral nervous system, which exists outside the brain – as a means of improving physical performance. I will call these *neurophysical* enhancements. Many of the available neurophysical enhancements are also effective for enhancing purely cognitive capacities. But the ethical considerations that must be made regarding their use as neurophysical enhancements are unique. In the following sections I will demonstrate why neurophysical enhancements deserve an ethical assessment which is independent of those relating to physical and cognitive enhancements.

I will focus almost exclusively on the use of neurophysical enhancements in the sporting arena, where they are for the most part prohibited. Of course neurophysical enhancements are useful in amateur sports and in skill-based pursuits outside of competitive sports, such as in aviation, musical performance, construction or in factory work. But sport is in many ways the bellwether case for this kind of ethical problem.

Enhancing Human Capacities, edited by Julian Savulescu, Ruud ter Meulen and Guy Kahane.
© 2011 Blackwell Publishing Ltd

Particularly at a professional level, sport is a competitive pursuit, where the rewards for the winners and losers are wildly disparate, but the differences in performance are vanishingly small. In such an environment, enhancements become much more significant, much more valuable to players, and players will hence accept much greater costs in order to use them. If it can be ethical to use an enhancement in professional sport, it will normally be ethical to use it outside of sport as well.

Before I can delve into ethical questions, however, it may be helpful to spend some time explaining what neuro-enhancements exist, and why they are effective.

What happens when you kick a ball?

Imagine you are a player on a football field, standing in position some distance from the start of play. The game is an important one, which will determine your team's qualification for the end-of-year playoffs. The weight of the moment excites you, and helps to bring your brain into a state of *arousal*, or generalized activation of the brain and the sympathetic nervous system. Your heart beats faster, pumping more blood to power your muscles. Being aroused, you are also more alert. Heightened alertness makes it possible to focus your *attention* on things (Andrewes, 2001).

Someone decides to kick the ball to you, making a loud "thump" noise which alerts you, causing your eye to seek out the source of the noise (Shepherd *et al.*, 1986). In your peripheral vision, you notice the motion of the ball, and your *attention* becomes focused on the ball. Your eyes rotate to focus and center on the ball's position. Neural systems filter away the irrelevant stimuli, like the spectators and irregularities in the playing field, selectively processing only information about the incoming ball. Combining information from the apparent motion of the ball, your perception of distance, and a guess about the ball's mass and elasticity, you judge that the ball is coming toward you. You react.

You don't have time to find a target for your kick. Instead you consult your *working memory*, where you have stored the locations of your teammates. You recall that Smith has bested his counterpart from the other team, and is open for a pass. You *decide* that Smith is the best option, so you *judge* the distance to him, and the power needed for the pass, and the right place to stand.

This complicated array of calculations takes time. Between the time it takes for you to see the ball and choose how to move, there might not have been time for you to make a successful return kick. But you are a trained athlete, and your reaction times are better than average. And, as it happens, the ball is approaching slowly enough that you make a decision with time enough to spare.

In fact, to kick the ball sweetly, you will need to wait a little until the ball reaches the ideal distance. You need to engage your capacity to judge *timing*, which depends on an unusual neural process which is distributed throughout your brain (Buhusi & Meck, 2005).

After a short and perfectly judged pause, you finally spring into action. But you do not consciously assess the motor mechanics involved in a successful kick. The motion of kicking is stored in your *motor memory* (popularly but misleadingly known as "muscle memory") which you have acquired through hours of repetitive training.

From these programmed instructions comes an instruction from your brain and spinal cord to your muscles, flinging you forward and making contact between the ball and the instep of your foot.

Midway through the kick, though, *anxiety* takes hold of you as you recognize the gravity of the situation. You worry that you might miss, and you momentarily make a conscious alteration in your movement, overriding your practiced motor memory. Suddenly unsure of your footing, your anxiety spikes, and you develop stage fright. *Physiologic tremor,* the natural involuntary oscillation in your skeletal muscles, becomes more pronounced. Your leg jerks involuntarily, throwing it slightly off course.

Now slightly off-balance, on your next step you roll your ankle, causing a stabbing *pain* which triggers a reflex in your spinal cord, causing the muscles in your leg to recoil involuntarily, distracting you from the task at hand. But the distraction is made complete when a photographic flash goes off in the crowd, and your heightened *impulsivity* causes you to turn your head towards it, putting you further off balance and finally making a good kick impossible.

You make contact with the ball, but it misses Smith entirely and flies directly to a player on the opposing team, who scores a goal.

The purpose of this story is to show how many neural processes are involved in the execution of physical actions. Even in producing a basic physical motion like a kick, a player needs to engage a large and complex web of neural mechanisms. Some of these mechanisms, like decision making and judgment, are confined to the central nervous system and the brain. Others, like stage fright and elevated heart rate, are primarily involved with the peripheral nervous system.

Each of these mechanisms can be targeted by pharmacological neuro-enhancements. And each can be slightly improved, to optimize the player's skill.

Neurophysical Enhancements

There is already a wide range of neurological enhancements which can be used to improve a person's physical performance.

The largest group of neurophysical enhancements, by a significant margin, are stimulants, such as amphetamines, caffeine, and cocaine. In broad strokes, stimulants increase the availability of neurotransmitters in the brain, causing it to function more rapidly.

Caffeine is the most available and widely used stimulant. It is thought that caffeine helps to mobilize fat stores during exercise in some individuals, increasing their endurance by making more fuel available for the muscles. It is currently unclear whether caffeine does this through neurological means, or by acting directly on the body's cells (Graham *et al.*, 2008).

But while it is unclear how it works to increase endurance, there is more certainty about the other effects of caffeine. Caffeine (like many other stimulants) stimulates both the central nervous system, increasing alertness and general brain activity, and the sympathetic nervous system, increasing heart rate, sweating, and blood pressure.

Outside of competitive sport, caffeine is most popular for its use in combating fatigue, which is reduced by nearly every stimulant. Fatigue can significantly reduce an athlete's ability to perform motor-memory tasks, and to track moving objects with the eye, but amphetamines and caffeine mitigate these effects significantly (Cochran *et al.*, 1994; Tedeschi *et al.*, 1983).

Amphetamines and "substituted amphetamines" such as methylphenidate (Ritalin) work by causing neurotransmitters to be released into the body and brain. The primary neurotransmitter involved is adrenaline, which is released from the adrenal glands above the kidney into the bloodstream of the athlete, in the so-called "fight-or-flight" response. Adrenaline activates various adrenergic receptors in the body's organs and in the brain. These receptors then act to increase heart rate, break down fats and glycogen for energy, and dilate blood vessels – all useful functions for athletic performance (Sulzer *et al.*, 2005).

Dextroamphetamine can also be used to reduce impulsivity – particularly useful for sports which involve inhibiting some action (de Wit *et al.*, 2002). For example, reduced impulsivity can make it easier to avoid swinging at a bad ball in baseball or cricket, or to avoid flinching in the face of an incoming projectile, or to avoid being fooled by a feint or a balk in boxing, fencing, or football.

Reaction time is not improved by amphetamines, but there are some indications that it can be improved by taking cocaine (Heinz *et al.*, 1994; Rasch *et al.*, 1960).

All these stimulants produce a constellation of unwanted side effects such as tremor and anxiety and physical dependence. But new stimulants known as "ampakines" provide many of the same benefits without the side effects.

For example, Modafinil is an ampakine which is usually prescribed to enhance wakefulness, but which also improves reaction time, pattern recognition, working memory, and spatial planning ability (Turner *et al.*, 2003). It improves the reaction time of rats by 25% – and is substantially more effective than amphetamines in this sense (Eagle *et al.*, 2007). It is currently banned in international athletics, despite the fact that the worst side effect it can produce is a headache.

Not every neurophysical enhancement involves increasing brain function; there are a number which enhance performance by inhibiting some unwanted neurological process. Most often in skill-based sport, the unwanted process in question is the activation of the body's "fight-or-flight" response, which occurs when the athlete is aroused, anxious, or stressed.

The activation of adrenergic receptors is useful for some sporting tasks, as I outlined above, but it is detrimental in tasks which require a cool head or a steady hand. In particular, it causes shallow breath, nausea, tremor, loss of muscular control and impulsivity (in other words, "choking" or stage fright) along with other symptoms like tunnel vision (Beilock & Carr, 2001).

The most basic way of reducing the release of adrenaline in sport is to use sedatives or anxiolytic drugs to reduce the levels of arousal and anxiety experienced by the athlete. For example, benzodiazepines like diazepam (Valium) work primarily by binding to the gamma-aminobutyric acid (GABA) receptors in the brain, which inhibit the function of the central nervous system, but they also reduce the activity of the sympathetic nervous system, which is responsible for most stage fright symptoms (Hossmann *et al.*, 1980).

Alcohol also binds to GABA receptors, and it can reduce physiological tremor, which helps to explain its popularity among darts and billiards players (Lakie *et al.*, 1994). For this reason athletes in sports governed by the World Anti-Doping Agency (WADA) are not permitted to have alcohol in their blood beyond a certain concentration in skill-based sports (WADA, 2008).

Another popular method of inhibiting the "fight-or-flight" response is to use beta-blocker drugs, which work by directly blocking adrenaline from stimulating the category of adrenergic receptors known as "beta receptors." These drugs have gained a great deal of popularity in sports like billiards, gymnastics, archery and shooting, and in all of these sports, they are now illegal.

The other important neurological mechanism which athletes try to inhibit is pain. Most professional athletes carry some sort of chronic painful injury. Pain causes an involuntary withdrawal reflex (seated in the spinal cord rather than the brain) which interferes with the voluntary movement of muscles and joints. All of the popular analgesics inhibit this reflex, allowing an athlete's performance to remain uninhibited by it (Skljarevski & Ramadan, 2001). Analgesics are not currently prohibited in sport, except for narcotic analgesics like morphine or heroin.

There are many other neurophysical enhancements on the horizon of medical research, which may have more pronounced enhancement effects than the currently available drugs. For example, GABA is involved in preventing the brain from breaking old connections and forming new ones – in essence, it helps us to remember old memories by stopping us from forming new ones. While there are as yet no enhancements which harness the effect, it seems that the GABA receptors can be blocked, making it easier to acquire new skills (Ziemann *et al.*, 2001). Drugs could be developed – at least in theory – to make a person learn more quickly during training, and forget less quickly once training is over.

I have focused thus far on pharmacological enhancements, but there is a range of non-pharmacological techniques for improving the neural mechanisms that underlie our physical abilities.

For example, when we learn physical skills, it works in two steps – first, we learn during training, and then what we learn is consolidated afterwards. Stimulants like caffeine prevent these skills from being consolidated, while sleep (including a post-training nap) enhances the consolidation effect (Korman *et al.*, 2007; Mednick *et al.*, 2008). Napping after training, therefore, can be considered a neurophysical enhancement. There is some indication that meditation may help to improve the results in competitive shooting by making shooters more relaxed (Solberg *et al.*, 1996). And in other sports, it is not relaxation but arousal that is desired, and players attempt to increase their level of arousal by "psyching up" or "firing up" using pep talks, inspirational music, and anger.

The list of available neurophysical enhancements is a long one, and one that is growing longer every year. No doubt I have only scratched the surface here. Yet while the list is long, there are fundamental similarities between all these enhancements, both in terms of their associated health risks and their other side effects, both wanted and unwanted. It is these side effects which ultimately will determine whether or not we ought to allow the use of these enhancements in sport.

Risks

Any enhancement technology has its risks. Most of the ethical questions surrounding any given enhancement depend on its capacity to cause harm as an unwanted side effect of its enhancing effects.

When athletes take anabolic steroids to grow muscle tissue more quickly, there are athletic benefits to taking doses that pose health risks. Steroids do not begin to become useful as a strength enhancer until they are taken at doses far in excess of their recommended medical dosage. Furthermore, many of the ill effects of steroid overuse do not counteract their effect as strength enhancements. The same is true of human growth hormone, human erythropoietin (EPO), and many other popular enhancements.

In the case of neurophysical enhancements, however, the range of useful dosages is narrower, and safer. Not many of these drugs are risky at an effective dose, and not many of them become more effective at unsafe doses. The risk profile of these enhancements is hence quite different from that of purely physical or purely neurological enhancements.

For example, while dextroamphetamine is effective at reducing impulsivity at doses of 10 and 20 mg, an overdose is closer to 1 mg per kilogram of bodyweight (de Wit *et al.*, 2002). The effective dose is similar to the dose prescribed to children with attention-deficit disorder, and at this dose the worst of the common side effects are weight loss and insomnia, neither of which is irreversible. Since the drug is not pleasurable at these doses, dependence is rare (Olson, 2004).

More importantly, as the dose is increased above 20 mg towards overdose, it ceases to be effective as a sporting enhancement: it begins by causing sweating and tremor, and then involuntary twitching and anxiety, long before more serious side effects such as heart attack and hyperthermia can assert themselves. No athlete would continue to increase their levels of anxiety, twitching and tremor just to obtain a small reduction in impulsivity.

The same goes for anxiolytics like diazepam (Valium). Use of benzodiazepines like diazepam can cause depression and dependence, so there are risks relating to people taking too high of a dose too frequently. But while an increased dose will produce an increased reduction in an athlete's anxiety, it will also reduce her arousal and alertness, making her substantially less skillful (Elia *et al.*, 1999). Worse still, long-term use of these drugs can lead to reduced visuospatial ability and slower cognitive processing, both of which would reduce performance in most sports (Kozena *et al.*, 1995).

Many people suffer from analgesic dependency, and many die from overdoses of analgesic drugs every year. But athletes – unlike the rest of us – cannot continue to increase their dose of analgesics until the pain is eliminated. For example, at a dose of 40 mg morphine reduces pain without impairing a person's physical or cognitive performance (Stewart, 2005). At a clinical dose such as this, almost nobody becomes addicted, even after weeks of constant drug use (Walker & Zacny, 1998). At higher doses, where the risk of dependence is significant, an athlete would be drowsy, inattentive, and slow.

Although anabolic steroids are in some senses safer than morphine and amphetamines, they are much worse in this sense than neuro-enhancements. None of the unwanted risks and side effects of steroids (other than death, which is extremely rare) stand in the way of the drug-taker's aims: enhancing their muscular strength. No amount of testicular atrophy can stand in the way of a sprinter's speed.

Of course, we use anxiolytics to treat anxiety, and analgesics to treat pain, and amphetamines to reduce bodyweight, and in these uses each of these drugs is dangerous in the same manner as steroids. Whenever the goal of drug use is not impeded by the side effects of overuse, it will always be tempting for users of the drug to continually increase the dose.

But when the goal is to maximize athletic performance – particularly skilled performance – by neurophysical means, the peak enhancement is constrained. As I hoped to illustrate with my opening vignette, even the most basic physical skills involve a multitude of neural tasks, many of which are at odds with one another.

There are exceptions to this rule. Stimulants are often also used in order to combat bodily fatigue in endurance sports such as cycling, which they do through a neural process involving the peripheral nervous system. In this capacity it becomes tempting to overuse them, since fatigue is constantly increasing during sporting activity – or indeed in any other demanding activity. That is why fighter pilots, who above all must stay active and awake, sometimes become dependent on stimulants (Lander, 1990). Tom Simpson famously died after taking amphetamines and alcohol in the Tour de France (Miller, 2003), although even in that sport, where amphetamine use has been so prevalent, there are few (if any) publicly known cases of addiction, and very few amphetamine-related deaths.

In most sports, however, such occurrences will be even rarer, since fatigue is not the primary determinant of performance, and since many other capacities are required beyond mere resistance to fatigue, and these other capacities are degraded by high doses of stimulants.

Perhaps there is also a risk of athletes using amphetamines to gain attention, and benzodiazepines to treat the side effects of the amphetamines, and so forth, creating a dangerous multi-drug cocktail. But we ought never to prohibit a substance just because it cannot safely be used in conjunction with other substances, so long as there are safe uses of the substance on its own. Otherwise, we must also prohibit alcohol (which interacts dangerously with a range of other legal prescription drugs).

Every substance is dangerous in a high enough dose, even water. But at least some neurophysical enhancements diminish performance when taken at a dangerous dose, and even WADA seems to agree that it is inappropriate to prohibit performance-enhancing substances from sport when athletes are unlikely to wish to take a dangerous dose. Caffeine used to be limited to concentrations of $12\,\mu\mathrm{g/ml}$ in international sports, and some athletes such as Australian pentathlete Alex Watson have been banned from competition for using caffeine above this limit. But in 2004 WADA, which performs all testing for enhancements in sports, removed caffeine from the banned list. Their reasoning was that caffeine is in fact performance *decreasing* above $12\,\mu\mathrm{g/ml}$. Subsequent monitoring has borne this out, indicating no health-threatening abuse of caffeine in sport after its legalization (Rasmussen, 2008).

Ethical Considerations

Neurophysical enhancements are used in sport for the same reasons as other enhancements, such as steroids or EPO. That is to say, they are used to improve absolute performance, and to provide a competitive advantage over other players.

A great deal has been written and said about the use of physical enhancements such as anabolic steroids in sport. In response to the doping scandals in the Olympics, the Tour de France, and other major events, the World Anti-Doping Agency was formed in 1999 to police the use of enhancements in nearly every professional sporting league worldwide.

The reasons for prohibiting enhancements are not financial, or political. Anti-doping programs do not save anyone any money, and they do not privilege one country or club over another. It was entirely for moral reasons that the anti-doping rules, and WADA, were developed.

But these moral reasons do not apply to neurophysical enhancements in the same way as they do to other types of enhancements. In what follows, I will show how the various moral arguments, which can be raised against the use of physical or cognitive enhancements, cannot be made to apply to neurophysical ones.

Harm and Benefit

Perhaps the most obvious objection to the use of anabolic steroids in sport is that athletes take such a high dose that the health risks are significant enough to warrant prohibition, in the interests of promoting athletes' health. Even if this argument succeeds in the case of steroids, it cannot succeed in the case of neurophysical enhancements, given that the risks they pose are not all that significant.

In any case, it seems that neurophysical enhancements are not prohibited primarily on the grounds that they are harmful, but on the grounds that they are beneficial.

First, some drugs such as Modafinil and beta-blockers are banned from sports even though they are known to be safe, because they are effective enhancements. It also appears that bottled oxygen has been banned in the newest revision of the prohibited list. WADA does not require a drug to be harmful in order for it to be banned (WADA, 2008).

Furthermore, no drug that is both harmful and ineffective as an enhancement is banned from competition, except for those that are also illegal for civilians (Rasmussen, 2008; WADA, 2008). WADA's approach to the risk seems to be focused much more strongly on addressing the enhancing effects of drugs rather than their dangers.

WADA does permit some drugs which are effective enhancements. Caffeine, as I mentioned above, is permitted on the rationale that it is ineffective at unsafe doses (and hence safe at an effective dose). This apparent confusion in the regulation of sporting competition reflects a deeper problem concerning the ethics of neurophysical enhancement in sporting competition.

The problem is this: Neurophysical enhancements do not push any one capacity to superhuman levels, but rather allow an athlete to seek out the optimal balance of neural functioning within normal limits. Athletes use training, environment, diet, and medical technologies to produce similar manipulations of their physical and cognitive capacities. Given this, how can we ground a claim that a neurophysical manipulation within physiological norms is unethical, while the physical and cognitive manipulations are allowed within physiological norms?

One way would be to appeal to an ideal conception of sport which excluded manipulations of athlete biology. But what are the ideal conditions of athlete neurobiology? Here there is a conflict between the athletes' interests and the interests of the spectators.

Some weaknesses are weaknesses which we spectators would not wish to remove. Many of the best aspects of sports spectatorship depend on the physical correlates of neural processes. Choking, stage fright, emotionality, aggression – all these things can be treated, and treating them would increase performance but it would probably diminish much of the human interest in sports. Interest in sports would be increased by making athletes *more* jittery, rather than more relaxed.

By contrast, athletes stand to gain little from the presence of anxiety and stage fright. They would mostly prefer to compete on voluntary components of skill rather than on the basis of involuntary neurological processes. Now, there are players who wish to capitalize on the neurological weaknesses of others, such as cricket players who insult or "sledge" opposing players in order to elicit a loss of concentration and attention. But even these players would probably prefer it if their own stage fright, and choking, and stress symptoms could be eliminated.

The problem is that a purely skill-based competition, free of emotionality and the symptoms of stress, would look robotic and inhuman to the crowd, however rewarding it was for the athletes.

Some drugs will, on balance, present benefits for both spectators and athletes. If, for example, GABA-inhibitors can be used to make training more efficient, it is hard to see how anybody will be disadvantaged. Spectators will enjoy a greater display of skill, while athletes will need to perform less arduous hours of practice to achieve the same level of motor memorization.

But when the worst thing about a drug is that it benefits one group more than the other, this seems like weak grounds for prohibition, unless it can be shown that the interests of the athletes clearly outweigh the interests of the spectators, or vice versa.

Fairness and Cheating

One of the most frequently made objections to the use of enhancements in sport is that taking them is a form of cheating. We can understand cheating as any illegitimate means of gaining an advantage over other players.

Now, competitive sport is entirely focused on gaining an advantage over other players, but these advantages become illegitimate if they are gained in ways which are not available to other players under the rules. The most basic way that this can happen is if a given advantage is explicitly prohibited by the rules so that they are not available to rule-abiding players.

The rules of sport are not set in stone, of course, and it was not until 1928 that new rules began to be invented in order to control the use of performance enhancements. While it is certainly unfair to break a rule which other players abide by, we still need to be able to decide whether fairness (or some other consideration such as harm) can justify the rule in the first place.

Nevertheless, it is possible for an advantage to be unfair even when it is permitted under the rules of a sport. While most of the effective neurophysical enhancements are prohibited in international competition, some, such as caffeine are not (WADA, 2008).

If a widely used, legal enhancement turns out to be unreasonably risky, then athletes may object that in order to remain competitive, they are forced to take on unacceptable risks. This objection is often made against the legalization of anabolic steroids.

But this kind of objection cannot apply to neurophysical enhancements, since their risk profile is so different. Nobody thinks that using safe, legal enhancements like coffee or caffeinated soft drinks is unfair, because even though they can be very effective, they are cheap, widely available, and *safe enough*. No method of athletic enhancement, least of all training, is completely free of risk.

Suppose an enhancement is freely available, cheap, and safe enough, just as caffeine is, and just as methylphenidate and Modafinil are. Suppose that the drug is prohibited in sport. In such a case, while it might be unfair to use the drug in contravention of the rules, the prohibition itself does not increase fairness at all. Since it serves neither the ends of fairness nor harm reduction, such a prohibition would need to be justified on other grounds. I will now consider two alternative options for the justification of prohibiting neurophysical enhancements.

Authenticity

Some philosophers have expressed concerns that enhancements which affect one's cognitive capabilities or mood will create inauthentic personalities (Elliott, 1999). This argument applies to some neurophysical enhancements, particularly those which seek to address the physical side effects of mood.

On this sort of view, Cullinan ought to feel nervous when he goes out on the playing field because he is an authentically nervous person, while Warne ought to feel confident, if that is what his personality is like. Correspondingly, Cullinan ought to sweat and shake, and Warne ought to be steady and cool.

Levy has argued that there is no reason why the enhanced self cannot be viewed as authentic, provided that it is an ongoing enhancement and not just a momentary one (Levy, 2007)). After all, Cullinan might repudiate the nervous, shaky version of himself as the inauthentic byproduct of a biological weakness. If Cullinan takes anxiolytic drugs to address his stage fright, we might say that this new, calm Cullinan is the authentic, "real" one.

Levy's argument cuts deeper when it is made about neurophysical enhancements than when it is made about cognitive enhancements. It seems highly plausible that an athlete would repudiate his tremor, or his nausea, or his perspiration in this manner. To tell him that his tremulous, sweaty, and nauseated self is his true self seems no more reasonable than telling dieters that it would be more authentic for them to remain overweight.

Dehumanization

Carol Freedman (1998) has argued that psychopharmacological drugs may lead us to conceive of ourselves in dehumanized, mechanistic terms. Her concern is that by making certain deliberate modifications to one's own mind we treat it as a mere means to an end.

By contrast, nobody objects when we see purely physical traits in mechanistic terms. When an athlete does sit-ups to improve her abdominal strength, or when she trains at high altitude to increase her hematocrit, we applaud her commitment to peak physical performance.

Now, it is a matter of fact that there is a mechanistic link between our neurological states – including our mental states – and our physical capacities. Boredom decreases attention, anxiety increases tremor and sweating, and anger increases arousal.

Not every neurological intervention involves the brain. For example, thoracic sympathectomy is a procedure in which some of the sympathetic nerve trunk in the chest is destroyed surgically, usually as a means to defeat excessive sweating. But the mind is not immune to such interventions – patients who undergo this treatment feel less anxious, though presumably in part because they no longer have to worry about excessive sweating (Kumagai *et al.*, 2005).

Even purely physical interventions on purely physical capacities affect the mind. For example, anabolic steroids can generate feelings of euphoria, energy, or aggression (Pope *et al.*, 2000; Yates *et al.*, 1999). Even sit-ups can affect a person's cognitive capacity and mood (Steptoe & Cox, 1988; Tomporowski, 2003).

Since it is not possible to deliberately improve any aspect of human functioning without affecting the mind and other neurological systems, the only possible concern is that neurological enhancements *intentionally* change a person's mind, while other more mundane interventions such as sit-ups do so only as an unintended side effect. But if we put Freedman's dehumanization argument thus, it cannot apply to neurophysical enhancements, which aim only to improve physical function.

Conclusion

WADA, which polices the great majority of professional sporting federations world-wide, has taken a doggedly prohibitive approach when it comes to new pharmacological enhancements. There are many reasons to resist this approach, which have been written about elsewhere at length (Savulescu *et al.*, 2004).

But even if one accepts that there is a need to hunt down every user of steroids, EPO and growth hormone, the category of neurophysical enhancements deserves separate consideration, since these enhancements are exempt from nearly all of the ethical objections which are made against purely physical and purely neurological enhancements.

Suppose we accept that we should continue to prohibit steroids for strength in athletics, amphetamines for endurance in cycling, and Ritalin for concentration among students. Even then, it could be ethical to allow beta-blockers for steady hands in archery, amphetamines for decreased impulsivity in baseball, and Valium for reduced anxiety-induced clumsiness in gymnastics.

It makes little sense to ban every performance enhancer from sporting competition, no matter what it is used for, and what the risks are, since sport is essentially a project of performance enhancement. If every form of enhancement is to be considered unethical, competitive sport must be abandoned.

References

Andrewes, D.G. (2001). *Neuropsychology: From Theory to Practice.* New York: Taylor and Francis.

Beilock, S.L. & Carr, T.H. (2001). On the fragility of skilled performance: What governs choking under pressure? *Journal of Experimental Psychology: General,* **130**(4), 701–25.

Buhusi, C.V. & Meck, W.H. (2005). What makes us tick? Functional and neural mechanisms of interval timing. *Nature Reviews Neuroscience,* **6**(10), 755–65.

Cochran, J.C. *et al.* (1994). Decoupling motor memory strategies: Effects of sleep deprivation and amphetamine. *International Journal of Neuroscience,* **74**(1–4), 45–54.

de Wit, H., Engasser, J.L. & Richards, J.B. (2002). Acute administration of D-amphetamine decreases impulsivity in healthy volunteers. *Neuropsychopharmacology,* **27**, 813–25.

Eagle, D.M. *et al.* (2007). Differential effects of Modafinil and methylphenidate on stop-signal reaction time task performance in the rat, and interactions with the dopamine receptor antagonist cis-flupenthixol. *Psychopharmacology (Berlin),* **192**(2), 193–206.

Elia, J., Ambrosini, P.J. & Rapoport, J.L. (1999). Treatment of attention-deficit-hyperactivity disorder. *New England Journal of Medicine,* **340**(10), 780–8.

Elliott, C. (1999). *A Philosophical Disease: Bioethics, Culture, and Identity. Reflective Bioethics,* New York: Routledge.

Freedman, C. (1998). Aspirin for the mind: Some ethical worries about psychopharmacology. In E. Parens (ed.), *Enhancing Human Traits: Ethical and Social Implications* (pp. 135–50). Washington, DC: Georgetown University Press.

Graham, T.E. *et al.* (2008). Does caffeine alter muscle carbohydrate and fat metabolism during exercise? *Applied Physiology, Nutrition, and Metabolism,* **33**(6), 1311–18.

Heinz, R.D., Spear, D.J. & Bowers, D.A. (1994). Effects of cocaine on simple reaction times and sensory thresholds in baboons. *Journal of the Experimental Analysis of Behavior,* **61**(2), 231–46.

Hossmann, V. *et al.* (1980). Sedative and cardiovascular effects of clonidine and nitrazepam. *Clinical Pharmacology and Therapeutics,* **28**(2), 167–76.

Korman, M. *et al.* (2007). Daytime sleep condenses the time course of motor memory consolidation. *Nature Neuroscience,* **10**(9), 1206–13.

Kozena, L., Frantik, E. & Horvath, M. (1995). Vigilance impairment after a single dose of benzodiazepines. *Psychopharmacology (Berlin),* **119**(1), 39–45.

Kumagai, K., Kawase, H. & Kawanishi, M. (2005). Health-related quality of life after thoracoscopic sympathectomy for palmar hyperhidrosis. *Annals of Thoracic Surgery,* **80**(2), 461–6.

Lakie, M. *et al.* (1994). The effect of alcohol on physiological tremor. *Experimental Physiology,* **79**(2), 273–76.

Lander, J. (1990). Fallacies and phobias about addiction and pain. *British Journal of Addiction,* **85**(6), 803–9.

Levy, N. (2007). *Neuroethics.* Cambridge: Cambridge University Press.

Mednick, S.C. *et al.* (2008). Comparing the benefits of caffeine, naps and placebo on verbal, motor and perceptual memory. *Behavioural Brain Research,* **193**(1), 79–86.

Miller, G. (2003). "Go" pills for F-16 pilots get close look: Amphetamines prescribed in mission that killed Canadians. *Los Angeles Times.*

Olson, K.R. (2004). California Poison Control System and Knovel (Firm), *Poisoning & Drug Overdose.* In *Lange Clinical Manual* (pp. xvi, 718). New York: Lange Medical Books/McGraw-Hill.

Pope, H.G., Kouri, E.M. & Hudson, J.I. (2000). The effects of supraphysiological doses of testosterone on mood aggression in normal men. *Archives of General Psychiatry,* **57**, 133–40.

Rasch, P.J., Pierson, W.R. & Brubaker, M.L. (1960). The effect of amphetamine sulfate and meprobamate on reaction time and movement time. *European Journal of Applied Physiology*, **18**(3), 280–4.

Rasmussen, N. (2008). *On Speed: The Many Lives of Amphetamine*. New York: NYU Press.

Savulescu, J., Foddy, B. & Clayton, M. (2004). Why we should allow performance enhancing drugs in sport," *British Journal of Sports Medicine*, **38**(6), 666–70.

Shepherd, M., Findlay, J.M. & Hockey, R.J. (1986). The relationship between eye-movements and spatial attention. *Quarterly Journal of Experimental Psychology Section a, Human Experimental Psychology*, **38**(3), 475–91.

Skljarevski, V. & Ramadan, N.M. (2001). The nociceptive flexion reflex in humans – Review article. *Pain*, **96**(1–2), 3–8.

Solberg, E.E. *et al.* (1996). The effect of meditation on shooting performance. *British Journal of Sports Medicine*, **30**(4), 342–6.

Steptoe, A. & Cox, S. (1988). Acute effects of aerobic exercise on mood. *Health Psychology*, 7(4), 329–40.

Stewart, S.A. (2005). The effects of benzodiazepines on cognition. *Journal of Clinical Psychiatry*, **66** (Suppl 2), 9–13.

Sulzer, D. *et al.* (2005). Mechanisms of neurotransmitter release by amphetamines: A review. *Progress in Neurobiology*, **75**(6), 406–33.

Tedeschi, G. *et al.* (1983). Effect of amphetamine on saccadic and smooth pursuit eye movements. *Psychopharmacology*, **79**(2–3), 190–2.

Tomporowski, P.D. (2003). Effects of acute bouts of exercise on cognition. *Acta Psychologica (Amsterdam)*, **112**(3), 297–324.

Turner, D.C. *et al.* (2003). Cognitive enhancing effects of Modafinil in healthy volunteers. *Psychopharmacology (Berlin)*, **165**(3), 260–9.

WADA (2008). *The 2009 Prohibited List*. Montreal: World Anti-Doping Agency.

Walker, D.J. & Zacny, J.P. (1998). Subjective, psychomotor, and analgesic effects of oral codeine and morphine in healthy volunteers. *Psychopharmacology (Berlin)*, **140**(2), 191–201.

Yates, R. *et al.* (1999). Psychosexual effects of three doses of testosterone in cycling and normal men. *Biological Psychiatry*, **45**, 254–60.

Ziemann, U. *et al.* (2001). Modulation of practice-dependent plasticity in human motor cortex. *Brain*, **124**(6), 1171–81.

24

Can a Ban on Doping in Sport be Morally Justified?

Sigmund Loland

Can a ban on the use of performance-enhancing drugs or doping in sport be morally justified? In a setting in which sport organizations and public authorities have joined forces in the World Anti-doping Agency (WADA) in a global fight against doping, the question may seem irrelevant. However, political consensus is no guarantee for moral justification. The fact is that doping is a complex and challenging moral dilemma that has to be handled with care. Some scholars hold that the ban is problematic and even unjustifiable (Black & Pape, 1997; Brown, 1991; Tamburrini, 2000). And, as is evident from extensive doping cases in international elite sports such as athletics and professional cycling, some athletes and coaches seem to accept and indeed practice doping.

In this chapter I will take a critical look at the moral reasons for banning the use of performance-enhancing drugs in sport and examine whether a ban can be properly justified from a moral point of view. First, I will sketch how intuitively appealing arguments in support of the ban need modification. Second, I will propose a framework in which traditional arguments can be combined in a systematic way to justify the ban on doping in sport.

The Fairness Argument

A frequently used argument in favor of the doping ban is that doping is unfair. The underlying understanding of fairness seems to be a neo-Kantian Rawlsian one: Fairness is a moral obligation on rule adherence that arises when we are voluntarily engaged in rule-governed practices (Rawls, 1971). Dopers break the rules to get an exclusive advantage. For doping to be efficient, dopers depend upon the rule adherence of others. In this way dopers enjoy the benefits of the cooperation of others without doing their fair share. They are free-riders of the sports system and treat other competitors as a means only in the striving towards their own success.

In a situation in which doping is banned, dopers who are not caught get away with a rule violation and an exclusive and unfair advantage. They cheat. However, the fairness argument does not really help in the justification of the ban itself. We cannot justify a

Enhancing Human Capacities, edited by Julian Savulescu, Ruud ter Meulen and Guy Kahane.
© 2011 Blackwell Publishing Ltd

rule by reference to the wrongness of breaking it. What is at stake here is the very rationale for banning doping in sport. In fact, the fairness argument is sometimes used to support lifting the doping ban (Tamburrini, 2000). If a significant number of athletes break the rules without being caught a minority of rule-adhering athletes have a disadvantage. Morality does not pay. The situation is unjust and the obligation of fairness becomes problematic. To restore justice, an alternative could be to make doping open to all.

The Health Argument

Stronger arguments in favor of the ban can be found in the view of doping as a health hazard and as implying a significant risk of harm. Indeed, although solid scientific evidence might be lacking in some cases, there are strong indications that extensive use of performance-enhancing drugs implies serious health risks. I take as a premise here the significant hazards and even the risk of death due to extensive use of, for instance, erythropoietin (EPO) and anabolic steroids.

However, competitive sport at elite levels involves significant risks of harm. Long-term and hard training implies a constant balancing of the anabolic and catabolic processes of the body. Imbalances can result in overtraining and injuries. Similarly, the intensity of competition can lead to acute injury. In fact, in some sports risks are constitutive elements of the activity. In parachute jumping and downhill skiing there is always the possibility for serious harm and death. In boxing, avoidance of pain and harm is a critical technical and tactical challenge. An argument on banning doping due to health risks could be developed into a more general argument against the practice of elite sport as a whole.

This conclusion is unreasonable, however, as no distinctions are made here on the relevance of health risks as related to the values of sport. Health is not the primary value in all circumstances. Risks of harm must be weighed against other values of the activity in question. Athletes take their chances in training and competition. In elite sport there is a strong drive to improve, to realize athletic potential, to test the possibilities of individual talent. The challenge of the training process is to strike the optimal balance between anabolic and catabolic processes. The challenge of competing is to put in the necessary effort to succeed and at the same time be smart and avoid injuries. One of the important challenges in both downhill skiing and boxing is the proper calculation and taking of risk. Health risks linked to doping seem to be of a different kind. Why?

An idea often expressed by sport leaders and athletes is that drug-enhanced performance comes about without training and individual effort – the enhancement is somehow "undeserved." Doping is considered "unnatural" and "artificial" and the risk involved is considered an unnecessary and non-relevant one. However, ideas of the "natural" and the "artificial" are to a large extent social and cultural constructions that change over time. There are countless examples of what was considered "unnatural" yesterday has now become common practice today. One predominant example is that during most of the 20th century there has been a strong and enduring resistance against women's sports as they were considered against nature and artificial (Guttmann, 1991).

Still, the idea of drug-enhanced performance as contradictory to sport values and somehow undeserved indicates that the question of a ban goes straight to the heart of discourses around the meaning of sport. A moral standpoint towards doping needs to build on an interpretation of what sports or more precisely what athletic performances are all about. In what follows, and based on previous work (Loland, 2001, 2002), I will critically review two such interpretations.

Athletic Performance

An athletic performance is the complex product of a high number of genetic and non-genetic influences from the moment of conception to the moment of performance. As with all human phenotypes, a clear-cut distinction between genetic and environmental factors is impossible. For analytic purposes, however, the distinction makes sense.

Genetic factors are the predisposition for developing the relevant phenotypes for good performances in a sport. A person with a good predisposition is usually characterized as having "talent." Talent in this sense is distributed in the so-called natural lottery and is based on chance.

Athletes develop talent through gene–gene–environment interaction. These are influences from the very first nurture via development of general abilities and skills, to specific training and the learning of the particular techniques and tactics of sports. Environmental influences are based in part on chance and luck: athletes are born next to a public pool with a good coach and have a talent for swimming; and in part on own effort, athletes realize their talent through hard training over many years.

The critical question is whether all kinds of inequalities linked to performance (including those caused by performance-enhancing drugs) are of relevance in sports, or whether some of them ought to be eliminated or compensated for.

The thin interpretation

One answer is that anything goes. Within the competition itself there are rules to be kept such as those against hands in soccer, or kicking in handball, or pushing in track and field races. These are constitutive rules that make up the sport and without which athletic performances cannot be evaluated. However, any restrictions on performance enhancement outside of competitions, such as the Olympic amateur rules or the current ban on drugs, are considered irrelevant. In this thin interpretation of athletic performance, sport is seen to be about the maximization of human performance potential with whatever means the individual athlete finds appropriate. The view is often linked to anti-paternalistic conceptualizations of autonomy and individual freedom and responsibility. In a free society, individuals ought to be able to choose whatever performance-enhancing methods and substances they want (Tamburrini 2000).

On the critical side this view can be seen as sociologically naive and contra-productive (Loland, 2001). No athlete is an island with full freedom to choose. Without clear rules and regulations, athletes, especially in early stages of their career, easily become even more dependent upon external expertise than what is the situation today. The control over and responsibility for performance is moved gradually from athletes and teams towards external expert systems. This, then, is contra-productive to the idea of athletes as free and autonomous persons and puts them in a vulnerable position. High-performance sport might turn into something like grand scientific experiments of human performance with athletes as the guinea pigs. In this sense, the thin interpretation of athletic performance is problematic.

The thick interpretation

The alternative is a thick interpretation in which concern for athlete autonomy, freedom, and responsibility leads to further regulations. Let me go into some more detail.

Inequalities in genetic predispositions for performance based on chance are not just or unjust in themselves. However, social interpretations and regulations (or the lack of it) of the consequences of such inequalities can be problematic indeed. A general l principle found in many moral theories (and which in Rawlsian terms can be labeled the fair opportunity principle) goes as follows:

> Persons should not be treated unequally based on inequalities that they cannot influence or control in any significant way and for which they therefore cannot be claimed responsible.

In democratic societies, the distribution of basic goods and burdens are built upon this principle to a large extent. For example, physical and mental handicaps or other unfortunate conditions in life are compensated, for instance in terms of financial support and integrative efforts in work and leisure.

This principle seems to have implications in sport as well. The rule systems of sport are full of attempts to eliminate, or at least compensate, a series of inequalities with impact on performance and upon which the individual has little influence or control. Athletes are classified according to sex, age, and sometimes body size. A lightweight boxer is not matched with a heavyweight as the outcome is usually based on inequality in body size. Similarly, female sprint runners do not compete with male runners as there seems to be significant inequalities in genetic predispositions for speed to the advantage of men. Mixed races among elite sprinters seem unfair and become predictable. The basic idea appears to be to evaluate inequalities in performances that are primarily the responsibility of the athlete. By following this line of reasoning athletes can be said to be treated as free and responsible moral agents and therefore sport can be admired as a sphere of human perfectionism and be morally defended as part of a good life.

There is of course much room for improvement of fair opportunities in sport. In some sports, there is a need for more classification, other sports classify too much. For instance, in basketball and volleyball where body height is crucially important, there is a rationale for classification according to height. In other sports such as in rifle shooting or archery, biological sex seems to be irrelevant to performance and sex classification ought to be abandoned. In spite of this, however, most sports seem to be structured with the thick interpretation of athletic performance as a regulative idea.

Doping Revisited

Let me now return to the case of doping. What would be the implications of the thick theory of athletic performance when it comes to doping in sport?

Drugs are biochemical substances that are intended to have ergogenic, that is work-enhancing effects such as EPO, or anabolic effects, such as steroids that stimulate muscle growth. Some substances are agonists. They mimic the action of substances that occur naturally in the body (steroids). Others have antagonist effects. They are not produced by the body and prevent biochemical agents produced in the body to interact with their receptors (beta-blockers). In general, it can be said that drugs interact with their biological targets and lead to changes in the biochemical systems of the body.

To a certain extent it makes sense to say that doping enhances performance independent of talent and without individual athletic effort. Inequalities due to doping are not the results of chance, nor are they expressions of athletic merit. Therefore performance-enhancing effects of drugs can be considered non-relevant and should be eliminated. To legalize doping would decrease athletes' responsibility for their own performance, often in favor of an external expert system, and hence athletes' potential of acting as a free and responsible moral agents. From the thick theory perspective, the use of performance-enhancing drugs implies unnecessary and non-relevant health risks in sport and should be banned.

Based on this premise, the fairness argument becomes valid, too. The ban on drugs is justified without reference to the wrongness of breaking it. Dopers violate the rules to get an exclusive advantage. For their drug use to be efficient they rely upon the rule adherence of others without doing their fair share. They cheat and therefore doping is unfair. If the situation is unjust in the sense that too many dopers are not caught and get away with an unfair advantage, the problem is not the doping ban but the weakness of the control system. From the thick theory, then, the WADA initiative is highly welcomed.

Concluding Comments

I have presented an argument so cut to the bone here that there is a need for a couple of additional comments.

I have argued that the doping issue goes straight to the heart of questions of the value and meaning of sport and that a ban cannot be based on fairness and health arguments alone but ultimately on a normative view of sport. In my view the thick interpretation is the superior one in this respect. The clarification of a normative basis for the doping ban is not just philosophically challenging. A ban will always meet the challenges of distinguishing in practice between acceptable and non-acceptable performance-enhancing methods and substances. The doping field is full of gray areas and there is a strong need for systematic and good casuistry to navigate in informed and reasonable ways. Good casuistry implies walking back and forth between general principles and the particularities of the case under consideration. The thick interpretation of athletic performance and the idea of unnecessary health risks offer a principled basis whereas biomedical facts on effects and health risks of the substance and method under consideration provide the particularities. I believe the WADA system is strong on the latter. What is presented here is an attempt to strengthen the principled level defined by WADA somewhat vaguely as "the spirit of sport."

A final comment is that the thick interpretation has considerable critical force beyond the doping issue (Loland, 2002). As indicated above, if taken seriously it could radically change some of the classification regimes in sport. In general, I believe there is too much sex classification and too little classification in terms of body size. Moreover, it would have radical consequences for the regulation of inequalities in financial, scientific, and technological resources. But his belongs to a more extensive discussion about fairness and justice in sport that is beyond the scope of this chapter.

References

Black, T. & Pape, A. (1997). The ban on drugs in sport: The solution or the problem? *Journal of Sport and Social Issues*, **21**(1), 83–92.

Brown, M.L. (1990). Practices and prudence. *Journal of the Philosophy of Sport*, **17**, 71–84.

Guttmann, A. (1991). *Womens Sport: A History.* New York: Columbia University Press.

Loland, S. (2001). Technology in sport: Three ideal-typical views and their implications. *European Journal of Sport Science*, **2**(1), 1–10.

Loland, S. (2002). *Fair Play in Sport. A Moral Norm System.* London: Routledge.

Rawls, J. (1971). *A Theory of Justice.* Cambridge, MA: Harvard University Press.

Tamburrini, C. (2000). *"The Hand of God." Essays in the Philosophy of Sport.* Gothenburg: Acta Universitatis Gothoburgensis.

Part V
Lifespan Extension

25

Looking for the Fountain of Youth
Scientific, Ethical, and Social Issues in the Extension of Human Lifespan

Gaia Barazzetti

Extending Human Lifespan: Demographic, Epidemiological, and Scientific Perspectives

Demographic data show that the average human lifespan has nearly tripled over the course of human history (Wilmoth, 1998). As a consequence of the industrial era, the complex interplay of improvements in income, nutrition, and sanitation brought about a progressive reduction of infant and child mortality which eventually resulted in the increase in life expectancy at birth. Mortality risks gradually shifted to older ages and became attributable to age-related disorders such as cancer, stroke, and degenerative diseases (Riley, 2001).

Many attempts have been made by demographers, epidemiologists, and biologists towards an understanding of the factors influencing human life expectancy today, and several contrasting hypotheses have been formulated on the future trends of human longevity and on the existence of biological limits for average human lifespan. From the second half of the 20th century, mortality rates at older ages have been declining exponentially at a roughly constant rate in industrialized countries and have not shown any noticeable sign of slowing down (Tuljapurkar *et al.*, 2000). These findings on the constant decline of mortality rates suggest that the reduction in death rates has changed its typology (Horiuchi, 2000; Wilmoth, 1998, 2000). Life expectancy is now driven by the extension of life to later stages and by the phenomenon known as "compression of morbidity": chronic illness and disability are postponed and morbidity is compressed into a shorter span at older ages.

Nowadays, the average length of life in wealthy countries is around 75–80 years, and projections of future trends predict even longer average lifespans. Data from national populations show an increase in life expectancy that provides a basis for a life expectancy forecasting which will eventually exceed the age of 85 (Kannisto, 1994; Kannisto *et al.*, 1994; Manton & Vaupel, 1995; Vaupel & Lundström, 1994).

Enhancing Human Capacities, edited by Julian Savulescu, Ruud ter Meulen and Guy Kahane.
© 2011 Blackwell Publishing Ltd

These forecasts, based on mathematical extrapolation from demographic data (Oeppen & Vaupel, 2002), have been recently criticized by biodemographers suggesting that the biological duration of life results from the complex interaction of genetic, behavioral, and environmental factors (Olshansky & Carnes, 2004). These opponents of the mathematical approach contend that forecasts on the future of human lifespan cannot ignore the biological evidence of the phenomenon of senescence, characterized by the inevitable and progressive decrease in the capacity to respond to environmental stresses, together with an increased susceptibility and vulnerability to disease. According to this view, human organisms operate under "biological warranty periods" that inevitably limit life duration. Even if age-related diseases were eliminated, life expectancy would never exceed its insurmountable biological constraints (Carnes *et al.*, 2003; Olshansky *et al.*, 1990). Hence, projections based on a biodemographic perspective should support more pessimistic and "realistic" forecasts of human life expectancy (Olshansky *et al.*, 2001).

However, the debate on the future trends of human life expectancy is still open and is further thickened by hypotheses on the determinants of decline in death rates at older ages. Recent studies, which are based on available demographic and epidemiological evidence, cautiously suggested that a significant proportion of the decline of death rates among the elderly in the last few decades might be due to medical progress (Christensen & Vaupel, 1996). Indeed, the development of many new pharmaceutical interventions validated through clinically controlled trials, as well as the improvements achieved in the treatment of potentially fatal age-related diseases, has played an important role in the increase of life expectancy. Moreover, advancements in geriatric medicine, which are directed both to intervention and to prevention, are likely to result in a further reduction in the incidence of premature deaths among the elderly. However, such results are not enough to support reliable predictions about the future trends of average lifespan extension. Biodemographic and epidemiological data available nowadays can only suggest that the hypothesis of a further reduction of mortality at older ages is highly plausible. Indeed, this prospect is not unconditional, since possible future decline of death rates among the elderly in developed countries depends on the complex interplay of medical advancements and environmental/genetic factors (Christensen & Vaupel, 1996).

Nevertheless, the hypothesis that foreseeable developments in interventions directed to forestall and to treat the disabilities of aging might result in the extension of the human lifespan may be further supported by the "evolutionary theory of aging." The basic assumption of this theory is that the forces of natural selection are blind to the effects of gene expression on the post-reproductive physiology of an organism (Kirkwood & Rose, 1991; Rose, 1991; Rose & Graves, 1989). As a consequence, aging can be viewed as a byproduct of selective forces, which are effective only in the optimization for early fitness. The evolutionary theory of aging provides strong scientific evidence that aging is not genetically programmed since specific genes selected to promote aging are unlikely to exist (Kirkwood & Austad, 2000). Besides its relevant implications for the study of the genetic factors that influence longevity and age-related diseases, the evolutionary theory of aging has been used to justify the idea that if aging is an accidental and not an intrinsic component of evolution, it could be manipulated just like any other process regarded as unnatural or pathological (Caplan, 2004). Following this idea, evolutionary biologists have developed successful techniques to postpone aging in a variety of species, such as insects and rodents, by delaying the onset of reproduction (Rose, 2004). Others have hypothesized the enhancement of healthy aging through interventions aimed at improving metabolic resources that can be invested in soma maintenance and repair when evolutionary pressure for early fitness and reproduction decreases (Westendorp, 2006). In short, by considering aging as neither natural nor inevitable brings it into the domain of medicine, thus leaving the door open for the prevention, the cure, or the elimination of the aging process.

Contrary to the idea that the phenomenon of senescence can be conceptualized in the language of pathology, Leonard Hayflick (1998, 2000) proposed several criteria to distinguish aging from disease: unlike any disease, aging occurs in every human being at some point in adulthood; unlike any known disease, aging appears in nearly all species and only after the reproductive period; and, unlike any disease, aging befalls all animals removed from the wild. In particular, biological aging in humans may have arisen as an artifact of civilization: unlike feral animals, humans have learned how to escape the causes of death long after the reproductive period, thus experiencing a process that they would have never encountered in the wild. If aging is not a disease, research on biological basis of aging, namely "biogerontology," should be distinguished from research on age-related diseases, namely "geriatric medicine" (Hayflick, 2000). According to this view, age-related diseases should be disentangled from the aging process, which is not a disease as such, and should not be considered as a pathological phenomenon that calls for a cure.

However, it is still questionable whether the process of aging can be identified and studied independently from age-related disease (Butler *et al.*, 2004). While it is agreed that there are age-related risk factors for disease which overlap aging risk factors, it is still not clear whether age-related diseases should be viewed as a mere byproduct of aging, or as an essential component of the aging process.

One of the most ambitious attempts to find out a viable distinction between a disease-free pattern of aging and the overlapping development of age-related diseases, such as diabetes, osteoporosis, cardiovascular disease, cancer, and a large variety of neurodegenerative diseases, is the *Baltimore Longitudinal Study of Aging* (BLSA; 1958, www.grc.nia.nih.gov/branches/blsa/blsa.htm).

This still ongoing National Institute on Aging research program, which was started nearly 50 years ago, aims to describe age-related changes by making successive measurements over a period of time. Many facts have emerged from the BLSA, the foremost of which is that it is extremely difficult to gain a definition of "normal" aging, and to separate the overlapping occurrence of changes related to senescence which do not threaten health (such as gray hair or wrinkled skin), from other changes which may eventually contribute to age-related diseases (such as accumulation of oxidative damage), and the others which may cause pathological phenomena (such as plaques and tangles in the brain as risk factors for Alzheimer's disease).

Since age-related pathologies and the aging process as such can hardly be distinguished, determining whether medical interventions aimed at preventing age-related risk factors for disease or at curing age-related diseases are to be considered as "treatments" or as "enhancements" still remains an extremely difficult task (Juengst, 2004). As far as medical interventions that contrast the morbidities of aging may delay the onset of age-related ailments and extend healthy lifespan, their life-extending consequences could always be condemned as enhancements, rather than be considered as side effects of appropriate treatments. Indeed, the extension of lifespan is generally conceived as a form of enhancement and it is often stressed that, lacking the resources to satisfy all health care needs, therapeutic interventions should have priority over enhancements of the normal functioning of the species (Buchanan *et al.*, 2000). However, the rise in technological possibilities makes it more difficult to define a clear division line between therapy and enhancement since it is not reasonable simply to assume that everything that counts as therapy should be prioritized and everything that counts as enhancement should be rejected (Parens, 1998). Some medical interventions that have life-extending effects are no doubt therapeutic and for those who classify aging as a pathologic process, all arguments based on the therapy/enhancement division should be rejected.

In a similar way, our working knowledge of the mechanisms of senescence seems to have a tremendous potential for the development of life-extension interventions. However, within the scientific community the debate on whether research on aging will eventually result in the enhancement of human lifespan is still open, and scholars seem to be divided into two opposite factions (Turner, 2003). On the one hand, optimistic proponents of life-extension technologies claim that existing knowledge of human aging provides a basis for the manipulation of the aging process itself, which will eventually enhance human longevity (de Grey *et al.*, 2002). On the other hand, more cautious scientists believe that aging is a complex and multifaceted process which cannot be easily manipulated or controlled (Warner *et al.*, 2005).

Though this controversy is still undecided and the appropriate limits of preventive medicine remain questioned, it is possible to foresee at least three scenarios of lifespan-extension research, which can be described under the following labels: "compression of morbidity," "decelerated aging," and "arrested aging" (Post & Binstock, 2004). The aspiration to the compression of morbidity pictures a scenario in which humans may experience longer healthy lifespans, until the sharp advent of senescence is followed rather quickly by death. The prospect of the compression of morbidity assumes that although infirmities associated with aging may be postponed and shortened, the maximum duration of human lifespan cannot be exceeded. As a consequence, the compression of morbidity may eventually result in the moderate increase in average life expectancy, but not in the extension of maximum human lifespan. A more ambitious prospect is the deceleration of aging, which envisages the slowing down of the aging process, thus postponing the morbidities of senescence and eventually increasing both life expectancy and/or maximum lifespan. Finally, the arrested aging scenario suggests the most radical paradigm of lifespan extension. Indeed, this scenario foresees a reversal of the aging process through strategies that forestall or remove the damage caused by the inexorable metabolic mechanisms of senescence. If successful, the reversal of the aging process would result in the absence of senescence and the achievement of a perpetually youthful physiological state. The prospect of arrested aging would also imply the achievement of "virtual immortality," since death would come from accidents, homicides or suicides, rather than from progressive decline in performance and fitness with advancing age. Should that come true, such a scenario might be the most challenging for our experience of human condition, since, for the first time in history, human beings would go beyond the limits imposed by finitude and mortality. An overview of the most promising foreseeable interventions aimed at lifespan extension may help to clarify the feasibility of these scenarios, and may provide a basis for further discussion on the ethical and social implications of such interventions.

Foreseeable Progresses in the Extension of Lifespan: The State of the Art

A significant lengthening of lifespan in a variety of species (e.g. yeast, worms, fish, rats, and mice), can be induced by caloric restriction (Masoro & Austad, 1996). The caloric restriction protocol differs from starvation in that it consists in lower caloric intake (by 30–70%), associated with fully adequate amounts of proteins, vitamins and minerals, fatty acids, and other nutrients. Basically, this experimental intervention increases longevity patterns through the extension of healthy lifespan and the delay in the onset of senescence (Arking, 2004). In order to understand if caloric restriction may have the same impact on human aging, and how long it should last to produce effects on humans, studies on rhesus monkeys have been carried out to investigate the effects of a 30% dietary restriction. Preliminary results demonstrate that caloric restriction might slow down or reduce some age-related physiological changes (Ramsey *et al.*, 2000; Roth *et al.*, 2001, 2002; Zainai *et al.*, 2000). Moreover, a few observational studies suggest that caloric restriction has beneficial effects on human health and aging (Nikolich-Zugich & Messaoudi, 2005). These include natural experiments such as the one conducted by a Spanish nursing home where patients who underwent a 35% reduction in caloric intake over three years reported fewer visits to the infirmary and a slight decrease in death rate (Hursting *et al.*, 2003). Data from a pilot caloric restriction experiment using human subjects (e.g. the Biosphere 2 project), have also suggested that the caloric restriction regimen improves several physiological functions (Weyer *et al.*, 2000).

These observations are highly encouraging and strongly suggest that caloric restriction, regardless of the fact that it may increase longevity, is likely to improve general health and well-being in elderly human beings. However, a few studies are currently investigating the quality of life and potential "pitfalls" of long-term caloric restriction in human beings (Dirks & Leeuwenburgh, 2006). Potential negative side effects may include hypotension, infertility, bone thinning and osteoporosis, and psychological conditions such as depression and irritability. Thus, the caloric restriction regimen used experimentally may not be feasible for most humans. The development of interventions mimicking the effect of caloric restriction seems to be promising in providing the same health benefits and in slowing the aging process as a rigorous caloric restriction regimen, while avoiding the need to reduce food and caloric intake. Possible caloric restriction mimics may imply pharmaceutical, hormone, or genetic manipulation, but would not include interventions involving appetite suppression or procedures such as stomach stapling (Guo *et al.*, 2001; Ingram *et al.*, 2004; Kirpichnikov *et al.*, 2002; Oliver *et al.*, 2001; Spindler *et al.*, 2003).

Besides caloric restriction, several hormone supply or replacement strategies are considered to contrast the functional decline associated with aging (Lamberts *et al.*, 1997). Hormone treatments may include growth hormone (GH), insulin-like growth factor I (IGF-I) signaling, dehydroepiandrosterone (DHEA), melatonin, testosterone, progesterone, and estrogen.

Amongst these, the "anti-aging" action of GH has been widely underlined. In 1990, a renowned study reported the effect on body composition after a six-month administration of human GH to 12 elderly men (Rudman *et al.*, 1990). This study incited a proliferation of a number of publications extolling the benefits of growth hormone in reversing or preventing aging. Beyond these claims for GH miraculous effects, research on GH continues to be promising. The release of GH by the pituitary gland decreases with age and reduced levels of GH almost certainly contribute to age-related loss of muscle mass, increase in adiposity, and loss of bone mineral (Corpas *et al.*, 1993; Rudman *et al.*, 1990). These changes resemble those observed in adult GH deficiency, and may be reduced or reversed by GH therapy.

However, there is no evidence for effects of GH therapy on life expectancy. It was claimed that although GH supplementation has shown to improve some of the physiological changes associated with aging, GH therapy has not proved to extend lifespan (Olshansky *et al.*, 2002). Indeed, it has been suggested that the "anti-aging" action of GH relates to its effects on body composition and functioning in elderly individuals, rather than to its role in determining longer lifespan (Bartke *et al.*, 2001; Laron, 2004). More recent studies have demonstrated the role of insulin-like growth factor I (IGF-I) in modulating age-related diseases (Yang *et al.*, 2005). These findings provide a strong basis for the hypothesis that healthy human lifespan depends on the maintenance of optimal IGF-I action in order to prevent morbidities associated with aging (Yang *et al.*, 2005).

Further uncertainty remains about the goals of foreseeable treatments based on GH and IGF-I (Kann, 2003). It is questionable whether these treatments should also retain the ability to work, avoid the need of care, increase vitality, or simply reduce morbidity. Finally, scientific knowledge of the possible individual risks or unwanted side effects for the GH-treated patients is still sparse, and should deserve further research. In fact, it is not known whether long-term administration of growth hormone in the elderly is potentially harmful particularly with regard to the risk of cancer (Kann, 2003; Vance, 2003). Therefore, further investigation on the safety of the use of foreseeable GH and IGF-I based treatments in healthy elderly persons is strongly needed (Kann, 2004).

Several experiments on animals have shown that dehydroepiandrosterone (DHEA) is a multifunctional adrenal steroid with immune function enhancement, anti-diabetic, anti-cancer, and anti-aging effects. In particular, DHEA seems to play a relevant role in the functional decline that involves memory and cognitive abilities which may occur with aging (Racchi *et al.*, 2003). In the 1990s, DHEA was exalted as a possible candidate for the "fountain of youth" (Baulieu, 1996). Today, the original enthusiasm about the potential anti-aging effects of DHEA has weakened, since studies on the replacement of DHEA in aging populations has produced results that are favorable in most studies but not in others (Yen, 2001). So far these contradictory results suggest that extrapolation for longevity is premature, and that investigation on possible anti-aging effects and potential risks of DHEA administration should deserve further research (Celec & Starka, 2003).

Research on interventions aimed at prolonging healthy lifespan and delaying the aging process includes the reduction of oxidative damage, telomerase activation, genetic manipulations, and potential cellular therapies from stem cell research. Recent studies have demonstrated that oxidative stress is a major determinant of lifespan in worms and flies, and that it can be counteracted by pharmacological intervention or genetic engineering techniques (Arking *et al.*, 2000; Kang *et al.*, 2002; Larsen & Clarke, 2002; Melov *et al.*, 2000). These studies have proved that strategies designed to contrast oxidative damage postpone the onset of senescence in invertebrate model organisms and significantly extend their lifespan. However, these strategies have not induced a similar extension of the lifespan in mammals, where a more complex control system working over the aging process might probably need more specific and elaborate interventions (Arking, 2004). As reviewed by Harman, more sophisticated measures to reduce oxidative damage may include, among others, caloric restriction, antioxidants enzymes, superoxide dismutase (SOD), mimics, and dietary antioxidants (Harman, 2001). However, at present, evidence from human studies that interventions aimed at reducing oxidative stress damage might lead to a reduction of the rate of aging is still sparse.

There is growing evidence that telomere shortening limits the regenerative potential of organ cells during aging and chronic disease (Djojosubroto *et al.*, 2003). Telomere shortening affects organ regeneration at cellular level and limits the pool of regenerating cells by activation of a senescence program in cells with critically short telomeres. The possibility of using telomerase activation, to extend the regenerative potential of cells during aging and chronic disease, depends on the effects of telomerase activity on tumor formation (Djojosubroto *et al.*, 2003; Geserick & Blasco, 2006). Studies from telomerase-deficient mice have suggested a dual role of telomere shortening and telomerase activation during cancer initiation and progression.

Since genes seem to play a relevant role in all biological processes, it has been suggested that specific genes should be involved in aging. However, to avoid any misinterpretation, it should be noted that there are no genes which have been specifically selected to cause aging. According to the evolutionary theory of aging, no genetic instructions to age animals are likely to exist. Yet, aging appears to have a genetic component, and it is possible that specific genes may influence longevity, even if the aging process itself is not genetically programmed (De Benedictis *et al.*, 2001; Finch & Tanzi, 1997). Although gene therapy directed towards the overall aging process seems to hold little promise, what is more likely to be achieved is that the manipulation of such genes, which seem to be involved in aging and lifespan, will prevent the onset of various age-related diseases (Rattan, 1998). Targets of gene therapy may include cardiovascular diseases, cancer, diabetes, osteoporosis, Alzheimer's disease, Parkinson's disease, and loss of renal function. Further knowledge of the genetic mechanisms involved in the maintenance and repair of cellular and sub-cellular components, such as the structural and functional integrity of nuclear and mitochondrial genome, may provide a basis for the development of interventions aimed at healthier and longer lifespans (Rattan, 1998). Indeed, if effective, these interventions may lead to preventive and treatment strategies for age-related diseases, which will have a relevant impact on enhancing the quality of life of the elderly population (Barzilai & Shuldiner, 2001).

However, Browner *et al.* have reviewed several genetic pathways that may extend lifespan through effects on aging, rather than through effects on age-related diseases such as atherosclerosis or cancer (Browner *et al.*, 2004). Therefore, the identification of genetic pathways that regulate longevity may enable the development of treatments that increase lifespan and improve health.

Such a possibility has been shown in mammals: p66ShcA-deficient mice were more resistant to oxidative stress and lived longer than the wild-type animals (Migliaccio *et al.*, 1999). Further studies have suggested that the level of p66ShcA could be modulated by a putative longevity-promoting agent aurintricarboxylic acid, also known as ATA (Fraifeld *et al.*, 2002). As reported by Sagi *et al.*, the lifespan-prolongation effect of ATA in a *Drosophila* model has been further validated, and results have supported the suggested role of p66ShcA as one of the lifespan determinants in mammals (Sagi *et al.*, 2005). Thus, p66ShcA may represent a potential target for pharmacological longevity-promoting intervention.

Stem cells have recently been isolated and have tremendous potential to treat a variety of age-related degenerative diseases (Gearhart, 1998). However, there remain many technical and conceptual hurdles to control the differentiation of such cells once they have been transplanted (Butler *et al.*, 2004).

Technology applications to reverse the adverse effects of aging will have significant potential if and when the above-mentioned hurdles will be overcome. Indeed, advances in embryonic stem cell technology may make the replacement of tissues and organs possible. However, possible cellular therapies of age-related diseases would not imply a treatment for the aging process itself (Kassem, 2006).

Ethical and Social Issues under Discussion

The ethical questions concerning the extension of the lifespan belong to two distinct areas: the area of individual morality and the area of social morality. In both areas, several arguments have been raised; most of them are highly problematic, and none seems to be definitive. Arguments related to individual morality can be distinguished into two types: those aiming to show that a huge increase in the lifespan is not a rationally desirable aim; and those aiming to show that it is against nature and therefore morally questionable.

The first idea is often argued for on the basis of a psychological account of personal identity, such as Derek Parfit's (1984), according to which the identity of a person is not guaranteed by the continuity of the same body but rather by the connectedness or continuity of one's mental states. In this respect, the lack of sufficient psychological continuity between my present self and the one I might become within the next century shows that aiming at such a long survival cannot be the object of my egoistic concern: in fact, that individual will not be me, rather a new self that will be "inhabiting" the human organism which now constitutes my body (Glannon, 2002a). The argument is, however, controversial, since the psychological view of personal identity is questionable, for it implies that an individual who undergoes a cerebral trauma that eradicates all of his memories, is thereby another person. It has also been maintained that, once we drop the idea that being a person is our substantial sortal and we accept that we are basically human animals, there is no longer any need for psychological connectedness to guarantee personal identity (DeGrazia, 2005; Olson, 1997). Hence, arguments for and against the desirability of lifespan extension for the individual are often grounded in different conceptions of personal identity.

The second and more radical critical attitude towards the extension of lifespan builds on the notion of *naturalness* of aging. That is, it aims to show that aging serves some kind of purpose or function, typically that of pursuing the evolutionary success of our species, eliminating elderly individuals to make room for younger ones. However, as already hinted above, aging is but the side effect of processes aiming to guarantee the best chance of reproducing oneself at a younger age, and can be viewed as a disease (Caplan, 2004).

The argument from unnaturalness can also be cast in ethical, rather than evolutionary, terms. It may be speculated that mortality is an inherent aspect of human experience and that the consciousness of having a set limit gives seriousness and depth to our projects. As noted by Kass (2004), while the Homeric gods waste their time in futile passions, as if spectators to the real life, mortal men commit themselves most seriously to their endeavors. What is highest and most elevated in life is in relation to death, its fear and avoidance, and it is naive to believe that higher aspirations of human beings could be satisfied by endlessly prolonging their lives. The least that can be said of this view is that it is highly speculative, and does not provide sufficient evidence for its main tenets.

Arguments related to social morality are perhaps stronger. For one thing, it has been noted that nature's aim of transmitting individuals' genes to their progeny is furthered by a particular protection against certain pathologies during the reproductive age. Because of the evolutionary tradeoff between reproductive capacity and longevity, manipulating our genetic endowment in order to increase longevity may increase vulnerability to diseases in the reproductive age (Glannon, 2002b). We should therefore be very careful before starting any experimentation on human subjects. However, this conclusion is not accepted by those who disqualify the precautionary principle, both as a principle of rational choice and as a moral one, in view of its tendency to irrationally emphasize highly hypothetical risks while underrating possible benefits (Harris & Holm, 2002).

Other worries are tied to the questions of distributive justice generated by the likely increase in the world population following the dissemination of life-extension treatments. While, in the compression of morbidity hypothesis, a relevant increase in health care needs of the elderly is not to be expected, problems may nonetheless arise for other basic resources, such as water or food. Thus, it seems likely that the scientific success of life-extending technologies would impose an unbearable burden on the environment and its resources. Moreover, in all probability, technologies would be implemented for a relatively long time only in the more affluent countries that already have a high life expectancy. This would further increase the difference of resources and opportunities among areas of the world population (Chapman, 2004).

Some scholars have objected to these considerations by saying that all scientific developments have first been implemented in a small part of the world, and only with time they have found widespread diffusion. Anti-aging techniques would follow the same path (Harris, 2002). A possible rejoinder is that, unlike other cases, what is at issue is a qualitatively new benefit, to be conferred on a small part, while a large part of the world population still lacks the resources even to get to the condition that would be "cured" by the new technologies. Moreover, the fact that partly analogous situations have been underrated in the past, when the injustice of the differences in life conditions was not perceived, may not justify a similar attitude today, when we have a clear consciousness of interdependency in the globalized world.

Some, however, are skeptical with regard to the likelihood of a demographic increase (Gems, 2003). Birth rates are declining in most advanced nations and the same may become true for the rest of the world if reliable means of birth control will diffuse. Therefore, a relevant increase in the average life expectancy would not sensibly affect the overall population. To this, it may be replied that new and sometimes strange procreative desires are ever increasing, along with the capacities of reproductive medicine to satisfy them. This may pose, in the long run, a displeasing dilemma between satisfying the reproductive desires of some and the desires of others to live longer lives.

In any case, even with a lack in the increase of global population, the unbalance between the young and old may pose problems of intergenerational justice (Callahan, 1990). The most evident one is tied to pensions: the more the ratio between the generations is in favor of the older ones, the more the younger will have to contribute to guarantee the social security of the former. Of course, the younger will eventually be repaid of their sacrifices by engaging a longer life, and the increase in the lifespan should also determine a prolongation of active and working life for the elderly. However, prolonging the working life of people with increased lifespans may not be beneficial for them, and may itself pose further problems of justice. Large numbers of still working, much elderly people might create serious problems for the new genera-tions trying to reach success or to gain acknowledgment of their capacities. In the political field, this may generate dramatic obstacles to any social and political reform.

Other concerns regarding policy interventions have been extensively discussed. Binstock suggested that, among the different older age groups that are generally recognized (i.e. the "young old," aged 65–74; the "old old," aged 75–84; and the "oldest old," aged 85 and older), life-extending interventions may produce a new cohort of "prolonged old," aged 95 and older (Binstock, 1996, 2004). On the basis of what is known about the politics of aging in the 20th and early 21st century, it is possible to speculate about the foreseeable impact of a growing population of "prolonged old" on future political and governmental interventions in a long-lived society (Binstock, 2004). Perhaps, the most relevant consequence may spring from an increase in the already higher voting participation of older people. However, new electoral rules may be introduced to avoid the specter of a "voting majority" comprised by older members of society. Moreover, it is questionable whether a higher percentage of older voters will influence policy decisions (Binstock, 2004). Contrary to what is assumed by the "senior power model" of the politics of age, older people have different political attitudes and do not represent a homogenous group of interest. Their voting decisions may vary considerably, depending on economic, social, gender, racial, and other factors that commonly affect voting behavior. In spite of the fact that age-group consciousness may not be a major factor influencing policy interventions, the economic burdens of sustaining old-age welfare programs may play an important role in the electoral campaigns taken on by politicians (Binstock, 2004). As a consequence, arguments for and against the protection of old-age interests put forward by political candidates may emphasize the rhetoric of warfare between generations. However, it would be more likely and desirable that old-age policies in a long-lived society make distinctions between the members of older population, thus distributing benefits on the basis of old persons' real economic status and needs, guaranteeing more equitable welfare programs, and eventually reducing possible conflicts between the young and the elderly population groups (Binstock, 2000).

References

Arking, R. (2004). Extending human longevity: A biological probability. In S.G. Post & R.H. Binstock (eds.), *The Fountain of Youth. Cultural, Scientific, and Ethical Perspectives on a Biomedical Goal* (pp. 177–200). Oxford: Oxford University Press.

Arking, R., Burde, V., Graves, K. *et al.* (2000). Selection for longevity specifically alters antioxidant gene expression and oxidative damage patterns in Drosophila. *Experimental Gerontology*, **35**, 167–85.

Bartke, A., Coschignano, K., Kopchick, J. *et al.* (2001). Genes that prolong life: Relationships of growth hormone and growth to aging and lifespan. *Journals of Gerontology. Series A: Biological Sciences and Medical Sciences*, **56**, B340–B349.

Barzilai, N. & Shuldiner, A.R. (2001). Searching for human longevity genes: The future history of gerontology in the post-genomic era. *Journal of Gerontology: Medical Sciences*, **56A**, M83–M87.

Baulieu, E.E. (1996). Dehydroepiandrosterone (DHEA): A fountain of youth? *Journal of Clinical Endocrinology and Metabolism*, **81**, 3147–51.

Binstock, R.H. (1996). Continuities and discontinuities in public policy and aging. In V.L. Bengston (ed.), *Adulthood and Aging: Research on Continuities and Discontinuities* (pp. 308–24). New York: Springer.

Binstock, R.H. (2000). Older people and voting participation: Past and future. *Gerontologist*, **40**, 18–31.

Binstock, R.H. (2004). The prolonged old, the long-lived society and the politics of age. In S.G. Post & R.H. Binstock (eds.), *The Fountain of Youth. Cultural, Scientific, and Ethical Perspectives on a Biomedical Goal* (pp. 362–86). Oxford: Oxford University Press.

Browner, W.S., Kahn, A.J., Ziv, E. *et al.* (2004). The genetics of human longevity. *American Journal of Medicine*, **117**, 851–60.

Buchanan A. *et al.* (2000). *From Chance to Choice: Genetics and Justice*. Cambridge: Cambridge University Press.

Butler, R.N., Sprott, R., Warner, H. *et al.* (2004). Biomarkers of aging: from primitive organisms to humans. *Gerontology*, **6**, 560–7.

Callahan, D. (1990). *What Kind of Life? The Limits of Medical Progress*. New York: Simon & Schuster.

Caplan, A.L. (2004). An unnatural process: Why it is not inherently wrong to seek a cure for aging. In S.G. Post & R.H. Binstock (eds.), *The Fountain of Youth. Cultural, Scientific, and Ethical Perspectives on a Biomedical Goal* (pp. 271–85). Oxford: Oxford University Press.

Carnes, B.A., Olshansky, S.J. & Grahn, D. (2003). Biological evidence for limits to the duration of life. *Biogerontology*, **4**, 31–45.

Celec, P. & Starka, L. (2003). Dehydroepiandrosterone – Is the fountain of youth drying out? *Physiology Research*, **52**, 397–407.

Chapman, A.R. (2004). The social and justice implications of extending the human lifespan. In S.G. Post & R.H. Binstock (eds.), *The Fountain of Youth. Cultural, Scientific, and Ethical Perspectives on a Biomedical Goal* (pp. 340–61). Oxford: Oxford University Press.

Christensen, K. & Vaupel, J.W. (1996). Determinants of longevity: genetic, environmental and medical factors. *Journal of Internal Medicine*, **240**, 333–41.

Corpas, E., Harman, S.M. & Blackman, M.R. (1993). Human growth hormone and human aging. *Endocrine Reviews*, **14**, 20–39.

De Benedictis, G., Tan, Q., Jeune, B. *et al.* (2001). Recent advances in human gene – Longevity association studies. *Mechanisms of Aging and Development*, **122**, 909–20.

de Grey, A.D.N.J., Ames, B.N., Andersen, J.K. *et al.* (2002). Time to talk SENS: Critiquing the immutability of human aging. *Annals of the New York Academy of Sciences*, **959**, 452–62.

DeGrazia, D. (2005). *Human Identity and Bioethics.* Cambridge: Cambridge University Press.

Dirks, A.J. & Leeuwenburgh, C. (2006). Caloric restriction in humans: Potential pitfalls and health concerns. *Mechanisms of Aging and Development*, **127**, 1–7.

Djojosubroto, M.W., Choi, Y.S., Lee, H.W. *et al.* (2003). Telomeres and telomerase in aging, regeneration and cancer. *Molecules and Cells*, **15**, 164–75.

Finch, C.E. & Tanzi, R.E. (1997). Genetics of Aging. *Science*, **278**, 407–11.

Fraifeld, V., Wolfson, M., Sagi, O. *et al.* (2002). Effects of anti-apoptotic agent aurintricarboxylic acid on longevity and longevity-associated processes. *Biogerontology*, **3**, 48.

Gearhart, J. (1998). New potential for human embryonic stem cells. *Science*, **282**, 1061–2.

Gems, D. (2003). Is more life always better? the new biology of aging and the meaning of life. *Hastings Center Report*, **33**, 31–9.

Geserick, C. & Blasco, M.A. (2006). Novels roles for telomere in aging. *Mechanisms of Aging and Development*, **127**, 579–83.

Glannon, W. (2002a). Extending the human lifespan. *Journal of Medicine and Philosophy*, **27**, 339–54.

Glannon, W. (2002b). Identity, prudential concern, and extending lives. *Bioethics*, **16**, 266–83.

Guo, Z., Lee, J., Lane, M. *et al.* (2001). Iodoacetate protects hippocampal neurons against excitotoxic and oxidative injury: Involvement of heat-shock proteins and Bcl-2. *Journal of Neurochemistry*, **79**, 361–70.

Harman, D. (2001). Aging: overview. *Annals of the New York Academy of Sciences*, **928**, 1–21.

Harris, J. (2002). A response to Walter Glannon. *Bioethics*, **16**, 284–91.

Harris, J. & Holm, S. (2002). Extending human lifespan and the precautionary paradox., *Journal of Medicine and Philosophy*, **27**, 355–68.

Hayflick, L. (1998). How and why we age. *Experimental Gerontology*, **33**, 639–53.

Hayflick, L. (2000). The future of aging. *Nature*, **408**, 267–69.

Horiuchi, S. (2000). Greater lifetime expectations. *Nature*, **405**, 744–5.

Hursting, S.D., Lavigne, J.A., Berrigan, D. *et al.* (2003). Calorie restriction, aging, and cancer prevention: Mechanisms of action and applicability to humans. *Annual Review of Medicine*, **54**, 131–52.

Ingram, D.K., Anson, R.M., de Cabo, R. *et al.* (2004). Development of calorie restriction mimetics as a prolongevity strategy. *Annals of the New York Academy of Sciences*, **1019**, 412–23.

Juengst, E.T. (2004). Anti-aging research and the limits of medicine. In S.G. Post & R.H. Binstock (eds.), *The Fountain of Youth. Cultural, Scientific, and Ethical Perspectives on a Biomedical Goal* (pp. 321–39) Oxford: Oxford University Press.

Kang, H.L., Benzer, S. & Min, K.T. (2002). Life extension in Drosophila by feeding a drug. *Proceedings of the National Academy of Sciences USA*, **99**, 838–43.

Kann, P.H. (2003). Growth hormone in anti-aging medicine: A critical review. *The Aging Male*, **6**, 257–63.

Kann, P.H. (2004). Clinical effects of growth hormone on bone: A review. *The Aging Male*, 7, 290–6.

Kannisto, V. (1994). *Development of Oldest-Old Mortality, 1950–1990: Evidence from 28 Countries*. Odense, Denmark: Odense University Press.

Kannisto, V., Lauritsen, J., Thatcher, A.R. *et al.* (1994). Reduction in mortality at advanced ages: Several decades of evidence from 27 countries. *Population and Development Review*, **20**, 793–810.

Kass, L.R. (2004). L'Chaim and its limits. In S.G. Post & R.H. Binstock (eds.), *The Fountain of Youth. Cultural, Scientific, and Ethical Perspectives on a Biomedical Goal* (pp. 304–20). Oxford: Oxford University Press.

Kassem, M. (2006). Stem Cells. Potential therapy for age-related diseases. *Annals of the New York Academy of Sciences*, **1067**, 436–42.

Kirkwood, T.B.L. & Austad, S.N. (2000). Why do we age? *Nature*, **408**, 233–8.

Kirkwood, T.B.L. & Rose, M.R. (1991). Evolution of senescence: Late survival sacrificed for reproduction. *Philosophical Transactions of the Royal Society of Medicine*, **332**, 15–24.

Kirpichnikov, D., McFarlane, S.I. & Sowers, J.R. (2002). Metformin: an update. *Annals of Internal Medicine*, **137**, 25–33.

Lamberts, S.W.J., van den Beld, A.W. & van der Lely, A. (1997). The endocrinology of aging. *Science*, **278**, 419–24.

Laron, Z. (2004). Do deficiencies in growth hormone and insulin-like growth factor-1 (IGF-1), shorten or prolong longevity? *Mechanisms of Aging and Development*, **126**, 305–7.

Larsen, P.L. & Clarke, C.F. (2002). Extension of life-span in *Caenorhabditis elegans* by a diet lacking coenzyme Q. *Science*, **295**, 120–3.

Manton, K.G. & Vaupel, J.W. (1995). Survival after age of 80 in the United States, Sweden, France, England and Japan. *New England Journal of Medicine*, **333**, 1232–5.

Masoro, E.J. & Austad, S.N. (1996). The evolution of antiaging action of dietary restriction: A hypothesis. *Journal of Gerontolology Series A: Biological Sciences and Medical Sciences*, **51**, B387–B391.

Melov, S., Ravenscroft, J., Malik, S. *et al.* (2000). Extension of life-span with superoxide dismutase/catalase mimetics. *Science*, **289**, 1567–9.

Migliaccio, E., Giorgio, M., Mele, S. *et al.* (1999). The p66shc adaptor protein controls oxidative stress response and lifespan in mammals. *Nature*, **415**, 26–7.

Nikolich-Zugich, J. & Messaoudi, I. (2005). Mice and flies and monkeys too: Caloric restriction rejuvenates the aging immune system of non-human primates. *Experimental Gerontology*, **40**, 884–93.

Oeppen, J. & Vaupel, J.W. (2002). Broken limits to life expectancy. *Science*, **296**, 1029–31.

Oliver, W.R., Shenk, J.L., Snaith, M.R. *et al.* (2001). A selective peroxisome proliferator-activated receptor delta agonist promotes reverse cholesterol transport. *Proceedings of the National Academy of Sciences USA*, **98**, 5306–11.

Olshansky, S.J. & Carnes, B.A. (2004). In Search of the Holy Grail of senescence. In S.G. Post & R.H. Binstock (eds.), *The Fountain of Youth. Cultural, Scientific, and Ethical Perspectives on a Biomedical Goal* (pp. 133–59). Oxford: Oxford University Press.

Olshansky, S.J., Carnes, B.A. & Cassel, C. (1990). In search of Methuselah: The upper limits to human longevity. *Science*, **250**, 634–40.

Olshansky, S.J., Carnes, B.A. & Désesquelles, A. (2001). Prospects for human longevity. *Science*, **291**, 1491–2.

Olshansky, S.J., Hayflick, L. & Carnes, B.A. (2002). Position statement on human aging. *Journals of Gerontology Series A: Biological Sciences and Medical Sciences*, **57A**, B292–B297.

Olson, E. (1997). *The Human Animal: Personal Identity Without Psychology*. New York: Oxford University Press.

Parens, E. (1998). Is better always good? The enhancement project. In E. Parens (ed.), *Enhancing Human Traits: Ethical and Social Implications* (pp. 1–28). Washington, DC: Georgetown University Press.

Parfit, D. (1984). *Reasons and Persons*. Oxford: Clarendon Press.

Post, S.G. & Binstock, R.H. (2004). Introduction. In S.G. Post & R.H. Binstock (eds.), *The Fountain of Youth. Cultural, Scientific, and Ethical Perspectives on a Biomedical Goal* (pp. 1–8). Oxford: Oxford University Press.

Racchi, M., Balduzzi, C. & Corsini, E. (2003). Dehydroepiandrosterone (DHEA), and the aging brain: Flipping a coin in the "fountain of youth." *CNS Drugs Review*, **9**, 21–40.

Ramsey, J.J., Colmana, R.J., Binkleya, N.C. *et al.* (2000). Dietary restriction and aging in rhesus monkeys: The University of Wisconsin study. *Experimental Gerontology*, **35**, 1131–49.

Rattan, S.I.S. (1998). Is gene therapy for aging possible? *Indian Journal of Experimental Biology*, **36**, 233–6.

Riley, J. (2001). *Rising Life Expectancy: A Global History*. Cambridge: Cambridge University Press.

Rose, M.R. (1991). *Evolutionary Biology of Aging*. Oxford: Oxford University Press.

Rose, M.R. (2004). The metabiology of life extension. In S.G. Post & R.H. Binstock, (eds.), *The Fountain of Youth. Cultural, Scientific, and Ethical Perspectives on a Biomedical Goal* (pp. 160–76). Oxford: Oxford University Press.

Rose, M.R. & Graves, J.L. (1989). What evolutionary biology can do for gerontology. *Journal of Gerontology*, **44**, B27–B29.

Roth, G.S., Lane, M.A., Ingram, D.K. *et al.* (2002). Biomarkers of caloric restriction may predict longevity in humans. *Science*, **297**, 811.

Roth, G.S., Lesnikov, V., Lesnikov M. *et al.* (2001). Dietary caloric restriction prevents the age-related decline in plasma melatonin levels of rhesus monkeys. *Journal of Clinical Endocrinology and Metabolism*, **86**, 3292–5.

Rudman, D., Feller, A.G., Nagraj, H.S. *et al.* (1990). Effects of human growth hormone in men over 60 years old. *New England Journal of Medicine*, **323**, 1–6.

Sagi, O., Wolfson, M., Utko, N. *et al.* (2005). p66ShcA and aging: Modulation by longevity-promoting agent aurintricarboxylic acid. *Mechanisms of Aging and Development*, **126**, 249–54.

Spindler, S.R., Dhahbi, J.D., Mote, P.L. *et al.* (2003). Rapid identification of candidate CR mimetics using microarray. *Biogerontology*, **4**(Suppl. 1), 89.

Tuljapurkar, S., Li, N. & Boe, C. (2000). A universal pattern of mortality decline in the G7 countries. *Science*, **405**, 789–92.

Turner, L. (2003). Life extension technologies: Economic, psychological, and social considerations. *HEC Forum*, **15**, 258–73.

Vance, M.L. (2003). Can growth hormone prevent aging? *New England Journal of Medicine*, **348**, 779–80.

Vaupel, J.W. & Lundström, H. (1994). The future of mortality at older ages in developed countries. In W. Lutz (ed.), *The Future Population of the World*. London: Earthscan.

Warner, H., Anderson, J., Austad, S. *et al.* (2005). Science fact and the SENS agenda. What can we reasonably expect from aging research? *EMBO Reports*, **6**, 1006–8.

Westendorp, R.G. (2006). What is healthy aging in the 21st century? *American Journal of Clinical Nutrition*, **83**(Suppl.), 404S–409S.

Weyer, C., Walford, R.L., Harper, I.T. *et al.* (2000). Energy metabolism after 2 y of energy restriction: The Biosphere 2 experiment. *American Journal of Clinical Nutrition*, **72**, 946–53.

Wilmoth, J.R. (1998). The future of human longevity: A demographer's perspective. *Science*, **280**, 395–7.

Wilmoth, J.R. (2000). Demography of longevity: Past, present, and future trends. *Experimental Gerontology*, **35**, 1111–29.

Yang, J., Anzo, M. & Cohen, P. (2005). Control of aging and longevity by IGF-I signalling. *Experimental Gerontology*, **40**, 867–72.

Yen, S.S.C. (2001). Dehydroepiandrosterone sulfate and longevity: Mew clues for an old friend. *Proceedings of the National Academy of Sciences USA*, **98**, 8167–9.

Zainai, T.A., Oberley, T.D., Allison, D.B. *et al.* (2000). Caloric restriction of rhesus monkeys lowers oxidative damage in skeletal muscle. *FASEB Journal*, **14**, 1825–36.

26

Is Living Longer Living Better?

Larry Temkin

Introduction

Is living longer living better? "Yes!" At least under favorable conditions of good health and such. But how *much* longer would it be good to live? Ten years? Undoubtedly. Fifty? Probably. But what about 1,000 years? What about *forever*? And even if it would be good for *me* to live forever and, more generally, good for *each individual* to live forever, would an outcome in which society's members lived forever be ideal? Would it even be as good as an outcome where society's members were continually replaced every 100 years, or perhaps every couple of centuries?

Unfortunately, like everyone else, my views on this topic are based not on *experience*, but on mere speculation and imagination. Clearly, then, anything I, or anyone else, writes on this topic should be taken with a large grain of salt. Nevertheless, the topic is exceedingly interesting, and it behooves us to think about it. Doing so may yield important insights about what we do care about, and what we should care about, both individually and collectively.

This chapter does not argue for a single thesis. Rather, it contains many disparate thoughts relevant to the issues. It is divided into six further sections. Section two comments on some current longevity research. Section three indicates the attitudes towards death and science with which I approach these questions. Sections four and five, respectively, discuss some worries about immortality raised by Leon Kass and Bernard Williams. Section six points to some practical, social, and moral concerns that might arise if society's members lived super long lives. I end by suggesting that we should favor living well over living longer, and ongoing reproduction over immortality; correspondingly, I suggest that we should think long and hard before proceeding with certain lines of longevity research.

Two preliminary comments before proceeding.[1] First, since most assume, unthinkingly, that immortality would be desirable, I emphasize some worries about immortality. But, in doing this, I am decidedly *not* offering an all-things considered judgment about the value of immortality, and I am acutely aware that many other considerations may also be relevant to these issues.

Second, much of my discussion presumes human nature and psychology as it exists today. But our natures and psychologies would surely change if we lived forever. Moreover,

Enhancing Human Capacities, edited by Julian Savulescu, Ruud ter Meulen and Guy Kahane.
© 2011 Blackwell Publishing Ltd

we might actively seek genetic and pharmacological solutions to some of my worries. I recognize the importance of these points, and have discussed them in a longer draft; unfortunately, space limitations prevent me from adequately addressing them here.

Longevity Research

We live in an amazing age. Events and objects that would have been regarded as pipedreams, or even miracles, a scant 50 or 100 years ago, are now routine, everyday, realities: transcontinental air flights, computers, cell phones, the internet, and so on. In the early 1980s I was told that my computer's 197K floppy disk contained more storage space than *all* of the Pentagon's many floors of computer banks *combined* back in the 1950s. Now, a scant 25 years later, a tiny, 93 gram, flash drive contains *10,000* times the storage capacity of my original floppy disk.

Advances in medicine are no less breathtaking. Entire diseases have been eradicated, and countless maladies that were previously crippling are now controllable or preventable. In addition to attacking illnesses afflicting the human condition, we can now improve the human condition *itself*, via a wide range of environmental, pharmaceutical, and genetic enhancements. Disease itself may one day be a thing of the past.

In this context, is it too farfetched to wonder whether we might eventually conquer old age itself? Might mortality be just another human condition remediable by human intervention? Is this thought any more implausible than a cell phone, a 93 gram two-gigabyte flash drive, a kidney transplant, or a "routine" triple bypass surgery would have seemed a scant 100 years ago? And if, as many contend, the pace of knowledge and innovation is increasing exponentially, is it too soon to be thinking about the possible ramifications of extending our lifespans significantly?

Michael Rose is one of many scientists currently engaged in longevity research. Professor of Evolutionary Biology at the University of California, Irvine, Dr. Rose directs the Intercampus Research Program on Experimental Evolution for the University of California system. For Rose, increasing the lifespan of a species is much more than a pipedream. It is a reality he obtained in the laboratory, where "through selective breeding, Dr. Rose ... create[d] a long-lived line of creatures he called Methuselah flies."[2] According to Rose, "natural selection [i]s really the ultimate controller of aging, not some piece of biochemistry." Hence he believes that "Aging is an optional feature of life. And it can be slowed or postponed." Asked whether "there was such a thing as a limited life span for humans?" Rose answered "No. Life span is totally tunable. In my lab, we tune it up and down all the time."

Rose is not alone in his views. Geneticist Aubrey de Grey leads the SENS (Strategies for Engineered Negligible Senescence) Project at Cambridge University, and is the Chairman and Chief Science Officer of the Methuselah Foundation. De Grey claims that the SENS project has "a very detailed plan to repair all the types of molecular and cellular damage that happen to us over time. And each method to do this is either already working in a preliminary form (in clinical trials) or is based on technologies that already exist and just need to be combined. This means that all parts of the project should be fully working in mice within just 10 years and we might need only another 10 years to get them all working in humans."[3] Thus, de Grey believes that the capacity to "prevent and cure ageing" is on the horizon, and suggests that "the first person to live to 1,000, might be 60 already."[4]

Rose and De Grey are not crazed, modern day, Dr. Frankensteins. They are serious, first-rate, scientists with major ongoing research programs. If they are right, we are not required *biologically* to die of old age.

I suspect they *are* right. Consider the famous philosophical example of the Ship of Theseus. During its voyage, as each plank wears out it is replaced with a fresh one. Continually replenished, one plank at a time, the Ship of Theseus could sail the oceans, in tip-top shape, in perpetuity. The same could, perhaps, be true of us. When young, many of our cells naturally duplicate themselves, replacing dead or damaged cells. But this process tends to slow or stop as we age. Moreover, some cells remain in a phase of development where they don't replicate, notably heart, muscle, eye, and brain cells. But many biologists believe that these features of cell biology, including the aging process itself, simply reflect a particular evolutionary strategy for species survival, one that is neither necessary nor immutable.

In principle, then, it seems that we could manipulate our DNA, so that *all* of our cells continually replaced themselves as older ones were damaged, wore out, or died; or that we could employ stem cells to perform such functions. In this way, we might become biological versions of the Ship of Theseus, maintaining ourselves in peak condition, presumably at a developmental stage of our choosing. This seems to me no more farfetched – in terms of its antecedent likelihood of proving possible – than any of a multitude of "modern miracles" would have seemed to my grandparents. I think, then, that we should take seriously the possibility that Rose, De Grey, and other longevity researchers are not merely tilting at windmills.

Perhaps, ultimately, they won't succeed. But perhaps they might. And perhaps they might much sooner than any of us, including they, now realize.[5] This is, I think, a possibility to take seriously. In any event, even if the eventual goal of conquering the aging process remains elusive, I think it can be illuminating to enquire whether it is a goal worth pursuing. Addressing this question may reveal important insights about our values.

In this chapter, then, I want to proceed on the assumption that the ultimate aim of longevity research is to stop the aging process, so that none of us need die of old age. I shall also assume that we will be able to choose the biological stage of development where we wish to remain; presumably, different people might choose to remain at different stages of development. So, in this chapter, living longer will not be correlated with a decline in physical or psychological capacities. I will focus, often, on the desirability of living *forever*; but most of my points would also apply, in varying degrees, to finite lifespans of great length.

Preliminary Confessions

Let me begin by confessing that I am as afraid of death as most people. As my son Daniel powerfully put it when he was three, "I don't want to lie, underground, in a box, *forever*." Nor am I consoled by the thought that the worms will have devoured my body long before forever arrives, that I could be cremated instead, or that I will have left the scene as soon as my brain stops functioning. My worry isn't really about what will happen to me *after* I die, since I assume there will *be* no *me*, for anything *to* happen to, once I am dead. Rather, the simple truth is that I don't want to be dead. I *like* being alive. And, other things equal, I would like to keep on living; *forever*, if possible. Thus, I frankly confess that if the pharmaceutical companies were to one day produce immortality pills, I, like most, would eagerly clamor to get my hands on them, for myself and those I love.

Let me also confess that I endorse Francis Bacon's (1605) Enlightenment project which seeks "the conquest of nature for the relief of man's estate" (*Advancement of Learning*, Book I.i.11). To be sure, I would put more constraints on our treatment of nature than Bacon would; still, I share his fundamental goal of ameliorating the human condition. And my hopes for achieving that goal rest squarely on reason and, especially, science. Thus, I am no fan of scientology, creationism, anti-rationalism, or post-modernism in any of their various guises.

Moreover, I believe that the philosopher should be the patron saint of Pandora, Eve, Ulysses, and the builders of the Tower of Babel (subject to the small problem of canonization!). After all, Pandora is vilified for the crime of exercising her curiosity, which according to the myth is responsible for all the world's evils; Eve is banished from Eden and cursed with the pains of childbirth, because she dared to eat fruit from the Tree of Knowledge; Ulysses is condemned to the eighth circle of Hell, in part for the hubris of leading his men past the Pillars of Hercules, which separated the safety of the human world from the dangerous open seas leading towards the home of the gods; and the builders of the Tower of Babel are confounded with multiple languages and "scattered ... upon the face of all the earth," because as a united humanity with a common language they had the ability and effrontery to build a tower that approached heaven itself.

The word "philosopher" comes from the Greek *philosophos* which means "lover or pursuer of wisdom." Ideally, a philosopher revels in exercising her curiosity in pursuit of fundamental truths. Given this, how could a philosopher *not* applaud the efforts of such great exemplars of humanity as Pandora, Eve, Ulysses, and the builders of the Tower of Babel?

Together, the myths in question warn that it is dangerous to try to transform ourselves into gods, either by acquiring their knowledge, or occupying their domain. And, indeed, the lesson is a fair one. Such actions *are* dangerous. Still, Aristotle claimed that man is *essentially* a rational animal; that Reason is the *highest* part of man, the *God*-like part of man; that Reason, more than anything else, *is*, man.[6] In light of such thinking, is it not the case, as Ulysses put it in Dante's *Inferno*, that if we are to be truly *men*, and not merely sheep, we must venture out into the dangerous open sea, away from the sheltered coves, exploring the unknown in our search for knowledge, and thereby fulfilling our true, divine-like, destiny (Dante, 1308–1321, *Inferno*, Canto XXVI, *Divine Comedy*)?

Putting these thoughts together, one might reason as follows. Death is surely one of the greatest evils that men face. So, the amelioration of the human condition should seek, if possible, to conquer death. To be sure, seeking immortality may strike some as pure hubris, as seeking to transcend our humanity and make ourselves as gods. But is that not what a patron saint of Eve, Pandora, Ulysses, and the builders of the Tower of Babel should approve of? Should we not use our Reason, the highest part of man, the god-like part of man, to seek the knowledge that will enable us to improve our estate, even to the point of transforming ourselves into even more god-like beings, if we can? This line of reasoning is powerfully attractive. Still, the questions must be asked: Is living *longer*, living *better*? *Would* it be better if the adamantine link between aging and death were finally broken?

I confess, on reflection, I'm not sure what the answers to these questions are. But I am certain that they are deserving of much more thought than they are typically given. In what follows, I broach a few of the many factors relevant to answering them thoughtfully. Unfortunately, each factor deserves much more consideration than I can give it here.

Kass's Worries

In "Mortality and Morality: The Virtues of Finitude," Leon Kass (1985, pp. 292–317), former Chair of the President's Commission on Bioethics, raised many deep worries about immortality. One was that many of our greatest creations resulted from the recognition of our own mortality. Kass believes that many people who fear death – understood, here, as the end of their earthly existence, and perhaps utter annihilation – have been spurred by that fear to great accomplishments. The idea, roughly, is that, consciously or not, many have hoped to achieve a *kind* of immortality, in the form of lasting recognition here on earth, through great achievements. Moreover, many of these achievements are among humankind's most lasting, inspiring, and ennobling feats. Thus, Kass suggests that some of the components that make our lives and our civilization most valuable would never have existed but for our mortality. Additionally, Kass suggests, our very recognition and appreciation of beauty, and life itself, may to some extent be conditioned by, and hence depend on, our awareness of our finitude.

It is hard to deny such claims. No doubt many of our most beautiful and inspiring monuments and cathedrals, as well as many of our most important literary, artistic, and philosophical works sprang, at least in part, from an acute sense of mortality. But for death, there would be no Pyramids, no Keats's "Ode on a Grecian Urn," and no Mozart's "Requiem."

Moreover, it is often true that we don't fully appreciate what we have until we've lost it, or unless there was a prior period where we lacked it. Thus, unless we have been hungry, homeless, sick, or unemployed, it is easy to take for granted food, shelter, health, and a job. Similarly, most take life itself for granted, until we have lost a loved one, or faced the prospect of death for ourselves or someone close. Given this, we almost certainly *wouldn't* appreciate the glory of being alive – and for most of us, it *is* glorious, is it not? – in the absence of death. For many, life seems incredibly precious precisely because it is so fleeting and fragile. Surely, Kass is right about this.

Still, there is reason to worry about how much weight to put on such claims. First, since people *have* died up to now, we already have numerous great works spurred by the fear of death. Perhaps we could quite reasonably forego the creation of even *more* mortality-inspired works, for the prospect of conquering the aging process?[7]

Second, Kass's argument seems to be making a virtue of necessity. It smacks of sour grapes, and the strong human proclivity for adaptive preference formation. Our *first* choice would be to live forever; but given the impossibility of that, we convince ourselves of the virtues of finitude – telling ourselves that living forever wouldn't be all that great anyway, and would cost us the Pyramids and the "Requiem." But as wonderful as the Pyramids and the "Requiem" are, if we could exchange them for *immortality*, mightn't it be worth doing so? After all, if we created such artifacts in our quest for a *kind* of immortality when the real thing was not available, why stick with our *second* choice, if our *first* becomes available?

Third, even if we don't *fully* appreciate food, shelter, health, or a loved one until we have lost them, isn't it actually better to *have* such things for a long time, underappreciated, than to fully appreciate them, perhaps after the fact, because, having had them, one has lost them? Even if we grant that it is better to have loved, and lost love, than to never have loved at all, we needn't grant that it is better to have loved, and lost love, than to have loved, and never lost love! Similarly, even if we wouldn't fully appreciate the glory of life, in the absence of death, that doesn't show that a fully appreciated mortal life would actually be *better*, all things considered, than an immortal life. The latter might be vastly more valuable than the former, even if it were underappreciated.

Finally, even if many of humankind's greatest achievements were spurred by the fear of death, many others were not. So, even if conquering mortality would cost us *some* great achievements, surely many others would be produced for the usual motivations of creativity, pride, recognition, reward, and self-realization. Moreover, presumably many unfinished masterpieces would be completed if people didn't die of old age, and many others would be begun and completed that would otherwise never be attempted. In addition, the possibility of far grander achievements that are currently unimaginable would open up – including, perhaps, achievements that could only be accomplished, or appreciated, over the course of centuries or millennia. I think, then, that the loss of some great achievements that would accompany the conquering of death would almost certainly be compensated by gains, including some great achievements that would otherwise not be possible.

Another point needs to be made about Kass's contention. Even if Kass is right about the virtues of *finitude*, that wouldn't be enough, by itself, to undermine the value of research whose ultimate aim is to stop aging. After all, a solution to *aging* wouldn't make us immortal. Thus, even if our bodies didn't naturally wear out, people could still die from murders, accidents, war, famine, or disease. Eventually, of course, we might hope to end famine and disease. But for the foreseeable future, at least, we would still confront death, and this might be enough to provide ample inspiration for the great achievements that Kass fears we would otherwise lose if we conquered death entirely.

But another of Kass's worries remains. Suppose enhancements enabled us to remain in an aesthetically pleasing body in peak physical and mental condition. For the reasons suggested above, we might lack an appreciation for the beauty, strength, and value of our condition. The fear, of course, is that our appreciation of the bloom of youth depends on the withering of the aged, so that in a world without the latter, we would simply take our "ideal" minds and bodies for granted, and fail to fully appreciate or value our healthy, vigorous, vital condition. Of course, what is most important is not that we *value* our lives, but that our lives *be* valuable and, arguably, vastly longer lives lived in peak condition *would be* much more valuable than our current lives. Still, Kass rightly reminds us that there might be important losses in our appreciation of life, vigor, youth, and health, were we to conquer the problem of aging. So, while such losses might be offset by substantial gains, this needs to be determined. One shouldn't assume that conquering aging *has* to be a net good, let alone an unalloyed good.

There is another worry Kass raises. Suppose we did, indeed, conquer aging, without conquering death. That would radically transform the implications and impact of death. In today's world, family and friends are frequently consoled about the passing of an elderly loved one, by the knowledge that their last years were difficult, debilitating, dehumanizing, or painful. For the infirmed elderly, death need not seem tragic. It may even be welcomed by the family, friends, and, most importantly, the elderly person herself. But if aging were arrested this would no longer be true. In such a world, each death would rob its victim of an open-ended future; one that might involve thousands, or perhaps millions more years of vital life. Assuming that all the extra years of lost life would have been valuable – which is the reason why we might want all those years in the first place – each death might indeed be tragic, at least for its victim and her loved ones.[8]

On a related note, in today's world, fortunately, most parents die before their children. Thus, relatively few people face one of the most tragic of human events – the burying of their own child. This would not be so in the envisaged world, where death comes not from aging, but from murder, accident, war or disease. In such a world, there is no reason to presume that a parent would die before its child. Now, as we will see later, the significance of this fact might be mitigated by loosened bonds between parents and children that might obtain in such a world. But I don't find that much consolation. If the bonds between parents and children weaken sufficiently that the burying of one's own child is no longer particularly tragic – that itself would be a tragedy. Or so I think, anyway. Thus, I, for one, abhor the thought of living in a world where it would no longer particularly bother me if one of my children died before me. I shall return to this point later.

Here, as elsewhere, these considerations are hardly conclusive. Arguably, it is much better that most die "tragically" at, say, age 1,000, than that most die at age 90 after some years of infirmities. Likewise, perhaps it is clearly better for my child to be buried by me, after 1,000 years of life, than for him to outlive me, but die at 90. My point, simply, is that there are *costs* to curing aging, as well as benefits. And we need to think carefully about *both*.

Williams's Worry

Bernard Williams notes that if our lives persisted unendingly through time, then there would either be significant alterations in a person's deepest projects, commitments, and character, or there would not. Either alternative, Williams argues, would be deeply problematic for the value of immortality *for us*. Following Williams, let us discuss each alternative in term.

Consider first the view that if one lived forever, eventually there would be thoroughgoing changes in one's deepest projects, commitments, and character. Williams wonders whether I have any reason to *care* about a future life of "mine" that is so utterly different from my current life in those respects that matter to me *most*? Williams (1981, p.1–19) elaborates on this theme in "Persons, Character, and Morality," where he contends that "my *present* projects are the condition of my existence, in the sense that unless I am propelled forward by the conatus of desire, project and interest, it is unclear *why I should go on at all*"(emphases added). Famously claiming that "the correct perspective on one's life is *from now*," Williams (1981, p.13) goes on to add that "a man's ground projects . . . [provide] the motive force which propels him into the future, and gives him a reason for living."

In sum, Williams suggests that in the absence of sufficient constancy in my deepest projects, commitments, and character, I would have no reason to care about my future self; no reason to go on at all; no reason, in other words, to find immortality, under such conditions, desirable. This claim is interesting; but dubious. Let me explain why.

First, Williams adopts a desire-based view of reasons in propounding his argument. Indeed, he adopts a particular desire-based view that grounds *all* reasons for agents in features of their current "subjective motivational set;" features tied, in one way or another, to such factors as their current hopes, beliefs, desires, and intentions.[9] This is why Williams contends, as noted above, that "my present projects are the condition of my existence," that "I am propelled forward by the conatus of desire, project and interest," and that "the correct perspective on one's life is *from now*." But on this view, I *could* have reason to care about my future self, *even if* my future projects, commitments, and character would be radically different than my present ones. What matters, on this view, is *not* constancy of character and commitments across time, but whether I currently have, as part of my subjective motivational set, an unconditional desire that I *have* a future flourishing self (one, perhaps, that is flourishing by *its* lights) even if its radically different than my current self. But there is nothing to rule out the presence of such a desire in someone's subjective motivational set. Thus, on Williams's desire-based view, for such a person immortality would be desirable.

Williams might retort that immortality will only *remain* desirable for such a person as long as the desire in question stays constant over time, in which case there is constancy of the relevant sort after all. But on Williams's view, the question of whether immortality would be desirable for myself is the question we need to address. The question, for Williams, is whether immortality would be valuable, *here and now*, and the answer to *that* is determined by my *current* subjective motivational set, not my future one. Of course, this line wouldn't establish that immortality would be valuable for everyone. It wouldn't. But it would show how, on Williams's view, immortality *could* be valuable for some, contrary to what he implies.

But in any event, I reject Williams's desire-based account of reasons, at least as a full account of reasons. Like Nagel, Parfit, and others, I believe there can be value-based reasons for caring and acting.[10] I also believe in both an objective theory of the good for individuals – according to which certain things are good for individuals, whether or not they want them; and an objective theory of the goodness of outcomes – according to which certain things make an outcome better, whether or not people want them. On my view, I *may* have value-based reasons to seek immortality even *if* my deepest projects, commitments, and character changed over time. This would be so if my living forever were better for me, or the outcome, according to the best value-based theory.

So, I reject Williams's view about practical reason which underlies his claim that unless our projects, commitments, and character were highly consistent throughout our lives, we would have no reason to want to live forever. I suspect that Williams's view may seem more plausible than it is, because it seems to be a natural extension of a view about the afterlife that many hold. Let me explain.

On some views, heaven involves disembodied souls basking in God's knowledge and glory. But some want to know why *they* should care about such an afterlife. They want to survive with recognizably human form, attachments, and ends. Moreover, they don't just want *any* old "recognizably human" attachments and ends; they want *their* attachments and ends. For example, they want to share the afterlife with *their* loved ones. Thus, for many, merely *surviving* death isn't enough, they want to survive pretty much intact (though presumably with a few upgrades!). Otherwise, they fail to see why they should take much interest in an afterlife, even if it involves a much higher form of celestial existence. This is a natural view, and it may seem to lend support to Williams's position which, though he puts his claims in terms of projects, commitments, and character, seems to generalize the view in question to *all* future lives and, in particular, to a distant future life that isn't a *after*life.

But there is an important disanalogy between the two views. In the afterlife case, we die one moment, and "awaken" the next in a *totally* different state. There is good reason to wonder whether we would even survive such an abrupt transformation, and even if we did, why we should care about such a future self so totally discontinuous with our current one. But regarding immortal life, we can assume that one's character is continuously and gradually evolving so that there is no abrupt, radical, discontinuity in one's deepest projects, commitments, and character. In this case, there will be a continuity of character from period to period that will both preserve our identity and give us reason to care about our future selves. And this is so even if, as a result of an ongoing series of gradual changes, eventually our distant selves are radically different from our present ones.

Here is a rough analogy. Suppose I leave home one morning, and return to find my home has been replaced with an entirely different one. I might rightly say "*that* isn't my home, what happened to *my* home?" But suppose, over many years, *I* steadily alter my home, one room at a time, until eventually, say 20 years later, the home is exactly like the one that would have appeared in the other scenario. I would, throughout the transformation, rightly regard it as my home, and have an interest in its being maintained. As indicated, the analogy is rough, but Williams's mistake is in declining to take an interest in my future self, *purely* because it is so different from my present self. He ignores whether my distant self steadily evolved from my current one. As long as there is significant continuity of character from period to period, that is enough for us to be self-interestedly concerned about the preservation and well-being of our evolving self. Thus, as indicated, there could well be reason to seek immortality, even if there would not be constancy of one's deepest projects, commitments, and character over time.[11]

Let me add a final point on this topic. Arguably, there are many cases where there is no constancy of projects, commitments, and character across a normal lifespan. In particular, in the relevant sense a child, a teenager, a 40 year old, and an octogenarian may be radically different from each other. But that does not suffice, I think, to establish that a child or young adult, has no reason to want to live to 80. Even if one recognizes that throughout one's life that there will be a continual and thorough evolution of one's character and commitments, it is perfectly reasonable to want to live to 80. But if this is so, then lack of constancy of character and such can't be a sufficient reason to not want immortality.

I conclude that the desirability of immortality is compatible with a thoroughgoing transformation, over time, of one's deepest projects, commitment, and character. So, contra Williams, even if such transformations resulted from our living forever, this would not be sufficient to make immortality lack value for *us*.

Let us next turn to Williams's second concern. Suppose that even if we lived forever, our deepest projects, commitments, and character remained constant. Williams then suggests that immortality would be undesirable, because it would inevitably result in a life of unbearable *boredom*. Indeed, one might believe that tedium looms even if one allows for radical character change across time. After all, arguably, there are only so many *desirable* life plans; that is, only so many combinations of projects, commitments, and character that would be rationally *worth* possessing. And forever is a *very* long time! So eventually, immortality might doom us to reliving desirable life plans *ad infinitum*, until ultimately our life become one of endless and depressingly boring repetition.

Is Williams right? Must an immortal life maintaining constancy of projects, commitments, and character necessarily be *so* tedious as to be unbearable? And might the same consequence loom, albeit millennia later, even if we allow for changes in one's projects, commitments, and character? I confess, when I first read Williams's article, at 22, I found his claim utterly preposterous. When I thought of *all* the many things I would like to do with my life – all the places to visit, the classics to read, the jobs I'd enjoy, the projects worth doing, the information to learn, and so on – I couldn't *imagine* ever getting tired of it all. But I'm a bit older now, and although I believe that Williams has almost certainly overstated his position, I suspect that for many, including me, there is much more to his position than we might like to admit.

My son, Daniel, sometimes likes to call me "tired old man," which for him is obviously redundant! For the most part, he's just kidding, affectionately giving me a hard time. But while I'm not especially old, or tired, I admit that I don't get as excited about things as I once did. To my son, in his early twenties, *everything* seems fresh, interesting, and terribly important. I recognize that outlook. It was *my* outlook – at his age. But I'm no longer his age, and I confess that I no longer have it.

The fact is that I've been around the block a few times now, and I'm a lot more jaded than my son, and most of his peers. Yet, crucially, I'm only 53! What if I'd been around the block not just a *few* times, but a *million* times, or more? And even a *billion* times doesn't *begin* to approach the number of blocks I would circle if I were immortal! If I lived forever, would anything still strike me as new, exciting, or bewitching?

Sometimes I find myself in a new city with a fine art museum. But though I really *like* art, I won't bother going. Why not? Well, I've already seen the Louvre, Prado, Hermitage, Tate, Rodin Museum, Riksmuseum, National Gallery, Frick, Guggenheim, Getty, and many other world-class museums – some of them many times. I've also seen scores of "lesser" museums. So now, when I visit a "fine" art museum, as often as not I'm bored. I wish it weren't true. But it is. I find myself comparing the art to the great works I've already seen, and I'm usually disappointed. So, I wonder, if I were a million years old, would I still be interested in going to an art museum, or seeing the "latest" and "greatest" developments in art?

Here is another example. I find talk radio terribly boring. But recently, I find myself turning it on while driving. I'll listen to it briefly, and then usually turn it off and ride in silence. But this is odd, since for most of my life I've loved music, and I could easily be listening to music instead. So why don't I? The reason is this. Most music pales in comparison to the great music I really love: Led Zeppelin's *Stairway to Heaven*, Jimi Hendrix's *Hey Joe*, Bob Dylan's *Highway 61*, Beethoven's *Ninth Symphony*, and Mozart's *The Marriage of Figaro*. But I have now listened to each piece on my all-time favorite list literally hundreds, and perhaps thousands, of times. So, sometimes, rather than listen to a favorite yet again, or an inferior, even if pretty good, song, I listen to boring talk radio, or simply ride in silence. Again, I wonder what my attitude to music would be after a million years?

Likewise, I once thought it would be fantastic if I lived long enough to pursue numerous careers. But I'm much less sure about that now. Would I *really* enjoy doing all the work necessary to start over again as a historian, and then do English, astronomy, physics, law, medicine, psychology, and sociology? Would I *really* want to continually restart at the bottom, reproving myself, each time, to my new peers? Unfortunately, having now graded thousands of papers and exams, I can easily imagine becoming bored with *all* of those subjects long before I reached my first millennium. And those are the subjects that interest me most! Having rotated through each of them, perhaps many times, would I really want to try my hand at accounting, or perhaps sales? And how many different jobs might I endure over the course of eternity, before I had had enough of *all* positions?

Mind you, I have trouble believing that I'd ever get bored making love, and I never tire of eating ice cream. But such activities don't constitute a life. So, even if there are activities that would never become stale, that wouldn't be enough to ensure that our lives, as a whole, wouldn't become tedious, were we to live forever.

I tentatively conclude that while Williams's argument is not convincing, I fear there is more to it than many of us might like to admit. Eternity is a *long* time, and many might be bored to tears *long* before that.

Before going on, let me offer several caveats regarding the foregoing considerations. First, Frances Kamm informs me that *she* never tires of visiting art museums, and Derek Parfit tells me that *he* never tires of hearing *The Marriage of Figaro*, *Goldberg Variations*, or *Tristan and Isolde*. So they find the preceding considerations unconvincing. Of course, both have lived less than 70 years, and might well feel differently after a million years, much less eternity! But let me not insist on this. Some people bore easily, and others do not. So perhaps some people, like Williams and me, would find eternal life boring, but others, like Kamm and Parfit, would not. So, while Williams suggests that for people whose projects, commitments, and character are constant, eternal life must, inevitably, be boring, I offer a more modest conclusion. I suggest that, for many, eternal life might not be as appealing as they might initially assume, because ultimately it may not be as interesting, exciting, or fresh as they might want.

Second, my argument focuses on how we might regard immortality if we maintained our current psychologies and present constellations of interests and life plans. But I grant that if we lived forever our psychologies would probably evolve, and we might find whole new life plans available to us that we can't currently conceptualize, and that we would then, with our evolved psychologies, never tire of. I certainly can't rule out that if we lived forever we might evolve in such ways, and we might come to regard our development as unambiguously good. But I confess that considering such a scenario in *prospect*, I begin to share some of Williams's doubts as to whether I have much reason to care about, or pursue, an eternal life whose psychology and pursuits would be *so* utterly different from those of my *current* life, which is the one I cherish and wish to prolong. Moreover, while I *might* eventually evolve in desirable ways, I might also eventually evolve in *un*desirable ways. Suffice it to say, I believe more thought needs to be given to such issues.

Third, it might be thought that if we can solve the problem of immortality, *surely* we can solve the problem of boredom. Perhaps we will develop "freshness," "rejuvenation," or "selective memory" pills or enhancements, so that no matter *how* many times we visit a museum, listen to a song, or perform a given task, we will find it just as fresh and exciting as we did originally. Again, I can't rule out this possibility, but I have some worries about it akin to Robert Nozick's worries about the experience machine.[12] Do such pills or enhancements simply improve my reality, change my reality, or distort reality? Am I in "contact with reality," to use Nozick's expression, if *Stairway to Heaven* sounds as fresh after listening to it a million times as it did the first 10 times, if the only *reason* it sounds so fresh is that I have taken the freshness pill, or been genetically altered to ensure that each experience of a pleasurable activity remained fresh and exciting, no matter *how many* times I engaged in that activity? I'm not sure what the answers to these questions are. But until we have such pills or enhancements, and have figured out the answers, is there not some reason to be cautious about a headlong rush towards immortality?

Finally, let me emphasize an important difference between Williams's view and mine. Williams implies that if we were immortal, eventually our lives would become *so* tedious that suicide would become an attractive option.[13] This is not my view. I believe that few would find suicide attractive because their lives were tedious. Even an incredibly boring life may yet be *worth living*, and better than no life at all. Correspondingly, it may well be better, from an individual's perspective, to live an exciting life for several hundred years that eventually becomes boring, but continues endlessly at a still worthwhile level, than to simply live an exciting life for a hundred years followed by death. The point of my discussion, inspired by Williams, is simply to remind us that living forever may not be as interesting, exciting, and valuable as one might unthinkingly assume it to be. If this is right, it is important to bear in mind when considering the overall consequences that immortality might have, some of which I turn to next.

Other Concerns

I have addressed some reasons to be concerned about the prospect of immortality. It may, indeed, not be all it is cracked up to be. But so far we haven't come up with sufficient reason to worry about longevity research, especially if we assume that we could later reverse course or opt out if we found our lives too tedious or unsatisfying. Still, there are many practical, social, political, or moral reasons for worrying about the quest to conquer aging. Let me mention just a few of these. Unfortunately, a full exploration of them must await another day.

First, we live in a horribly unequal world. It has been claimed, for example, that a mere one-half of 1% of the income of the top 20% of income earners would be more than sufficient to double the income of *everyone* in the bottom 20%.[14] Given this, and given that millions of innocent children "die [each year] from easy to beat disease, from malnutrition, and from bad drinking water" (Unger, 1996, p.3), is there not a moral imperative to address the plight of the world's needy, and try to give them something of a *normal* human lifespan, *before* we engage in longevity research? Surely, the benefits of longevity, if successful, would almost certainly go *first* to the world's best off, who would willingly pay handsomely for them, and would only "trickle down" to the world's less fortunate, if it later became easy and cheap to do so. Are there not strong considerations of justice, equality, humanitarianism, and prioritarianism to worry about this predictable result?

Second, in the United States, social security is already facing collapse. Clearly, then, if we slowed the aging process, the retirement age for social benefits would need to be extended proportionally. *A fortiori*, as matters currently stand, if we actually halted aging, retirement would need to be postponed indefinitely. Moreover, all countries will eventually face this predicament if they manage to successfully combine efforts to prolong life with effective population control. Of course, having stopped the aging process, we will be perfectly *capable* of working indefinitely. But do we really relish the prospect of working indefinitely, much less *forever*? I have my worries about this. After all, I *already* find myself looking forward to retirement – especially when I am grading papers! – and I have only been at it 27 years.

To be sure, at some point we may no longer need to work to live. That will raise the different question of what to do with ourselves in a life of perpetual "retirement." But I will not address that question here. Until we have reached the stage where we no longer need to support ourselves, the question of prolonged life must be inevitably tied to the issue of prolonged work.

Third, Winston Churchill once said that if a man wasn't a liberal at 20 he didn't have a heart, if he wasn't a conservative at 40 he didn't have a brain. I think Churchill was wrong, but his point is well taken. Often it is the youth who generate new ideas, take risks, and idealistically tilt at windmills trying to right the world's wrongs. Imagine the dynamics of a population overwhelmingly composed of 80 year olds – then imagine what it might be like if there were a population overwhelmingly composed of individuals who had lived millions of years. Even at an arrested stage of "youthful" biological development, the predominant social and political outlook of people who had lived *so* long might resemble that of the most apathetic or jaundiced amongst us! Or worse.

It is, of course, impossible for us to accurately predict the social, cultural, and psychological effects on a population with unending years of experiences. But the world already has more than its share of people suffering ennui and Weltschmerz. I worry, as Williams did, that having seen and experienced "it all" for a few million years, ennui and Weltschmerz might be a prevailing attitude, and this might manifest itself in a natural tendency to resist "yet another round" of change or new ideas.

Fourth, consider next the impact on the family structure. As things stand today, the physical, psychological, and experiential gap between a grandmother at 60, a mother at

35, and a daughter at 9 is enormous. But the physical, psychological, and experiential gaps between a grandmother at 10,060, a mother at 10,035, and a daughter at 10,009 would be practically inconsequential; as would be, I suspect, the gaps between a million-year-old parent and, say, her 900,000-year-old child. With such changes the lines between generations might well be blurred, and the relations inevitably and profoundly changed.

Of course, not all change is for the worse. But, speaking for myself, I think it would be terrible if I came to regard my mother or daughter, not so much as a mother or daughter, but as a peer. Likewise, as lifespans have increased, the desirability of lifelong monogamy has been increasingly challenged, and many have started second families in their 50s. If we lived indefinitely, mightn't we naturally have 100s or 1000s of spouses over the years? And then, depending on the rules of procreation in play, 100s or 1000s of children or stepchildren? What impact would this have on our notions of familial loyalty and duty?

I, for one, don't relish the prospect that if only I lived long enough, I might no longer care about, or even remember, my *first* set of children, Daniel, Andrea, and Rebecca. Nor am I excited by the thought that in a relatively fixed population enduring forever, one might eventually cycle and recycle through the whole population in choosing partners, including, probably, the generations of one's parents and children, grand-parents and grandchildren, great-grandparents and great-grandchildren, and so on. Indeed, I suspect the taboo against incest would disappear, and that eventually everyone be "fair game" as possible partners in such a world.

Fifth, if we succeed in extending lifespans indefinitely, where would everyone live, and from where would the resources come to support them? Perhaps the resource problem will ultimately have a feasible technological solution. But the space question cannot be easily ignored. The problem of overpopulation already looms large. Even if we grant that the earth could comfortably sustain several times its current population, slowing the aging process would, in a very short time, inevitably carry with it a commitment to slowing the birth rate.

This is not a deep philosophical point about the meaning of life or the nature of man. It is a simple practical point. One day, it, too, may admit of a technological solution; perhaps, in a limited form, via super skyscrapers, or colonies beneath the oceans or the earth's surface, but ultimately, and inevitably, in the form of interplanetary and intergalactic travel. Correspondingly, if such technological advances are realized, we may revisit the advantages of perpetual youth. But until then, the following seems undeniable. Were we to succeed in stopping our biological clocks, at some point we would only be able to permit new births to offset those deaths due to murders, accident, war, and disease. Imagine the centralized power and bureaucracy that would be required, on a global scale, to enforce such a worldwide population policy. It staggers the mind, and even if it were desirable – a highly dubious proposition – at this stage it isn't even remotely on the horizon.

Sixth, suppose that, in time, civilization significantly advanced Bacon's Enlighten-ment project by ending all deaths due to aging, war, murder, and disease. Virtually everyone today would hail this development. Then death – and hence, if there were limited space, extra room for new births – might only come in the form of accidents and natural disasters. Were this to happen, I suspect that accidents and natural disasters would come to be regarded as natural blessings that were eagerly hoped for!

I am grateful to my mother – thankfully not my peer! – for pointing out that some of my worries are put nicely in the Yisgor Service on the Jewish Day of Atonement. During that service, the following words are spoken in consolation to those who have lost loved ones:

> If some messenger were to come to us with the offer that death should be overthrown, but with the one inseparable condition that birth should also cease; if the existing generations were given the chance to live forever, but on the clear understanding that never again would there be a child, or a youth, or a first love, never again new persons with new hopes, new ideas, new achievement; ourselves for always and never any others – could the answer be in doubt?[15]

I share the view implied above that such a tradeoff would be abominable. Nor would it be enough if a limited number of "replacement" children were permitted to offset correspondingly losses due to accidents or disasters.

Conclusion

In a fascinating short story, "The Ephemera," Benjamin Franklin considers the meaning of life.[16] He describes a group of people-like flies who only live for seven or eight hours, and he wryly notes how most waste their short lives arguing about trivial matters, such as the merits of various foreign-born musicians.[17] Franklin wonders whether instead of frittering away their short lives in trivial pursuits, they should address issues of good government and morals, or focus on deep friendships. Franklin's point, of course, is that *we* are ephemera. On a cosmic scale, or even a geological one, our lives are but a few seconds or minutes.

But notice, Franklin's point is just as telling, whether our lives are seven hours, 70 years, or 7,000 years. Ultimately, what matters is not so much whether we are living *long*, but whether we are living *well*. And a life which is frivolous at 70 years, wouldn't acquire significance if it persisted for 7,000 years.[18]

In *King Lear*, Shakespeare's Fool poignantly admonishes Lear: "Thou shouldst not have been old till thou hadst been wise."[19] I feel the same way about our society. In the United States, people revel in shows like *Nip/Tuck*, *Fear Factor*, and *Desperate Housewives*. By all accounts, Americans can't get enough of gossip about Jessica Simpson, Paris Hilton, or Brad Pitt – though undoubtedly these celebrities will be old news soon after this chapter is in print, if not before. Worse, our society can fund hundreds of millions for athletic stadiums, but can't properly fund inner city education. Likewise, infant mortality rates for disadvantaged Americans *exceed* that of many developing nations, even as, but a few miles away, global elites enjoy world-class medical care from hospitals resembling five star hotels. I think our society "shouldst not become old till we've become wise." Let us *first* learn to live *well*, *before* we learn to live *long*. Perhaps once we've learned to live well, if we ever do, it may no longer seem so pressing to live long.

In sum, even if it would be better for *each* of us, *individually*, to live as long as possible, it may not be better for *all* of us, *collectively*, to do so. But even if it *would* be better for all of us, collectively, to live forever, I still doubt whether that outcome would be most desirable. Specifically, I believe that an outcome with a fixed, immortal, population, would be significantly worse than one involving regular regeneration.

Consider two outcomes. In one, two groups of n people live 150 years each. In a second, one group of n people live 300 years each. I grant that each person in the second outcome might be better off than each person in the first. Even so, I believe the first outcome would almost certainly be better than the second. Why? Well, in part it is because I believe that in many cases, though certainly not all, once people have experienced certain kinds of events "enough" times in their lives, there will be a diminishing marginal value to subsequent similar experiences. If this is right, then even if a 300-year life would be better than a 150-year life, it may not be, globally, *much* better. Consider the joy and significance of a first wedding, overseas trip, child, grandchild, and so on; or the first *really* meaningful kiss, love, job, paycheck, or publication. There will be twice as many such events in the first outcome as the second. Of course, there will be some possibilities for happiness and achievement that are only available in the second; but, even so, I doubt that all things considered the second outcome would be better than the first.

The preceding has direct implications for Narveson's (1967, 1973) famous person-affecting view, that from a moral perspective "We are in favor of making people happy, but neutral about making happy people." Narveson's view has great plausibility, but in thinking about the future of humanity and the question of immortality it seems clear that it must be rejected. Surely, if we developed a pill enabling each of us to live wonderful lives for 120 years, it would be terrible for us to take the pill if the cost of doing so were the extinction of humanity. This is so even *if* taking the pill were better for each individual who took it, and hence everyone who ever lived, collectively. If right, this undermines Narveson's contention.

Similarly, though less obviously true, I think if the cost of immortality would be a world without infants and children, without regeneration and rejuvenation, it wouldn't be worth it. And this is so even *if* each immortal would be better off than each mortal. Here, too, we should care about *more* than just "making people happy," we should *also* care about "making happy people."

This chapter's considerations are hardly conclusive. But they should give us pause. Indeed, I think they are sufficiently worrisome that we should think long and hard about supporting longevity research that might ultimately end aging. I do not say this lightly. As indicated previously, I subscribe to the Enlightenment project of science ameliorating the human condition. The last thing I favor is philosophy standing in the way of human progress. But the stakes in this area are so huge that it is imperative to carefully determine whether stopping aging really *would* be progress. And I fear we must have this debate *before* the research goes too far. After all, given our powerful fear of death, and the overwhelming human propensity to use whatever technologies become available, it is almost certain that any anti-aging technology that is developed *will* be used once it becomes available. And make no mistake, once research points the way to a feasible anti-aging technology, such technology *will* be made available.[20]

I conclude with a second quote from the Yom Kippur service:

> Alas for those who cannot sing, but die with all their music in them. Let us treasure the time we have, and resolve to use it well, counting each moment precious – a chance to apprehend

some truth, to experience some beauty, to conquer some evil, to relieve some suffering, to love and be loved, to achieve something of lasting worth. . . . [Let] us . . . fulfill the promise that is in each of us, and so to conduct ourselves that, generations hence, it will be true to say of us: the world is better because, for a brief space, they lived in it.[21]

Acknowledgments

I would like to thank the editors of this volume, Julian Savulescu, Ruud ter Meulen, and Guy Kahane. I would also like to thank the organizers of the Seventh Annual Joint Applied and Urban Ethics Conference, *"Perfect" Bodies in "Perfect" Minds*, held at the Newark campus of Rutgers, the State University of New Jersey, Spring 2006, and Julian Savulescu and Matthew Liao for the opportunities they provided me to originally explore this topic. Additionally, I am extremely grateful to Ruth Chang, Shelly Kagan, Frances Kamm, Jeff McMahan, and Derek Parfit for many excellent suggestions. Finally, I owe a special debt to Leon Kass, who first convinced me to rethink my views about this topic.

Notes

1. Ruth Chang alerted me to the importance of emphasizing the following two comments.
2. All quotes in this paragraph are from Claudia Dreifus's *A Conversation with Michael R. Rose: Live Longer with Evolution? Evidence May Lie in Fruit Flies* (*Science* section, *New York Times*, December 6, 2005, available at www.nytimes.com/2005/12/06/science/ 06conv.html?ex=1181361600&en=70585c6051d4b398&ei=5070). Rose reaffirmed these views at the *"Perfect" Bodies in "Perfect" Minds* conference where we were co-panelists.
3. See "We will be able to live to 1,000," BBC News, December 3, 2004, available at http:// news.bbc.co.uk/2/hi/uk_news/4003063.stm. Ruth Chang brought this article to my attention.
4. Ibid.
5. Princeton University's molecular biologist, Lee. M. Silver dramatically illustrated this point at the 10th Annual Mates David and Hinna Stahl Memorial Lecture in Bioethics, *Remaking Human Nature: The Ethics of Genetic Enhancement* (Robert Wood Johnson Medical School, New Brunswick, New Jersey, March 28, 2007). Silver presented slides containing predictions by famous scientists, including Nobel Laureates, that certain developments in their fields would probably *never* occur, or not occur for *many* years, where *in fact* the developments occurred within *10* years after the predictions were made. Thus, even scientific experts tend to notoriously underestimate the speed and possibilities of scientific progress and technological breakthroughs.
6. See Aristotle's *Nicomachean Ethics*, especially Book X, chapter 7.
7. Derek Parfit suggested this point.
8. For reasons discussed below, such deaths would probably *not* be tragic for society.
9. See "Internal and External Reasons," in *Moral Luck*, (Williams, 1981, pp.101–13); the notion of a subjective motivational set is introduced on p. 102.
10. Value-based reasons are extensively treated and defended in Derek Parfit's unpublished manuscript *On What Matters* (forthcoming, Oxford University Press).
11. Jeff McMahan (2002, pp.102–3) offers some similar criticisms of Williams's position.

12. The experience machine is famously discussed in Nozick (1974, pp. 42–5).
13. As with the main character in Capek's play, *The Makropulos Affair*. The Czeck composer Leos Janacek Sarka turned Capek's play into an opera, *The Makropulos Case*, from which Williams's article takes its name.
14. Thomas Pogge claimed this in correspondence, based on information contained in the 1998 United Nations's *Human Development Report*.
15. This frequently cited quotation, often attributed to Herbert Samuel, appears in the "Yom Kippur Memorial Service" of the Machzor, the Jewish prayer book for the High Holy Days (*New Union Prayer Book for the Days of Awe*, Central Conference of American Rabbis, 1978, p. 484).
16. Franklin's 1778 essay was reprinted in *The Oxford Book of American Essays*, edited by Matthews, Brander (Oxford University Press, 1914). See www.bartleby.com/109/1.html.
17. There is a delightful (anachronistic) irony in Franklin's choice of beings, given Michael Rose's manipulation of the lifespan of certain flies.
18. Thomas Nagel (1979, pp.11–23) made this point in his wonderful article "The Absurd."
19. Act I, Scene 5, lines 44–45.
20. These sentiments were strongly endorsed at the Stahl Memorial Lecture in Bioethics (see note 5) by both Princeton's molecular biologist, Lee Silver, and Harvard's philosopher and bioethicist Dan Brock. Brock was especially vehement that once enhancements were possible they *would* become available and they *would* be used.
21. This quote appears shortly after the one cited previously from the Yom Kippur Memorial Service (see note 20). It, too, was brought to my attention by my mother, Lee Temkin.

References

Kass, L. (1985). *Toward a More Natural Science*. New York: Free Press.

McMahan, J. (2002). *The Ethics of Killing: Problems at the Margins of Life*. Oxford: Oxford University Press.

Nagel, T. (1979). The absurd. *Mortal Questions*. Cambridge: Cambridge University Press.

Narveson, J. (1967). Utilitarianism and new generations. *Mind*, 76, 62–72.

Narveson, J. (1973). Moral problems of population. *Monist*, 57, 62–86.

Nozick, R. (1974). *Anarchy, State, and Utopia*. New York: Basic Books.

Unger, P. (1996). *Living High and Letting Die*. Oxford: Oxford University Press.

Williams, B. (1981). *Moral Luck*. Cambridge: Cambridge University Press.

27

Life Extension versus Replacement*

Gustaf Arrhenius

Introduction

It seems to be a widespread opinion that increasing the length of existing happy lives is better than creating new happy lives although the total welfare is the same in both cases, and that it may be better even when the total welfare is lower in the outcome with extended lives. I shall discuss two interesting suggestions that seem to support this idea. Firstly, the idea there is a positive level of well-being above which a life has to reach to have positive contributive value to a population. This view is usually called critical level utilitarianism. Secondly, the view that it makes an outcome worse if people are worse off than they otherwise could have been. I shall call this view comparativism.

Firstly, I shall describe what I call the pure case of life extension versus replacement. Then I shall very briefly describe some different views about the value of life extension and indicate why I think some of the arguments in favor and against life extension fail. I shall then turn to the implications of critical level utilitarianism and comparativism in regards to life extension versus replacement, which is the main topic of this chapter.

Life Extension versus Replacement: The Pure Case

Figure 27.1 shows two outcomes (or populations as I shall sometimes say): A and B. The width of each block represents the number of people, and the height represents their lifetime welfare. These outcomes could consist of all the lives that are causally affected by, or consequences of, a certain action or series of actions (a policy). All the lives in Figure 27.1 have positive welfare, or, as we also could put it, have lives worth living.[1]

In outcome A, there are five billion people, the x-people, who live for 100 years, then another five billion people, the y-people, who live for 100 years. In outcome B, there are five billion people, the x-people, who live for 200 years. There is the same welfare per year for everybody, thus the same total temporal welfare in both outcomes.

Outcome A is a case of replacement, since the x-people are being replaced by the y-people, whereas outcome B is a case of life extension, since the x-lives are extended. This

Enhancing Human Capacities, edited by Julian Savulescu, Ruud ter Meulen and Guy Kahane.
© 2011 Blackwell Publishing Ltd

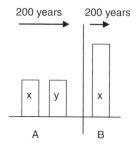

Figure 27.1

is, of course, a very simplified and unrealistic case but it will make our discussion take a clearer form and work as a test case for different theories.

The outcomes above involve the same total amount of temporal welfare. According to some theories, it follows that there is the same total welfare in the outcomes, since total welfare is just a sum of temporal welfare. This is controversial, however, since it might be that some welfare components don't have a temporal location. The standard examples are accomplishments and posthumous fame. Such welfare components do increase an individual's lifetime welfare but not at any specific date, or so it is sometimes argued. However, for our current discussion this doesn't matter much since we could just assume that the cases considered here are equally good in regards to such welfare components.[2] Hence, we are going to assume that the lifetime welfare of the B-people is double that of the A-people, and that the total welfare is the same in both outcomes.

Longevity could be non-instrumentally valuable in two ways: as an independent value apart from welfare or as a welfare component. In the latter case, longevity is another non-dated welfare component that will not show up if we only look at people's temporal welfare. Since the value of longevity is what we are investigating in this chapter, we cannot assume that it is the same in the compared cases and we don't want to include it in the welfare depicted in the figures. So the welfare depicted doesn't include the eventual contribution of longevity to people's lifetime welfare. Thus, in the following when we refer to "welfare," we have in mind temporal welfare and welfare from non-dated welfare sources other than longevity.

Which outcome, if any, is better? According to hedonistic total utilitarianism, A and B are equally good since they involve the same amount of total temporal welfare, and according to hedonism, all welfare components (pains and pleasures) are dated. Likewise for many consequentialist and deontological theories since they satisfy the following condition:

Neutrality: If there is the same total welfare in two outcomes A and B, and there is perfect equality in A and B, then A and B are equally good (or choiceworthy), other things being equal.[3]

According to such theories, whether we should choose life extension or replacement depends only on empirical considerations regarding the probable effect of different policies on the total welfare, given that no other values are at stake. If life extension increases the total welfare, other things being equal, then that should be our policy, if it doesn't, then it shouldn't be. Of course, such estimates are likely to be very difficult since life extension with 100 years or more over the average life expectancy in the affluent societies today might arguably alter the structure of those societies in quite a far-reaching way, not to talk about radical life extension and eternal life. I think neutrality has much in its favor but I shall not consider it further in this chapter.

According to some theories and suggestions, the *ceteris paribus* clause in neutrality cannot be satisfied since there are some other values or structural features involved in the comparison between A and B that makes a difference between them. For example, some have argued in favor of life extension by appealing to a positive right to carry on living. Aubrey de Grey (2005), for example, writes that "[h]uman rights do not get any more fundamental than the right to carry on living" and "...there is no moral distinction between ... acting to shorten someone's life and not acting to extend it."

Just postulating such a positive human right seems quite unsatisfactory, however, and it relies on an especially controversial denial of the act and omission doctrine. In essence, according to de Grey, we are complicit in mass murder of old people by not providing them with the means for life extension. As he writes elsewhere (2007), "[t]here may well be some sort of population explosion [from eliminating all deaths caused by ageing] ... but the first priority is to end the slaughter. Everything else is detail."

Some argue in favor of replacement by claiming that a too long life or a life without death is a nonhuman life. Leon Kass (2001), for example, claims that "... to argue that human life would be better without death is, I submit, to argue that human life would be better being something other than human." Clearly, such an argument doesn't touch moderate life extension. Moreover, it is unclear why an eternal life would be a nonhuman life and, if it is, why we should consider it a worse life than a human life. Arguably, such a nonhuman life could be better than a human life.

Average utilitarianism yields that B is better than A since the average well-being is higher, and likewise for so-called compromise theories, which are combinations of average and total utilitarianism and give some weight to the average utility in the compared outcomes. As I and others have showed elsewhere, however, average utilitarianism and its relatives have a number of very counterintuitive implications in different number cases so we can safely put them to the side (Arrhenius, 2000a, section 3.3, 2000b; Parfit, 1984, p.143). For example, average utilitarianism implies that one can make a population better by adding very bad lives since such an addition might increases the average well-being.

Critical Level Utilitarianism

A better developed effort in support of life extension is critical level utilitarianism (CLU), as propounded by John Broome (2004) in a recent book. In its simplest form, CLU is a modified version of total utilitarianism (Broome, 2004).[4] The contributive value of a person's life is her lifetime welfare minus a positive critical level. The value of a population is calculated by summing these differences for all individuals in the population. CLU could thus be written in the following form:

$$CLU(X) = \sum_{i=1}^{n}(u_i - k) \quad n > 0$$

In the above formula, n is the population size of X and u_i is the numerical representation of the welfare of the ith life in population X, and k is the critical level.

The critical level k is supposed to be the level at which it is axiologically neutral whether a life is created or not, what Broome calls "the neutral level for existence." Broome doesn't equate this level with the welfare level of a life that is neutral *for* a person, that is, neutral welfare – an option that the classical utilitarian would use. As he writes (2004, p.259), "…the neutral level for existence is positive, once the zero of lifetime well-being is normalized at the level of a constantly neutral life." Hence, since the critical level is positive, the contributive value of lives with positive welfare below the critical level is negative.

What does CLU imply in regards to the case in Figure 27.1? Let w and $2w$ represent the lifetime welfare of the people in A and B, respectively, and let $2n$ and n be the population size of A and B, respectively. Then $CLU(A) - CLU(B) = 2n(w - k) - n$ $(2w - k) = - nk$, that is, $[CLU(B) > CLU(A)]$. Hence, CLU ranks B as better than A and thus supports life extension.

Notice that it is not essential to CLU's ranking of A and B that the x-people's extra welfare in outcome B appears in the form of longer lives. Even if the x-people only lived for 100 years in outcome B, but with the same lifetime welfare as in the original case, CLU would still prefer B over A. In general, CLU favors that a given amount of welfare is spread among as few people as possible, and its implication in regards to life extension is a corollary of this general feature.[5]

Broome illustrates CLU's implications in respect to life extension with a choice between extending an already existing person's life or creating a new person. In his example, a couple can choose between extending their already existing child's life or having one more baby (Broome, 2004, pp. 8–9, 259). This can be seen as a micro-version of the case in Figure 27.1.[6] I take it to be a widespread view that we should extend the existing child's life instead of creating a new life, even if the total welfare would be the same in both cases. CLU seems to capture this intuition.

Nevertheless, I don't think CLU captures most people's intuition in the case of the couple's choice and life extension in general. For many people I think that the fundamental intuition is, roughly stated, that we should avoid making people worse off when no one else would benefit from it.[7] Let's call it the pointless harm intuition.

In the case of the couple's choice, if they don't extend their existing child's life, then she would be worse off. According to a commonly shared intuition, however, the new child doesn't benefit from being brought into existence. As Broome himself (1999, p.168, emphasis in original) eloquently puts it in another context:

> …[I]t cannot ever be *true* that it is better for a person that she lives than that she should never have lived at all. If it were better for a person that she lives than that she should never have lived at all, then if she had never lived at all, that would have been worse for her than if she had lived. But if she had never lived at all, there would have been no her for it to be worse for, so it could not have been worse for her.[8]

Broome's account of the value of longevity doesn't capture the pointless harm intuition, however, since it applies also to cases in which only the well-being of uniquely realizable people (that is, people who only exist in one of the possible outcomes) are at stake. In such cases, no one will be made worse or better off depending on our choice since their existence also depends on it. This could be the case, for example, when we evaluate future outcomes consisting of different people. CLU, however, would still prefer B over A even if there was no overlap and thus different people in A and B.[9]

The difference can be seen more clearly if we consider the following version of the couple's choice. Assume a couple can choose between extending their already existing child's life and having one more child with a short life (as short as the non-extended life of the existing child would be), or not extending their existing child's life and having a different extra child with a long life (as long as the extended life of the existing child would be). CLU is indifferent between these choices whereas most people, I surmise, would prefer the first option since then no one is made worse off.

Secondly, as Krister Bykvist (2007, p.104) has pointed out, the intuition involved in Broome's example about the couple's choice probably draws on our commonsense idea about parental duties. According to this, we have a special duty towards our already existing children which doesn't apply to the children we have not yet created. Hence, the intuition seems to be deontic rather than axiological in nature and is thus not an appropriate test case for an axiological theory.

Another aspect of CLU's support for life extension that some might like and other might find peculiar is its generality. For example, it prefers extremely long lives over very long lives. Assume that the people in outcome A in Figure 27.1 live for 500 years whereas the people in B lives for 1,000 years. Still, CLU ranks B as better than A. Actually, Broome (2004, p.108) seems a bit hesitant here since he writes that "[t]here may be limits to this intuition [the intuition that extension is better than replacement]. I am not sure we would think it better to prolong a 100-year-old person's life for another 100 years, rather than have a new person live for 100 years." But CLU doesn't leave room for such doubts, as its implication in the case in Figure 27.1 shows.

Moreover, CLU prefers long lives with horrible suffering rather than more lives with less suffering. Assume that the height of the blocks in Figure 27.1 represents people's negative welfare, their pain and suffering, so that the people in B suffer the most whereas the people in A suffer much less since they have shorter lives. Still, CLU would rank B as the best outcome. Actually, this could still be the case even if there was more total suffering in B. Those who believe that we should give extra moral weight to suffering, or to those that are worse off, will find this implication unacceptable. Although not all of us are convinced negativists who regard suffering as morally more important than happiness, surely an acceptable theory of beneficence must at least give as much weight to suffering as it gives to happiness.

Finally, there is a general problem with CLU which I think gives us a decisive reason to reject it, and this problem becomes extra pressing in the current context. CLU will only give the intuitively right result in the couple's choice if the critical level of existence is set very high. Even if the new child would have a very good life, many would think that this is not enough to make it better to let the existing child die, if the existing child would have a good future life.[10] Assume, for example, that if the couple doesn't have another baby, then their existing child will enjoy 80 very good years. If they do have

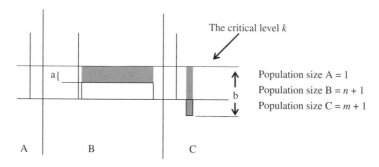

Figure 27.2

another baby, then she will enjoy 80 very good years whereas the first child will only live for 40 years. Still, even if the critical level is set as high as 39 very good years, CLU will recommend that the couple has another baby. Hence, the critical level has to be well above 40 very good years to preserve our intuition in the couple's choice.

It is easy to show, however, that CLU has a very counterintuitive conclusion which is especially disturbing if the critical level is set high. CLU implies that a population with negative welfare may be better than a population with positive welfare, a conclusion I have called the sadistic conclusion (Arrhenius, 2000a, 2000b, forthcoming):

In Figure 27.2, the width of each block shows the number of people, and the height shows their welfare. Outcome A consists of one person with welfare well above the critical level. In outcome B, we have added n people with positive welfare x. Their welfare is a units below the critical level k, as indicated in the diagram. The negative value of this addition is thus $n(x - k) = -na$ which is represented by the gray area in outcome B. In outcome C, m people with negative welfare y have been added. Their welfare is b units below the critical level, as indicated in the diagram. The negative value of this addition is $m(-y - k) = -mb$ which is represented by the gray area in outcome C. Since $mb < na$ (the gray area in outcome C is smaller than the gray area in outcome B), it is better to add the people with negative welfare rather than the people with positive welfare, a clear case of the sadistic conclusion.

CLU implies especially troublesome versions of the sadistic conclusion:

> *The very sadistic conclusion*: For any population of lives with very negative welfare, there is a population of lives with positive welfare which is *worse*, other things being equal.

There is always a population with sufficiently many people with positive welfare slightly below the critical level such that the total negative value of these people is greater than that of a given population made up of people with negative welfare. This holds irrespective of how much people suffer and of how many they are. Thus, CLU implies the very sadistic conclusion. If the critical level is set above 40 very good years, then I find this implication utterly counterintuitive.

Comparativism

Let's turn to a more promising idea that several people have proposed to me in conversation in defense of the superiority of life extension over replacement: It makes an outcome worse if people are worse off than they otherwise could have been.[11] Another way to put it is to say that such people have a legitimate complaint or grievance and this makes the outcome worse. In addition to the well-being of everybody, we should take the badness of legitimate complaints, or what we will call comparative harms, into account. Moreover, a person is not harmed by not coming into existence since you have to exist in both of the compared outcomes to be harmed or to have a legitimate complaint. Let's call this view comparativism. It can be more exactly described by the following two principles:

> *The principle of comparative harm*: If a person exists in two alternative outcomes A and B, and if she would be worse off in terms of welfare in A as compared to B, then she would be comparatively harmed if A rather than B came about.

> *Comparativism*: The value of an outcome is determined by the total welfare and the comparative harm in the outcome.

Notice that the notion of "comparative harm" is a technical notion that doesn't completely map onto our everyday use of "harm." For example, if you will enjoy an excellent life in both outcome A and B but you are slightly less happy in B, then you are comparatively harmed if B came about, but many would hesitate to say that you are harmed in the ordinary language sense of "harm" (there are many other examples). I could have used some other term to capture the idea that it makes an outcome worse if people are worse off than they otherwise could have been, but I think the technical notion of "comparative harm" is sufficiently related to the ordinary notion of harm to justify its name.[12] For brevity, I will in the following sometimes use the term "harm" and its cognates although I always have in mind "comparative harm" in the above sense.

Moreover, nothing is yet said about how to calculate and aggregate the value of total welfare and comparative harm. The above formulation is open to many different ways of doing this. Intuitively, all such extension will imply that the more welfare, the better the outcome, other things being equal; and the more comparative harm, the worse the outcome, other things being equal.

Comparativism seems to give us an argument in favor of life extension. Consider again outcome A and B in Figure 27.1. In A, the x-people are harmed since they have only half of the welfare they enjoy in B. The y-people are not harmed in B since they don't exist in that outcome, and according to comparativism, a person is not harmed by not coming into existence (recall that according to the principle of comparative harm, you have to exist in both of the compared outcomes to be a candidate for harm). Consequently, although the total welfare is the same in both outcomes, A is worse in one respect since if it comes about, some people will be worse off than they could have been and thus there will be people who are harmed and can legitimately complain. Hence, since A and B are equally good in terms of people's well-being, but B is better in terms of comparative harms, B is better than A all things considered. In other words, life extension is better than replacement.

Notice that comparativism not only gives support to extending lives that exist now, which I guess is the fundamental intuition in the pro life extension camp, but also future lives which exist in both of the compared future scenarios. In practice, this will not be a very common situation but consider the following case: A woman has the choice of either implanting two fertilized eggs or just one of them. If she implants both eggs, then her offspring are likely to live for 100 years each. If she implants only one of them, then, because of a new therapy that can only safely be used when one egg is implanted, her child is likely to live for 200 years. This case only involves future people but comparativism would still recommend the latter option, given that the total well-being is roughly the same in both outcomes.

As with CLU, comparativism's ranking of A and B doesn't turn on the fact that the x-people's extra welfare in outcome B appears in the form of longer lives. Again, if the x-people only lived for 100 years in outcome B, but with the same lifetime welfare as in the original case, comparativism would still prefer B over A. In general, comparativism favors that a given amount of welfare is spread only among non-uniquely realizable people and not shared with uniquely realizable people.[13] Its implication in regards to life extension is a consequence of this general feature.[14]

Non-transitivity

As we have so far formulated comparativism, it has a serious flaw. Consider Figure 27.3.

The x- and y-people exist in outcome A, the y- and z-people exist in B, and the z- and x-people exist in C. Assume that all of these people have positive welfare, but that the y-people are better off in B as compared to A, the z-people are better off in C as compared to B, and the x-people are better off in A as compared to C.[15] All the outcomes in the diagram are equally good in respect to the amounts of people's well-being. However, since the y-people are worse off in A as compared to B, the y-people would have a complaint if A came about. In this respect, A is worse than B. Consequently, all things considered, A is worse than B. The same reasoning yields that B is worse than C, and C is worse than A. But if A is worse than B, and B is worse than C, then transitivity yields that A is worse than C. Consequently, A is both better and worse than C, which cannot be true.

To meet this objection, one could argue that we should abandon transitivity of the relation "better than," or that comparativism should be couched in normative rather than axiological terms, and add the claim that there is no analogue to the transitivity of "better than" for normative concepts. This wouldn't help much, partly because non-transitivity in the above case is just plainly counterintuitive (the intuitively correct result

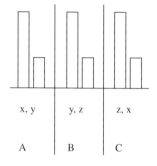

x, y   y, z   z, x

A | B | C

Figure 27.3

is that all the outcomes are equally good) and partly because non-transitive value orderings easily translate to moral dilemmas on the normative level. However, since I've discussed these latter problems at length elsewhere, and since there is another way of explicating comparativism which doesn't imply non-transitive orderings, I shall not dwell on those details here.[16]

Here's one way to formulate comparativism to avoid non-transitivity. When determining the value of an outcome we should consider both people's well-being and whether they are harmed in the sense of being worse off than they could have been. The value of an outcome is determined by the value of the total well-being in the outcome reduced by a factor that reflects whether people are harmed in the sense of being worse off than they could have been.[17]

Here's how this could be done. Assume that we represent well-being on a numerical scale and that the total well-being of the best-off people in Figure 27.3 is 10 units and the total well-being of the worst-off people is 5 units. Assume also that all the possible outcomes in the choice situation considered are those depicted in Figure 27.3. The value of outcome A would then be 15 minus some factor h that represents the fact that the y-people are worse off than they could have been. Intuitively, this factor should correspond to how much worse off the y-people are in A as compared to B. Similarly, the value of outcome B and C would be 15 minus h. Consequently, on this view all the outcomes in Figure 27.3 are ranked as equally good which seems to be the intuitively correct all things considered ranking in this case.

However, in regard to replacement versus life extension, this version of comparativism picks B since the two outcomes are equally good in regard to people's welfare but A is worse in one respect since in A, some people are worse off than they otherwise could have been.

Dominated Outcomes

Although the reformulated version of comparativism neatly captures some people intuitions regarding the value of life extension as compared to replacement and avoids the threat of non-transitivity, it also has implications which some might consider counterintuitive. Consider the three outcomes shown in Figure 27.4.

There is the same number of people in all three outcomes in Figure 27.4. Everyone in A is better off than everyone in B, and everyone in B is better off than everyone in C.

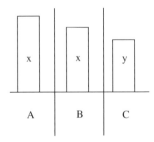

Figure 27.4

Again, the x-people would be harmed if outcome B came about since they would be worse off than they otherwise could have been, i.e., if A would have been the case instead. Let h represent the total value of the harm done to the x-people in B. Let d represent the total difference in well-being between the x-people in B and the y-people in C. The difference in value between outcome B and C will then be d minus h.[18] Consequently, if h is greater than d, then comparativism will rank C as better than B although everyone in the latter outcome is better off than everyone in the former. This seems a bit counterintuitive.

Yet, this result might not perturb the comparativists. They might say that since they believe in the negative value of comparative harm, they're willing to trade off some welfare to avoid such comparative harm. They might point to other non-welfarist axiologies such as desert theories where the value of an outcome is determined both by the receipt of welfare and the fit between receipt and desert. On such theories, it might be cases where we have to forego some welfare to achieve a better fit between receipt and desert (Arrhenius, 2003a, 2006, 2007; Feldman, 1997). Likewise for other pluralist axiologies.

Nevertheless, there are further related problems with this view if we turn to its normative implications. Assume some weak form of consequentialism, or consequentialist part of a deontological theory, to the effect that we ought to choose the best outcome in the cases currently under discussion.[19] Assume further that A is a very unlikely outcome. If we try to achieve A, we are most likely to fail and end up with C. If we aim at B or C, we will succeed. Still, comparativism tells us that it would be wrong to choose B, just because there is an unlikely outcome A in the choice set.[20]

One might think that this problem can be fixed by letting the harm factor depend on the probability of the better alternative. Instead of letting h represent the total value of the harm done to the x-people if we were to choose outcome B, it should be represented by ph, where p is the probability that A will be the case given that we choose A, and h is the harm done to the x-people were we to choose outcome B when we could have chosen A with certainty of success. The difference in value between outcome B and C will now be d minus ph so still, if ph is greater than d, which is clearly possible, then comparativism will rank C as better than B although everyone is better off in B.

A better solution might be to let the harm factor depend on people's expected welfare given a certain action which with certain probabilities brings about certain outcomes. On this view, people are harmed if their expected welfare is lower than it could have been given a different choice of action. Assume that if we choose an action a_A aiming at bringing about A, then the probability that A will be the case is 0.10 and the probability that C will be the case is 0.90, whereas if we choose action a_B, then B will be the case with certainty. Assume further that the total well-being in A is 10 and in B is 8. Then the x-people's expected welfare if we choose a_A is $0.10 \times 10 = 1$, whereas it is 1×8 were we to choose action a_B. Hence, on this formulation of comparativism, the x-people are not harmed if we choose a_B since their expected welfare is higher if we choose that action rather than a_A. Hence, by switching to expected welfare and defining harm in terms of expected welfare, the problem of unlikely outcomes disappears.

On the other hand, if we went for a_A and A actually came about, then we would still have harmed the x-people and done the wrong thing since their expected welfare (at the time of the choice) was lower than it would have been had we chosen a_B, although they are better off since A rather than B actually came about. This might strike some as implausible but a possible rejoinder is to claim that it was wrong to choose a_A since that action exposed the x-people to a risk of getting nothing.[21]

This problem, however, is not peculiar to comparativism but analogous to the old dispute among consequentialists regarding whether one should go for a formulation of consequentialism in terms of the actual or probable outcomes of actions, so I shall not discuss it further here (Carlson, 1995; Feldman, 2006). It is noteworthy, however, that comparativism seems more compatible with a probabilistic rather than an actualistic formulation of consequentialism.

Let me end this section with two other objections to comparativism.[22] In Figure 27.3, comparativism correctly ranked all the outcomes as equally good. One might object, however, that we cannot know this without knowing that exactly these three outcomes are the only ones available in the situation since, according to comparativism, the value of an outcome depends on the set of possible outcomes in the situation. Suppose, for example, that there was another outcome D with only the x-people at level 15. This would not only yield that D was the best outcome in the situation but also change the ranking of A, B, and C, since the x-people in C will be more harmed than the y-people in A and the z-people in B. Hence, C will be ranked as worse than A and B.

The first objection is that it is absurd that one and the same outcome can both be worse than and equally as good as another outcome. This seems to be the case here since when D is not present in the set of outcomes, C is ranked as equally as good as A and B, whereas when D is present, C is ranked as worse than A and B. Hence, it looks like the same outcome, C, is both worse than and equally as good as A and B.

This would surely be absurd but the obvious rejoinder is to deny that these outcomes are the same outcomes. We can just partly individuate outcomes by the situation to which they belong. Hence, if we add another outcome to the situation described in Figure 27.3, then we have a new situation with, say, alternatives A', B', C' and D and it is B' which is better than C' which doesn't contradict that outcome B and C in the original situation are equally good.

The second objection is that in practice, we could never be epistemically justified in limiting the number of possible outcomes as we have done in the examples above. Hence, since the comparativist ranking depends on the possible outcomes in the situation, we cannot be justified in believing in the ranking.

It is true that this makes comparativism a bit special as an axiology since most axiologies, such as the axiological component of classical utilitarianism, yield context-insensitive rankings of outcomes. However, this problem appears for these theories on the normative level, since which outcome is the best one, and thus the one we ought to choose, depends on which other outcomes are available in the situation. Hence, this alleged particular problem with comparativism reduces to the old problem of whether consequentialist theories ought to be and can be action guiding and is thus no special problem for comparativism. The same standard responses come in handy here. For example, we could make a sharp distinction between criterion theories and decision methods and claim that comparativism is a criterion theory that has no claim to be used as a decision method other than indirectly in the choice of which decision methods that we should use.[23]

Anti-Egalitarianism

Here's a more problematic case for the comparativist:

The energy policy case: A country is facing a choice between implementing a certain energy policy (alternative A) or not (alternative B). Were this country to implement this policy, then there would be an increase in the welfare of the presently existing people of this country (the x-people) since they will live for a longer time. On the other hand, this increase would be counterbalanced by the harm the waste from this energy system will cause in the lives of people in the future (the y-people) by shortening their lives. The existence of these future people is contingent upon the implementation of this energy policy. If the country doesn't implement this energy policy, other people will exist in the future (the z-people) with the same good quality and length of life as the x-people. The advantages and disadvantages of other effects of this policy balance out (cf. Parfit, 1984, pp. 371–2).

In the above energy policy case, assume that the total difference in well-being for the x-people in the two outcomes equals the difference in well-being for the y- and z-people. We can also assume that the total (and thus average) length of life is the same in both outcomes. In other words, A and B involve the same number of people, the same total sum of well-being, and the same total length of life.

A reasonable and modest egalitarian (or prioritarian) consideration implies that B is better than A since they are equally good in regards to the total (and average) well-being but there is perfect equality in B whereas there is inequality in A. Comparativism implies, however, that A is better than B because the x-people would be harmed if we were to choose outcome B rather than A since they then would be worse off than they otherwise could have been. The y- and z-people, on the other hand, cannot be harmed in this way since they are uniquely realizable (i.e., their existence depends on our choice and you cannot be harmed by not coming into existence according to comparativism). Consequently, there is a tension between comparativism and a reasonable egalitarian consideration.

Even if we lower the total welfare in A by reducing the longevity, and thus the welfare, of the y-people, comparativism would rank A as better than B as long as the lower total welfare in A is counteracted by the comparative harm in B. Hence, comparativism yields that an outcome with lower total well-being, lower total (and average) length of life,

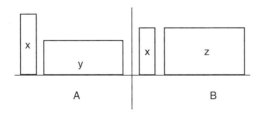

Figure 27.5

and inequality can be better than an outcome with higher total well-being and perfect equality.

Again, however, I think the comparativist can reply that since they believe in the negative value of comparative harm, they're willing to trade off some welfare to avoid such comparative harm. Moreover, if we also take comparative harm into account, then outcome B is also an unequal outcome since although people have the same welfare, the x-people are harmed.

Nevertheless, the point is that as a support for life extension, the above implication is a bit odd. If we are in favor of life extension, why should we opt for the alternative with less total and average longevity and with an unequal distribution of longevity? So this case shows that there is a conflict between intuitions regarding life extension and comparativism.[24]

Future Populations and Tradeoffs

Lastly, comparativism might not deliver all the goods that the life extension proponents want. For instance, in all cases involving only uniquely realizable people, that is, situations in which there are different people in all outcomes, comparativism determines the ranking by the total sum of people's welfare since such cases don't involve any comparative harm. Consequently, like total utilitarianism, in respect to future populations where there is no overlap of individuals in the compared populations, it will imply that A and B in Figure 27.1 are equally good. Moreover, it implies that for any population of 200-year lives, there is a better population in which, say, everybody has 50-year lives, since with enough people, there will be a greater total sum of well-being in such a population.

These might be acceptable implications for some life extension proponents, however, since what matters to them is that if lives are not extended, some existing people will be worse off than they otherwise could have been. This is of course exactly the intuition that comparativism tries to capture. Nevertheless, it will imply similar conclusions even in cases that involve overlaps and thus involve great losses in longevity for non-uniquely realizable people, including existing people.

Here is a numerical illustration of this point (see Figure 27.6).[25] Assume that we have a choice between outcome A with 10 persons, the presently existing x-people, and outcome B with the x-people and an additional 200 persons, the y-people. In outcome A, the x-people have very high lifetime welfare because of their long lives. Assume that

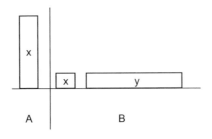

Figure 27.6

this high welfare corresponds to 10 units of welfare. Consequently, the value of outcome A is $10 \times 10 = 100$.

In outcome B, the x- and y-people have very low positive lifetime welfare because of their short lives. Assume that this very low welfare corresponds to one unit of welfare. Since the x-people have much lower welfare in B, they are harmed in B. Assume that the harm factor for each x-person corresponds to her difference in welfare between outcome A and B. Thus, the value of the harm to the x-people in B is $10 \times (-9) = -90$ whereas the value of their welfare is $10 \times 1 = 10$. Taken all together, the value of the x-people in outcome B is $10 - 90 = -80$. However, since there are also 200 y-persons in outcome B, the total value of outcome B, according to comparativism, is $200 - 80 = 120$ which is greater than the value of A. Hence, comparativism here opts for the outcome with short lives, outcome B, although it involves a great loss in welfare and longevity for the existing people. In this respect comparativism doesn't give a strong support for life extension over replacement.

One might think that this result depends on the weight given to comparative harm. However, as long as the harm factor is represented by a finite number (that is, as long as we don't give lexical priority to comparative harm), comparativism will have the above implication. Here's a general demonstration: Assume that h is a positive finite number that represents the weight given to the comparative harm of an individual due to the fact that she is worse off than she could have been. Let A consist of n non-uniquely realizable persons with very high welfare u_1 (because of their long lives). Let B consist of a mixed population of n uniquely and m non-uniquely realizable people with very low positive welfare u_2 (because of their short lives). The value of A is thus nu_1 and the value of B is $n(u_2 - h) + mu_2$. Now, for any value of h, there is an m such that $nu_1 < n(u_2 - h) + mu_2$, that is, a value of m that makes B better than A, namely $m > n(u_1 - u_2 + h)/u_2$.

Of course, how strong support comparativism will give for life extension over replacement depends on the negative weight given to comparative harm. If we give lexical priority to avoiding comparative harm, then life extension will always be better than replacement. Given such an extreme negative weight on comparative harms, however, we will face extremely counterintuitive versions of the cases described in Figures 27.4 and 27.5.

For example, consider Figure 27.5 again and assume that there is only one x-person (or only one x-person with lower welfare in B as compared to A) but a vast number of y- and z-people. Assume further that the y-people in A only have lives barely worth living, and that the x-person's welfare in B is just slightly lower than in A (for example, one extra pin prick in her left thumb on her fifth birthday). The z-people in B have the same welfare as the x-people, that is, very high welfare. Still, if we give lexical priority to avoiding comparative harms, A is better than B.[26]

Likewise, consider a version of the case depicted in Figure 27.4 in which the y-people in C have lives barely worth living and only one of the x-people have slightly lower welfare in outcome B as compared to outcome A. Again, if we give lexical priority to avoiding comparative harms, C is better than B.

Comparativism as a support for life extension might be caught in a dilemma here. If it gives a great negative weight to comparative harm, then it will give a strong support for life extension but imply clearly unacceptable versions of the cases described in Figures 27.4 and 5. It can avoid these counterintuitive implications if it puts a small negative weight on comparative harm, but then it will give a very weak support for life extension. It seems hard to find an acceptable way out of this dilemma.

Acknowledgments

I would like to thank Margaret Battin, Nick Boström, Dan Brock, Speranta Dumitru, Nir Eyal, Frances Kamm, Julian Savulescu, Torbjörn Tännsjö, Dan Wikler, and especially John Broome and Krister Bykvist for fruitful discussions and comments. The comments from the editors and one of the anonymous reviewers were also very useful. Earlier versions of this chapter were presented at *Enhance: The Ethics of Human Enhancement*, IAB Satellite Conference, 8th World Congress of Bioethics, Beijing, August 2006; *Oxford Medical Humanities Forum*, Oxford University, November 2006; *James Martin Advanced Research Seminar*, Faculty of Philosophy, Oxford University, December 2006; and at *Ethical Issues in the Measurement of Health and The Global Burden of Disease*, The Harvard University Program in Ethics and Health: Third Annual International Conference, Harvard University, April 2008. I would like to thank the participants at these occasions for their stimulating criticism. Thanks also to Oxford Uehiro Centre for Practical Ethics for being such a generous host during some of the time when this chapter was written. Financial support from the Bank of Sweden Tercentenary Foundation and the Swedish Collegium for Advanced Study is gratefully acknowledged.

Notes

*   This chapter is a reprint (with minor changes) of an already published paper: Life Extension versus Replacement. *Journal of Applied Philosophy*, **25**(3).

1.   We shall say that a life has neutral welfare if and only if it has the same welfare as a life without any good or bad welfare components, and that a life has positive (negative) welfare if and only if it has higher (lower) welfare than a life with neutral welfare. A hedonist, for example, would typically say that pain is bad and pleasure is good for a person, and that a life without any pain and pleasure has neutral welfare. This definition can be combined with other welfarist axiologies, such as desire and objective list theories. There is a number of alternative definitions of a life with positive (negative, neutral) welfare in the literature. For a discussion of these see Arrhenius, 2000a, forthcoming; Broome, 1999; Parfit, 1984, p.358. Notice also that the welfare shown by the height of the blocks in the figures incorporates all possible sources of welfare in life, including the eventual loss of welfare due to the frustration of future oriented preferences that death brings about, or the happiness generated by having children, and so forth. See also the discussion below.

2.   Alternatively, we could disperse the value of such components evenly throughout a person's life (Broome 2004). Another reason to resist making a person's lifetime welfare a mere sum of temporal welfare is that this view yields counterintuitive results when one compares lives where both the length and the temporal welfare vary (Arrhenius, 2005a). I don't have space to consider these problems further here.

3.   We have included a *ceteris paribus* clause in the formulation of the above condition. The idea is that people's welfare and longevity is the only axiologically and deontically relevant aspect

which may be different in the compared populations, and that the compared populations are roughly equally good in regard to other axiologically and deontically relevant aspects. There are neither constraints (e.g. promise keeping) nor options (e.g. great personal sacrifice for the agent which is beyond the call of duty), nor non-welfarist values in the outcomes (e.g. cultural diversity) that give us a reason to (not) choose one or the other of the involved outcomes. The only reasons for choosing one or the other of the involved outcomes arise from the welfare and the longevity of the lives in the involved populations.

4. This theory was first proposed by Blackorby and Donaldson (1984) and Blackorby *et al.* (1997). These authors also propose a more refined version of CLU according to which the contributive value of people's welfare is dampened by a strictly concave function. Another version introduces incommensurability among some populations. These modifications have no relevance for the arguments made here.

5. For more on CLU's implications in population ethics see Arrhenius 2000a, 2000b, forthcoming.

6. I'll point out a crucial difference below.

7. Three other possibilities are that we should give priority to presently, necessarily, or actually existing people just because they are presently, necessarily, or actually existing. I discuss these views at length in the context of population ethics in Arrhenius (2000a) and Arrhenius (forthcoming) and shall say nothing more of them here due to space constraint. In a comment on Broome's example, Bykvist (2007, p.104) suggests that "... it is crucial to many people that the case is about extending the life of an *already existing* individual. This means that if the life is not extended then there is someone who will be worse off" (emphasis in original). The first sentence seems to indicate that Bykvist thinks that the intuition is about presently existing individuals, whereas the second expresses what I think is the source of the intuition.

8. See also Parfit (1984, pp. 395, 489), Heyd (1988), Bykvist (2006), and Narveson (1967). I actually don't think Broome's argument is valid and I have criticized it in Arrhenius (forthcoming) and Arrhenius and Rabinowicz (2010).

9. For the same point, see Bykvist (2007, p. 104).

10. The same point is made, I think, in Bykvist (2007, p. 104).

11. Private communication with, among others, Julian Savulescu and Nick Boström. Andrew Williams also suggested this possibility to handle certain problems in population ethics. Similar ideas are put forward in Hope (2003), Meyer (2003), Roberts (1998, 2007).

12. An analogy would be the difference between the notion of the "consequence of an action" in ordinary language and in the formulation of consequentialism (usually the whole possible world that would be the case if the action were performed).

13. For more on comparativism's implications in population ethics, see Arrhenius (2000a, 2003a, forthcoming).

14. Comparativism also shares with CLU that it favors extremely long lives over long lives, although only in respect to non-uniquely realizable lives.

15. Temkin (1987) uses a similar example to illustrate the intransitivity of the so-called "person affecting restriction."

16. See Arrhenius (2005b). Another option is to claim that the only thing we can say about this case is that B is better than A for the y-people, C is better than B for the z-people, and so forth, and that we cannot say anything at all about the all-things considered ranking of these outcomes. In other words, extensive incomparability would appear in all cases involving uniquely realizable people (people that exist in some but not all of the compared outcomes). Apart from counterintuitive implications of this move (it seems reasonable to claim that the outcomes above are equally good and it seems daft to claim that the outcomes involved in the energy policy case are incomparable), it wouldn't be very helpful in the context of medical ethics and other practical contexts where we have to make a choice.

17.   Alternatively, we could represent the value of an outcome with an ordered pair (w, h) in which w represents the total well-being in the outcome and h represents the total harm in the outcome. Such a representation would leave open the possibility that comparative harm has lexical priority over total welfare in the ranking of outcomes. As I shall discuss below, such a view is not very attractive.

18.   Assume that the total well-being in C is m and in B thus $m + d$. The difference in value between B and C is then $(m + d - h) - m = d - h$.

19.   The kind of consequentialism I have in mind is what we could call *ceteris paribus* act consequentialism: Other things being equal, an action is right (obligatory) if and only if its outcome is at least as good as (better than) that of every alternative. An action is wrong if and only if it is not right. In other words, if a choice situation doesn't involve actions that are right or wrong by virtue of a certain deontic constraint or option, then the normative status of the actions are determined by the value of their respective outcomes. Most deontologists accept this form of consequentialism. For a discussion, see Arrhenius (2005b).

20.   Strictly speaking, comparativism in conjunction with consequentialism has this implication. For the sake of brevity, I omit this qualification below.

21.   Another interesting possibility, suggested to me by an anonymous referee, is to claim that people are comparatively harmed if and only if they are worse off than they could have been both in terms of expected and actual welfare. According to this view, if we choose a_A and A actually came about, then the x-people are not harmed since their actual welfare is maximized. A problem for such a theory, however, is that its normative prescriptions are a bit unclear. Does it direct us to choose a_A or a_B?

22.   I'm indebted to John Broome for pressing these two points.

23.   See Bales (1971) for an excellent treatment of this issue. See also Brink (1986).

24.   I'm grateful to Speranta Dumitru for pressing this point.

25.   This is basically a micro-version of Parfit's famous "repugnant conclusion." See Parfit (1984, chapter 17).

26.   One could also construct examples in which the y-people have horrible tormented lives. However, such counterexamples could be avoided by revising comparativism such that it counts as being comparatively harmed if you are born into a life not worth living and there is an alternative in which you're not brought into existence. I'm grateful to an anonymous referee for pressing this point.

References

Arrhenius, G. (2000a). *Future Generations: A Challenge for Moral Theory.* Uppsala: University Printers.

Arrhenius, G. (2000b). An impossibility theorem for welfarist axiologies. *Economics & Philosophy*, **16**.

Arrhenius, G. (2003a). The person affecting restriction, comparativism, and the moral status of potential people. *Ethical Perspectives*, **10**(3–4), 185–95.

Arrhenius, G. (2003b). Feldman's desert-adjusted utilitarianism and population ethics. *Utilitas*, **15**(2).

Arrhenius, G. (2005a). Superiority in value. *Philosophical Studies*, **123**, 97–114.

Arrhenius, G. (2005b). The paradoxes of future generations and normative theory. In J. Ryberg & T. Tännsjö (eds.), *The Repugnant Conclusion*. Dordrecht: Kluwer.

Arrhenius, G. (2006). Desert as fit: An axiomatic analysis. In R. Feldman, K. McDaniel, J.R. Raibley & M.J. Zimmerman (eds.), *The Good, the Right, Life and Death: Essays in Honor of Fred Feldman*. London: Ashgate.

Arrhenius, G. (2007). Meritarian axiologies and distributive justice. In T. Rønnow-Rasmussen, B. Petersson, P. Josefsson & D. Egonsson (eds.), *Hommage à Wlodek: Philosophical Papers Dedicated to Wlodek Rabinowicz* (www.fil.lu.se/hommageawlodek/).

Arrhenius G. (forthcoming). *Population Ethics*. Oxford: Oxford University Press.

Arrhenius G. & Rabinowicz, W. (2010). Better to be than not to be? in *The Benefit of Broad Horizons. Intellectual and Institutional Preconditions for a Global Social Science*. Leiden: Brill.

Bales, R.E. (1971). Act-utilitarianism: Account of right-making characteristic or decision-making procedure? *American Philosophical Quarterly*, **8**(3), 257–65.

Blackorby, C., Bossert, W. & Donaldson, D. (1997). Critical-level utilitarianism and the population-ethics dilemma. *Economics & Philosophy*, **13**.

Blackorby, C. & Donaldson, D. (1984). Social criteria for evaluating population change. *Journal of Public Economics*, **25**.

Brink, D. (1986). Utilitarian morality and the personal point of view. *Journal of Philosophy*, **83**(8), 421–7.

Broome, J. (1999). *Ethics Out of Economics*. Cambridge: Cambridge University Press.

Broome, J. (2004). *Weighing Lives*. Oxford: Oxford University Press.

Bykvist, K. (2006). The benefits of coming into existence. *Philosophical Studies*, **135**.

Bykvist, K. (2007). The good, the bad, and the ethically neutral. *Economics & Philosophy*, **23**.

Carlson, E. (1995). *Consequentialism Reconsidered*. Dordrecht: Kluwer.

de Grey, A. (2005). Life extension, human rights, and the rational refinement of repugnance. *Journal of Medical Ethics*, **31**(11), 659–63.

de Grey, A. (2007). Why we should do all we can to hasten the defeat of human aging. www.sens.org/concerns.htm#opop (accessed July 25, 2007).

Feldman, F. (1997). *Utilitarianism, Hedonism, and Desert: Essays in Moral Philosophy*. Cambridge: Cambridge University Press.

Feldman, F. (2006). Actual utility, the objection from impracticality, and the move to expected utility. *Philosophical Studies*, **129**(1), 49–79.

Heyd (1988). Procreation and value: Can ethics deal with futurity problems? *Philosophia* (Israel), **18**.

Hope, T. (2003). Physicians' duties and the non-identity problem, mimeo, Oxford University.

Kass, L. (2001). L'Chaim and its limits: Why not immortality? *First Things: Journal of Religion, Culture, and Public Life*, May.

Meyer, L. (2003). Intergenerational justice. In Edward N. Zalta (ed.), *The Stanford Encyclopedia of Philosophy* (Summer 2003 Edition), http://plato.stanford.edu/archives/sum2003/entries/justice-intergenerational/.

Narveson, J. (1967). Utilitarianism and new generations. *Mind*, **76**, 69–72.

Parfit, D. (1984). *Reasons and Persons*. Oxford: Clarendon Press.

Roberts, M. (1998). *Child versus Childmaker: Future Persons and Present Duties in Ethics and the Law*. Rowman & Littlefield.

Roberts, M. (2007). The non-identity fallacy: Harm, probability and another look at Parfit's depletion example. *Utilitas*, **19**(3), 267–311.

Temkin L.S. (1987). Intransitivity and the mere addition paradox. *Philosophy & Public Affairs*, **16**(2), 168–9.

28

Lifespan Extension: Metaphysical Basis and Ethical Outcomes

Christine Overall

Introduction

*"**Live long and prosper**"* (Vulcan greeting from the original *Star Trek* "First Contact" series).

Any inquiry into the meaning and implications of the prolongation of the human lifespan requires an investigation of its metaphysical basis and its ethical outcomes. In this chapter I state and explain a series of metaphysical and ethical claims about lifespan extension (see also Overall, 2003a, 2003b, 2004a, 2004b, 2006a, 2006b, 2006c, 2008). Along the way I highlight a number of arguments that are typically put forward against these claims, and I show the ways in which they are mistaken.

> *Metaphysical Claim #1: Aging and life stages are neither wholly constituted by biological givens, nor wholly understandable in terms of biological parameters. Instead, aging and life stages are, in crucial ways, socially constructed.*

Aging – what it is and how it is experienced – is affected by social action and inaction: access to health care or not, water and nourishing food, housing, education, and work, whether paid or unpaid. All of these features are the result of human action and inaction. Moreover, aging is also affected by attitudes: whether the society in which one lives welcomes or shuns, values or rejects people as they age, and whether aging people are fully integrated into society and experience loving, respectful, supportive relationships.

Aging is therefore not a unitary, monolithic state, condition, or experience. What it is and how it is experienced are determined by the social conditions within which it occurs. This is not to deny the reality of the body or the immediacy of some changing capacities that may accompany the process of aging for some, though not all, persons. But within different social contexts, characteristics of the aging person may or may not be recognized as liabilities and defects – rather than as, for example, reserves of wisdom or the fruits of years of experience.

Enhancing Human Capacities, edited by Julian Savulescu, Ruud ter Meulen and Guy Kahane.
© 2011 Blackwell Publishing Ltd

Moreover, aging is socially constructed insofar as there is no definite, biologically given number of years lived that, by itself, constitutes being old in any transcultural sense, or that provides an immutable and inevitable foundation on the basis of which social aging processes are built. Years lived do not, of themselves, constitute one's age – whether it be in youth, middle age, or old age. Different cultures, at different times, *pick out* a certain number of years and *attribute* biological and cultural significance to that number as constituting the state of being old, physically and mentally worn out, no longer in one's prime, and near the end of one's life. "Old age" can also be *redefined* or expanded, by picking out different numbers of years lived and/or new arrays of features and defining them as constituting oldness.

The state that was regarded as being "old age" came much earlier a century or even half a century ago than it does now. Sixty-five, sixty, or even fifty-five was once considered definitively, inevitably, and unavoidably old, even though there were always some individuals who lived much longer than these ages, into their eighties and nineties. But over the past century, with improvements in health, nutrition, and education, and as more people work, both with and without pay, well after the normative date for retirement, none of these ages is considered as "old" as it once was. The social and medical changes that enable people to live longer and healthier lives create an environment in which human beings can redefine and reschedule former life milestones. Oldness has gotten older, so to speak, and is probably now around seventy-five or eighty. All life-stage concepts are not just empirical reflections of the actual duration of objectively given human life stages, but the product of socially shaped material conditions. They also incorporate and reduplicate normative judgments about how long both the parts and the whole of human life *ought* to be (Overall, 2006a).

Nonetheless, opponents of lifespan increases often argue there is an inherent "rhythm" to human life. Eric T. Juengst calls this view "life-cycle traditionalism" (Juengst, 2004, p.331). It is a deeply conservative theory, according to which "nature" provides us with the moral message that human beings should simply accept their aging and death, not resist it or rail against it. "Whether or not the biological changes of aging are beneficial or harmful, they are meaningful: they and their natural timing constitute part of the normal life cycle for human beings and thus part of what it means to be human" (Juengst, 2004, p.328).

But as Betty Friedan wisely notes, "The very concept of 'normal aging' denies the *developmental possibilities* of age as a unique period of human life" (Friedan, 1993, p.84, her emphasis). The history of humanity is, in part, a history of creative response and resistance to the apparent facticity of our existence. Through medicine, social policy, education, engineering, and art we have consistently changed our supposed biological inheritance. Without eye glasses, most middle-aged and elderly people would have varying degrees of visual impairment. Society does not refuse to provide eye glasses to such people just because it is "normal" for them to suffer from near-sightedness or far-sightedness. Instead, society happily makes such people's vision "better than normal," through the availability of eye care, regular vision examinations, and eye glasses and contact lenses. And just as humankind has not acquiesced in the supposed biological imperative that compelled women to experience constant pregnancies, so also human-kind need not accept our current lifespan but can choose to make deliberate attempts to improve it.

Skeptics about the value of a longer life sometimes write, mistakenly, as if human beings have never before taken action, individually or collectively, to increase the human lifespan. Thus, bioethicist Leon Kass,[1] in an argument that he attributes to unidentified "critics" of lifespan extension, suggests that "the retardation of aging will present a classic instance of the Tragedy of the Commons, in which genuine and sought-for gains to individuals are nullified or worse, owing to the social consequences of granting them to everyone" (Kass, 2004, p.308). But such an argument overlooks the fact that "the retardation of aging" has been going on for at least two centuries, with no resulting tragedy from the extension of life that has been produced by reduced infant and maternal mortality, better hygiene, improved nutrition, and the use of preventive medicine such as vaccines against deadly diseases.[2]

Metaphysical Claim #2: *Aging, life stages, and death are gendered.*

Given that aging, life stages, and death are socially constructed, they are in no way immune to the effects of the social categories that shape the lives of all of us. As a result, aging, life stages, and death are not gender neutral.

James Lindemann Nelson argues, for example, that the significance of death is not merely a function of an individual's age, but must be understood more broadly, by reference to the burdens and benefits, duties and responsibilities, that are available to or even enforced upon individuals. Two persons who die at seventy-five are not necessarily similarly situated if they are of different genders, for their gender helps to determine the kind of life they had. One may have had a full and rewarding life, and the other may not. Both the goods that they receive (or do not receive) and the moral obligations that are incumbent upon them are dependent upon society's interpretation of their gender (Nelson, 1999, p.116). Similarly, Norah Kizer Bell argues that the belief that a person's life is complete at a particular age fails to take account of the ways in which women, in contrast to men, may have experienced a diminishment of their goals, indifference to their "life possibilities," and an irresistible requirement that they occupy service roles (Bell, 1992, p.85). The existence of gendered expectations about women's biological and cultural roles makes it less likely that women will have had a full human life than many men may have had, and more likely that the quality of their lives may be lower than those of men (Bell, 1992, p.86).

Moreover, gender stereotyping inflicts upon many women a two-fold liability. On the one hand, women are often valued primarily for their role as caregivers, and therefore may have had fewer opportunities than men to explore a broader range of personal and work-related goals. On the other hand, as they age, women may not be valued if they give up the care-giving role, or if they become, themselves, the subjects of care. In a culture that is accustomed to taking for granted the self-effacing care-giving behavior of women, the prospect of losing that care giving and instead having to care for and support old women may help to generate an implicitly gender-biased argument against prolonging human life, since such prolongation in fact may primarily benefit women. As Bell says, the perceived absence of value for very old people, and reluctance to provide the services to sustain their lives, may be "due in large measure to the fact that there are few male competitors for these services" (Bell, 1992, p.88).

It is also important to remember that gender affects the aging of males. Worldwide, men have a lower life expectancy than women. The list of causes for men's lower life expectancy includes a mix of what appear to be physical and social factors. But since human beings are thoroughly social animals, no aspect of our physical being is immune to social influence. For example, men's greater tendency to heart disease is exacerbated by cultural conditions that promote and support smoking and alcohol consumption. Men also receive strong encouragement, even the requirement, to engage in risk-taking behavior, to labor in difficult and dangerous jobs, to fight, and to serve as cannon-fodder. Because all of these characteristics are social, they may – despite the difficulties of altering the socialization process – be open to change.

Hence, the features of aging and our reactions to it, the construction of life stages, resistance to lifespan extension, and even death itself have a deeply gendered dimension.

Metaphysical Claim #3: *The extension of lifespan need not threaten personal identity and integrity.*

Philosopher Bernard Williams believes there is a danger that greatly lengthened life will threaten one's personal identity. Beyond a certain point, new experiences and further development would change a person so utterly as to yield the result that she is literally no longer the same person, and will feel no attachment to that person (Williams, 1975). Similarly, Kass argues that there is a "deep confusion" in "choosing to have some great good only on the condition of turning into someone else" (Kass, 2004, p.311). He thinks there is something irrational about selecting a particular condition or goal that we know will make us very different.

Williams may be right to be concerned about the preservation of personal identity under (the impossible) conditions of immortality. But if what is at issue is simply an *increase* in the human lifespan by fifty or even one hundred years, then worries about the persistence of personal identity are unjustified. Personal identity will be preserved even if a longer lifespan entails the opportunity for human beings to choose to make major changes – psychological, intellectual, spiritual, physical, and material – in their lives.

Given that personality changes usually take place gradually, over a period of time, and that sudden discontinuities in the evolution of character are not inevitable, it is difficult to see why an individual who is developing and changing over a large number of years would necessarily cease to be the same person. To the degree that the individual is different from her previous self, yet that difference was desired and sought by her previous self, the change may be good, not bad, and rationally chosen. Indeed, it may be more valuable than remaining unchanged. Even within our existing lifespan, a person may rationally choose to immigrate to a nation very different from her own, to become a mother, or to convert to a new religion. In each case, the individual has good reason to believe she will be different after acting on her choice. But there is nothing that is inevitably "confused" about making such choices, and the individual's identity is not thereby shattered.

Convinced that a substantial extension of lifespan would compromise personal identity, Walter Glannon (2002, p.268) argues,

[T]he connections between earlier and later mental states in a life of roughly 200 years would be so weak that there would not be any good reason to care about the future selves who had these states. The selves would exist at a future time that would not matter to us, given the nature of our present mental states and the limit to which their contents can extend into the future.

But the reality is that very few people create grand plans that cover a lifetime of activities. Nor should we be expected to. Our connection to our future states is not direct, but only via the intervening stages. Almost everyone looks forward, at most, to just the next stage of her or his life. Each new stage of one's life is a product of the previous one. One's current self at time T can rationally aspire to become one's self at time T+1, which can then aspire to become one's self at time T+2, and so on indefinitely. The person herself persists throughout these transformations because each transformed version of the self is desired and actively sought by the previous one, so that the transformed self grows out of the previous self and can be understood in terms of characteristics of the previous self (Nozick, 1981, p.35). In this way, the future experiences that one has as a transformed self can be anticipated to be as much one's own as would be the future experiences that one would have had if one had not gone through the process of transformation.

Moreover, the continuity of personal identity over large periods of time is supported by sources in addition to our own memories. The ongoing presence of other people in one's life – friends, neighbors, family members, co-workers – provide continuity. It might be objected that it is very unlikely that one person will be present throughout one's life. This is true, but the continuity of just one person is unnecessary to obtaining the sense of personal identity. People overlap in one's life. Some family members are present from one's earliest memories; friends and new family members come into one's life; they in turn are overlapped by co-workers, and so on. We also get a sense of personal identity via the memories that others have of us (Scheman, 1997, p.126). People narrate their memories, which provide a confirmation of and a correction and supplement to our own. Finally, for almost everyone there are material records that help to confirm and contain our identity. They can include childhood drawings, school records, diaries, letters sent and received, photographs, and all the many videos, recordings, e-mail messages, computer files, memos, minutes of meetings, and text messages that one either created or in which one participated. In the future, technology may provide additional methods for sustaining identity, for example, via "neuron-computer interfacing or even the gradual replacement of biological memory by more reliable, artificial structures" (Schloendorn, 2006, p.200).

Ethical Claim #1: Death is bad, and other things being equal, a longer life is a better life.

Despite contemporary attempts to glamorize death, and frequent excoriations in the press of Westerners who supposedly, in contrast to people in the East, fear death and try to banish it from their lives, it is reasonable to resist death and wish to postpone it. Death is not our little friend, to be welcomed as a savior or hailed as that which allegedly gives meaning to life. Kass repeats the usual platitude when he says, "To know and to feel that one goes around only once, and that the deadline is not out of sight, is for many people the necessary spur to the pursuit of something worthwhile" (Kass, 2004, p.313). If that were true, then young people – who notoriously have little or no sense of their own mortality – would never be able to engage in worthwhile activities.

Those who advocate increasing lifespan wish to prolong human life not because they dread the state of being dead, but because they value the state of being alive. As Thomas Nagel (1975, p.407, his emphasis) expresses it,

> [T]he time after [a person's] death is time of which his death deprives him. It is time in which, had he not died then, he would be alive. Therefore any death entails the loss of *some* life that its victim would have led had he not died at that or any earlier point.

Those who fear death are not fearing some supposed state of nothingness after death, but rather are dreading, and reasonably so, the end of their existence. Other things being equal (that is, in the absence of severe, unremitting, and incurable pain, or [possibly] total incapacitation) it is always (on balance?) a benefit to have a longer life.

Opponents of lifespan extension insist that the current lifespan is entirely adequate for human beings. The vociferous opponent of lifespan extension Daniel Callahan argues that "at some point it [life] *will* end, and, in light of the infinite number of years we will be dead, a few years longer of life seems inconsequential, particularly after we have already lived a full life" (Callahan, 2006, p.572, his emphasis). Moreover, "a life of eighty years or so is sufficiently long to experience most of the goods of human life" (Callahan, 2006, p.573). But first, it's unlikely that anyone assesses her life by reference to the infinite number of years she will be dead. What matters are the years during which she is alive, and their value is not the least compromised by the number of years she will be dead. Second, many of the lucky minority who live to eighty have not experienced a "full life". And third, it is not self-evident that eighty years, even under the best conditions, constitute a full life.

The case for valuing longer life is not based upon claims about the supposed intrinsic value of longevity, of life itself, or of individual human lives (Overall, 2003a). Instead, it is founded upon respect for human potential, and an appreciation of what people want within their lives and are capable of doing and experiencing when given more time and more opportunities. An increased lifespan provides individual human beings with the chance for activities and experiences that they would not otherwise have enjoyed. Collectively, extending the lifespan provides for the society in which it occurs the value of increased experience, know-how, labor, loving relationships, and so on – that is, everything that healthy old(er) people can contribute.

Some have stated that even a modest extension of the lifespan would result in tedium and boredom. According to Kass (2004, p.313),

> If the human lifespan were increased even by only twenty years, would the pleasures of life increase proportionately? Would professional tennis players really enjoy playing 25 per cent more games of tennis? Would the Don Juans of our world feel better for having seduced 1250 women rather than 1000? Having experienced the joys and tribulations of raising a family until the last left for college, how many parents would like to extend the experience by another ten years? Likewise, those whose satisfaction comes from climbing the career ladder might well ask what there would be to do for fifteen years after one had been CEO of Microsoft, a member of Congress, or the president of Harvard for a quarter of a century.

This remarkable argument betrays a singular lack of imagination. Kass fails to recognize that the vast majority of people will never be professional tennis players, CEOs, or politicians. So, even if such jobs may become tiresome, they are not a problem for any but a minute fraction of 1% of the population. Indeed, poor and working-class people, members of racial minorities, and people with disabilities, who are likely to miss out on a lot of life's goods, might welcome the challenges and financial rewards of professional work.

What is important in extended life is the exploration of one's talents, capacities, and potential. It is likely that as lives get longer, the content of individuals' goals will change, and people will play a larger variety of roles (familial, domestic, community, work, and volunteer functions) during their lifetimes. Like today, people will undertake new tasks, projects, and interests at different life stages, but if those life stages are longer, then the range of tasks, projects, relationships, and interests can become broader.

But extended life also provides more opportunities for small pleasures, repeated activities, and renewed connections. These are the sorts of things that Kass and others who worry about the alleged boredom of lifespan extension fail to value.[3] They include spending time with family and friends, listening to music, planting a garden, or enjoying a meal. Life need not consist of one grand project after another. While the stressful (but materially rewarding) life of a university president is open to very few and may in any case lose its allure, the small satisfactions of life are available to almost everyone and often do not lose their value. Moreover, they are renewable resources: Human beings can go on enjoying them almost until death. The claim that a longer life will inevitably be boring and unrewarding is highly implausible.

Ethical Claim #2: *The lifespan should be extended, in accord with carefully considered moral guidelines.*

The human lifespan is not just a matter of "nature," of what is given and must be accepted. If we opt not to extend the lifespan, then we are simply submitting to the exigencies of particular phase of human history. We are saying, in effect, "So far and no further. Scientists, educators, and governments have assisted human beings (at least many of us in the privileged West) to double our life expectancy over the past century. But we will accept the situation at which we have now arrived and not strive for more." At the very least, the burden of proof for such a decision must rest upon those who advocate and defend it, for they are, in effect, calling for a halt in the various human ongoing projects that have enabled human beings in the West to enjoy a healthier and longer life.

Of course, the mere availability of technology for life extension does not, in itself, constitute a case for life extension. Opponents of lifespan extension such as Kass appear to believe, incorrectly, that the technological imperative is the main argument put forward by those who support lifespan extension. Kass (2004, p.308) writes,

> [A] new moral sensibility has developed that serves precisely medicine's crusade against mortality: anything is permitted if it saves life, cures disease, prevents death. … [E]verything should be done to preserve health and prolong life as much as possible, and … all other values must bow before the biomedical gods of better health, greater vigor, and longer life.

Technological capacity alone exerts no moral imperative, and those who wish to press forward with further attempts at life extension merely because it is medically possible are doing so on wholly inadequate grounds. Just as our seemingly biological nature is socially constructed, so also is, of course, technology. What we do with them is a matter of moral decision, and how we act with respect to them must be the subject of ethical debate. Neither biology nor technology tells us what to do, or what we ought to do.

There is, therefore, a legitimate need for debate about means and ends with respect to lifespan extension. How much longer life should we be aiming for? For whom should longer life be available? What are the appropriate steps for increasing the human lifespan? What limitations on the means are morally justified?

Now, Kass (2004, p.309) disparages any such attempts at discussion, and suggests that there is no principled way to answer these questions:

> Which of us would find unreasonable or unwelcome the addition of ten healthy and vigorous years to his or her life . . .? . . . Maybe we should ask for five years on top of that? Or ten? Why not fifteen, or twenty, or more? If we can't immediately land on the reasonable number of added years, perhaps we can locate the principle. What is the principle of reasonableness? . . . We have no answer to this question.

Here we have a classic slippery-slope argument, intended to show that there is no rational way of arriving at a good answer to the question, How much longer should the human lifespan be? It provides no evidence to show that the question cannot be answered. But it is only via systematically searching for potential principles and then evaluating them that we can decide whether or not there are significant criteria by means of which questions of means and ends can be answered.

One possible criterion is justice. Hence the third ethical claim.

Ethical Claim #3: Social policy with respect to lifespan extension should take into account the gendering of aging and death and should be shaped by concerns for justice and human well-being.

Kass says that a criticism of lifespan extension is the worry that "technology's gift" of long life "will not be granted to everyone, especially if, as is likely, the treatments turn out to be expensive" (Kass 2004, p.308). Surely, then, it is worthwhile to consider how increases in lifespan may be made compatible with fairness to everyone. We already know that life expectancy varies by gender, race, and socioeconomic class. We have a moral responsibility to erase or at least reduce these disparities, and then avoid reintroducing them via any new methods of lifespan increase.

Roberto Mordacci distinguishes between extending the number of long lives and extending the human lifespan. "More of long lives does not imply longer lives" (Mordacci, 2007, p.1). He is correct. But in extending the lifespan, we should also not neglect to create more long lives. We should not favor a longer lifespan for only a privileged few, especially if it is to the neglect of the well-being of the many. Moreover, what works to extend the lifespan may also contribute to lengthening the lives of everyone.

Because not every person has enjoyed fair and equal opportunities, it is false to assume that all elderly persons – and especially those who are female, who have disabilities, who are poor, and/or who are racially identified – have already experienced all of life's goods and should be ready to die. Therefore, research and support for the extension of lifespan should place a special emphasis on benefiting members of disadvantaged groups, who seldom have much prospect of living out a long life.

Juengst, however, pessimistically worries that the experience of a debilitating old age may be needed both to enable elderly people to develop wisdom and to enable their offspring to manifest "filial maturity" in caring for their parents (Juengst, 2004, p.333). Hence, attempts to prolong life and ameliorate aging would have a spoiler effect upon family relations. But having aging, increasingly dependent parents does not necessarily evoke a caring response from their children. If it did, there would be no elderly people warehoused in old people's residences. In any case, treating frail old people as a means to the moral development of their offspring violates the basic principle that individuals should not be used as means to the ends of other people.

Juengst also cites, without entirely endorsing, a claim that "the anti-aging enterprise is complicitous with prejudicial social attitudes toward aging and the elderly, and would feed discrimination against those who do age normally. On this view, an anti-aging ideology within medicine could be just as pernicious as medical racism and sexism and should be similarly eschewed as a professional perversion" (Juengst, 2004, p.323). In other words, the project of lifespan extension is not beneficial to aging and elderly people, but will inevitably contribute to their oppression. But if this approach were justified, it would seem to imply that medicine should also do nothing to correct impairments and improve the health of persons with disabilities, lest doing so exacerbate ableism. It is not, in fact, inevitable that helping people to avoid the liabilities attendant upon their social identity will increase the oppression of people with that social identity. Instead, supporting and assisting individuals in a stigmatized group makes them better able to resist their oppression, and constitutes a powerful social message saying that persons in that group deserve fair treatment that promotes their well-being.

Some opponents of lifespan extension pessimistically claim both that the aspiration for lifespan increase and the effects of lifespan increase are and will be morally retrograde. Concomitant with a continuing search for the extension of human life, Kass predicts a weakening of our sense of beauty and our capacity to love (Kass, 2004, pp.313–14). He believes that all of "virtue and moral excellence" depend upon the fact of human mortality (Kass, 2004, p.314). The implication is that true morality is not an expression of compassion, justice, and human solidarity, but is occasioned primarily by the fact that we age and die. This is surely an *a priori* claim in no way testable by empirical observation, and it reflects an improbable notion of what motivates morality.

Kass also holds that the quest for lifespan extension is responsible for most of what is problematic in twenty-first-century Western life. He says that the pursuit of the conquest of death

> Threatens – already threatens, human happiness by distracting us from the goals toward which our souls naturally point. By diverting our aim, by misdirecting so much individual and social energy toward the goal of bodily immortality, we may seriously undermine our chances for living as well as we can and for satisfying to some extent, however incompletely, our deepest longings for what is best (Kass, 2004, p.316).

Given that Kass yet again provides no argument to support this claim, it is difficult to know what to make of it. In fact, very little individual and social energy is directed toward *immortality*. In most places in the world, individual energy is devoted to staying alive and ensuring that one's family stays alive. "*Social* energy," if there is such a thing, tends, regrettably, to be devoted to enhancing the well-being of members of the dominant group. A concern for justice and well-being for everyone, including the opportunity to live a longer life, is more likely to help satisfy "our deepest longings for what is best" than is abandoning any quest to extend the human lifespan. Indeed, the extension of the human lifespan provides the opportunity for more cultivation of our sense of beauty, our capacity to love, our moral excellence, and our individual and collective happiness.

Kass's final argument is perhaps his most troubling. He says, "in all higher animals, reproduction *as such* implies both the acceptance of the death of the self and participation in its transcendence. . . . Biological considerations aside, simply to covet a prolonged lifespan for ourselves is both a sign and a cause of our failure to open ourselves to procreation and to any higher purpose. . . . It is in principle hostile to children, because children, those who come after, are those who will take one's place . . ." (Kass, 2004, p.317, his emphasis).

It is hard to know what evidence could be given for the claim that procreation in itself implies the acceptance of death of the self. The claim is virtually meaningless. It's unlikely that most pregnant women contemplate the death of the self. It's unlikely that parents are obsessed with their own death – other than, perhaps, to try to ward it off because they want to care for their children and see them through to adulthood and beyond. Wanting to have a longer life is, in fact, a child-friendly goal, for it seeks to ensure that healthy adults will be around to care for children as they mature, to support and encourage their grandchildren, and to be part of their great-grandchildren's lives. It is also false that those who promote the extension of the human lifespan are not open to procreation; many of us have offspring. At the same time, it is wrong to imply that everyone must be "open to procreation". Such an exhortation is especially dangerous for women, who, both biologically and socially, bear most of the responsibility for the next generation. A woman who decides to have no children at all is not thereby closed to any "higher purpose". Her childlessness may, indeed, be a way to serve a higher purpose.[4]

There is no inevitable conflict between lifespan extension and morality. Indeed, living longer provides human beings with opportunities for greater moral growth.

"*Peace and long life*" (Vulcan response to "live long and prosper," from the original *Star Trek* "First Contact" series)

The extension of the human lifespan is of significant value because it provides human beings with opportunities for activities and experiences that they would not otherwise have enjoyed if their lives had ended sooner. This is not to say that every prolonged life is necessarily good, that no one may ever rationally reject a longer life, or that all persons will inevitably make good use of the years they have. But it is to say that what is evil about death, especially a death that is earlier than necessary, is that it terminates all possibilities for anything more. Lifespan extension therefore is, at its best, a deeply moral project whose value has already stood the test of two hundred years of human effort. It deserves to continue.

Acknowledgments

For their comments and suggestions I am grateful to Roberto Mordacci, of San Rafaelle University, and the other participants at the Second International Workshop on the Extension of Lifespan, Faculty of Philosophy, San Raffaele University, Cesano Maderno, May 17–18, 2007.

Notes

1. In what follows, I focus on many of Kass's arguments because they so clearly represent the views of the opponents of lifespan extension.
2. Walter Glannon says, "[I]f everyone were to live much longer than they actually do, and the availability of resources did not increase, then more people competing for the same amount of resources over an extended period of time likely would lower the overall quality of life for all people" (Glannon 2002, 274). That statement reflects the real Tragedy of the Commons: the short-sighted overconsumption of resources by privileged members of Western societies, and the assumption that such overconsumption is justified and should continue (or cannot be prevented from continuing).
3. Perhaps they are subject to an unconscious Puritanism that rejects the value of pleasure.
4. The more education women have, the fewer children they have. Thus, the education of women is one answer to the concerns of those who think that lifespan extension will contribute to overpopulation.

References

Bell, N.K. (1992). If age becomes a standard for rationing health care.... In H.B. Holmes & L.M. Purdy (eds.), *Feminist Perspectives in Medical Ethics* (pp. 82–90). Bloomington: Indiana University Press.

Callahan, D. (2006). Longer lives – Whose good? Part of a symposium on *Aging, Death, and Human Longevity: A Philosophical Inquiry. Dialogue*, **XLV**(3) 567–75.

Friedan, B. (1993). *The Fountain of Age*. New York: Simon & Schuster.

Glannon, W. (2002). Identity, prudential concern, and extended lives. *Bioethics*, 16(3), 266–83.

Juengst, E.T. (2004). Anti-aging research and the limits of medicine. In S.G. Post & R.H. Binstock (eds.), *The Fountain of Youth: Cultural, Scientific, and Ethical Perspectives on a Biomedical Goal* (pp. 321–39). New York: Oxford University Press.

Kass, L. (2004). L'Chaim and its limits: Why not immortality? In S.G. Post & R.H. Binstock (eds.), *The Fountain of Youth: Cultural, Scientific, and Ethical Perspectives on a Biomedical Goal* (pp. 304–20). New York: Oxford University Press.

Mordacci, R. (2007). Lifespan extension, living personally and social justice. Paper presented at the Second International Workshop on the Extension of Lifespan, San Raffaele University, Cesano Maderno, May 17, 2007.

Nagel, T. (1975). Death. In J. Rachels (ed.), *Moral Problems: A Collection of Philosophical Essays*, 2nd edition (pp. 401–9). New York: Harper & Row.

Nelson, J.L. (1999). Death's gender. In M.U. Walker (ed.), *Mother Time: Women, Aging, and Ethics* (pp. 113–29) Lanham, MD: Rowman & Littlefield.

Nozick, R. (1981). *Philosophical Explanations*. Cambridge, MA: Belknap Press.

Overall, C. (2003a). *Aging, Death, and Human Longevity: A Philosophical Inquiry*. Berkeley, CA: University of California Press.

Overall, C. (2003b). Concepts of lifespan and life-stages: Implications for ethics. In S. Brennan (ed.), *Feminist Moral Philosophy (Canadian Journal of Philosophy* Supplementary Volume 28, pp. 299–318). Calgary: University of Calgary Press.

Overall, C. (2004a). Longevity, identity, and moral character: A feminist approach. In S.G. Post & R.H. Binstock (eds.), *The Fountain of Youth: Cultural, Scientific, and Ethical Perspectives on a Biomedical Goal* (pp. 286–303). New York: Oxford University Press.

Overall, C. (2004b). Optimism, pessimism, and the desire for longer life, review essay of *A History of Ideas about the Prolongation of Life* by Gruman, G., and *The Prolongation of Life: Optimistic Studies* by Metchnikoff, I.I. *The Gerontologist*, **44**, 847–51.

Overall, C. (2006a). Old age and ageism, impairment and ableism: Exploring the conceptual and material connections. *National Women's Studies Association Journal Special Issue on Aging, Ageism, and Old Age*, **18**(1), 126–37.

Overall, C. (2006b). Précis of aging, death, and human longevity. *Dialogue*, **XLV**(3) 537–48.

Overall, C. (2006c). Staying alive (a response to commentators). *Dialogue*, **XLV**(3) 577–90.

Overall, C. (2008). Life enhancement technologies and the significance of social category membership. In N. Bostrom & J. Savulescu (eds.), *The Ethics of Human Enhancement*. Oxford: Oxford University Press.

Scheman, N. (1997). Queering the center by centering the queer. In D.T. Meyers (ed.), *Feminists Rethink the Self* (pp. 124–62) Boulder, CO: Westview Press.

Schloendorn, J. (2006). Making the case for human life extension: Personal arguments. *Bioethics*, **20**(4), 191–202.

Williams, B. (1975). The Makropulos case: Reflections on the tedium of immortality. In J. Rachels (ed.), *Moral Problems: A Collection of Philosophical Essays*, 2nd edition (pp. 410–28). New York: Harper & Row.

29

Life Extension and Personal Identity

Gaia Barazzetti and Massimo Reichlin

Life Extension, "Sameness" and "Selfhood"

There is growing public interest in developing biomedical technologies capable of extending the human lifespan (Turner, 2004). What lies behind this interest is what Robert Binstock and Stephen Post refer to as the search for "prolongevity," that is a "significant extension of the length of human life, free from the diseases and disabilities now associated with old age."[1] This is precisely what we will mean by life extension: a substantial increase in the human lifespan characterized by health and good quality of life. As a consequence, we will not consider the prospect of lengthening life without an appreciable reduction of the debilitations of aging, the so-called "prolonged senescence" scenario of life extension (Juengst *et al.*, 2003). Nor we will consider the possibility of a slowing down of the aging process that may result in only a moderate extension of healthy productive lifespan.[2]

We will assume the prospect of counteracting the aging process at the cellular and molecular level (de Grey *et al.*, 2002), thus prolonging human life far beyond the historical record of the maximum individual lifespan (i.e. age 122) (Robine & Allard, 1999). Should this become possible, such a scenario would impact our understanding of the human condition, since, for the first time in history, human beings would experience centenarians' lives, thus breaking the limits imposed by the natural process of aging. This raises the pivotal question whether this is a desirable prospect for the individual human being.

In particular, we will discuss the desirability of a substantial life extension with regard to its implications for personal identity over time.[3] The possibility of significant lifespan extension involves two different personal-identity questions. First, it raises the question of whether one is identifiable as the very same person throughout a lifetime; secondly, it challenges our self-conception. David DeGrazia (2005) claims that these two distinct questions are at issue when we examine the relationship between enhancement technologies and personal identity, and that they refer to at least two different views on personal identity over time, namely the "numerical" and the "narrative" views.

Enhancing Human Capacities, edited by Julian Savulescu, Ruud ter Meulen and Guy Kahane.
© 2011 Blackwell Publishing Ltd

This framework has been thoroughly reviewed by Marya Schechtman (1996) in terms of the distinction between the "reidentification" question and the "characterization" question, and can be traced back to Paul Ricoeur (1992), who first distinguished between the idea of personal identity as "sameness," and personal identity as "selfhood."

In general, an account of personal identity as "sameness" aims at providing criteria on the basis of which one can determine whether an individual at one time is identical to another individual at some later time. This approach to the concept of personal identity has been extensively discussed in the philosophical literature (Noonan, 2003). This notion of personal identity results in an inquiry into which criteria of persistence over time (namely: bodily, brain, physical, memory, psychological, etc.) determine whether changes, occurring over a lifetime, undermine the identity of an individual. Generally speaking, from this point of view personal identity is something that has to be conceptualized and explained in terms of intrinsic or causal relationships between an individual P1 at time t1 and an individual P2 at time t2.

Unlike the notion of personal identity over time as "sameness," the notion of personal identity as "selfhood" focuses on the individual's self-conception, self-evaluation, and self-development throughout a lifetime. Such an account of personal identity over time is methodologically different in that individuals are conceived as authors of their own identity over time by their capacity for agency. On this view, what matters in survival is not merely persistence as may be attested to by constitutive or evidential criteria, but that we, as authors of our present self-narratives, will continue to exist and to develop our self-narratives into the future.

Both of these notions of personal identity entail theoretical as well as practical consequences for our identity as persons. Indeed, they both involve the question of our identity as unitary continuing entities as well as the question of our concern for our future selves.

We will explore what each of these accounts of personal identity suggests for the prospect of radical life extension with a view to assessing the desirability of a centenarian life for the person concerned. First, we will consider the way in which personal identity as "sameness" might be affected by the prospect of substantial life extension. Then, we will turn our attention to the significance of the conception of personal identity as "selfhood" for radically extended lifespans. Finally, we will argue that a substantial life extension raises important concerns about the continuity of one's identity over time and is not straightforwardly desirable for the individual.

"What Matters" in Life Extension?

Let us assume the possibility of prolonging human lifespan up to 300 years. This substantial lifespan extension raises some fundamental questions concerning the 300-year-old person's identity. Will the person at age 300 be the very same person he/she was at age 30?

We will contend that what is at stake in the case of substantial life extension is not merely an assessment of whether a person at 30 is the same person at 300. Rather, life extension technologies question the very belief that what matters in survival is personal identity as "sameness."[4] We will start by considering Parfit's discussion of the so-called "psychological continuity criterion,"[5] since the Parfitian thesis on what matters in survival raises a somewhat counterintuitive but powerful argument in favor of substantial lifespan extension.

The general idea grounding this criterion is that the "continuity" of different kinds of strong psychological connections (memories, beliefs, desires, as well as the connection between an intention and a later act) is constitutive of the persistence of personal identity over time. On this view, direct links of causal dependence between a present mental state and each of the following mental states will result in strong psychological "connectedness," while "continuity" is defined as the existence of traceable overlapping chains of such strong psychological connections over time. It follows that, according to the "psychological continuity criterion" of personal identity, P2 at t2 is the same person as P1 at t1 if and only if P2 at t2 is psychologically continuous with P1 at t1.

As Derek Parfit observes, such a "psychological continuity criterion" of personal identity (which he calls "Relation-R") requires that personal identity is a one-one (i.e. transitive) relation, and that it does not admit of any degrees. However, according to Parfit, there are puzzle cases that may challenge this conception of personal identity over time. One of these cases is that of a population of "immortals" with everlasting but gradually changing bodies. Parfit argues that, in this case, direct mental connectedness may eventually fade away, since connectedness can weaken when it holds over long eons of time, and Relation-R may show intransitivity. We could easily conjecture a similar case, where individuals are not immortal but may survive to age 300 thanks to innovative life-extension technologies aimed at counteracting the aging process at the cellular and molecular level.

Confronted by the imaginary but logically persuasive case of the "immortals," Parfit (1984) claims that identity, as conceptualized by the "psychological continuity criterion," is not what matters in survival. Rather, he advocates a variant of the criterion which he refers to as "psychological connectedness and/or continuity" in a wide sense. Thus, Parfit proposes a new version of "Relation-R" as a non-transitive relation which admits of degrees in psychological connectedness, and in which continuity is no longer necessary. This new version of "Relation-R" is combined with a "reductionist view" of persons, according to which persons are nothing over and above their brains and bodies, and "the occurrence of a series of interrelated physical and mental events" (Parfit, 1984). Finally, Parfit argues that our brains and bodies are merely accidental causes of our "psychological connectedness and/or continuity," thus opening the possibility that "Relation-R" may be copied and transferred to another brain and body, or that it may hold in more than one body. In this respect, Christine Korsgaard (1996) points out that Parfit's "Relation-R" may be represented in Aristotelian terms as a "formal" relation, which ultimately consists in the way our physical matter is organized, rather than in the particular physical matter of our brains and bodies.

Parfit's arguments have two implications for what concerns us, that is, the relationship between personal identity over time and the prospect of a substantial life extension. The first implication is that, according to Parfit, what should matter to "me" in survival is not that "I" (myself) will survive, but that someone will exist who is R-related (in a Parfitian sense) to me. The implication is counterintuitive, since it means that "I" might survive as "someone else," and that this is something that should be desirable for me. The second main implication of Parfit's arguments – as pointed out by Noonan – is that both our concerns about our future existence and our concerns about our future well-being are merely derivative, that is, they are not directly related to an end, rather they are the means to an end. According to Parfit, we should aim at the existence and well-being of a future person who will be sufficiently R-related to us, but we mistakenly believe that the means to such an end is our own survival. In other words, instead of being concerned with the future existence and well-being of our "Parfitian survivors," we wrongly believe that the only way to achieve this is by ensuring our "literal" survival. Of course, we are not aware of this mistake and of the fact that our concerns are merely derivative.

Following Parfit, we can conclude that it would be irrational for us not to use life-extension technologies, where available and effective, simply on the basis that they would not be identity preserving. Indeed, my interest in "literal" survival is merely a derivative interest. Rather, it could be rational to be prudentially concerned about our future selves, even though they are "someone else," since they would be "quasi me" (although "not me"). My "Parfitian survivors" would carry on my life plans and projects as if they were me. In other words, my future selves would be the best guarantee of the "quasi survival" of my own desires, ideals, memories, and of any other psychological and mental trait that characterizes me. For this reason, I could regard my future selves' well-being, pains, and pleasures as if they were my own. Therefore, life extension as the survival of "someone else" who is sufficiently R-related to me is something that should be regarded as desirable.

On this view, the question is only whether my future selves, following radical life extension, would be sufficiently R-related to me to justify my concern for their well-being. While it is highly probable that, at the age of 270, my R-related successive self will retain no memory of my interests and life concerns at 50, he/she will have memories of a previous self aged 220, who in turn had memories of a previous self aged 170. In this way, it may be that there is sufficient overlap between successive selves in order to justify our concern towards them. Indeed, a sufficient psychological connectedness between present and future selves may resemble the degree of psychological information we usually share with close friends (e.g. common life experiences, memories, projects, etc.) (Schloendorn, 2006). This degree of psychological connectedness is the rational ground for our concern towards close friends. Similarly, a sufficient psychological connectedness may uphold a substantial concern towards our future selves and, consequently, towards their survival.

It is interesting to note that, though Parfit's psychological theory of personal identity is by no means undisputed, the main philosophical alternative to it is no counter argument to its pro-life extension implications. In fact, the biological approach developed by Olson (1997) and endorsed by DeGrazia, is itself a powerful argument in favor of life extension.[6] By assuming that psychological continuity plays no part in assuring personal identity, which is really guaranteed by the permanence of the same human organism (or "animal") supporting and coordinating the basic biological functions, the biological approach seems to justify any intervention aimed at extending biological life, as long as the same brain stem supports the life of the organism, even in the complete absence of psychological connection.

A "conditional" argument for life extension can also be advanced on the basis of Robert Nozick's "closest continuer" theory (1981). Nozick argues that one may have fundamental concerns for his/her future self not simply because such future self is a "sufficiently R-related" continuer, but because he/she is the "closest" of one's continuers. According to Nozick's theory, a future self B is the "closest continuer" of a present self A only if B's features develop from or are causally related to A, and if there is no other future self C who is "closer" or "as close" to A as B.[7] Nozick claims that our concerns about future selves are not merely dependent – *à la* Parfit – on the holding of "psychological connectedness and/or continuity" (in the wide sense). Rather, our degree of care towards future selves is directly proportional to the "qualitative closeness" of these future selves. Consequentially, our degree of care depends on an evaluation of the best candidate for the continuation of our identity through time (Nozick, 1981). Indeed, the "closest continuer" relation is nothing more than the best realization of the relation of identity: we care about our "closest continuer" because what we care about is exactly our "continued identity" over time. However, this continuation entails a "surrogate" (not "literal") survival: my "closest" continuer is not "me"; rather, he/she is "someone else" whom I might consider as "the best instantiated realization" of my identity over time.[8]

Although Parfit and Nozick agree that our "literal" survival is not what matters, Nozick's "closest continuer" theory provides an argument against the idea that survival (or we may say: "radical life extension as a form of survival") is "always" the preferable option. Indeed, Nozick argues that the fact that we care about our "closest continuers" as far as they exist, does not imply that we should care that they actually exist: "I do care especially that there be a continuer that continues me closely enough to be me when it is my single continuation, but, given this, I do not care that there be a closest continuer" (1981). Such a paradoxical structure of our "carings" is not infrequent, and can be found in our attitudes towards infanticide and non-conception. (Nozick, 1981, p. 65)[9] The fact that we may find it elsewhere shows that this pattern of concern about future selves is not incoherent and that, consequently, we only "may" (not "should") rationally be concerned with the future existence and well-being of our "closest continuer." In other words, the fact that I may desire to live longer as my "closest continuer" does not prove that such a prospect is always desirable for me. Although this is not an argument against substantial life extension *per se*, Nozick's discussion of the special concern that we have towards our future selves suggests that, notwithstanding Parfit, the desirability of a substantial extension of human lifespan is not beyond question.

Nozick's theory is itself doubtful, however, since it implies the counterintuitive idea that the relation of identity between two individuals A and B depends on the existence or non-existence of some individual C, who might show a greater psychological connectedness to A, thus qualifying as the "closest continuer" (Rudder Baker, 2000, p. 135). The theory is also exposed to counterintuitive consequences in the event of two equally close continuers: if we imagine the transplantation of A's two cerebral hemispheres, in two other individuals B and C, it seems that A's identity should be considered as equally continuing in both B and C. That, of course, requires the denial of the transitivity of identity, since B and C, *ex hypotesi*, are *not* identical. And, if we assume that a relation of "closest continuity" is only the basis of egoistic concern, while denying that it is constitutive of identity, it seems that we are committed to the strange conclusion that we may have *egoistic* concern for a *plurality* of people.

Of "Character', "Agency" and Extended Lives

In this section we will turn our attention to the idea of personal identity over time as "selfhood." Before going into the details, it is worth stressing a core trait of the Parfitian account of personal identity, since this may help to understand the reasons why we are turning to a different paradigm of personal identity.[10]

Let us recall Parfit's claim that identity is not what matters in survival. This thesis turns out to be paradoxical in itself: how is it possible to inquire on "what matters" without caring about "to whom" it should matter? This is precisely the reason why Parfit's claim seems counterintuitive and disturbing: The reductionist attitude towards persons implies that it is possible to give an "impersonal" description of a person's identity over time "without either presupposing the identity of this person, or explicitly claiming that the experiences in this person's life are had by this person, or even explicitly claiming that this person exists" (Ricoeur, 1992, p. 210). Such an impersonal description of personal identity, which necessarily rules out any reference to the person's self-awareness, self-conception, and self-evaluation, justifies Parfit's under-scoring of puzzle cases, where physical as well as mental states are described as events that befall to persons, rather than as experiences of a self. But, despite Parfit's puzzle cases, we can neither easily put aside the fact that we perceive ourselves as enduring over time, nor neutralize our belief that what matters in survival is our own identity. This is not because, as Parfit would say, we are naive "non-reductionists" who wrongly believe in the existence of a separate entity, something like a Cartesian pure ego or a spiritual substance holding over and above our physical and mental states. Instead, it is the very same experience of ourselves as individuals existing over time that makes Parfit's claim counterintuitive and disturbing. In other words, we cannot simply rule out the question of personal identity over time as selfhood, unless we deliberately exclude it from the beginning, as Parfit does. Of course, Parfit does concede that there are two perspectives from which identity can be viewed. But he seems to view the perspective centering on identity as selfhood as a mere psychological epiphenomenon of the "real" fact, which is his view of identity as sameness; and he tends to dismiss this psychological phenomenon as a metaphysical relic. However, to have shown the possibility of constructing a reductionist theory of personal identity entirely "from without," so to speak, is not to have really done away with the lived experience of being the continuing author of one's life, that is, the perspective "from within."

Therefore, it seems to us that an exhaustive examination of the issues that life-extension technologies raises with respect to personal identity should include a discussion of "selfhood" in the sense of self-conception, self-evaluation, and self-development over time. Such a discussion will mainly focus on two ways in which we experience our identity over time as "selfhood": our "character," and the conception of ourselves as "agents."

Let us take up the discussion with the famous argument against immortality presented by Bernard Williams (1973) in "The Makropulos Case." Rather than concentrating on Williams' arguments against immortality, we will focus on his account of personal character. Indeed, this issue will be extremely fruitful for our discussion on personal identity and life extension.

Confronted with the question whether the perspective of immortality is desirable, Williams claims that it is not, since it very likely would result in tedium and insensitivity. Williams contends that, in order to be conceivable, immortality should satisfy at least two requirements: it should be clear that it will be "me" (i.e. "I" at this present stage in my life) who lives forever; and my future immortal self should be strongly related to the aims I now have in wanting to survive.

At the core of Williams' argument is what he refers to as the spectrum of the "constancy of character," i.e. the idea that immortal persons may be trapped in their own somewhat fixed character, incapable of prizing an everlasting life because of their limited and possibly already exhausted capacities for enjoying it. Williams concludes that, due to the "constancy of character," the perspective of immortality would not be appealing for the present self, since it would appear as the mere eternal continuation of the present self's life, and may eventually lead to an endless sense of ennui.

Williams (1981) deepens his analysis of character in a later essay where he points to an intrinsic relationship between the "individual person" and his/her "character," and provides us with a definition of character as an individual's personal set of desires and concerns. To quote Williams (1981, p. 5), "an individual person has a set of desires, concerns or, as I shall often call them, projects, which help to constitute a *character*." Williams further claims that character plays a crucial role in a person's concerns towards his/her own future. Indeed, that a person "now" should have some interest towards his/her "future" depends on the fact that he/she "now" has projects that refer to that "future." Williams (1981, p. 12) claims that "the correct perspective on one's life is *from now*." What he means is that a person is pushed forward by the projects that constitute his/her character, and that without the "perspective from now" he/she would not know why to go on. In other words, the pattern of projects that constitute his/her character, also constitute the condition for the existence of his/her own future; and the "perspective from now" is what gives us reasons for living.

Williams' theses on "character" and on the "perspective from now" provide a strong argument against life-extension technologies. And they seem to imply that a radically extended lifespan would not be a desirable perspective, since it would inevitably be associated with the "constancy of character." Indeed, since concerns about the future originate in one's present character, which is strongly dependent on the "perspective from now," it will not be possible to imagine one's future life outside the pattern of desires and concerns that constitute one's present character. The consequence would be boredom and insensitivity.

According to Christine Overall (2003), however, Williams' argument on the "constancy of character" is hardly convincing. Williams' mistake is in the fact that he considers the "fixity" of character as a necessary condition for the preservation of a person's identity over time. Overall (2003, p. 160) suggests that there is another way to avoid the loss of personal self-identity over time in the case of radically extended lifespans, which involves considering personal transformation as the possible object of one's rational desire: an individual could, in effect, aspire to "undergo a series of transformations of self." As a consequence, it may be possible to conceive of an individual undergoing a potentially infinite series of "personal transformations" that do not undermine the individual's identity. Thus, Overall imagines a series of selves (i.e. Self 1, Self 2, Self 3, etc.), each one aspiring to undergo a personal transformation that will result in a later self. The identity of the person persists throughout the series of transformations because each self in the series is causally generated by the previous one's wish for personal transformation.[11]

One more reservation about the desirability of a substantial life extension may be drawn from Christine Korsgaard's (1996, p. 378) discussion on the relationship between personal identity and agency. Korsgaard rejects Parfit's claim that it does not matter whether or not I am the same person as the "subject of experiences" who will be sufficiently R-related to me and will occupy my body in the future. Against Parfit, she contends that there are powerful "practical" reasons to regard oneself as the same "agent" who will occupy that same body in the future.

Korsgaard points out that the "reductionist view" embraced by Parfit entails that a person is a mere "locus of experiences," and that within a Parfitian account of identity agency is considered as a particular form of experience. In contrast, Korsgaard embraces a "Kantian" conception of the human person, according to which we could regard ourselves as "agents," sources of our actions and "authors" of our lives.[15] From this standpoint, which Korsgaard refers to as the "practical point of view," the relationship between persons and their actions and choices is essentially "authorial": actions are originated by agents, and persons view them as their own, not simply as experiences that befall them. This is precisely the reason why "we think of living our lives, and even of having our experiences, as something that we *do*" (Korsgaard, 1996, p. 378).

On the basis of this assumption, Korsgaard claims that the identity of persons rests upon their capacity for agency since, when we do act, we regard ourselves as unified agents enduring over time. This does not mean that we should look at ourselves as separate existing entities holding over and above our brains and bodies. The "authorial" relationship between the person and his/her actions does not involve any further metaphysical fact. Instead, there are at least three "practical" (not "metaphysical") reasons for regarding ourselves as unified agents enduring over time. First, our conception of ourselves as unified agents is grounded on the basic necessity of choosing among the various conflicting motives that may motivate our actions. Second, every time we choose which motives to act on we deliberate on the basis of reasons for and against these motives, that is, we assume a "deliberative standpoint" from which we act (Williams, 1981, p. 5). This standpoint from which we choose how to act is expressive of ourselves as agents, and is what we identify with as unified agents. Third, we think of our actions and choices as related to each other in a coherent way, that is, we think of them within the life plans which we carry out over our lifetime. So, the phenomenon of devising a life plan itself presupposes the continuity of our identity as agents.

In this respect, Korsgaard observes that the idea of a series of rational agents who will occupy my body in the future is something misleading. Indeed, every time we choose and act "we"/"ourselves" are forthwith taken into the future. In other words, the raw pragmatic necessity of acting and leading our own lives requires that we identify with our future selves. On the basis of this assumption, Korsgaard concludes that this "authorial" continuity between my present and my future self is consistent with drastic changes, so long as these radical changes involve my agency and are not imposed from the outside.

Korsgaard's arguments have relevant implications for the prospect of life-extension technologies. Let us assume the imaginary case of a centenarian individual who, at age 300, regards himself as a different person than he was at age 30, when he decided to radically extend his lifespan by means of medical intervention. Following Korsgaard, we may argue that a substantial life extension which may turn myself into a different person would not be desirable, since the "authorial" continuity needed for my identity will not be preserved.

However, what if a substantial extension of the lifespan would not necessarily impinge my enduring identity as the single author of my life history? Nick Bostrom and Rebecca Roache (2007) imagine the possibility of embarking on life plans that extend over hundreds or thousands of years, such as mastering every musical instrument in the orchestra, or writing a book in each of all the major languages, or even traveling to Alpha Centauri. Such projected life plans, that would develop over vast eons of time, could provide to the radically extended life the sort of inner coherence needed for the "authorial" continuity criterion of personal identity.

However, we cannot rule out the possibility that the individual who began learning to play every musical instrument in the orchestra, or writing a book in several languages, or – were that feasible – travelling to Alpha Centauri, could one day deliberate that these projects are no more worth leading, thus rejecting them and starting to carry out new ones. In other words, we cannot exclude that, at a given point in their lives, centenarians may redirect their life plans from the beginning. Will centenarians be the same individuals who began the former rejected life plans? Or, will they regard themselves as new individuals, incapable of integrating the former rejected life plans in their sense of themselves? Will this radical change still be consistent with the "authorial" continuity which holds over the former rejected life plans? Or, will this radical redirection of their life plans mean that these individuals are now different persons?

In the case of substantial life extension, the mere possibility of embarking on life plans that extend over great reaches of time does not provide sufficient evidence for "authorial" continuity over time. Instead, as Korsgaard's arguments show, only a "factual" ability of carrying out unified plans and projects over extremely long lifespans would guarantee the "authorial" continuity needed for identity. But, such a "factual" ability of implementing unified plans and projects over radically extended lifespans is something that, at present, we can only hypothesize. As a consequence, we shall argue that given that substantial life extension is just a "prospect" and not a "reality" that we can experience as agents, any assumption about our enduring identity over time must be cautious and cannot provide the basis for sanctioning a straightforward desirability of implementing life-extension technologies.

Closing Remarks

From the discussion in the previous sections we can conclude that an account of personal identity as "sameness" is not a conclusive argument for the straightforward desirability of lifespan extension. If we understand personal identity in terms of strong relationships of psychological connectedness and continuity, a radical life extension would be achievable only at the price of a "surrogate" survival as "someone else" (a

"Parfitian survivor," or a "closest continuer"). As Nozick's "continuers" show, the idea that we should have prudential concerns about the existence and well-being of our future selves is disputable. There is evidence to suggest that we have no fundamental concern about the existence of our "closest continuer": what we primarily care about is the persistence of our identity over time, not the existence of our future self *per se*. As a consequence, there may be cases in which we do not judge such a "surrogate" continuation of our identity as worth having.

We have also contended that it is not possible to gain a full perspective on the relationship between personal identity and life extension unless we consider identity as "selfhood" as well. And we have shown that, in this perspective, the desirability of a radical life extension for the individual is doubtable. Indeed, following Korsgaard, we may argue that what matters to me in survival is the "authorial" continuity holding between myself now and myself in the future. However, in the case of radically extended lifespans, we cannot rule out the possibility that the "authorial" continuity which my identity is bound to will fade away over eons of time. Hence, so long as we accept that the persistence of "authorial" continuity is what matters to the individual in survival, the desirability of life extension is something which should be cautiously assessed.

We may conclude that, with regard to its implications for personal identity over time, the prospect of a radically extended lifespan would not be straightforwardly and unquestionably alluring for the individual concerned.

Acknowledgments

We acknowledge with gratitude the helpful comments that we have received on earlier drafts from Françoise Baylis, Thomas Douglas, and Rebecca Roache. We also thank the colleagues and the experts involved in the ENHANCE Project, for they urged us to sharpen our argument on some crucial points.

Notes

1. As Binstock explains, the historian Gerald Gruman (1966) first coined the term "prolongevity."
2. Such a scenario is not far from what Post and Binstock (2004) term the "decelerated aging" model, and Richard Miller (2002) and Denham Harman (1998) envisage as a likely achievable increase of the "functional lifespan."
3. This issue has been recently discussed by Walter Glannon (2002a, 2002b), whose arguments opened up a heated debate with John Harris (2002) in the journal *Bioethics*.
4. The presentation and discussion of these arguments draw on the inspiring work of H.W. Noonan (2003).
5. For a presentation of the "psychological continuity criterion" we will refer to D. Parfit (1971, 1984).
6. As Lynne Rudder Baker (2000, p.135) points out: "On the closest continuer view, whether or not I am person S depends on whether or not there is some other person who is a closer continuer to S than I am."

7. Here is the way Nozick states his theory: "y at t2 is the same person as x at t1 only if, first, y's properties at t2 stem from, grow out of, are causally dependent on x's properties at t1 and, second, there is no other z at t2 that stands in a closer (or as close) relationship to x at t1 than y at t2 does" (1981, pp. 36–7).

8. Nozick's "closest continuer" theory has been recently put forward as an argument for the desirability of the extension of human lifespan. However, it is worth noticing that there is a widespread tendency to report Nozick's theory without explicitly mentioning that it implies the idea of survival as "someone else" (Harris, 2004).

9. "(…) the infant, once it exists, has a certain moral status and exerts certain moral claims, yet we are not similarly required to bring something with this status into existence."

10. The following remarks draw on Ricoeur's (1992) criticism of Parfit.

11. As Overall herself asserts, she borrows her argument from Nozick's "closest continuer" theory.

References

Bostrom, N. & Roache, R. (2007). Ethical issues in human enhancement. In J. Ryberg, T.S. Petersen & C. Wolf (eds.), *New Waves in Applied Ethics*. Palgrave Macmillian.

Darwall, S. (1983). Unified agency. In S. Darwall, *Impartial Reason* (pp. 101–13). New York: Cornell University Press.

de Grey, A.D.N.J., Ames, B.N., Andersen, J.K. *et al.* (2002). Time to talk SENS: Critiquing the immutability of human aging. *Annals of the New York Academy of Sciences*, **959**, 452–62.

DeGrazia, D. (2005). *Human Identity and Bioethics*. New York: Cambridge University Press.

Glannon, W. (2002a). Identity, prudential concern, and extended lives. *Bioethics*, **16**, 266–83.

Glannon, W. (2002b). Reply to Harris. *Bioethics*, **16**, 292–7.

Gruman, G. (1966). A history of ideas about prolongation of life: The evolution of prolongevity hypothesis to 1800. *Transcriptions of the American Philosophical Society*, **56**, 1–102.

Harman, D. (1998). Extending functional lifespan. *Experimental Gerontology*, **33**, 95–112.

Harris, J. (2002). A response to Walter Glannon. *Bioethics*, **16**, 284–91.

Harris, J. (2004). Immortal ethics. *Annals of the New York Academy of Sciences*, **1019**, 527–34.

Juengst, E.T., Binstock, R.H., Mehlman, M. *et al.* (2003). Biogerontology, "anti-aging medicine," and the challenges of human enhancement. *Hastings Center Report*, **33**, 21–30.

Korsgaard, C.M. (1996). Personal identity and the unity of agency: A Kantian Response to Parfit. In C.M. Korsgaard (ed.), *Creating the Kingdom of Ends* (pp. 366–7) Cambridge: Cambridge University Press.

Miller, R.A. (2002). Extending life: Scientific prospects and political obstacles. *The Milbank Quarterly*, **80**, 155–74.

Noonan, H.W. (2003). *Personal Identity*, 2nd edition. New York: Routledge.

Nozick, R. (1981). *Philosophical Explanations*. Cambridge, MA: The Belknap Press.

Olson, E.T. (1997). *The Human Animal. Personal Identity without Psychology*. New York: Oxford University Press.

Overall, C. (2003). *Aging, Death, and Human Longevity. A Philosophical Inquiry*. Berkeley, CA: University of California Press.

Parfit, D. (1971). Personal identity. *The Philosophical Review*, **81**, 3–27.

Parfit, D. (1984). *Reasons and Persons*. Oxford: Clarendon Press.

Post, S.G. & Binstock, R.H. (2004). Introduction. In S.G. Post & R.H. Binstock (eds.), *The Fountain of Youth. Cultural, Scientific, and Ethical Perspectives on a Biomedical Goal* (pp. 1–8). Oxford: Oxford University Press.

Ricoeur, P. (1992). *Oneself as Another*. Chicago: University of Chicago Press.

Robine, J.M. & Allard, M. (1999). Jeanne Calment: Validation of the duration of her life. In B. Jeune & J.W. Vaupel (eds.), *Validation of Exceptional Longevity* (pp. 145–72) Odense: Odense University Press.

Rudder Baker, L. (2000). *Persons and Bodies. A Constitution View*. Cambridge: Cambridge University Press.

Schetchtman, M. (1996). *The Constitution of Selves*. Ithaca: Cornell University Press.

Schloendorn, J. (2006). Making the case for human life extension: Personal arguments. *Bioethics*, **4**, 199–200.

Turner, L (2004). Life extension research: Health, illness, and death. *Health Care Analysis*, **12**, 117–29.

Williams, B. (1973). The Makropulos case: Reflections on the tedium of immortality. In B. Williams (ed.), *Problems of the Self* (pp. 82–100). Cambridge: Cambridge University Press.

Williams, B. (1981). Persons, character and morality. In B. Williams (ed.), *Moral Luck. Philosophical Papers 1973–1980* (pp. 1–19) Cambridge: Cambridge University Press.

30

Intergenerational Justice
and Lifespan Extension

Roberto Mordacci

> Certainly no one will dispute the propriety of
> that partition of goods which separates them into three classes,
> viz., external goods, goods of the body, and goods of the soul,
> or deny that the happy man must have all three.
>
> (Aristotle, *Politics*, 1323 a 24–27, tr. B. Jowett)

Money, health, and justice have always been deemed fundamental for happiness at every stage of life. Aristotle makes this uncontroversial point in various works.[1] He also declares that the moral value of a life cannot be assessed on the basis of isolated actions, but that a whole lifespan perspective is needed:

> Human good turns out to be activity of soul in accordance with virtue, and if there are more than one virtue, in accordance with the best and most complete. But we must add "in a complete life". For one swallow does not make a summer, nor does one day; and so too one day, or a short time, does not make a man blessed and happy (*NE* I, 7 1098 a 18–20, tr. W.D. Ross)

A whole lifespan perspective on happiness implies that we not only consider virtue – and justice in particular – but also an adequate presence, during all the stages of life, of those goods which indeed make virtue possible, such as enough money and good health. Without these external and bodily goods during a whole life, on Aristotle's account, a just man can hardly be happy (Nussbaum, 1986).

These external goods in Aristotle's times were mainly dependent on good genealogy, as was money, good luck, and health. Today such goods still resist our complete control, but they are nevertheless the object of intensive social and political strategies aiming to reduce disparities between people with respect to access to equal economic opportunities and fairly decent health care.

Difference in age often makes a difference in having access to those opportunities and services, but it seems that the idea of a *just* distribution of these goods has become a commonly shared principle in modern societies. This obviously cannot mean that all people, young and old, have equal access to the *same* kinds of opportunities and care,

Enhancing Human Capacities, edited by Julian Savulescu, Ruud ter Meulen and Guy Kahane.
© 2011 Blackwell Publishing Ltd

since needs vary greatly during a lifespan, e.g. the young need more opportunities, the old need more long-term health care. Therefore, since we have limited resources, a problem of allocation arises: At which stage of life should we allocate more of a determinate good or service or opportunity? The role of *prudence* in a lifespan is as obvious as it is the fact that in time we age.

Problems of distributive justice throughout the lifespan are therefore not new. Yet, the increased aging rate of contemporary societies and an array of new life-extending technologies (LETs) make these problems more and more urgent and complicated. Distributing scarce resources along a lifespan of 55 years as an average, as it was in 1930 (in developed countries), or doing so when the average lifespan is around 80, as it is now, or even when LET will have brought "normal" lifespan as far as 100 years or more, are quite different matters. What would a prudent distribution of resources during a lifespan look like, if we are supposed to live up to 120 years and more? What would be *fair* to allocate to the young and the old, if we are going to have more people above 90 in our societies? Can we afford offering free and equal access to, say, public health care services and income support, to all age groups for present and future generations as well? Can it be right that some age groups bear the burden of benefits to other age groups, or that a birth cohort pays for services that will be available only to another birth cohort, or that future generations pay the costs of imprudent and unwise behavior of past generations?

These problems tend to be treated under the rather generic heading of *intergenerational justice*. Yet, we must clearly distinguish between the very different questions just mentioned, especially if our aim is to assess the moral and political impact of the LET, as it is here.

The Varieties of Intergenerational Justice

By "intergenerational justice" we may mean quite different things. We can distinguish between issues of justice between distant generations, between birth cohorts, and between age groups (Gosseries, 2003). This distinction could be reframed so that the notion of a "generation" appears in all of them. Let us assume that a "generation" is a birth cohort comprising those born within a determinate time span, usually 15–20 years. The assumption is that a new generation appears when the members of the previous one start to have children, that is by the time they are around childbearing age. We already have a problem here: there is a clear trend, at least in some countries, to postpone having children until 30 years of age or even more. The effect on the notion of a generation is that we should progressively postpone its start later than 15 and extend its duration up to 35–40 years, at least when the trend is going in this direction. The LET will very likely increase the speed of this process and will probably stretch even more the temporal width of a generation. It might be suggested that this shift is going to make the notion of generation more fuzzy and less useful for analyzing problems.

The ideas of "birth cohort" and "age group" seem more precise. A birth cohort is made up of the people born within a determinate period, arbitrarily defined: there is no reference to the idea of "generation," so the assumption concerning childbearing age is not necessary. A birth cohort can be made, e.g. of those born between 1965 and 1974.

For issues of justice we confront similar birth cohorts in terms of opportunities and resources available, for example what a baby-boom child (those born in the 1960s) can expect for his retirement years in comparison with what the children-of-the-war (born in the 1940s) cohort is having now.

An age group is made of people of about the same age, say their thirties. They obviously are a birth cohort as well, but they are considered at a certain moment in their lives, so that in time the age group is made of different persons, while the birth cohort members remain the same while they move from one age group to another. No reference to the idea of "generating" people is implied here, though it is obviously assumed that some age groups are generating and others not. LETs are creating new age groups and enlarging already existing ones: the young old (aged 65–74), the old old (aged 75–84), the older old (aged 85–94), and possibly the prolonged old (aged 95 and more) (Binstock, 2004). When greater groups and new ones enter the picture, the figures of a just distributive frame change dramatically.

Therefore, we have three kinds of "intergenerational" justice. First, we have issues of justice between *non-coexisting generations*. There is quite a long and disputed tradition of debate concerning this issue, usually called the issue of justice towards *future* generations (Laslett & Fishkin, 1992; Sikora & Barry, 1978): Since past generations clearly cannot claim any right towards the present ones, the issue seem to be whether we have obligations concerning not-yet-existing people, such as those who will come when our depletion of resources and spoiling of the environment will have reached irreversible deleterious effects. These issues typically rise first within consequentialist frameworks (Heyd, 1992; Mulgan, 2006), where they merge with questions concerning the "non-identity problem," i.e. the possibility that we may have no prudential reasons concerning "our" future since by then we will be different people (DeGrazia, 2005; Parfit, 1984).

LETs obviously bear on this debate, but they do not change the *kind* of issues of justice between generations. Even if the precautionary principle and the non-identity problem can be applied to this debate, the fact that we could live longer and even enlarge our notion of a "generation" does not seem to alter the data and the concepts concerning justice between *distant* generations. *Whether* we owe a decent life on this planet to our descendants or not does not depend on how long our lives can be. Yet, if we *do* owe this to next generations, the fact that longer lives of present people can be a threat to future people of course is an issue and we should take it into account. Anyway, we should first have answered the general questions about justice towards future generations before we consider whether life-extending technologies would be unjust in this respect. Devoting too many resources to the project of indefinitely long lives might be considered an infringement of the precautionary principle, since it would create unsustainable conditions for the generations to come (Glannon, 2002). Those who oppose the precautionary principle (often from a consequentialist standpoint) would object to such a conclusion (Harris & Holm, 2002), but this does not depend *directly* on the effects of LETs.

Second, we have problems of justice between *partially co-existing generations*. In this case, what is at issue is justice between birth cohorts. If those born in a certain period, let us say the baby-boom years, are likely to suffer serious side effects because of the disparity between their number and the highly reduced number of those whose work is needed to maintain the welfare system, this is a problem of justice between birth cohorts. It is likely that the new birth cohort will have to pay higher taxes if the present system is to be maintained or that the baby-boom people will suffer a great reduction in available health care services and income support in comparison with their elders. Deciding policies concerning these issues is the core of present welfare politics, and a number of possible solutions have been proposed both in theory and practice (Gosseries, 2003).

Rawls's early proposal, the *just savings principle* (Rawls, 1971, p.287), defines the rate of savings which contractors (behind the veil of ignorance) would be willing to accept at each stage in order to let all the other generations have at least as much as they have. The proposal has raised extended discussion (Dasgupta, 2005; English 1977, 1991; Mulgan 2006). Utilitarians tend to reject this principle because their goal is to increase overall benefit over time, so that the savings rates will have to be strongly positive in order to let subsequent generations have more than preceding ones. This results in an *inequality* of resources between birth cohorts, supposedly justified by the overall increase of welfare among subsequent generations, though at the expense of previous ones.

LETs indirectly affect these issues. If we invest in such technologies and significantly raise the normally expected lifespan, the various birth cohorts will experience different levels of available resources and different ranges of opportunities. Older generations (birth cohorts arriving at old age) will benefit from longer lives, if the treatments are successful, and will claim for prolonged working time, more health care resources and more income support. Younger generations (birth cohorts at young age), will have either to suffer higher savings rates, up to severe restrictions of their ability to have access to opportunities and to develop personal projects, or to face a harsh fight with the older birth cohort, which is still in power and does not seem willing or in the condition of renouncing the use of such resources. When the latter will be dead, quite later on, the former will likely be in a *poorer* condition in all respects.

Since this is an ongoing problem, the issue is better understood as a third kind of problem of intergenerational justice: justice *between coexisting generations*, that is, between age groups. Problems of justice between age groups are different from problems of justice between non-coexisting generations. Issues of intergenerational justice are often identified with the latter, but a real and present challenge is in the area of justice between contemporary age groups. For reasons of simplicity, I will include these issues into the general heading of "intergenerational justice" and treat them in this contribution as such. Yet, it should be clear that here we are not dealing with problems of justice towards future generations. No "repugnant conclusion" (Parfit, 1984) is involved in the prospects of fairly distributing resources between contemporary age groups. For the same reason, the non-identity problem posed by Parfit and others is irrelevant to the point at issue. Even if we were different persons in different stages of life, this would not change the fact that different age groups need to respond now to the requirements of justice between each other. This is suggested by a prudential lifespan approach (Daniels, 1988), which is based on the idea that it would be prudent to save resources *for oneself* while one is active and productive in order to be able to support one's needs in the old age. Since the assumption is that the contractors in the original situation are *blind to their age*, they simply cannot think of themselves as just young or just old: who was before I came up and will be after I'm gone is just a contiguous entity to whatever stage of life I am in. Therefore, all stages are for me equivalent in value: they remain different in problems and perspectives, but since I do not know in which I am in at the moment, I treat them equally, in order not to be in too bad conditions when the veil of ignorance is taken away.

It is clear that the problems of distributive justice between different age groups will change in the future and that the prospects of a significant extension of the human lifespan will greatly affect how *in the future* the issues of justice between different age groups will need to be faced. But obviously it will be a problem of justice between *coexisting* generations, so the usual objections to the notion of intergenerational justice understood as justice between *distant* generations do not arise. We *do* have rights and obligations towards our contemporaries who belong to a different age group: these are *existing* people and the utilitarian objection concerning the emptiness of the notion of right of future people or of duties towards future persons does not apply. If the lifespan extension will dramatically change the societal setting in the (near) future, this will *then* raise problems of justice without further qualifications, because it will be a problem of fairness in the distribution of present goods to present people. So, justice between age groups is an ongoing matter and the perspectives open by the life-extending technologies pose problems of justice now as well as in the future. We already have a number of problems deriving from the different needs and desires of different age groups, as well as from the same people at different stages of their lives.

Justice Between Age Groups and the Extension of Life

Prospects of greatly extending the human lifespan raises serious problems of justice between age groups. If lives are longer and healthier, a number of side effects will affect society: higher public expenditure for retirement wages, reduction of job opportunities for young people, and higher costs for health care systems. At the same time, the variety of ideas, fresh energies, and creative activities will be reduced. These problems involve distributive justice as well as general welfare.

Proposals so far have concerned ideas like postponing having children, a later entrance to jobs (preceded by a longer education), the alternation of working and leisure time during a lifetime (compartmentalized working/retirement periods). Assuming that the *principle of fair equality of opportunities* (Rawls, 1971) also applies to matters of justice between age groups (Daniels, 1988), we might suggest that the extension of lifespan should not negatively affect the access of young people to opportunities for improvement and personal projects such as having a family or starting a career. At the same time, this cannot result in a reduction of the opportunities of a satisfactory life and a good care when necessary in the old age. This implies a more flexible social distribution of tasks and possibilities, which might lead to great changes in present models of family, instruction, higher education, working regulation, leisure time, and retirement policies.

These prospects have raised some general objections to LETs, leading some to argue that we should not aim at radical life extension owing to its intrinsic badness

(Kass, 2004) or that an upper limit to access to medical and other resources should be established at a certain age (Callahan, 1987). This is also called "rationing by age" and there is evidence that some health care systems are already applying it (Daniels, 1988).

The general objection to LETs on a social-moral basis has been addressed by Christine Overall (Overall, 2003; see also chapter 28, this volume). One can basically agree with her main line of argument. The arguments offered by the opponents lack cogency and disregard some fundamental facts about aging: its cultural as well as biological nature, its being connected with normative judgments about what constitutes a "good" human life, and its moral relevance as a stage of life in which experience should have generated more responsible people. A few remarks of a rather general kind on her arguments seem nonetheless to be in order.

First, it seems that Overall's thesis in a way avoids the main theoretical question posed by the lifespan extension project. In response to Callahan's argument that 80 years seem to be enough "to experience most of the goods of human life," Overall replies that "on this planet many hundreds of millions of people never reach eighty" and that therefore it is "patronizing" to stop the search for longer lives. Although one can agree with the objection, the answer just seems to beg the question.

The point at issue here is not whether we should "extend the number of long lives" (which can be considered a duty of justice), but whether we should "extend the human lifespan," which is a different problem: more of long lives does not imply longer lives. On a statistical view, of course, more of long lives means that human life, as a statistical entity, will become longer; but this does not mean that we have extended the human lifespan. The latter is measured in relation with the "current outside limit for the human lifespan," or the "maximum human lifespan," which Overall recognizes at about 120 years. She seems to be quite happy with that limit, but strongly emphasizes the issues of fairness and paternalism which seem to be underpinning some of the objections against the extension of the human lifespan.

With respect to the *maximum* human lifespan, a way of formulating the question might be as follows: "How much can be enough in order to fully express one's human potential?" We must bear in mind that the question must be posed concerning *individuals* and not just a general conception of "the human potential," because this can have much wider limits than those which a single individual has: even if I live eternally, I will only have the capacities to develop *certain* human potentialities. My bodily constitution and my intellectual abilities (lest we accept the idea of genetically engineering ourselves, which poses different problems) make available to me certain potentialities, which I could exploit up to high levels of excellence if I just had more time to live and a good health to let me work for a long time. But certain projects are clearly not open to me from the very beginning: as long as I could live, I would never be able to win a weightlifting championship.

So the point is "how long can be enough in order to exploit *my* potentialities?" and this is tied up with the issue of personal identity. As said earlier, the objections coming from this direction do not seem to oppose enhancing the human lifespan *as such*. In a dynamic conception of personal identity, one in which personal identity is conceived of as a task and not as a given, there is no reason to oppose the idea of having more time to fulfill one's life projects. Yet, the idea loses its grip if we think that living too long a life might mean losing contact with the original source and author of those projects. If we take a broadly Kantian stance, for example the "authorial view" of personal identity (Korsgaard, 1996), we might argue that sustaining the "practical point of view" requires the possibility of recognizing oneself as the continuous author of one's life, and this gradually fades away with time. It is true that the "deliberative point of view" travels with me over time, and that I am brought forth as a full person by my successive deliberations. Yet, in order to be *my* deliberations, they need to keep some contact with the *history* that has generated them, even if I undergo a number of cultural or personal conversions. It must still be "me" the one who operates changes, and *I am my history*. Now, this connection is not a given fact, it is the result of a constant recollection of memories and projects which come from all of my life. This effort might become, at a certain point, too difficult to be sustained by a single individual. Beyond a certain age (120, or 150? Not much more than that, I suspect) it may be too hard to feel in contact with those far away memories and hopes, so that living longer, at that time, loses its appeal as a *personal* experience: it may mean continuing to live while losing oneself. At that point, I can deliver my projects to someone else, but they will not be *my* projects any more.

A third issue which would seem underdetermined in Overall's essay is exactly that of *intergenerational justice* in our third meaning, i.e. justice between age groups. Overall states that "living longer provides human beings with opportunities for greater moral growth" so that "responsibilities may last longer" and people can bring their projects over an extended time (chapter 28, this volume). In principle, I think, everyone would agree. But there is more that needs to be said: Older people will be ever more eager to keep their responsibilities over time, since they are in good health and claim to be wiser than younger people. In keeping power, the old can be very aggressive and younger people will be carefully kept out of the control room for the longest time possible.

This is clearly unfair. If longer lives means more power to the old, this will inevitably deprive young people of the possibility of having their "fair equality of opportunities" for living their lives. They will also live longer, but those opportunities which can be exploited only in young years will be forever lost. Furthermore, they may never reach the top positions, if the old manage to become immortal and get rid of these vociferous and inexpert rebels.

This raises a tremendous issue of justice between age groups. Even if we imagine practices of "coercive retirement," with a life of 120 years such a retirement could not reasonably be earlier than 90 or 100. Why should one retire at 100 if the assumption is that he will live in good health until 120? Furthermore, we also know very well that it is unwise to increase the number of the retired when we do not have enough resources to pay pensions for all. There are good reasons to promote healthy and long lives, but we must be aware that this will inevitably raise very deep conflicts between age groups (Scharlach & Kaye, 1997).

The advantage of considering LETs in the light of justice between age groups is that we can assume a *complete-life view*. Aging is a process which affects everyone. In this sense, there is no possible analogy between discrimination by age and discrimination by skin color. In the perspective of a whole life, every person arriving at old age will have passed through each stage of life. Therefore, egalitarian worries about discrimination do not arise in relation to age as far as it is guaranteed that a proportionate amount of certain goods are equally distributed over a whole lifespan (McKerlie, 1989,

1993). Even though different age groups receive different proportions of that good, each person reaching old age will have in the end received the same overall amount of that good.

This feature of age permits us to face the challenges it poses in the light of principles which do not need to invoke an immediate appeal to an intersubjective view. Since we *all* age, we do not need to think what others would want for themselves and to imagine how to regulate competition for goods. It is enough to think about how *we* would better distribute the available goods and opportunities across our lifespan, keeping in mind the fact that we need not assume that what we want now will still be what we want in the future. The general perspective on a just distribution of goods in different ages is what has been called a "keeping the options open" principle: It is imprudent to assume that what we now imagine we will want later in life will really be what we want in that stage of life. *Therefore*, we'd better not choose distributions which would impair certain stages in important respects in order to have much more in other stages (e.g. working very hard and saving all the possible resources, even beyond the limit of poverty in young years, in order to have huge amounts of money in the old age – which could be then spent in health care or leisure). A prudent agent, it is suggested, should define a savings rate to the effect that "at each stage of life I shall have a reasonable share of basic social goods which serve as the all-purpose means of pursuing what I think is good. Keeping options open implies that I must be neutral or unbiased toward the different stages of life that I shall go through" (Daniels, 1988, p.58).

This is why a prudential lifespan account seems to be the case in these issues. If we imagine ideal contractors, like in Rawls's original position, who assume they will live a normal lifespan, yet are blinded not only to their substantive conception of the good, but as well to their age, we obtain a picture in which a prudent agent tries to imagine how to distribute goods and opportunities along *his lifespan* without prejudice in favor of a certain age or a certain conception of the good. This picture will obviously take into account the different needs of different ages, since the contractors know that they are different. Yet, since they do not know what specific projects they would engage in at each stage, they will try to "keep the options open" for each stage, guaranteeing what is most needed for basic activities in each stage.

What becomes important in this stage is identifying the basic activities and needs that characterize each stage of life, though leaving enough space for flexibility. Typically, a standard conception of these stages assumes (albeit somewhat acritically) that a normal life has a profile where there is a rearing and education stage, a professional and family-creating stage, a mature, expert stage and a late, retired or reduced-activity stage. Each of these stages has different needs in terms of health care, job opportunities, training, income support, family and social support for childrearing, and so on.

In this respect, LETs raise issues concerning the *life profile* of persons (Gosseries, 2003, pp.475–7). Living much longer most likely implies stretching the duration of periods in life when certain features are prominent and others are, so to say, "silent" or less important. If life extension simply prolongs old age, though in good health conditions, we cannot assume that society could afford offering high levels of health care, income support, and retirement wages. This would have too high costs for younger age groups. Therefore, it is just obvious to think about age-based or seniority-based practices such as raising the eligibility age for retirement. What is more likely to be required is a certain willingness to redesign the standard profile of lives, adjusting them to the extended lifespan profile, a reality which is anyway imposing itself.

The "complete-life view" has been criticized on utilitarian and egalitarian grounds. It is objected that we change our identity in time, so that it would be better to consider a life profile using "segments" of lifespan rather than whole lives (McKerlie, 1993). Such an objection would be analogous to Parfit's approach when he suggests if one is willing to sacrifice parts of his life, this is like sacrificing oneself for the good of other people. Therefore, a utilitarian perspective would favor such a segment view, since what counts in it is the total amount of happiness lived overall, discounting prudence and rational self-interest.

This view has been criticized on contractarian grounds (Daniels, 1996, pp.264–9). The "keeping the options open principle," as we observed, is applied to justice between age groups and the non-identity objection does not apply to this area. If a prudent agent's *actual age* is concealed behind a veil of ignorance, then, even assuming that he will not care for his future selves, he still cannot know his actual age. So he has to think about fixing a distributive policy to the effect that at every stage there will be at least a normal opportunity range. This is a prudent choice not in terms of future prospects, but in terms of present choices, since the agent does not know to which age group he belongs.

I would simply add that we cannot avoid considering differences in the kind and range of opportunities needed for each stage of life. This is why a "sufficientarian" approach (Gosseries, 2003, p.481) is not enough: The suggestion that some goods (food and shelter, basic rights, minimal income opportunities and so on) are needed at *every* stage of life and therefore should be guaranteed to every age group is obviously right, and it is implicit in a "keeping the options open principle." Yet, the latter further suggests that the options which need to be open for different age groups can indeed be quite different and that therefore we have to elaborate on an image of each stage of life in terms of *specific* needs and opportunities.

Conclusions

LETs significantly modify the duration and the features of each stage of life. Lower mortality rates at birth and in infancy, longer education, intermediate periods at home with parents while working, postponed creation of families or of making a life of one's own, longer working periods, continuous training, retarded eligibility for retirement, a long period after working age still in good health, increasing needs of long-term health care in the very old and prolonged old age are only but a few of the already visible effects of better health care and medical progress. Enhancement techniques will make these changes even more rapid and extensive.

It seems that at present we do not possess the cultural, theoretical, and political tools to face these changes. An essential feature of an approach to the problems posed by these changes is *flexibility*: we will have to change our settings and therefore our own life profiles. But flexibility needs to be built into the criterion of our decisional procedures concerning these issues. The idea of a *normal opportunity range,* which changes through age groups and is designed so that, beyond just sufficient goods for any age, it would offer the possibility of taking the opportunities and facing the different needs that any age group faces, must be understood as a way of inserting a greater amount of flexibility into our life profiles. In terms of health care services, policies already recognize that age can be a reason for offering or not offering some kinds of treatment (e.g. cardiopulmonary resuscitation, heart transplants) and age rationing is not *per se* opposed to an egalitarian approach, while it is clearly built into utilitarian perspectives through the instrument of quality adjusted life years (QALYs) (but see Harris, 1987 for an internal critique of this criterion). It is clear that age rationing becomes less crude if it is included into a framework of overall fair institutions and interpersonal relations (Daniels, 1988, pp.47–52). A consideration of the specific needs and features of each stage of life in a lifespan-enhanced society is therefore needed to regulate policies and offer fair equality of opportunity to each age group.

Notes

1. See also e.g. *Nichomachean Ethics* 1098 b, 9–18, *Magna Moralia* 1184 b 1–5. For a comment on this see Annas 1996, pp. 246–8.

References

Annas, J. (1996). Aristotle and Kant on morality and practical reason. In S. Engstrom & J. Whiting (eds.), *Aristotle, Kant, and the Stoics* (pp. 237–58). Cambridge: Cambridge University Press.

Binstock, R.H. (2004). The prolonged old, the long-lived society and the politics of age. In S.G. Post & R.H. Binstock (eds.), *The Fountain of Youth. Cultural, Scientific, and Ethical Perspectives on a Biomedical Goal* (pp. 362–84). Oxford: Oxford University Press.

Callahan, D. (1987). *Setting Limits: Medical Goals in an Aging Society.* New York: Simon & Schuster.

Daniels, N. (1988). *Am I My Parents' Keeper?* New York: Oxford University Press.

Daniels, N. (1996). *Justice and Justification: Reflective Equilibrium in Theory and Practice.* Cambridge MA: Cambridge University Press.

Dasgupta, P. (2005). Three conceptions of intergenerational justice. In H. Lillehammer & D.H. Mellor (eds.), *Ramsey's Legacy* (pp. 149–69). Oxford: Clarendon Press.

DeGrazia, D. (2005). *Human Identity and Bioethics.* Cambridge, MA: Cambridge University Press.

English, J. (1977). Justice between generations. *Philosophical Studies*, **31**, 91–104.

English, J. (1991). What do grown children owe their parents? In N. Jecker (ed.), *Aging and Ethics: Philosophical Problems in Gerontology* (pp. 147–70). Totowa, NJ: Humana Press.

Glannon, W. (2002). Identity, prudential concern, and extending lives. *Bioethics*, **16**, 266–83.

Gosseries, A. (2003). Intergenerational justice. In H. La Follette (ed.), *The Oxford Handbook of Practical Ethics* (pp. 459–84). Oxford: Oxford University Press.

Harris, J. (1987). QALYfying the value of life. *Journal of Medical Ethics*, **13**, 117–23.

Harris, J. & Holm, S. (2002). Extending human lifespan and the precautionary paradox. *Journal of Medicine and Philosophy*, **27**, 355–68.

Heyd, D. (1992). *Genethics. Moral Issues in the Creation of People*. Berkeley: University of California Press.

Kass, L. (2004). L'Chaim and its limits: Why not immortality? In S.G. Post & R.H. Binstock (eds.), *The Fountain of Youth: Cultural, Scientific, and Ethical Perspectives on a Biomedical Goal*. (pp. 304–20). New York: Oxford University Press.

Korsgaard, C. (1996). *The Sources of Normativity*. Cambridge: Cambridge University Press.

Laslett, P. & Fishkin, J.S. (eds.) (1992). *Justice between Age Groups and Generations*. New Haven: Yale University Press.

McKerlie, D. (1989). Equality and time. *Ethics*, **99**, 475–91.

McKerlie, D. (1993). Justice between neighboring generations. In L. Cohen (ed.), *Justice Across Generations: What Does it Mean?* (pp. 215–25). Washington, DC: American Association of Retired Persons.

Mulgan, T. (2002). Neutrality, rebirth and intergenerational justice. *Journal of Applied Philosophy*, **19**(1), 3–15.

Mulgan, T. (2006). *Future People: A Moderate Consequentialist Account of Our Obligation to Future Generations*. Oxford: Clarendon Press.

Nussbaum, M.C. (1986). *The Fragility of Goodness: Luck and Ethics in Greek Tragedy and Philosophy*. Cambridge: Cambridge University Press.

Overall, C. (2003). *Aging, Death, and Human Longevity. A Philosophical Enquiry*. Berkeley: University of California Press.

Parfit, D. (1984). *Reasons and Persons*. New York: Oxford University Press.

Rawls, J. (1971). *A Theory of Justice*. Oxford: Oxford University Press.

Scharlach, A. & Kaye, L. (eds.) (1997). *Controversial Issues in Aging*. Boston: Allyn & Bacon.

Sikora, R.I. & Barry, B. (eds.) (1978). *Obligations to Future Generations*. Philadelphia: Temple University Press.

31

The Value of Life Extension to Persons as Conatively Driven Processes

Steven Horrobin

The Procrustean Lifespan: Lifespan as Natural History, Aging as Cultural Artifact

As the eminent biogerontologist Robin Holliday (2006) has asserted, "aging is no longer an unsolved problem in biology." While there is still some debate over the relative significances and interplay of its multi-factorial nature, there is no longer considerable doubt over its origins and fundamental predicates. There is a biogerontological consensus that aging serves no natural or biological "purpose" or "function." There appears no intelligible teleology of aging. There are no "gerontogenes" and aging is not regarded as some indispensable positive function of biology, qua biology and natural history themselves (Kirkwood, 2002; Rattan, 1995). Aging is rather principally a byproduct of the long-term diminished, null, or deleterious effects of alleles and processes whose short-term benefits are strongly selected for. The optimal reproductive age of an organism is calibrated by a complex interplay between its endogenous factors and its environment. Evolutionary selective "pressures" act upon the species to optimally calibrate its individuals' development and reproduction within the contexts in which the species happens ancestrally to have existed, and which its biology and activities helped to shape. Beyond this spontaneously ordered or emergently calibrated age of optimal reproductive efficiency, selective pressures tail off until they fall to zero. Simply put, evolution does not regard what occurs to the progenitors once they have successfully reproduced. There are no selective forces holding them together, and their biological program ceases to have positive functionality. Their systems of repair fail, their positive functions pass beyond optimal efficiency and can become antagonistic, and inexorable degeneration to death occurs (Kirkwood & Rose, 1991).

Attempts have been made by bioethical commentators to construct value arguments based upon reverence either or both for "natural" wild history, and the "normal" in human cultural history. I have elsewhere (Horrobin, 2006a) argued against the force of

Enhancing Human Capacities, edited by Julian Savulescu, Ruud ter Meulen and Guy Kahane.
© 2011 Blackwell Publishing Ltd

these quasi-sanctity, proto-conservative positions (most explicitly iterated by Dworkin (1993), though more directly by Kass (2003) and Sandel (2002) in the context of aging intervention and life extension). I will not rehearse these arguments here other than to say that in absence of any relevant teleology of aging, there is no *prima facie* case for respecting the calibration of lifespan, arising from the deep natural history of our distant precultural ancestors, in absence of the circumstances of its formation, any more than there would be a case to preserve the genotypes of sickle cell anemia given a culturally mediated neutralization of malaria.

The various uses of the concepts of the natural and the normal in a *normative* sense in context of arguments opposing aging intervention and life extension all reference some concept of the *factually* "appropriate" lifespan. There is some underlying notion that, whatever else aging and death within a *very particular* span of years may represent, the present situation is the *correct* one, and, whatever the other facts about individual persons or their desires, preferences, and plans may be there are fully normative matters of fact in the world which must be observed in preserving the status quo.

A discussion of the status of the "natural" and of human interventions and values in relation to it is beyond the scope of this chapter. However, suffice to say at this point that I assert that anything within the causal economy of the universe is entirely natural, including values,[1] humans themselves, together with their artifacts and products, and indeed, lifespans either as presently the case, or else radically extended. Further, normality of itself is no predicator of normativity.[2]

In view of this, such arguments concerning the "appropriate length" of life from naturalness or normalness are akin to the kind of hardened prejudice manifested by Procrustes in his beliefs concerning the appropriate length of beds, and the sleepers therein, and one whose consequences may be just as brutal.

The Value of Life to Persons as Conatively Driven Processes

The value of life: sanctity and life plans

I have elsewhere (Horrobin, 2005, 2006b) laid out in greater detail, arguments suggesting that neither the mainstream liberal nor conservative camps in bioethics supply sufficient groundings or explanations of the value of life *extension*. In summary, the conservatives' bases for what they call the "value of life" cash out as being ideas whose primary function and motivation is the denial of prerogative, rather than the establishment of a value of continued life for persons. Further, the idea of an intrinsic value *simpliciter* cannot of itself underwrite the value of life's *continuance*, since in the classic picture intrinsic value is bivalent,[3] and, given universal mortality, can tell us nothing whatever about why it is good to live a longer, rather than a shorter life (Horrobin, 2006b). An intrinsic value of life *simpliciter* cannot be *time incremental* (Horrobin, 2006b). In the case of subjectivist views, whether expressivist, constructivist or whatever, there seems to be a mismatch between the strength, pervasiveness and apparent stability of the ordinary sense of the value of life (extension) for persons, and the claim of irreducibility of subjective preference in relation to this value. More explicitly, there either seems to be a negative, or else there does not seem to be any answer to the simple question that is demanded by analysis of the value of life extension: Is there a basis for the value of the *continuance* of person-instantiated life, *simpliciter*, and *ceteris paribus* (in the sense of disregarding) of *all* particularizations of subjectively selected instrumental value which might or might not be held, from time to time?[4] Answering the latter question will form the focus of the remainder of the chapter.[5]

Personhood as process

While the classic liberal conception of personhood is correct in its broad requirements of self-consciousness, rationality, and autonomy, it is incomplete. What is missing from the picture is the fundamental requirement for *extendedness in time* of a person. But while mere extendedness in time is necessary, it is likewise insufficient. Required to make the picture both necessary *and* sufficient is an acknowledgment of the fundamentally and irreducibly processual nature of personhood. Persons are not substances, possessed of *unchanging* unique predicates, which are therefore importantly *timeless*, and for whom relative extension in time would thus be irrelevant. Rather, persons *are* processes, fully embedded in time, with *constitutive* forward-looking aspects. For without the constant interchange of future-directed elements of desiring, hoping for, wishing and planning, without the rational identification and shepherding of the objects of such desires into present experience, and the recollection of past mind-states, which in turn feed back into, sustain, and inform the future-directed aspects, then valuing activity, indeed all activity would cease. In such a case, our autonomy would be meaningless, our consciousness empty and without object even of self, our rationality fixed, idle, and impotent, and our very subjectivity impossible. Rationality itself fundamentally involves *movement* and the movement of rationality is *processual* in nature, proceeding from one concept to the next, or to the process of construction of the next. Autonomy without change is empty and meaningless. Self-consciousness *flows* from one object to the next, and the autonomous *proto*-rational directedness of this *flow* is what constitutes the process of personhood.

The value of life extension

Consider the following passage from Bernard Williams (1972):

> . . .a man might consider what lay before him, and decide whether he did or did not want to undergo it. If he does decide to undergo it, then some desire propels him on into the future, and *that* desire at least is not one that operates conditionally on being alive, since it itself resolves the question of whether he is going to be alive. He has an unconditional or (as I shall say) a *categorical* desire . . .It is not necessarily the prospect of pleasant times that create the motive against dying, but the existence of a categorical desire and categorical desire can drive through both the existence and the prospect of unpleasant times.

Williams is absolutely right in his characterization of what he terms a "categorical desire," insofar as its capacity to "drive through" facts and circumstances of particular person's lives, gives a "motive against dying," and so a value of life extension.

Consider the desiring for, wishing for, hoping for, and planning towards that form the obvious features in the landscape of valuing activity, and the movement towards whose subjectively underwritten objects form the *instrumental* value of continuing to live. Such affects form the quasi-objective furniture of the subjectivist view of value, and the rational *process* by which they are selected constitutes the construction of the value itself, according to constructivists such as Korsgaard (1996). It is this kind of desire which Williams appears to be putting forward as a possible candidate for the ascription of "categorical" desire, in that continuing to live, and thus continuing to be a person (as I would have it), having the forward-directed motivation that drives the process of personhood towards the future, is suggested by this to be a contingent object of personal will. It does not follow, however, that each and every such desire of necessity takes the form of an explicit desire towards or is contingent upon some objective, or the fulfillment of some existing project.

Williams' concept of a person's "ground projects providing the motive force which propels him into the future, and gives him reason for living" (1981) begs the further question of the nature of origin of those "ground projects," as well as the question of the origin of their less-developed but still explicit precursor subjective categorical desires. Do these projects or desires both arise and provide their motivating force of themselves? Are they driven into being somehow by and simultaneously sufficiently constituting the "motive force" which "propels"? Or are they themselves driven into being by a more basic psychological motivator, which is prior, and is not describable in terms of an explicit project towards anything in particular? After all, a person does not appear to be born with an explicit prior set of these, and once possessed of them does not typically carry the same set through life, but forms new ones, and discards the old along the way. Each person differs in their subjectively endorsed set, and none seems logically necessary to persons, else if it were, the question of whether we *always* have (at least some) reasons for continuing to live would be to that extent resolved. Certainly, Williams does not think the question is so resolved, and appears to think that persons may exist without any such whatever (1972, 1981). Thus it is open to question what *motivates the formation* of these projects at all, as well as to question whether this basic motivation towards the existence of such categorical desires is *itself* constitutive of personhood.

What is the *driver* of the subjectivity which then forms and selects these objects of the affective component of our psychology? Further, is the idea of the "categorical desire," which "drives through" the negative aspects of experience to underwrite the value of continuation in life as being subjectively contingent the best or only picture we may have of such a motivator? Is it even the ordinary picture which we do have, and which appears to us throughout our lives? Consider the following from Nagel (1979):

> The situation is this: there are elements which, if added to one's experience, make life better; there are other elements which, if added to one's experience, make life worse. But what remains when these are set aside is not merely *neutral*: it is emphatically positive. Therefore life is worth living even when the bad elements of experience are plentiful, and the good ones too meager to outweigh the bad ones on their own. The additional positive weight is supplied by existence itself. . .

This seems right. But this is, however intuitively right-seeming, also mysterious. For how can "mere existence" be positive in some sense? I agree with Nagel, that there is such a non-contingent positivity, but disagree with Williams to the extent that I assert that such a positivity can be considered to represent a kind of *non-contingent* categorical desire, such that the mere continuance of the *person* represents fulfillment of this desire.[6]

Discussing the gap between his account of the value of life's continuance and that of Nagel, Williams (1972, pp.87–8) himself appeared to acknowledge that further analysis would perhaps discover a more stable and less overtly subjective (perhaps even non-subjective) basis for the origin and persistence of such life-affirming, categorical desires:

> The difference is that the reasons which a man would have for avoiding death are, on the present account, grounded in desires – categorical desires – which he has... Nagel, however, ... does not see the misfortune that befalls a man who dies as necessarily grounded in the issue of what desires or sorts of desires he had; ... In fact, further and deeper thought about this sort of question seems likely to fill up the gap between the two sorts of argument; it is hard to believe, for one thing, that the supposed contingent fact that people have categorical desires can really be as contingent as all that.

So what is missing, to fill in the picture? What is missing, I propose, is the conception of persons as future-directed *processes*, whose process must be driven continually by something, some motivating force, or nisus. This force or nisus, or in Leibniz, for example, the "appetitive" feature of the monad, I identify as and with the conative aspect in our psychology. It is this desire, this fundamental driver of striving, this forward-directed motivating principle, this conation, that drives the process and processes of personhood, all other considerations and values aside.

Indeed it is from the conative that particular desires arise at all, for without the fundamental and constitutive aspect of the process of personhood that this represents, there would be no motivation for any desire to form, or to come into defined being as an object of the affective. The original motivating component of the formation of desire is conation itself. Further, since without the driving of conation the process itself would cease, there would be no person to form desires, at all.

But this fundamental conation is not open for negation by an action of the personal will, or some overriding desire. This is because the will is itself conative, and any desire that seeks to direct it, is driven by the conative, and in any case must locate within an originating person, who would not exist without the conatively driven process by which they are constituted. What "puzzles the will" (Shakespeare, 1601, Hamlet, Act III, Scene i) about death is not, to deny Hamlet, that there may be continuance of the person in "what dreams may come" beyond death, but rather that there may *not* be continuance at all. When thinking about one's own extinction, the attempt to imagine it results, involuntarily, in an attempt to "see beyond," to think of blackness, say, or of another world in which the process continues, but falsely or paradoxically, perhaps merely contemplating its own non-existence. What the will balks at is the cessation of personhood, and *why it does so is that personhood is an intrinsically future-driven open-ended process.* The fundamental future-directed element of the process of personhood, the root categorical desire represented by the inseparable conative aspect, *presupposes the continuation of a person into the future.*

From this point of view, then, there is no point in time at which the continuation of a person's life may be said not to be valuable, since these forward-directed elements are necessary to the process of being a person.

In this way, it would appear that there can be no arbitrary upper limit on the good of the extension of life to a person. There is no point at which being a person does not involve the future-directed elements and their involvement in the process of inter-change with the present and past elements. An attempt to set or discover such a general limit would appear to involve a misunderstanding of the nature of the process itself. That we may know some facts about human biology, which suggest that we indeed have an end in store, and even how far in the future that end is likely to be, in no way impinges upon the intrinsic nature of the future-directed elements that are fundamental to the process of being a person. These point toward the ever-distant horizon of the possible, irrespective of the actual personal circumstances, such as, say, a terminal disease, or else the biological limitation of the lifespan of our species.

If no general limit can be arbitrarily set or discovered, could one be set by a person upon themselves? That my desires, hopes, and plans may fix upon particular objectives does not in itself suggest that I can easily, or at all, fix these elements of myself purely upon and contained within some set of particular objectives, such that the categorical desire itself can be somehow brought to an end upon the completion of this set. No matter what I specifically plan for, desire, or hope for, *it seems that the conative aspect of my psychology overflows the limits of these particular objects without any particular second-order act of will on my part*, and indeed, in *defiance* of one attempted in opposition, giving rise willy-nilly to a continual stream of fresh particular desires. So, *willing* these aspects of ourselves to be contained within a fixed, time-limited framework would seem to be impossible. I may seek rationally to direct or curtail the objects of my first-order desires and affects (those that simply "I desire") with my second-order desires (those by which "I desire that I do or do not desire") (Frankfurt, 1982), but that a second-order desire to have *no* desires should be effective would seem impossibly self-defeating. For such a desire *is itself a future-directed desire*, and so arises from the inalienable categorical conation which is the fundamental driver of the process that itself enables the autonomous will to exist. We cannot *effectively* will ourselves not to be a person,[7] while also being one, since that will *itself requires us to be a person*. It is instructive to try to imagine a person setting a particular date beyond which she will be free of all desires. Such a picture strikes one as absurd. This is not to say that we may not, from time to time, harbor clearly conceived desires for personal annihilation.[8] It is just to say that these alone will never of themselves annihilate the primary conative driver, since this is required for their very being, and in the process of being a person such desires are unlikely permanently to be pre-eminent, since the very driver which gives them rise functions to form new desires and changes in character, in the process of personhood, which *ex hypothesi* cannot be static. That such a self-negating desire should be made effective by action of suicide appears to ignore this fact, and fails to respect the total process-person.

Further, if it is acknowledged that a person, in any particular moment of the extended process of their personhood, is rarely or never presently conscious of *all* the particular desires they themselves possess, much less the general driver of categorical desire that gives rise to them, as silently pervasive as gravity, this observation becomes greatly stronger. So it does not seem reasonable that a person may even set a limit to the good of *their own* future extension in time.

It should be recognized that the case for the constitutive drive for personal continuation is isomorphic with perhaps the most pervasive and universally recognized moral imperative throughout history and culture: do not kill persons (even yourself!). Of course constructivists will point to the pragmatic social aspects of this universality. But is it the case that we must assume that there are no related internal motivations as well?[9] While the connection between the normative value "pro-life" and against murder or suicide with the constitutive conative drive of personhood-as-process which comprises the conative categorical desire-driver spoken of here may seem questionable, it must surely be acknowledged that it is at least both plausible, and isomorphic. Further, if it is right that this drive gives rise and motion to all desires, and itself motivates rationality, in the process of personhood, then it is the motivational underwriter of all and any value, *including* the second-order desires held by some to be exclusively normative. In this way, it might be called the master value. And such a value could be expected to be pervasive, singularly powerful, and uniquely motivating. In this way, I suggest that this underlying, ubiquitous, and therefore often overlooked, generator of the value of life's continuance is far more akin to the "ordinary picture of life's value" which we intuitively perceive as being something which must be both very powerful, pervasive, and very stable, than is some value derived from a second-order endorsement of some further and subsidiary, rationally constructed object of desire. It need hardly be noted that, whatever else their philosophic or religious convictions, when suddenly confronted with the prospect of imminent death (however sotto-voce it has previously appeared on account of its very ubiquity) there are few indeed, if any, who would not feel the reality, subjective inaccessibility, and force of this value, most keenly.

Person-Processes and the Personal Condition

Mortality, person-processes, and existentialism

In his famous 1946 lecture "Existentialism is a Humanism," Sartre (1989) declared

> Man is nothing else but that which he makes of himself. That is the first principle of existentialism. And this is what people call its "subjectivity," using the word as a reproach against us. But what do we mean to say by this, but that man is of a greater dignity than a stone or a table? For we mean to say that man primarily exists – that man is, before all else, something which propels itself towards a future and is aware that it is doing so.[10] Man is, indeed, a project which possesses a subjective life, instead of being a kind of moss, or a fungus or a cauliflower. Before that projection of the self nothing exists; not even in the heaven of intelligence: man will only attain existence when he is what he purposes to be. Not, however, what he may wish to be. For what we usually understand by wishing or willing is a conscious decision taken – much more often than not – after we have made ourselves what we are. I may wish to join a party, to write a book or to marry – but in such a case what is usually called my will is probably a manifestation of a prior and more spontaneous decision.[11]

Here Sartre is very close indeed to a discussion of the subject matter of this chapter. In many ways, I accept the thrust of this passage, and its description of what has been termed the "human," though for the purposes of this chapter, the "*personal* condition." But there is one aspect in which I believe Sartre to be mistaken, or at least confused, and indeed the matter is significantly blurred or glossed over in this passage. This is whether persons, as Sartre appears to have it, "propel" (or "hurl" in Frechtman's translation) *themselves* toward the future in some subjective sense, for which they as persons are then responsible, as he appears later to suggest, or else whether they are *propelled*, by the very thing which he is describing (in Frechtman's translation) as a "will." I believe that Sartre was skating across the, admittedly difficult to disentangle, boundary between cognition, affect and conation. If so, I assert that he is wrong to suggest that there is some "decision" (Mairet) or "choice" (Frechtman) in the matter. Rather persons are helplessly and inevitably propelled towards the future by the very process that makes them persons at all. In this way, Sartre was right at one level, that it is something inherent in ourselves as persons that does the propelling, but wrong at another, since it is not something that is open to subjective, second-order re-evaluation. The "will," described as prior to "wish" or plan, is deeper, prior, and "more spontaneous" than the decisions or choices Sartre speaks of. I believe that in these words Sartre was feeling his way towards the idea of conation, and a conative driver of the person, without wishing, however, to surrender the notion of radical freedom or autonomy of responsibility that was central to his conception of the existential predicament, and ethic. In this way, Sartre and I disagree on the level of autonomy that persons have over their own natures, but we seem to agree that conation indeed gives rise to other desires, wishes, and later, projects towards these.[12] On this adjusted view, the *personal* condition[13] is indeed still a predicament, for surely what we feel in view of our mortality is a sincere and profound existential problem, a dissonance between what we are inevitably as beings and what we know to be our inevitable fate. And what are we to make of this helplessness, in relation to life extension, and its value, if it is indeed accepted that we are unavoidably *mortal* beings, however long we may live? For us, helplessly future-projected beings, the difficulty is *ex hypothesi* never alleviated, *so long as we are persons.*

Some symmetries and false solutions

In a post-hoc manner, after formulating the initial persons-as-process view with regard to the value of life extension, I noticed some similarities between certain aspects of this view, and the view described in the core Buddhist text known as the "Four Noble Truths." In this text, and in its later philosophic elucidations, it is asserted that desire is what predicates suffering, and desire is fundamental to persons. The project of Buddhism, in one sense, is to free the subject of this suffering by freeing the subject, ultimately, of their very personhood. The purpose of the "eightfold path" is to quiet particular desires or affects, and that of meditation is to allow, eventually, a kind of "first-hand" insight into the purportedly illusory nature of personhood, such that personhood, and the constitutive desire that propels it, along with the affects which form the furniture of "samsara," or the game of personal life, evaporates, or is "snuffed out" in nirvana.[14] The causes of future-directed coming-into-being, thus the personhood itself, in this manner ceases altogether on attainment of nirvana.

Now it is not at all self-evident that desires should, at base, be undesirable, whatever suffering may also come of them. A discussion of this latter is beyond the scope of this chapter, but suffice to say that I do not particularly accept the broader commitments of Buddhism. However, the strict focus is germane. The point here is that it is generally acknowledged that, for the vast majority, nirvana, or the cessation of personhood, whether desirable in itself or not, *is not attainable within the scope of an ordinary lifespan.* About this I can agree. About the Buddhist solution to this issue – reincarnation – I can only say that I do not, since it seems unlikely, unwarranted, unevidenced, and indeed irrelevant.[15] What we may take from this, then, is that the Buddhists agree that there is a problem, but pose a solution which is for the majority no solution at all, since in the meantime, the central problem, death, manifests. Something very similar may be said of the solutions offered by the other major religions, which do not take the view that persons should seek self-extinction through realization of the illusion of personhood, but, implicitly recognizing the fundamental problem, seek to compensate for it by conjecturing or constructing fantastic future worlds in which we do continue to live, in any case, beyond our own deaths. However, in absence of any clear warrant, or evidence for this, we may bracket such hopes as rather conveniently wishful, and focus instead on the problem, and the fact that whatever else may be true about these ideas, the real predicator of the problem – the occurrence of death to persons, occurs just as factually along the way as it does without such corrective cultural construction.

Indeed further problems are present in the picture of the "eternal" person, which ironically have been raised by canonical conservative theorists seeking mistakenly to criticize life extension, when in fact they are criticizing supernatural immortality. It is argued that far from being a problem in view of the conative, striving aspect of persons, mortality is what gives persons the drive they have. Of course I deny this on two levels. Firstly, *ex hypothesi,* conation is constitutive, and therefore the lack of striving for persons will never be a problem, and is not, in any case, derived at base from *awareness* of mortality at all. Secondly, natural physical persons are irrevocably mortal, and so even if such theorists were right about striving, they would be wrong.

Such arguments often tout, as one of the virtues of aging, that its suffering gradually overpowers our will to live. But of course aging does not do this except by a process of increasing impediment, discomfort, exhaustion, and humiliation, none of which impinge in any central way on the conative drive of personhood. And we should not welcome this any more than a person who seeks euthanasia in view of a terrible terminal illness welcomes, or should welcome the illness itself on the basis that it makes them more open to the idea of dying. This is repugnant because such a person does *not desire to die.* If they could, they would live. They *desire to live.* But they *know that* they will die, and *know that* nothing but suffering intervenes. This in no way whatever means that they have a diminished categorical drive of personhood towards the future. In view of this it likewise does not mean that, in absence of the sickness unto death, life extension would not, for them be a clear, categorical good! It is the desire to live which itself makes the suffering towards death *most* intolerable.

The Makropulos objection – boredom misused

Various modern commentators (e.g. Kass, 2001) have taken up the suggestion, initiated in the discourse by Williams (1981), using the example of Karel Capek's opera *The Makropulos Secret,* that we should not seek to extend life because it will end in boredom. Consider the following from Capek (1923) (the eponymous Elina Makropulos is speaking of her own radically extended life):

> Boredom. No, it isn't even boredom. (...) you have no name for it. One cannot stand it. For 100, 130 years, one can go on. But then (...) one's soul dies. (...) For you, everything has value because for the few years that you are here, you don't have time to live enough. (...) no one can love for 300 years – it cannot last. And then everything tires one. It tires to be good, it tires to be bad. The whole earth tires one. And then you find out there is nothing at all: no sin, no pain, no earth, nothing.

It is interesting to notice that Capek himself appears unsure what he is speaking about, in this passage: "No, it isn't even boredom." He is of course right, though, it is not boredom. Simply put, boredom presupposes affect, and conation. We are not bored *simpliciter.* Boredom without reference *to something we would rather be doing* is meaningless. When people are bored, they speak of boredom *in relation to* having nothing to do (or else an inability to do it), and having nothing to do is not, in itself, a problem, *unless one is feeling driven to do something!* The person who is bored is indeed still a person, still driven, and one who feels boredom in view of feeling aggrieved at not doing something!

The argument presupposes that persons have a *uniform* "natural" span within which they can have desires towards fulfillable projects, and outside which they will, by some *constitutive* element, *entirely unexplained in the argument,* be *inevitably* bored, regardless of whether they are in full possession of their faculties and abilities, or not. Any Makropulos-type objection depends upon boredom being *structurally inevitable,* given sufficient time. There are a few options here. In deep time, a human being may find that they are:

H1: A person with valuing and desiring processes, which settle upon objectives and develop into ground projects, in which case the situation is normal and boredom cannot be structurally inevitable.

H2: A living human no longer manifesting *psychological* conation giving rise to valuing and desire, in which case one is no longer a person, and boredom cannot exist.

H3: A person who has such desires and projects, but for whom these are frustrated either functionally by some disability or by external constraint.

H4: (At least conceivably) A person whose sole desire is towards the project of having projects, but yet finds this impossible.

A putative Makropulos must be either H3 or H4. In the case of H3, it appears clear that the problem is not inherently to do with temporal scope, but rather either an internal failure (of bodily capability, or of the likes of curiosity or imagination), or else some other external constraint (e.g. incarceration). The latter has, frankly, nothing whatever to do with longevity *per se,* and can be discounted. The former, if age-related, must be accounted among the pathologies of aging, and therefore cannot legitimately be used as an argument *against* aging intervention, as it would be a clear target of such intervention. It is a bad argument, sadly common among critics of aging intervention, to urge the horrors and degenerations experienced by the biologically aged as an argument *against* aging intervention and the prolongation of youthfulness! Any successful Makropulos argument must therefore hold *ceteris paribus* other conditions than simple extension of lifespan, and must assume continuation of full functionality of a person.

Therefore, the proponent of an Makropulos argument must urge the structural inevitability of H4, which in turn can only really obtain if either there is a functional failure (in which case it collapses into a case of H3, dealt with above), or else if there really are simply no further worthwhile projects to be had at all! Presumably, this will happen if and only if the sum total of all possible projects has been exhausted. If not, the Makropulos argument collapses into the argument from *laziness*. In any case, this seems a fatuous worry, given the mind-boggling, possibly infinite vastness of what there is to know, to experience, and to do, not to mention the constitutive and inalienable open-endedness and forward-directedness of persons as classes of being, necessarily *changeful* processes as they are. After all, a truly and comprehensively static mind cannot, *ex hypothesi,* actually manifest a person at all, and is merely a case of H2.

Is there, then, no merit at all to such an argument? It seems unlikely, surely, that such intellects as Williams were *wholly* mistaken. So what is the true character of this observation, and does its true construction in fact argue *against* radical life extension, or could it perhaps amount to an argument *for* it, instead?

The Makropulos argument inverted: Procrustes and the imperative for scope

Suppose, for a moment, that the solution to the muddled story of Elina Makropulos is that Karel Capek, and his followers, have not *fully* grasped the role of conation in the *process* of personhood. Suppose they have (incorrectly) thought of persons as fixed substances, and mistaken the *functionally mediated* boredom of the biologically aged, for the extinction of personhood that might come as a result of the true end of striving, conation, and therefore affect, and indeed, *ex hypothesi* reasoned cognition, perhaps as a natural consequence of person-processes running out, or self-resolving in deep time. I suggest, then, that it may be that what Capek really wished to describe was not boredom, but nirvana, or true personal quiescence. Nirvana not in the false, common mistaken conception, of some kind of bliss, but rather true nirvana, being the extinction, within the scope of being alive, of desire, *and* personhood, entire. Seen in this way, Capek simply did not have a full or clear conception of what he was attempting to express, and Elina's wailings and lamentings are therefore an absurd form of malingering, since by them she demonstrates entirely conclusively that she is most certainly not what she claims: wholly empty.

But should complete emptiness, should the end of conation, should the cessation of personhood in an unhindered, processual manner (if such processes can indeed work themselves out to equilibrium or standstill), should such true quiescence be considered *negative*? Is this what makes death bad? Is the death of the person, in such a manner of cessation *prior to biological death* bad of necessity? The Buddhists, and I, would certainly suggest that it is not.

In view of this, remembering Procrustes, death for the vast majority, whatever their circumstances of health, surely constitutes a shocking and brutal foreshortening of the self-defining *structure* of the process of their persons.

To allow some perspective upon what I here suggest, take the example of Aristotelian virtue ethics. Virtue ethics is processual in nature, and person-process regarding. From arête, through phronesis, towards Eudaimonia, the process continues through life. But since there are striking variations in the raw material of character (as identified with arête) and the opportunities for development afforded by life- and person-processes (as identified with phronesis), eudaimonia is unobtainable by most, indeed, by any but the happy few. But what if there were greater scope for phronesis? It seems reasonable to suppose that character development requires, in this picture, some *significant* and *non-uniform*-across-all-persons, but rather person-predicated extension in time, and that it is indeed true that for most, the present scope will be insufficient for the purpose. The one-size-fits-all approach to appropriate lifespan just seems to mistake or worse, ignore, what *various* structures person-processes are, and how they generate their own purposes and characters. Self-resolution seems a mirror image of such self-realization, and perhaps the latter is required before the former may occur.

For a person-process that has achieved self-resolution, and come to a processual end, for a true Makropulos, there would be no passion, no fear, no affect, no boredom, no disvalue, no wailing.[16] There would simply be no person. Life extension would have no value, and death no horror or disvalue, whatever. True quiescence of the person-process would have been achieved, and the structure of the person-process whole and complete. Such an outcome, if plausible at all, would appear to obviate the difficulty posed by death to person-processes.

But for a *person*, for one who still feels and is constituted by the powerful, primal conative drive, pervasive as gravity, and progenitor, sustainer, and motivator of all desires, rational plans, projects and values; in the ordinary way, *their* process unfolds the immeasurably variable body of their personal life upon the uniformly short iron frame of ancient and irrelevant biological circumstance,[17] continuously towards the relentless, purposeless Procrustean cleaver of decrepitude and death at its end.

Seen in this light, a Makropulos story told in full consistency would look, I suggest, more like an argument for life extension, than one for *false* and self-deceiving (ac) quiescence in the face of Procrustes.

Notes

1. In the case of values, the problems outlined by the likes of Hume, and in a separate mode, Moore, are thus to be regarded as pointing to an as yet unresolved relationship, as opposed to one unresolvable, and the thesis of this chapter suggests a direction towards their resolution. In forthcoming publications, the relationship of person-processes in value theory to systems biology and the physics of self-organization will be explored with a view to completion of this grounding.
2. For example, historically slavery was normal in most human societies.

3. So the intrinsic positive value, since nonderivative and conditional only upon the fact of being alive, is present in whole or not present at all, which being the case it will not be affected by the length of a person's life. A life of 5 years is intrinsically as valuable as a life of 55 years. To account for a difference one must turn to subjectively grounded instrumental value accounts, or otherwise abandon nonderivative value of life *simpliciter*.

4. A simple negative answer to this opens up the subjectivist camp to a (in my opinion justifiable) charge of excessive whimsicality regarding this surely gravely serious value.

5. In so doing, however, it should be noted that I am in no way discounting the potency and importance of the ordinary subjective instrumental reasons, which perhaps more obviously underwrite the value of life extension.

6. It should be noted that in this sense, the "desire" represented, identified with nisus or conatus, is not of a subjective sort, but is basic, and profound. It is, then, a kind of *person-originating desire*. I may be accused, perhaps, of equivocating on the meaning of "desire," but at the extreme originating leading edge, it seems to me that the meaning of this term may in fact turn out to be rather equivocal. Further, I do not intend that this will of necessity override all other considerations such that we must strive to continue living whatever the circumstances at all. There may be other factors which are capable of defeating it in particular situations, say, of an overdetermination towards certain death with the sole prospect of intense suffering in between, or otherwise no prospect whatever other than suffering, or perhaps the desire towards self-sacrifice in order to save a loved one. But in none of these cases is the basic conative desire extinguished, rather it is generally what makes these kinds of situations *most* intolerable, and may be the ultimate source of the suffering, worse than any mere pain. To paraphrase Emily Dickinson: dying is not so pitiful as the frustrated desire to live.

7. In other words, one cannot cease being a person by a pure act of will alone.

8. Though I believe such desires are on analysis likely to be found to be predicated upon idealizations of existence, which are themselves desires for continuance of life, though in a different mode than that which happens to be the case, and so are unlikely to be clearly nihilistic, but only contingently so given presently prevailing facts in the person's circumstances.

9. To assume this would surely be akin to accepting Hamlet without the prince, and in any case would beg the question: for what, again, *motivates* the pragmatism?

10. For useful comparison, Frechtman's translation (1957) differs slightly, but carries an enlightening slant in this context: "For we mean that man first exists, that is, that man first of all is the being who hurls himself toward a future and who is conscious of imagining himself as being in the future."

11. Frechtman's translation again: "Because by the word 'will' we generally mean a conscious decision, which is subsequent to what we have already made of ourselves. I may want to belong to a political party, write a book, get married; but all that is only a manifestation of an earlier, more spontaneous choice that is called 'will'."

12. So Korsgaard's constructivist ethics, taking place as it does, in the "heaven of intelligence," is on Sartre's view also only secondary to this motivation.

13. For there is a crucial difference between the set of humans, and the set of persons, and it is very much the latter that the personhood as process view regards.

14. At its Sanskrit root, nirvana literally means nir- (out) vati (it blows).

15. To the particular instantiated person in question.

16. And also one might note, as one might mischievously suggest that Capek noted also: no action to the play, *no personal development*, and therefore, no opera!

17. The character identity of *process* resolving all questions of identity of person.

References

Capek, K. (1990; f.p. 1923). The Makropoulos secret. In P. Kussi (ed.), *Toward the Radical Center* (pp. 173–4). Catbird Press.

Dworkin, R. (1993). *What is sacred? Life's Dominion*. London: HarperCollins.

Frankfurt, H. (1982). Freedom of the will and the concept of a person. In G. Watson (ed.), *Free Will. Oxford Readings in Philosophy* (pp. 81–95). Oxford: Oxford University Press.

Frechtman, B. (1957), *Existentialism and Human Emotions*. New York: Philosophical Library.

Holliday, R. (2006). Aging is no longer an unsolved problem in biology. *Annals of the New York Academy of Sciences*, **1067**, 1–9.

Horrobin, S. (2005). The ethics of aging intervention and life extension. In S.I. Rattan (ed.), *Aging Interventions and Therapies*. Singapore: World Scientific Publishers. Available at: www.worldscibooks.com/lifesci/etextbook/5690/5690_chap01.pdf (Accessed October 30, 08).

Horrobin, S. (2006a). Immortality, human nature, the value of life and the value of life extension. *Bioethics*, **20**, 279–92.

Horrobin, S. (2006b). The value of life and the value of life extension, *Annals of the New York Academy of Sciences*, **1067**, 94–105.

Kass, L. (2001). L'Chaim and its limits: Why not immortality? *First Things*, **113**, 17–24.

Kass, L.R. (2003). Ageless bodies, happy souls: Biotechnology and the pursuit of perfection. *New Atlantis*. Spring, 9–28.

Kirkwood, T.B.L. (2002). Evolution of ageing. *Mechanisms of Ageing and Development*, **123**, 737–45.

Kirkwood, T.B.L. & Rose, M.R. (1991). Evolution of senescence: Late survival sacrificed for reproduction. *Philosophical Transactions of the Royal Society of London B*, **332**, 15–24.

Korsgaard, C. (1996). *The Sources of Normativity*. Cambridge: Cambridge University Press.

Nagel, T. (1979). Death. In T. Nagel (ed.), *Mortal Questions* (pp. 9–10). Cambridge: Cambridge University Press.

Rattan, S.I. (1995). Gerontogenes: Real or virtual? *FASEB Journal*, **9**, 284–6.

Sandel, M. (2002). What's wrong with enhancement? President's Council on Bioethics (PCBE). Available at: www.bioethics.gov/background/sandelpaper.html (accessed October 10, 2008).

Sartre, J.P. (1989), Mairet, P. (trans.). Existentialism is a humanism. In W. Kaufman (ed.), *Existentialism from Dostoyevsky to Sartre*. New York: Meridian.

Williams, B. (1972). The Makropolos case: Reflections on the tedium of immortality. In B. Williams (ed.), *Problems of the Self* (pp. 86–100). Cambridge: Cambridge University Press.

Williams, B. (1981). Persons, character and morality. In B. Williams (ed.), *Moral Luck: Philosophical Papers 1973–1980* (p. 13). Cambridge: Cambridge University Press.

32

Enhancing Human Aging: The Cultural and Psychosocial Context of Lifespan Extension

John Bond

Increasing Life Expectancy and the Human Lifespan

Life expectancy is increasing world wide (United Nations, 2003). Yet it is really only in the last 25 years that there has been general acknowledgment of increasing life expectancy and more recently that human lifespan is also increasing. Prior to this there was a general consensus among biologists, demographers, and social scientists that human lifespan had a fixed upper limit. General improvements in the built and social environments during the period of the industrial revolution have been recognized as contributing to an increase in life expectancy in European societies. But beliefs and attitudes about lifespan remained relatively fixed until life expectancy exceeded assumed average lifespan.

Over the last 150 years, since that period in European history when the industrial revolution was at its height and transforming the social and economic landscape, life expectancy has increased at a steady two years per decade. This was first clearly described by Oeppen and Vaupel (2002) in their influential paper in *Nature* that plotted life expectancy in the "record-breaking" countries since 1840. Figure 32.1 shows the linear rise in female life expectancy from about 45 years in 1840 to over 80 years at the millennium, an increase that corresponds to 2.3 years per decade. Male life expectancy has also increased but at a slightly slower rate such that at the millennium the life expectancy of men was some six years less than that of women (Oeppen & Vaupel, 2002). Also shown in Figure 32.1 are the projections of life expectancy made by demographers for the World Bank and United Nations in recent years; projections that have had to be increased upwards as new records in life expectancy and lifespan are achieved. The use of data based on the "record-breaking" countries provides a more dramatic presentation of the linear nature of the rise in life expectancy over the recorded period. Data plotted for individual countries show more uneven curves due to contingencies experienced in different countries such as the two world wars, economic

Enhancing Human Capacities, edited by Julian Savulescu, Ruud ter Meulen and Guy Kahane.
© 2011 Blackwell Publishing Ltd

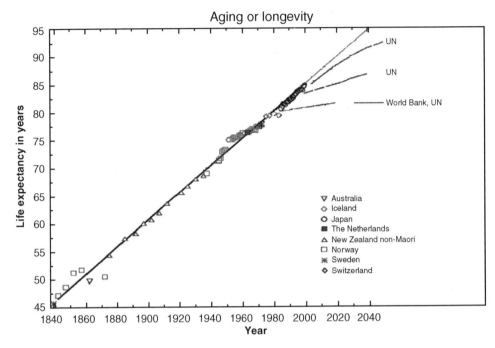

Figure 32.1   Recorded female life expectancy from 1840 to the present
Note: The dashed lines denote projections of female life expectancy in Japan as published by the United Nations in 1986, 1999 and 2001, respectively.
Source: Oeppen, J. & Vaupel, J.W. (2002). Demography. Broken limits to life expectancy. *Science*, **296**, 1029–31. The American Association for the Advancement of Science

recession, and disease pandemics. (See for example the cases of Japan and England and Wales, Westendorp & Kirkwood, 2007, pp.28–9.)

   Data and projections about lifespan are almost non-existent since these data are based on individual records reported in different countries and for which the authenticity of the claims are often open to challenge. However, the reality of increasing human lifespan is well illustrated by the increasing numbers of centenarians across European countries from 1840 onwards as recorded, for example, in Census data from Britain (Thatcher, 1997).

Healthy Active Life Expectancy

From an individual and a societal perspective increasing length of life requires a corresponding increase in the quality of life and particularly health-related quality of life. With increasing lifespan there has been an increasing burden of age-related disease and associated loss of function or increased disability. There is an increasing expectation that science and technology will play a major role in the prevention of age-related disease, in the development of cures and in the provision of technological enhancements to alleviate disability and functional limitations. Indeed the prevalence of functional limitation due to chronic disease has increased in the last 25 years (Freedman & Martin, 2000) although this may be partly explained by better recording methods and earlier diagnosis, as well as improved medical treatment. A reduction in the severity of disability (Deeg *et al.*, 1994; Robine *et al.*, 1998) may have also been a benefit of earlier diagnosis and improved medical treatment. But from the social model of disability perspective (Oliver, 1990), it may also be due to changing attitudes and expectations about disability or the impact of assisted technology that has reduced the disabling effects of the environment.

A key policy indicator of changes in health and life expectancy is the concept of healthy active life expectancy (Bone *et al.*, 1996) and the associated concept of disability-free life expectancy (Perenboom *et al.*, 2004). In the early 1980s the idea emerged that morbidity (and therefore disability) would be compressed in later life (Fries & Crapo, 1981). Evidence for whether this is happening is equivocal (Jeune, 2006; Robine & Michel, 2004). Much of the support for the compression of disability hypothesis and increased disability-free life expectancy comes from studies in the United States (Freedman *et al.*, 2002, Manton *et al.*, 2006) that show a decline in the prevalence of "less severe" disability since the 1980s (Freedman *et al.*, 2004). In European countries, however, both decreases and increases in disability have been reported (Parker *et al.*, 2005; Sagardui-Villamor *et al.*, 2005). Evidence about the experience of the oldest old (people aged 85 years or over), who have the highest rates of disability, is limited because of the absence of robust studies of this age group.[1]

Thus the optimistic idea produced by the compression of morbidity and disability hypotheses supported the desire to add life to years and not just years to life with the aim to increase health span as well as lifespan. However, for example, whereas in the United Kingdom over the last 20 years life expectancy has increased by some four years healthy active life expectancy has only increased by about two years (House of Lords Science and Technology Committee, 2005). Recent understandings from the new biology of aging has recognized the increasing malleability of lifespan but as yet we do not know whether health span will increase faster or slower than lifespan in the future (Westendorp & Kirkwood, 2007, p.31).

Inequalities in Life Extension and Healthy Aging

Life expectancy varies by nine years between European countries. Across Europe women live longer than men by four to eight years. Disability is estimated to be highest in Italy and Spain and lowest in Finland (Pluijm *et al.*, 2005; Van den Brink *et al.*, 2003) and there is a north–south gradient in hand-grip strength which is a strong predictor of both disability and mortality (Jeune *et al.*, 2006). Not only does life expectancy differ significantly between men and women but there are inequalities in healthy active life expectancy. Data from the UK MRC Cognitive Function and Ageing Study (MRC CFAS) highlight inequalities in healthy active life expectancy between men and women, socioeconomic group, and regions (Medical Research Council Cognitive Function and Ageing Study (MRC CFAS), 2001). At the age of 80 men could expect to live for 6.3 years, 5.5 years with a physical illness, 1.1 years with functional impairment, and 0.6 years with a cognitive impairment. In contrast women at the age of 80 could expect to live for a further 8 years, 7.3 years with a physical illness, 2.7 years with a functional impairment, and 1.5 years with a cognitive impairment.

The prevalence of disability is also associated with socioeconomic status (Ebrahim *et al.*, 2004). In MRC CFAS the number of disability-free life years is some 2 years more for men in higher socioeconomic groups than men in lower socioeconomic groups at 65 years of age and 1 year more at 85 years of age. Differences among women are less evident at older ages. At 65 years of age women in the higher socioeconomic groups could expect some 1.5 years longer disability-free life years than women in lower socioeconomic groups. By 85 years of age there is no difference between women from different socioeconomic groups. All women in this age group could expect 2.5 years of life free from disability.

Understanding Increasing Life Expectancy

The increasing of life expectancy since 1840 throughout Europe and other economically developed parts of the world has been too rapid for biological explanations such as genetics and is more to do with changes to the physical and social environments (Christensen *et al.*, 2006). However, there still exists within different birth cohorts considerable variation in life expectancy as can be seen from inspection of estimates for European countries, social groups within countries, and different groups of human behaviors such as smoking and not smoking. Understanding of this diversity is far from clear with genetics, environment, gene–environment interactions, and epigenetic or stochastic processes all likely to be involved. It is the complex interaction between genes, the physical and social environment, and chance that influences life expectancy of populations and the health and lifespan of individuals.

Different influences on changes in European life expectancy since 1840 have been highlighted for different historical periods (Vaupel & Romo, 2003). For example, between 1840–1900 a reduction in infant mortality led to increased life expectancy while after 1960 it was a reduction in premature mortality in mid-life (between 45 years and 65 years) that became the dominant driver of increased life expectancy. Since 1990 there is increasing evidence that changes in the patterns of late-life mortality (aged 65 years or over) from cardiovascular disease has continued the increase in life expectancy. These observations led Oeppen and Vaupel (2002) to argue that increases in life expectancy could be explained by "a regular stream of continuing progress" (p.1029) including increases in absolute income and wealth; improvements in education, nutrition, and sanitation; and developments in preventative and therapeutic medicine.

The contribution that different aspects of continuing human progress have made to improvements in population health and human longevity is hard to pinpoint because of the lack of concrete evidence on causality. However, some attempts have been made to understand the role of biological, economic, environmental, and social factors in the development of health span and lifespan. Perhaps the seminal analysis was the work of McKeown (1979) on the decline of mortality in England and Wales between 1848 and 1971. He estimated that about three-quarters of the decline in infant and adult mortality was due to a decline in infectious diseases particularly airborne diseases such as tuberculosis. This he attributed to improvements in living conditions such as the provision of clean water and sanitation, improved nutrition, and less overcrowding. In the Netherlands, Mackenbach (1996) also estimated that the decline in mortality between 1875 and 1970 was mainly due to a reduction in mortality from infectious diseases but suggested, contrary to McKeown, that medical science was also influential. This was in line with Szreter (1988) who reviewed the role of public health measures in Britain between 1850 and 1914 and suggested that measures that had reduced the onslaught of disease on the immune systems would probably increase resistance to other infections.

The contribution that medical science has made to increasing life expectancy remains contested. For example Bunker (2001) and Bunker *et al.* (1994) estimated that medicine has probably contributed to about 5 years of the about 30-year increase in life expectancy since 1900 and about 3–4 year gain since 1950. However, Wilkinson (1996, citing Mackenbach *et al.*, 1990) suggests that "the social and economic determinants of mortality remain substantially more powerful" (p.31).

Recent studies have highlighted the impact of medical intervention on contemporary increases in life expectancy. Analysis of data from the MONICA European study of middle-aged populations suggested that two-thirds of the changes in mortality rates due to coronary heart disease can be attributed to a decline in the risk factors that influence the incidence of the disease and one-third are due to treatments that influence case fatality (Kuulasmaa *et al.*, 2000; Tunstall-Pedoe *et al.*, 1999). It has been highlighted that the prevention of cancer and heart disease would lead to the greatest improvements in life expectancy (Bronnum-Hansen *et al.*, 2006). Jeune (2006) has argued that since more than half of the oldest old (people aged 80 or over) die from diseases of the circulatory system, that the mortality impact must have had a substantial impact on the recent increase in maximum lifespan.

Human Aging and the Future of Old Age

So far this chapter has focused on documenting the changes in life expectancy and human lifespan and reviewing current understandings of these demographic and epidemiological transitions. In so doing the chapter assumes shared understandings of the meaning of aging and old age.

Aging

From a social gerontological perspective aging is a concept that is less contested than the idea of old age. It is generally agreed within gerontology that human aging is a process that begins and ends. There is some discussion about the nature of the beginning and end, but insufficient contestation to not have a shared understanding. Much of that discussion is philosophical with debates about whether human aging begins at birth, conception, or at the point when the human egg is first created.

Biogerontologists generally take the view that the development of the fetus following conception is the start of the aging process. Psychogerontologists and social gerontologists are more likely to focus on the individual and the societies in which individuals are members and therefore define birth as the starting point of the aging process. Gerontologists probably generally agree that death is the endpoint of the aging process although this may be contested by some who accept the possibility of an afterlife and by those who see individuals' life histories surviving after their death. This, however, is probably where the broad consensus between gerontologists stops. For contemporary biogerontologists aging is "nothing more nor less than the gradual, lifelong accumulation of subtle faults in the cells and organs of the body" (Westendorp & Kirkwood, 2007, p.20). This is in contrast to the common stereotype of aging, dominant in Western cultures, reflected in everyday life, popular culture, and policy rhetoric that highlights the later life decline of bodily functions resulting in graying hair, changing skin texture, failing eyesight, waning muscular strength, or reduced vitality. Although biogerontology recognizes natural variation in the rate of accumulation of bodily faults and the impact of the environment on these processes, it is the generalization of biological decline in social discourse that ignores the diversity of the human aging experience. From lifespan or life-course perspectives in social science aging is an individualized and unique process that involves changes in many aspects of people's lives and not just declining health and vitality. Thus a contrasting viewpoint might be the idea of the accumulation of diverse experiences and knowledge over the life course.

Old age

In contrast to aging, "old age" is a more difficult concept to fix. In biogerontology, since aging is a gradual process there is no point at which the human organism has reached old age. Where biogerontologists talk about old age they are doing so as members of society and accepting taken-for-granted concepts of everyday life based on chronological age rather than the scientific concepts of biogerontology. Nowadays most social gerontologists would take a constructionist perspective[2] and avoid definitions based on chronological age, however convenient this may be for societies and their members. Rather old age is something that is created as a product of individual and societal processes and varies between different discourses. Understandings of the meanings of age or aging are constructed within different social spaces, social fields and institutions, for example within biomedicine, the making of public policy, media and the arts (Westerhof & Tulle, 2007). Each space provides us with different meanings of age and aging (although some overlaps are apparent).

The biomedicalization of aging (Estes & Binney, 1989) has been a major influence across these social spaces. In the biosciences, the notion of "natural" physiological and cognitive decline with age has been under steadily more effective assault, as novel biomedical theories and analytic techniques have been deployed to divide, fix, and define "normal" and "abnormal" aging. This has led to the characterization of aging in terms of boundary issues around the "normal" and "abnormal" organic processes that lead to mental and physical decline and the labeling of older people as a distinct biomedical category.

Chronological age has been used in public policy for demarcating between "older people" and others in society. Here the meaning of age is represented in terms of old age as a social problem to be solved (McIntyre, 1977), of dependency and decreasing economic productivity (Walker, 1982), and apocalyptic demography (Robertson, 1997). Early public policy discourse perceived older people as in need of financial, medical, and social support. More recent public policy discourse has been increasingly alarmist and has focused on the impact of the increasing demands of aging populations on social protection systems. The development of negative stereotypes of aging and the development of institutionalized ageism has been reinforced by the process of individualization within the biomedicalization of aging and the emphasis on individual responsibility within contemporary public policy. This has led to the blaming of older people for the largely societal impacts of population aging and also for the biological processes not within their own control.

The representation of later life in the media and the arts reflects the negative attitudes of society toward older people. Images of aging reflect the public's perception that aging is a bodily affair reinforced by society's preoccupation with health, illness, and mortality underpinned by commonsense knowledge of our own aging bodies and the biomedicalization of aging. Recently the emerging concept of the Third Age (Laslett, 1996) has been used to create a sharp distinction between the often idealized positive images of the freedom and wealth in the early years of retirement (Gilleard & Higgs, 2000), and the frailty and helplessness of the Fourth Age. These negative images are likely to create a fear of aging and injure the self-images of older people (Jolanki, 2004) as well as reinforcing negative stereotypes of later life.

The development and reinforcement of negative stereotypes of older people has led to discrimination against older people encapsulated in the concept of ageism – defined as the systematic stereotyping of and discrimination against people because they are old (Butler, 1969). Institutionalized ageism through the systematic exclusion of older people from the mainstream of everyday life by the institutions and structures of European societies has only recently been challenged and included within the equal opportunities framework. However, the experience of aging, old age, and ageism by individual older people is enormously heterogeneous with a diversity of experience based on gender, ethnicity, socioeconomic position, and country of residence. Those at the bottom of the social structure (the have nots) are more likely to have experienced ageism than those with higher social status (the haves and the have mores).

Inequalities in Later Life

In addition to the inequalities in health and vitality already highlighted there are significant inequalities between genders, generation, and socioeconomic position mediated by ethnic status. Despite claims that older people are increasingly affluent compared with adults with young families and that mobility between social classes is greater than ever, the evidence suggests otherwise.

Gender

Perhaps the starkest comparison is the difference between men and women (Arber & Ginn, 1991). Over the last 50 years the roles of men and women have remained remarkably consistent. In most European societies men remain the main wage earners, fewer women are in full-time paid work, and average incomes for those in full-time employment are less than their male colleagues; few women penetrate the "glass ceilings" within organizations and make it to the top jobs in industry or the public sector; and the role of home maker and main carer disproportionately falls upon women. Gender roles across the life course are a consequence of male domination (and oppression) reflected in the privileging of men (Acker, 1992). Although women may live longer in most other respects older women are worse off than men in general and men from their own socioeconomic position in particular. This reflects inequalities and oppression across the life course that persists into later life.

Older women are more likely than older men to live in poverty and have less access to a financially secure retirement (Estes *et al.*, 2003). This can be illustrated by data from the Commission of the European Communities (2003) that estimated the risk of poverty for different age groups and genders in 2001. The average risk of poverty for people aged 65 and over in the 15 states of the European Union (EU15) was 12% (men 12%; women 14%). In Ireland (total 31%; men 19%; women 40%), Greece (total 26%; men 24%; women 28%), and Portugal (total 24%; men 22%; women 25%) the risk of poverty is far greater than the EU15 average particularly in rural areas (Naegele & Walker, 2007: Table 7.2). Although on average the risk of poverty among older women is only slightly higher than that for men, in some countries gender differences are significant, particularly in Ireland (men 19%; women 40%), Austria (men 10%; women 24%), Finland (men 7%; women 21%), and the United Kingdom (men 12%; women 17%) (Naegele & Walker, 2007: Table 7.2). However, what is also evident is that across Europe the incidence of poverty in later life increases with advancing age particularly among older women and those who are widows (Walker & Maltby, 1997).

The burden of providing informal support falls to women. Data from the European Community Household Panel (Eurostat, 1999) shows that women in Europe are more likely to be the informal caregivers of older people (Nordic countries 64%; continental countries 60%; southern countries 75%; UK and Ireland 59%) (Bond & Cabrero, 2007). Data from the UK also shows that women will always be the first choice for informal caregiver (Qureshi & Walker, 1989; RIS MRC CFAS Resource Implications Study Group of the Medical Research Council Cognitive Function and Ageing Study, 1999).

Generation

In thinking of generation we need to go beyond the idea of population cohorts that share a social location based on chronological age but embrace Mannheim's (1952) ideas that generations share historical and sociocultural locations (Gilleard & Higgs, 2002; Vincent, 2005). For example, those generations who were children in the 1930s at the time of the Great Depression and survived the turmoil of the 1939–45 Second World War in Europe have very different values, attitudes, and lifestyles to the "baby-boomers" born in the post-war period of increasing economic prosperity and national reconciliation within states in the European Economic Community between 1945–65. Distinguishing between generations highlights further the diversity of experience of European citizens by placing all individuals in the context of their cultural, economic, and social environment. Future generations of older people will have aged through a period of increasing rapid technological change, the hegemony of consumerism, and widening economic inequality across populations.

Inequality occurs both within and between generations. Inequality within generations can be seen as an aspect of cumulative advantage or disadvantage across the life course described formally "as the systematic tendency for interindividual divergence in a given characteristic (e.g. money, health or status) with the passage of time" (Dannefer, 2003, p.S327). The idea of cumulative disadvantage focuses on collectivities rather than individuals and highlights the widening gap between the "haves" and "have nots" and increasingly the "have mores," not just in terms of income and wealth but also in terms of longevity, health, cultural activity, and social inclusion.

Inequality between generations has become an increasingly important political and social issue with the aging of the population. Two beliefs are important here. First the idea that the younger working population supports older people through social-protection mechanisms in terms of pensions, health care, and long-term care and that the demand for these is outstripping the ability of societies to support them. This has important implications at a time of increasing life expectancy and the development of new life-enhancing technologies. Second the beliefs that the younger generation, particularly children, are deprived of resources that are going to an increasingly affluent and wealthy generation of older people (Phillipson, 1998). Both these beliefs appear blind to the myth of the WOOPE (well off older people) (Falkingham & Victor, 1991) and the wide diversity of experience within later life that reflects the diversity of experience in earlier life. These two beliefs were reflected in the idea of increasing inequality and generational conflict between younger and older generations fueled by the aging of the population which it was argued would generate economic instability (Johnson *et al.*, 1989).

Commodification of Aging

From a political economy perspective[3] a further consequence of inequalities in later life and the biomedicalization of aging has been the commodification of aging and old age. "Commodification is the process of taking a good or service that has been produced and used, but not bought and sold, and turning it into an item that is exchanged for money" (Estes *et al.*, 2003, p.49). The commodification of aging and old age provides an example of the commodification of life-course experience and later-life lifestyle that is part of "the relentless commodification of everyday life"(Gilleard & Higgs, 2000, p.7). The rapid expansion of global capital and particularly increasing investment by markets in the services and retail industries has fueled the hegemony of consumerism and the search by capital investors for new markets. "Old age" may not itself be seen as a market for new cars or clothes but provides increasing opportunities for new later-life lifestyles and "anti-aging medicine."

Anti-Aging Medicine

Anti-aging medicine is a term that describes a wide range of human interventions that potentially influence the processes of human aging or increase longevity.

Vincent (2006) has described four categories of anti-aging medicine: symptom alleviation; life expectancy extension; lifespan extension; and abolition.

Symptom alleviation

Agents designed to "hide, postpone or relieve the effects of biological ageing" (Vincent, 2006, p.689) have been available for many years. Such agents can be categorized on the basis of their "scientific pedigree": traditional remedies based on folk medicine that have been past down through the generations; agents advertised as "miracle" treatments and sold by charlatans; and new agents that have been developed within the experimental paradigm that is central to the development, regulation, and marketing of modern pharmaceutical products. These agents fall into three classes of marketable products: cosmetics (e.g. anti-wrinkle creams); prophylactics (e.g. vitamin pills); and treatments (e.g. Viagra). As part of the commodification of aging these products are part of a large and increasing market.

Life expectancy extension

The extension of life expectancy through the eradication or control of age-associated diseases such as cancer and heart disease has been the traditional focus of anti-aging medicine in the latter half of the 20th century and has been credited with a reduction in late-life mortality (Kuulasmaa *et al.*, 2000, Tunstall-Pedoe *et al.*, 1999). With the decline in risks associated with many late-life medical interventions there is a demand by practitioners and patients alike for the routinization of effective interventions in the treatment of ever-older patients (Shim *et al.*, 2006). With increasing public expectations that are fueled by the media portrayal of health and illness (Seale, 2003) and of scientific breakthrough (Petersen, 2001) the demand for relatively low-risk and ineffective treatments is also increasing, for example the recent controversy over the use of cholinesterase inhibitors for patients with dementia (Alzheimer's Society, 2006). The international pharmaceutical industry plays a major role here through the direct marketing of products in some markets (e.g. the United States), the promotion of expectations (Brown & Michael, 2003), and the manufacturing of new diseases (Fishman, 2004). A recent trend has also been the closer involvement of academic scientists in the discovery, evaluation, production, and marketing of new pharmaceutical agents (Clarke *et al.*, 2003) for the alleviation of symptoms and life extension. This trend is clearly a challenge to the moral credence and scientific independence of the academic biomedical community.

Lifespan extension

It is only in the last few decades that the demographic evidence of lifespan extension has appeared. Yet the biology of aging is still contested (Binstock, 2004). As argued above, existing success with the extension of lifespan is clearly the outcome of old technologies – the public health measures of the 19th century, increasing education and affluence, lifestyle changes in the 20th century, and routinized biomedical interventions of the last couple of decades. But much of the debate in biogerontology focuses on the new biology of aging and the impact that future scientific breakthrough will have on both life expectancy and lifespan extension. In the laboratory the lifespan of worms, fruit flies, and rodents has been manipulated but as yet there have been no examples of lifespan being manipulated in humans.

Abolition

The fourth category of anti-aging medicine identified by Vincent (2006) is one that enters the cultural space of science fiction. Few scientists are claiming that aging can be abolished with the creation of immortality although some may, in private, be cautiously optimistic that such an outcome is a possibility for the future.

Forecasting the Future

The future of increasing life expectancy and life extension remains highly contested. For bioscience there is strong belief that human aging is a biological process that is capable of being controlled by human intervention. What remains unclear is whether current projections that life expectancy will increase on average by 2.5 years per decade are accurate. The analysis by Oeppen and Vaupel (2002) highlights the difficulty of estimating future life expectancy and maximum lifespan. The dramatic linear trend that they have plotted suggests that life expectancy will continue to rise steadily at the same rate for the foreseeable future. However, there is no theoretical reason either for or against this prediction. Their analysis of the different possible explanations for changes in life expectancy over the last 160 years should encourage caution. However, the prevailing view among some experts engaged in AGEACTION (Kirkwood, 2007) (a Specific Support Action of the EU Framework Programme 6) is that the steady increase in life expectancy is set to continue into the near future based on the knowledge of medical interventions that have recently been introduced into medical practice and those in the pipeline. The rate of increase in new biological and biomedical knowledge and the potential of new technologies could have a more dramatic impact on life expectancy. Equally as historical data indicate (for example the impact of the Second World War on life expectancy in the UK, Westendorp & Kirkwood, 2007) these trends can quite easily be transformed by economic, political, and social change.

Although the nature of human aging and the experience of later life have seen considerable change during the 20th century, individuals, organizations and states appear ill-equipped or unwilling to prepare for the economic and social changes likely in the 21st century. Without any dramatic increase in lifespan the proportion of the population defined as old will increase considerably with a tripling of people aged 80 years or over as the baby-boomer generation reach their eighth decade. This "graying" of society will have profound implications for individuals in all walks of life and how we organize our societies in the future. Of course, human aging is only one aspect of human experience that may change markedly in this century. If we take the last 100 years as a guide we should expect in the next 100 years continuing changes to the natural environment reflecting both the serendipity of nature and the impact of human activity; accelerating development of technological and scientific innovation that will change the way we organize our lives; and with increasing globalization changes in our cultural, political, and social institutions. It is within these contexts that individuals and societies will experience human aging.

Globalization

The inevitable march of globalization – the interconnectedness of global economic, political, and social orders characterized by global hierarchies of power and inequality that challenge the power of the nation state and individual citizenship – is a key economic and political context in which human aging will exist. The ideology of globalization has influenced the way that social policies in response to aging have privatized the risks of aging (Phillipson, 2006). The decline of collectivism and the sharing of risks have placed the responsibility of financial security and health and long-term care firmly on the individual and their social networks. In the future, increasing social exclusion and inequality between the "haves," "haves nots," and "haves more" is inevitable as there will be an accumulative disadvantage over the life course for those who are poor or less well-educated.

How will future generational cohorts be able to sustain current lifestyles? Some have argued that the "baby-boomer" generation of Third Agers will have the financial and political power to maintain their individualized consumer-oriented lifestyles (Higgs & Gilleard, 2006). However, in the longer term patterns of work are changing and those currently economically active will change jobs (as opposed to employers) many times in their lifetime and will require continuous retraining and life-long learning to keep up with changing production technologies and products. Greater flexibility in employment regulations associated with increasing portfolio working will increase the risks of unemployment and poverty in later life limiting the opportunities for consumption. Unless men and women can maintain relatively stable work patterns in full-time employment and above-average wages then their ability to achieve financial independence and maintain an acceptable lifestyle in a perhaps longer later life will be seriously limited.

Social protection

An enduring feature of the last 25 years of the 20th century was the decline of the Welfare State across the European Union. A key challenge for social protection in Europe has not simply been an increase in the numbers of older people demanding support but it has also been the nature of that support in terms of costly new treatments and services. In response to increasing demand a decline in collectivist solutions and the increasing acceptance of individualistic market-based solutions to managing individual health and long-term care and income provision in later life, is likely. The impact of this would be increased inequalities in income, health and social care and the provision of informal care. It would also mean that individuals would be responsible for funding anti-aging technologies with implications for wider inequalities in life expectancy between the "haves" and the "have nots."

Given the enduring inequalities that persist across the life course a key issue for policy makers will be how society pays for increasing health care costs that are the result of new technologies. Rationing of scarce health care resources is currently a reality. There is substantive evidence that rationing of health care resources has been based on age or through the use of waiting lists (Bond, 1997; Coulter & Ham, 2000; Shaw, 1996; Tsuchiya *et al.*, 2003). In the UK, even with the substantial investment in the National Health Service (NHS) since 2002, there remains a substantial market for the "haves" and the "have mores" as private patients outside the NHS. The increasing demand for the new therapies and technologies could conceivably lead to the breakdown of publicly funded health care in many European countries. However, there is no evidence to suggest that this is inevitable (Frankel *et al.*, 2000).

Social relations

A key question is whether the post-modern view of the fluidity of social relations will prevail within European societies. Traditional family and kinship structures, religious and political institutions, and the influence of the local "community" still remain strong in some parts of most countries, particularly in rural areas, and in some cultures. These may continue to underpin social networks and relationships in the future. But relationships are becomingly increasingly compartmentalized to specific contexts and settings in which they occur (Askham *et al.*, 2007). In the future, with the continuing feminization of later life, the decline in the size of family and kinship networks, the creation of "patchwork families" due to increasing divorce and separation rates, and the emergence of a sizable proportion of older people living independently alone, friendship relationships will become increasingly important. Fluidity in friendships are more likely with serial relationships developing in line with different later-life-course experiences around the interests and needs of older people. With the changing face of communication, particularly internet technology, more widespread social networks and individual relationships will be established and developed.

The Future of Later Life

The development of anti-aging technology, science, and practice challenges us to think about the enhancement of human aging and the future of later life. Although there is little evidence that life extension will be increased in the foreseeable future beyond the current human lifespan of some 120 years (Vincent *et al.*, 2008), the policy assumption of increasing life expectancy and the rhetoric of apocalyptic demography has required us to think about later life and the future roles of older people.

The future may see a greater contribution from older people to wealth creation in European economies. To achieve this ageism in employment will have to be overcome and the positive roles and functions of older workers will have to be recognized. Future demand for skilled labor might facilitate this to some extent. Although retirement will be delayed in the future, those who have retired from formal paid employment will have more time to spend on other activities. Aside from leisure and consumption this may often be in carer or grandparenting roles, active roles in political or religious organizations, and other forms of civic and community participation.

But what remains clear is that attitudes to aging remain essentially negative with little evidence to suggest that institutionalized ageism will disappear. If human life expectancy increases enormous challenges in the way that European societies organize the labor market and systems of social protection and manage social inequalities will remain. The reality of the effects of globalization on European economic productivity and disadvantaged "dependency" ratios will continue to give support to many of the alarmist prophesies of apocalyptic demography unless fundamental economic and social change responds to the "success" of the new biology of aging.

Acknowledgments

I would like to acknowledge the joint working with colleagues that have influenced my thinking on this topic. In particular I would like to thank Bernard Jeune, Marie Jylha and Dorly Deek who as members of the Social Science Panel of Age Action (a Specific Support Action of the EU Framework Programme 6) (Kirkwood, 2007) updated my knowledge and understanding of increasing life and healthy life expectancy; Freya Dittmann-Kohli, Sheila Peace and Gerben Westerhof with whom I spent many happy hours considering the future of aging (Bond *et al.*, 2007), and to John Vincent who first introduced me to thinking about these important issues (Vincent, 2003). Needless to say the content and presentation in this chapter is entirely my own responsibility.

Notes

1. Increasing evidence about the health of the oldest old will shortly be available with the publication of findings from the Newcastle 85+ Study (Collerton *et al.*, 2007) that will complement existing data from the Netherlands (Stek *et al.*, 2004).
2. A constructionist perspective in social science is concerned with understanding the constructions of personal meaning in the lives of older people and the cultural, economic, political, and social contexts in which meanings emerge and evolve.
3. Political economy is concerned with understanding the role of older people in contemporary society and the impact that economic, political, and social structures have on their everyday lives.

References

Acker, J. (1992). Gendered institutions – From sex roles to gendered institutions. *Contemporary Sociology, 21*, 565–9.

Alzheimer's Society (2006). *Action on Alzheimer's Drugs Alliance*. Available at www.handsoff-dementiadrugs.org/ (Accessed December 2006).

Arber, S. & Ginn, J. (1991). *Gender and Later Life. A Sociological Analysis of Resources and Constraints*. London: Sage.

Askham, J., Ferring, D. & Lamura, G. (2007). Personal relationships in later life. In J. Bond, S. Peace, F. Dittmann-Kohli & G.J. Westerhof (eds.), *Ageing in Society: European Perspectives on Gerontology* (pp. 186–208). London: Sage.

Binstock, R.H. (2004). Anti-aging medicine and research: A realm of conflict and profound societal implications. *Journal of Gerontology*, **59A**, 523–33.

Bond, J. (1997). Health care reform in the UK: Unrealistic or broken promises to older citizens. *Journal of Aging Studies*, **11**(3), 195–210.

Bond, J. & Cabrero, G.R. (2007). Health and dependency in later life. In J. Bond, S. Peace, F. Dittmann-Kohli& G.J. Westerhof (eds.), *Ageing in Society: European Perspectives on Gerontology* (pp. 113–41) London: Sage.

Bond, J., Dittmann-Kohli, F., Westerhof, G. & Peace, S. (2007). Ageing into the future. In J. Bond, S. Peace, F. Dittmann-Kohli& G.J. Westerhof (eds.), *Ageing in Society: European Perspectives on Gerontology*. London: Sage.

Bone, M., Bebbington, A., Jagger, C., Morgan, K. & Nicolaas, G. (1996). *Health Expectancy and its Uses*. London: HMSO.

Bronnum-Hansen, H., Juel, K. & Davidsen, M. (2006). The burden of selected diseases among older people in Denmark. *Journal of Aging and Health*, **18**, 491–506.

Brown, N. & Michael, M. (2003). A sociology of expectations: retrospecting prospects and prospecting retrospects. *Technology Analysis and Strategic Management*, **15**(1), 3–18.

Bunker, J. (2001). *Medicine matters after all. Measuring the benefits of medical care, a healthy lifestyle, and a just social environment*. Nuffield Trust Series no. 15. London.

Bunker, J.P., Frazier, H.S. & Mosteller, F. (1994). Improving health: Measuring effects of medical care. *Milbank Quarterly*, **72**(2), 225–58.

Butler, R.N. (1969). Age-ism: Another form of bigotry. *Gerontologist*, **9**, 243–6.

Christensen, K., Johnson, T.E. & Vaupel, J.W. (2006). The quest for genetic determinants of human longevity: challenges and insights. *Nature Reviews. Genetics*, **7**, 436–48.

Clarke, A.E., Shim, J.K., Mamo, L., Fosket, J.R. & Fishman, J.R. (2003). Biomedicalization: Technoscientific transformations of health, illness, and US biomedicine. *American Sociological Review*, **68**, 161–94.

Collerton, J., Barrass, K., Bond, J., Eccles, M., Jagger, C., James, O. *et al.* (2007). The Newcastle 85 + Study: biological, clinical and psychosocial factors associated with health ageing: study protocol. *BMC Geriatrics*, 7, 14.

Commission of the European Communities (2003). Commission Staff Working Paper 'Draft Joint Inclusion Report', Statistical Annex. Brussels: Commission of the European Communities (COM (2003) 773 final).

Coulter, A.& Ham, C. (eds). (2000). *The Global Challenge of Health Care Rationing*. Buckingham: Open University Press.

Dannefer, D. (2003). Cumulative advantage/disadvantage and the life course: Cross-fertilizing age and social science theory. *Journal of Gerontology*, **58B**(6) S327–37.

Deeg, D.J.H., Kriegsman, D.M.W. & van Zonneveld, R.J. (1994). Prevalence of four chronic diseases and their impact on health in older persons in the Netherlands between 1956-1993 [In Dutch, abstract in English]. *Tijdschr Soc Gezondheidsz*, **72**, 434–41.

Ebrahim, S., Papacosta, O., Wannamethee, G. & Adamson, J. (2004). British Heart Study. Social inequalities and disability in older men: Prospective findings from the British regional heart study. *Social Science and Medicine*, **59**, 2109–20.

Estes, C.L. & Binney, E. (1989). The biomedicalisation of aging: dangers and dilemmas. *Gerontologist*, **29**(5), 587–96.

Estes, C.L., Biggs, S. & Phillipson, C. (2003). *Social Theory, Social Policy and Ageing: A Critical Introduction*. London: Open University Press.

Eurostat (1999) European Community Household Panel (ECHP) wave 6. Available at http://forum.europa.eu.int/irc/dsis/echpanel/info/data/information.html (accessed May 30, 2006).

Falkingham, J. & Victor, C. (1991). The myth of the Woopie?: Incomes, the elderly and targeting welfare. *Ageing and Society*, **11**, 471–93.

Fishman, J.R. (2004). Manufacturing desire: The commodification of female sexual dysfunction. *Social Studies of Science*, **34**(2), 187–218.

Frankel, S., Ebrahim, S. & Davey Smith, G. (2000). The limits to demand for health care. *British Medical Journal*, **321**, 40–5.

Freedman, V.A., Crimmins, E., Schoeni, R.F., Spillman, B.C., Aykan, H., Kramarow, E. *et al.* (2004). Resolving inconsistencies in trends in old-age disability: Report from a technical working group. *Demography*, **41**, 417–41.

Freedman, V.A. & Martin, L.G. (2000). Contribution of chronic conditions to aggregate changes in old-age functioning. *American Journal of Public Health*, **90**, 1755–60.

Freedman, V.A., Martin, L.G. & Schoeni, R.F. (2002). Recent trends in disability and functioning among older US adults. *Journal of the American Medical Assocation*, **2888**, 3137–46.

Fries, J.F. & Crapo, L.M. (1981). *Vitality and Aging. Implications of the Rectangular Curve.* San Francisco: W.H. Freeman.

Gilleard, C. & Higgs, P. (2000). *Cultures of Ageing: Self, Citizen and the Body.* Harlow: Prentice Hall.

Gilleard, C. & Higgs, P. (2002). Concept Forum. The third age: Class, cohort or generation? *Ageing and Society*, **22**(3), 369–82.

Higgs, P. & Gilleard, C. (2006). Departing the margins: social class and later life in a second modernity. *Journal of Sociology*, **42**(3), 219–41.

House of Lords Science and Technology Committee (2005). *Ageing: Scientific aspects. Volume I: Report.* London: The Stationery Office.

Jeune, B. (2006). Explanation of the decline in mortality among the oldest-old: The impact of circulatory diseases. In J.M. Robine, E.M. Crimmins, S. Horiuchi & Z. Yi (eds.), *Human Longevity, Individual Life Duration, and the Growth of the Oldest-Old Population.* Springer.

Jeune, B., Skytthe, A., Cournil, A., Greco, V., Gampe, J., Berardelli, M. *et al.* (2006). Handgrip strength among nonagenarians and centenarians in three European regions. *Journals of Gerontology*, **61A**, B707–12.

Johnson, P., Conrad, C. & Thomson, D. (1989). *Workers versus Pensioners.* Manchester: Manchester University Press.

Jolanki, O. (2004). Moral argumentation in talk about health and old age. *Health (London)*, **8**(4), 483–503.

Kirkwood, T. (ed.) (2007). *Age Action: "Changing Expectations of Life".* Institute for Ageing and Health, Newcastle University, Newcastle upon Tyne.

Kuulasmaa, K., Tunstall-Pedoe, H., Dobson, A., Fortmann, S., Tolonen, H., Evans, A. *et al.* (2000). Estimation of contribution of changes in classic risk factors to trends in coronary-event rates across the WHO MONICA Project populations. *The Lancet*, **355**(9205), 675–87.

Laslett, P. (1996). *A Fresh Map of Life: The Emergence of the Third Age.* London: Weidenfeld and Nicolson.

Mackenbach, J.P. (1996). The contribution of medical care to mortality decline: McKeown revisited. *Journal of Clinical Epidemiology*, **49**, 1207–13.

Mackenbach, J.P., Bouvier-Colle, M.H. & Jougla, E. (1990). "Avoidable" mortality and health services: A review of aggregate data studies. *Journal of Epidemiology and Community Health*, **44**, 106–11.

Mannheim, K. (1952). The problem of generations. In P. Kecskemeti (ed.), *Essays on the Sociology of Knowledge* (pp. 276–320). London: Routledge & Kegan Paul.

Manton, K.G., Gu, X. & Lamb, V.L. (2006). Change in chronic disability from 1982 to 2004/ 2005 as measured by long-term changes in function and health in the US elderly population. *Proceedings of the National Academy of Sciences of the United States of America*, **103**(48), 18374–9.

McIntyre, S. (1977). Old age as a social problem. In R. Dingwall, C. Health, M. Reid& M. Stacey (eds.), *Health Care and Health Knowledge* (pp. 41–63). London: Croom Helm.

McKeown, T. (1979). *The Role of Medicine: Dream, Mirage or Nemesis?* Oxford: Basil Blackwell.

Medical Research Council Cognitive Function and Ageing Study, (MRC CFAS) (2001). Health and ill-health in the older population in England and Wales. *Age and Ageing*, **30**, 53–62.

Naegele, G. & Walker, A. (2007). Social protection: Incomes, poverty and the reform of the pension systems. In J. Bond, S. Peace, F. Dittmann-Kohli& G.J. Westerhof (eds.), *Ageing in Society: European Perspectives on Gerontology* (pp. 142–66). London: Sage.

Oeppen, J. & Vaupel, J.W. (2002). Demography. Broken limits to life expectancy. *Science*, **296**, 1029–31.

Oliver, M. (1990). *The Politics of Disablement*. Basingstoke: Macmillan.

Parker, M.G., Ahacic, K. & Thorslund, M. (2005). Health changes among Swedish oldest old: Prevalence rates from 1992 and 2002 show increasing health problems. *Journals of Gerontology*, **60A**, B1351–5.

Perenboom, R.J.M., van Herten, L.M., Boshuizen, H.C. & van den Bos, G.A.M. (2004). Trends in disability-free life expectancy. *Disability and Rehabilitation*, **26**(7), 377–86.

Petersen, A. (2001). Biofantasies: Genetics and medicine in the print news media. *Social Science and Medicine*, **52**(8), 1255–68.

Phillipson, C. (1998). *Reconstructing Old Age: New Agendas in Social Theory and Practice*. London: Sage.

Phillipson, C. (2006). Aging and globalization: Issues for critical gerontology and political economy. In J. Baars, D. Dannefer, C. Phillipson& A. Walker (eds), *Aging, Globalization and Inequality*. New York: Baywood.

Pluijm, S.M.F., Bardage, C., Nikula, S., Blumstein, T., Jylha, M., Minicuci, N. *et al.* (2005). A harmonized measure of activities of daily living was a reliable and valid instrument for comparing disability in older people across countries. *Journal of Clinical Epidemiology*, **58**, 1018–23.

Qureshi, H. & Walker, A. (1989). *The Caring Relationship. Elderly People and their Families*. London: MacMillan.

RIS MRC CFAS Resource Implications Study Group of the Medical Research Council Cognitive Function and Ageing Study. (1999). Informal caregiving for frail older people at home and in long-term care institutions: Who are the key supporters? *Health and Social Care in the Community*, 7(6), 434–44.

Robertson, A. (1997). Beyond apocalyptic demography: towards a moral economy of interdependence. *Ageing and Society*, **17**, 425–46.

Robine, J.-M., Mormiche, P. & Sermet, C. (1998). Examination of the causes and mechanisms of the increase in disability-free life expectancy. *Journal of Aging and Health*, **10**(2), 171–91.

Robine, J.M. & Michel, J.P. (2004). Looking forward to a general theory on population aging. *Journals of Gerontology*, **59A**, M590–7.

Sagardui-Villamor, J., Guallar-Castillon, P., Garcia-Ferruelo, M., Banegas, J.R. & Rodriguez-Artalejo, F. (2005). Trends in disability and disability-free life expectancy among elderly people in Spain. *Journals of Gerontology*, **60A**, B1028–34.

Seale, C. (2003). Health and media: An overview. *Sociology of Health and Illness*, **25**(6), 513–31.

Shaw, A.B. (1996). Age as a basis for healthcare rationing. *Drugs and Aging*, 9(6), 403–5.

Shim, J.K., Russ, A.J. & Kaufman, S.R. (2006). Risk, life extension and the pursuit of medical possibility. *Sociology of Health and Illness*, **28**(4), 479–502.

Stek, M.L., Gussekloo, J., Beekman, A.T., van Tilburg, W. & Westendorp, R.G. (2004). Prevalence, correlates and recognition of depression in the oldest old: The Leiden 85-plus study. *Journal of Affective Disorders*, **78**(3), 193–200.

Szreter, S. (1988). The importance of social intervention in Britain's mortality decline c. 1850–1914: A re-interpretation of the role of public health. *Social History of Medicine*, **1**, 1–37.

Thatcher, R. (1997). Trends and prospects at very high ages. In J. Charlton & M. Murphy (eds.), *The Health of Adult Britain 1841–1994, Volume 2* (pp. 204–10). London: The Stationery Office.

Tsuchiya, A., Dolan, P. & Shaw, R. (2003). Measuring people's preferences regarding ageism in health: Some methodological issues and some fresh evidence. *Social Science and Medicine*, **57**, 687–96.

Tunstall-Pedoe, H., Kuulasmaa, K., Mahonen, M., Tolonen, H., Ruokokoski, E. & Amoouyel, P. for the WHO MONICA Project. (1999). Contribution of trends in survival and coronary-event rates to changes in coronary heart disease mortality: 10-year results from 37 WHO MONICA project population. Monitoring trends and determinants in cardiovascular disease. *Lancet*, **353**, 1547–57.

United Nations (2003). The ageing of the world's population. Available at www.un.org/esa/socdev/ageing/agewpop.htm (accessed January 2004).

Van den Brink, C.L., Tijhuis, M., Kalmijn, S., Klazinga, N.S., Nissinen, A., Giampaoli, S. *et al.* (2003). Self-reported disability and its associates with performance-based limitation in elderly men: A comparison of three European countries. *Journal of the American Geriatrics Society*, **51**, 782–8.

Vaupel, J.W. & Romo, C. (2003). Decomposing change in life expectancy. *Demography*, **40**, 201–16.

Vincent, J.A. (2003). What is at stake in the "war on anti-ageing medicine" [review]. *Ageing and Society*, **23**(5), 675–84.

Vincent, J.A. (2005). Understanding generations: Political economy and culture in an ageing society. *British Journal of Sociology*, **56**(4), 579–99.

Vincent, J.A. (2006). Ageing contested: Anti-ageing science and the cultural construction of old age. *Sociology*, **40**(4), 681–98.

Vincent, J.A., Tulle, E. & Bond, J. (2008). The anti-ageing enterprise: Science, knowledge, expertise, rhetoric and values. *Journal of Ageing Studies*, **22**, 291–4.

Walker, A. (1982). Dependency and old age. *Social Policy and Administration*, **16**, 115–35.

Walker, A. & Maltby, T. (1997). *Ageing Europe*. Buckingham: Open University Press.

Westendorp, R.G.J. & Kirkwood, T.B.L. (2007). The biology of ageing. In J. Bond, S. Peace, F. Dittmann-Kohli & G.J. Westerhof (eds.), *Ageing in Society: European Perspectives on Gerontology* (pp. 15–37). London: Sage.

Westerhof, G.J. & Tulle, E. (2007). Meanings of ageing and old age: discursive contexts, social attitudes and personal identities. In J. Bond, S. Peace, S., G.J. Westerhof & F. Dittmann-Kohli (eds.), *Ageing in Society* (pp. 235–54). London: Sage.

Wilkinson, R. (1996). *Unhealthy Societies: The Afflictions of Inequality*. London: Routledge.

33

Policy-Making for a New Generation of Interventions in Age-Related Disease and Decline

Kenneth Howse

Introduction

There is a broad consensus about the desirability of an enhanced capability to prevent age-related disease that appears to dissipate when we come to consider the prospect of an enhanced capability to extend survival. Current research efforts to understand the biological mechanisms involved in aging open up the prospect of a new generation of health technologies that would be much more effective at achieving both these outcomes than anything now available; and as a consequence the future direction of this research – and its eventual application – has become a matter of disagreement. The magnitude of the gains in life expectancy that are now being touted as feasible in the foreseeable future are large enough for some commentators to argue not only that we might find ourselves with more lifetime than it is reasonable for anyone to want – but also that we would be introducing into society a technology that could change the conditions of social life for the worse.

In this chapter I consider how we should frame and deal with the policy decisions that are raised by the prospect of a new generation of technologies with enhanced capabilities for changing and extending the normal human lifespan. What kinds of ethical consideration should we bring to bear in making these decisions – and how exactly do they feed into the decision-making process? Do they require us to amend, extend, or elaborate existing frameworks for decision making?

The focus on policy decisions is intended to emphasize a contrast with a related set of questions about the desirability of what we stand to gain as individuals by an enhanced capability to intervene in the aging process. Instead of asking whether greatly increased longevity would enhance or detract from individual well-being, I will frame the issue in the way that analogous decisions about potentially beneficial technologies are standardly presented for collective deliberation in a liberal democracy. Should public funds be committed to support the development or use of this capability to intervene in the

Enhancing Human Capacities, edited by Julian Savulescu, Ruud ter Meulen and Guy Kahane.
© 2011 Blackwell Publishing Ltd

aging process in humans? Should legal restraints be imposed on private attempts to develop or use such a capability?

The importance of the difference between these two different kinds of decision is well recognized. The kind of reasoning to which we appeal in assessing the case for public investment or spending is quite different from the kind of reasoning to which we appeal in assessing the case against permitting corporations or individuals to use their own private resources for similar purposes. In the first case, we look for benefits that would justify the expenditure involved in supporting the relevant activity. Are they sufficiently worthwhile to justify the claim on our collective resources? In the second case, we look for harms and risks that would justify imposing restrictions on highly valued liberties; and it is, as a general rule, much harder in liberal democracies to justify a curtailment of freedom than a refusal to approve public expenditure. This is not to say that there is complete consensus about the nature of the tests to be applied in making either kind of decision, but it is nonetheless characteristic of liberal democracies that the reasoning involved tends to follow a common pattern. This pair of decisions defines, furthermore, the range of possible "verdicts." It is only if the case for collective funding fails that we need to consider whether or not there might be a case for restricting the freedom of individuals to pursue the relevant activities.

Policy Decisions Now or in the Future?

At present, the only serious candidate for a decision that might require our present attention concerns the commitment of public funds for research and development. To ask whether we should prevent private individuals and corporations from committing their own resources and energies to developing technologies that would radically change the aging process could be of interest as a way of exploring the boundaries of our ethical reasoning, but it is implausible to suggest that we should treat such an extreme proposal as a live policy issue.[1]

The case for making research into the mechanisms of biological aging a priority for public funding will appeal to the same kind of reasoning that is used to justify large-scale public investment in any biomedical research: it offers the prospect of improved technologies for alleviating suffering and saving lives. Hence we either accept or reject an appeal for a level of public investment commensurate with the magnitude of the potential benefits – and the view that the potential benefits in this instance are enormous is easy enough to understand.

It is arguable that any such appeal is premature, that the frontiers of knowledge have not yet advanced far enough for us to be confident that large amounts of additional funding will be well spent; claims about the scale of the potential benefits should be assessed in the light of our ignorance about what is really feasible. It is quite a different matter, however, to argue that the appeal for a large-scale collective effort should be rejected in principle, on the grounds that public funds should not be used to develop technologies that offer us the prospect of a substantial extension of the human lifespan. If this is the benefit that is intended to justify the additional expenditure, then, so the argument goes, we should reject the appeal. The focus of the rejection is the prospect of maintaining – even perhaps accelerating – the extraordinary improvements in life expectancy that have been seen in the more developed countries of the world over the last 100 years.

Two quite different kinds of counter-argument have been made against this "principled" rejection of support for a "War Against Aging."[2] On the one hand, there are those (mainly philosophers) who challenge the view that a pay-off specified in terms of increased lifespan would not justify the additional investment in research. And on the other hand, there are those who sidestep this issue, and argue that the investment is justified because this line of research offers the best chance of alleviating the impact of age-related disease and functional loss on well-being (Olshansky *et al.*, 2006). They appeal to what I have already characterized as a consensus view.

Should usable technologies eventually emerge from these various research efforts, there will be other decisions to be made – decisions, for example, about the use of public funds to purchase and deploy the technology. How do these future decisions about technologies that do not yet exist relate to decisions about what to do now? Although it seems clear that any practical decisions we make now about the funding or restraint of research must rely ultimately on assessments of the potential impact of the actual use of the capability to manipulate the aging process in humans, we should be wary of eliding altogether the distinction between policy decisions that can and should be made now and hypothetical policy decisions that may have to be taken in the future. In the rest of this chapter I propose to put current policy decisions to one side in order to speculate about how we might tackle future policy decisions about a new generation of health technologies with much enhanced capabilities to postpone age-related disease and decline.

It is sometimes assumed that we will be presented with these possible future decisions as a result of a number of convergent scientific breakthroughs which will radically and comprehensively transform our ability to intervene in the aging process in humans (President's Council on Bioethics, 2003). What I have to say should, however, be quite compatible with a somewhat different scenario in which successive piecemeal enhancements in our ability to prevent age-related disease and decline together extend the average human lifespan beyond what is now seen in the most exceptionally long-lived individuals. Even when a particular decision refers to the deployment of the next in a series of progressively improving technologies (with none of them perhaps having a much larger effect than its predecessor), there is still an important underlying issue to consider, namely how to handle the prospect of continuing incremental improvements in technologies that enable us to buy more healthy life years for ourselves.

I will assume, furthermore, that this issue is raised in the context of a system of publicly subsidized health care. A system of publicly subsidized health care is able to ask whether to use public funds to purchase these technologies for use as a standard therapy within the system – and it is this purchasing decision that I wish to explore, not least because when governments provide publicly subsidized health care, they are making a direct public "investment" in the health of their population and look for more immediate returns than can be expected from research.

Fairness and the Restriction of Freedoms

The case for committing public funds to purchase these innovative technologies will turn essentially on the health benefits to be expected from their use. The issue is not whether it is reasonable for individuals to want what the technology has to offer, but rather their claim on collective funds for this purpose. Recognizing the technology as a "valid candidate" for public subsidy – on the grounds that we expect from it the kind of benefits that we agree should be paid for out of our collective resources – doesn't by itself imply, however, that the technology should be provided to individuals at public cost. We would also want to be reasonably confident that these benefits are sufficiently worthwhile to justify both the risks to the user and the cost to the public purse.

In this section I consider the fairness of allowing some individuals to purchase for themselves technologies that could substantially extend their lifespan if it is decided not to make public funds available for this purpose. Would we, in these circumstances, have any reason to deny individuals the right to purchase the technologies at their own expense? The answer must depend at least in part on the nature of the case against a public subsidy.

Suppose first that the case for a public subsidy is rejected on the grounds that the technology is not a valid candidate for public funds. We take the view that life expectancy for the average individual in the wealthy countries of the world is fast approaching the point at which claims on collective support for assistance in achieving a longer life should cease to have any force. Surely the presumption must be that individuals should still be free to purchase it at their own expense? To challenge this conclusion we would have to argue – as some commentators have tried to do – that what these technologies have to offer is so special that unless everyone has access to it, no one should. Since we are assuming, however, that what these technologies have to offer is not the right sort of good to be a candidate for a public subsidy, we can hardly argue that possession or non-possession of this kind of benefit is so important for human well-being that no one should have access to it unless everyone has. We would be treating it as an expensive and much coveted luxury – in a quite distinct category of goods from basic health care or education.

The case is somewhat different if we suppose that the basic problem with the proposal for a public subsidy is that the technologies are simply too expensive to represent a cost-effective use of public funds. The problem is not that they fail to offer bona fide health benefits. It is rather that they are beyond our collective means. This is quite compatible with the view that what these technologies have to offer is so important that everyone should "ideally" have access to them, which suggests that the subsidy should be provided if and when our society became rich enough. But what should we do in the meantime? The case would be similar to that of a low-income country today in which wealthier citizens are able to purchase at their own cost very expensive forms of life-saving therapy which are excluded from its menu of publicly subsidized health care.

Would it make any difference to our judgment on this position if the technologies proved effective in giving individuals what they wanted (more years of healthy life and more years of life), but at the cost of more years of dependency? Should individuals who could afford to purchase these technologies in the private sector be allowed to assess this tradeoff for themselves if their dependency imposes costs on other people? The point here is not that unprecedented success in extending survival in humans might lead to the kind of absolute expansion of morbidity which some analysts discern in existing trends in population health – that it could exacerbate an already difficult situation. Although the problem does indeed lie with the risk that these technologies will prove more effective at extending survival than they are at reducing the burden of age-related disease, in other words, that they will be only partially successful, the argument does not require us to assess the consequences of achieving only partial success on the assumption that there is widespread use in the population. The suggestion is rather that any individuals who buy these technologies should not be allowed to pass on to others the costs of achieving only partial success – and the problem would seem to be resolved by requiring purchasers to take out some form of long-term care insurance, which would effectively protect the public against the risk of this kind of free-riding.

The argument is different again if we appeal to the worry that enhanced capabilities for extending human survival would give a powerful extra impetus to demographic trends that are already a cause of serious concern. The widespread uptake of technologies which are effective in extending human lifespan would constitute a large-scale social experiment – and the likelihood of it turning out badly is sufficiently great to justify us in refraining from making it. Although there is no problem if only a few people use the technology, the risk of unwanted demographic effects increases with the spread of use through the population, and hence the case for a public subsidy, which would allow everyone who wanted to take advantage of the technology to do so, is rejected because it is likely to bring about the situation we want to avert. The problem, therefore, is that a behavior that has no discernible impact when it is limited to a few people has a serious impact when it becomes widespread. Does this supply us with a reason for denying individuals the right to purchase the technologies at their own expense? Perhaps this is a little like the choice between imposing a general hosepipe ban (when we know that there's no problem if only a few people use their hosepipes) and allowing a few wealthy people to pay for the privilege of use. However this may be, it is clear that the issue of this version of the argument turns on our assessment of the case for a public subsidy, and it is into this decision that we have to channel an assessment of the social risks of widespread use.

Demographic Change and Social Costs

Once we accept that the widespread use of technologies which are effective in extending the human lifespan constitutes a social experiment which *may* turn out badly, we are bound to incorporate an assessment of this risk into our decision about what to do. If we decide that these technologies are valid candidates for a public subsidy, we will have to find some way of weighing the risks against the potential benefits; and should this decision go the other way, we can still ask whether the risks of widespread use would give us good reason for restricting individual freedoms. Either way, because of what is at stake, we are likely to be very demanding about assessments of the likelihood and magnitude of any supposed "social costs." And if we are inclined to set a high value on the potential benefits, we are also likely to argue that we should make the experiment anyway; trusting to our ingenuity and capacity for social innovation to devise institutions that will enable us to adapt to radically different demographic circumstances. So what can we say about the likely social impact of the kind of demographic change that would result from making the experiment?

In its most general form the problem that concerns us is the possibility that some kinds of demographic change may exceed our capacity as a society to adapt and adjust. It is, for example, widely thought that, under conditions, persistent high fertility can lead to unsustainable rates of population growth. The variable to be considered in this case, however, is different: the driver of demographic change that is of interest is not fertility, but mortality; the demographic outcomes include changes in population age structure as well as changes in population size; and it is arguable that we should recognize the potential relevance of other social outcomes besides population survival to our assessment.

Consider first what appears to be the worst-case outcome – the possibility that a large increase in life expectancy would add significantly to the population pressures that already give us serious cause for concern. What would be the impact of a very large increase in life expectancy on population growth? Population growth depends on what happens to fertility as well as what happens to mortality – and in our world as things are now, the main determinant of long-term population growth is going to be fertility. The impact of falling mortality on population growth varies with the age groups in which rate changes occur. A decline in infant and child mortality has a large impact on population growth – since this determines the proportion of individuals that will survive to adulthood and be capable of reproduction. A decline in mortality rates in the post-reproductive age groups has a much smaller impact. In our current global demographic situation – and in the short term – a very large increase in life expectancy would slow down the effect of fertility decline on population growth.[3] Below-replacement level fertility heralds the end of population growth (Lutz *et al.*, 2004), and although substantial increases in life expectancy will delay this transition, they are unlikely to do so indefinitely.

Most developing countries are now experiencing changes in their population age structure that are a serious cause of concern for policy-makers, and it might seem folly to give an additional impetus to these trends – and so exacerbate what are already substantial policy challenges. It is important, however, to keep these matters in perspective, and also to be clear about what it is in these trends that gives cause for concern. The fear that population aging might cause the "burden of dependency" to become "unaffordable" has been replaced by a more tempered recognition that institutional reforms and changes in individual behavior are needed not only to minimize the strain on public finances, but also to maintain the sort of economic growth to which developed countries have become accustomed.[4] Our assessment of the impact of age-retarding technologies on this situation depends crucially on the distinction between "partial" and "unqualified" success. If the widespread use of these technologies did not merely shift the age structure of the population but also led to an expansion of morbidity, it could well make an already difficult situation worse. We would incur the social costs of an increased burden of dependency, though it is possible that concomitant gains in healthy life expectancy (HLE) would enable us to bear these cost increases without too much strain. Much would depend presumably on our ability to turn gains in HLE into gains in labor force participation; and the balance between gains in HLE and gains in overall life expectancy.

The distinction between "partial" and "unqualified" success points us, furthermore, to what is probably the second-worst outcome, namely that these technologies will prove to be only partially successful. We have to ask ourselves, therefore, whether this is a risk worth running. We should perhaps decline to take the risk if we thought that the probability of unqualified success was low and the costs of partial success very high. But we are not really in any position to say anything quite as definite as this. It depends, as I have said, on the balance between gains in HLE and gains in overall life expectancy, and on our ability to turn gains in HLE into gains in labor force participation.

This leaves us with the possibility of a negative social impact as a result of unqualified success. Could "more of the same" – further substantial increases in life expectancy – make it more difficult to manage the adjustments that are needed to pay for increased longevity? If there is a problem here, it would seem to lie mainly in the extent to which future gains in life expectancy are turned into gains in leisure. Other things being equal, one clear limit on our ability to pay for greater longevity is the limit that old age places on our ability to remain economically active – and to the extent that increasing life expectancy is accompanied by increasing healthy life expectancy, this should make it that much easier to promote the longer working lives that would help pay for more leisure. What is required is a set of social arrangements that limit – and place conditions on – the extent to which we can turn gains in life expectancy into gains in leisure. Such adjustments may well prove difficult to achieve, but this hardly gives us a reason to deplore further substantial gains in life expectancy – always provided of course that our success in engineering greater longevity in the population is not associated with any expansion of morbidity.

Given that population aging challenges us to make major adjustments to important social arrangements, it is reasonable to suggest that if we are to get these arrangements right, we should consider the way in which the costs of adjustment (such as working longer or saving more) are apportioned between successive generations. Although it is not easy to say anything very precise about the generational impact of any substantial increases in life expectancy without knowing, firstly, how substantial they might be, and secondly, how the prevalent arrangements for managing intergenerational transfers might have changed from what they are now, there is an analogy at hand. Suppose, for example, that the first generation to benefit from this technology passed on to future generations the costs of their general consumption over many more non-working years.[5] They would be in a position similar to that of the first beneficiaries from U.S. Old Age Social Security – who paid in very little and got out a great deal – but without the kind of justification that can be offered for providing windfall benefits to a generation of Americans who mostly lacked the resources to pay for their own retirement. Should we regard this as a "generationally unfair" outcome? Would subsequent generations – especially their immediate descendants who would bear most of the burden of paying for their increased longevity – have a legitimate grievance against them? Even if we suppose that it is a condition of introducing the technology that the first generation to benefit makes this kind of windfall gain, the problem of cost-shifting seems to diminish to negligible proportions if we think that subsequent generations would much prefer to have the technology – even on these terms – than to be without it.

There is one final aspect to the generational impact of a substantial increase in life expectancy which we should consider. Along with changes in dependency ratios (which are the source of concern about the "burden of dependency"), there will also be changes in the patterns of generational succession. If there is a problem here, it is based on the assumption that the continual turnover of generations – the replacement of old generations by new generations – has an important role to play in maintaining different social institutions (e.g. the family, the workplace, housing). Radical change in established patterns of generational succession may therefore lead to radical disruption in these institutions and have adverse effects on intergenerational solidarity. In other words, a slowdown in the generational turnover of (i) power and influence and (ii) private wealth seems quite likely to increase intergenerational conflict. This may well be true – but it's not altogether unreasonable to suppose that we might devise institutional solutions to such difficulties.

Assessing Benefits

Since the case for committing public funds to support a particular activity will appeal to both the nature and the magnitude of the expected benefits, what should we require of the technologies under consideration here? Interventions which are effective at (i) delaying the onset of an age-related and severely disabling degenerative medical condition or (ii) slowing down its progression or (iii) alleviating its symptoms provide us with acknowledged health benefits. The increase in healthy (or active or disability-free) life expectancy for the at-risk population would confirm that the intervention produced "health gain" in that population. As a rule, in order to reach this conclusion, we do not also require evidence that the intervention will produce "*net* lifetime health gain" (or no *net* lifetime health loss) – i.e. that the gain in "healthy life years" is not offset by an increase in the number of life years spent in a frail and disabled state at the end of life. As things now stand, therefore, although success in compressing morbidity/ preventing an expansion of morbidity is accepted as an important goal for population health, progress towards this goal does not supply us with a criterion that may be used in assessing health technologies.

Let us now suppose ourselves to be convinced that current gains in life expectancy (and HLE)[6] are associated with an absolute expansion of the period of severe morbidity at the end of life. This is not an implausible reading of the available epidemiological evidence (Robine & Michel, 2004), and lends support to the view that the health gains achieved as a result of the cumulative effect of all currently effective interventions come at the cost of an absolute expansion of morbidity. What policy conclusions should we draw from this assessment?

We could reject the reading of the evidence by reaffirming and updating James Fries' (2004) views on the compression of morbidity. In others words, we regard our present situation as a temporary phase in a process of evolving population health – and remain confident that matters will improve if we continue to make improvements in the primary and secondary prevention of age-related disease. We rely on the limits that our biological natures place on our capacity for extended survival to get us out of our collective fix. Essentially we carry on as we now are. Given continuing improvements in

HLE, the fact that there are limits to human longevity implies that there has eventually to be a compression of mortality, and hence also a compression of morbidity.

Even, however, if we have lost our faith in claims about the limits to human longevity (Oeppen & Vaupel, 2002), it is still open to us to ignore the evidence for an expansion of morbidity as irrelevant to our collective decisions about the publicly subsidized deployment of health technologies. We insist that for this purpose it is enough that there should be gains of the kind we currently recognize as evidence of effectiveness in our assessments of particular interventions. In other words, we do not attempt collectively to set against these gains any additional life-years spent in poor health to determine whether or not there is *net* gain or loss. This is not to say that individuals should not try to assess the tradeoff for themselves, but that of course is a different matter. The expansion of morbidity may be of concern, but as far as our collective decision making goes, we should simply accept it as an unfortunate consequence – at a population level – of legitimate processes of decision making about interventions in late-life disease.

The alternative is to accept the need for a strategy that gives us more healthy life years without also giving us more life years spent in poor health; and for this there seem to be two main options. Either we stop spending money on the development and use of technologies which seem likely to contribute to an increase in life expectancy; or we look for a "win-win" solution in the development and deployment of a new generation of technologies which offer the prospect of increased HLE without any offsetting expansion of late-life morbidity and disability.

The first option would have us reconsider our whole approach to the assessment of medical interventions that deliver benefits in late-life health. We become more selective, and prioritize interventions that seem most likely to improve health/active life expectancy without also producing large gains in life expectancy. We step back not merely from those interventions which deal with the potentially fatal complications of severe disease – but also look very carefully at late-life secondary intervention of life-threatening disease. The best interventions would be those which give us most gains in healthy/active/disability-free life expectancy with least impact on life expectancy. In effect, we make a collective decision to set additional life-years spent in poor health against gains in HLE. Public funds should not be spent on interventions which increase the social burden of dependency even if individuals gain HLE as a result of their use.

The second option would have us press on with the development of a new generation of technologies which offer the prospect of a much enhanced capability to prevent age-related disease and decline. Since these technologies promise a much enhanced capability to extend survival, we acknowledge that their use enables us to extend the limits to human longevity rather than approach them ever more closely. From the point of view of the strategy, this is not a "problem" – provided that the gains in HLE delivered by the new generation of technology satisfy the test implicit in its adoption, namely that the increase in life expectancy should not lead to an expansion of morbidity.

There are two important issues that arise in this brief outline of policy options, and they both concern the relevance of evidence about the expansion of morbidity to our collective decisions about the publicly subsidized deployment of health technologies. Does the prospect of an expansion of unhealthy lifespan give us good reason to turn off the flow of public expenditure into technologies which promise more healthy life years?

And are more healthy life years always worth having provided we can be reasonably confident that they will not lead to such an unwanted outcome? Is there any reason in principle (apart that is from the sheer monetary cost) to desist from continuing to improve and apply the technologies which produce this outcome?[7]

Let me conclude by distinguishing three different positions we might adopt on these issues:

1. The case for spending our collective resources on increasing the healthy lifespan only fails if the expenditure produces (or seems likely to produce) an expansion of unhealthy lifespan.

On this view, we accept that our strategic commitment has implications for our spending decisions. We think ourselves justified in trying to balance gains in health (more healthy life years) against losses (more unhealthy life years) in our decisions about public spending on health care. There is, however, no other reason (apart that is from cost) to desist from continuing to improve and apply the technologies which give us more healthy lifespan without any expansion of morbidity/disability at the end of life. Current HLE should have no bearing on our valuation of the benefits we get from technologies that promise to give us more.

2. The case for spending our collective resources on increasing the healthy lifespan fails once a certain level of healthy lifespan has been reached.

This brings into play the first case against a public subsidy (see above), namely that our entitlement to collective support for a further "upgrading" of medical assistance in order to secure more healthy life years depends on how much healthy lifespan we can expect without it. If we consider this suggestion from the point of view of the individual "consumer" of health care, and ask whether it is reasonable for this consumer to want (and pay for) these gains, everything presumably turns on the marginal utility of healthy life years for the individual. And if we assume that they do not show diminishing marginal utility (one more healthy life year is not like one more Mercedes), then from the economist's point that would appear to be the end of the argument. In order therefore to make anything of this suggestion at all, we must consider the issue, not from the point of view of the individual consumer, but from the point of view of the claim that individuals have on collective support and collective funds for the purchase of these additional healthy life years. Does this give us a perspective from which the marginal utility of healthy life years to the individual becomes irrelevant to the decision whether the "package" counts as the kind of benefit which should exert a claim on the use of our collective resources? Only if we deploy something like a distinction between (i) interventions that would enable individuals to achieve the full potential of our species for a long and healthy life; and (ii) interventions that would enhance this potential. Additional healthy life years would cease to count as the kind of benefit which should exert a claim on the use of our collective resources when they take us across the line from (i) to (ii). Why? Presumably because we can be said to "need" type (i) interventions in a way that we do not "need" type (ii) interventions; and this category of "need" is essential to making the case for the collective provision of health care.

3.   The case fails once a certain level has been reached unless the technology is (promises to be) effective in compressing the period of severe morbidity of disability at the end of life (or in reducing its intensity).

The rationale for qualifying the previous position in this way is that it avoids the implication that once a certain level of healthy lifespan has been reached, we should refrain from purchasing a additional increment in healthy life years even if we had good reason to think that the technology would produce an absolute compression of morbidity. If we think that spending decisions should reflect a strategic commitment to the compression of severe morbidity – and not just the prevention of an expansion of morbidity – then a reduction in the burden of ill-health in late life is something that should always exert a claim on our collective resources. It also seems to suggest a kind of theoretical limit to our commitment to fund increases in healthy lifespan at public cost. It stops when it looks as though we have taken the process of compressing morbidity as far as we can – when the gap between HLE and LE has been reduced to such an extent than any further gains are going to be negligible.

Whereas the first of these positions deals with the prospect of partial success, and accepts the legitimacy of an attempt to counterbalance gains in healthy lifespan with increases in unhealthy lifespan, the second and third positions focus on the weight we should assign to these benefits (no weight/reduced weight/same weight?) in our deliberations about public spending. They both rest on the idea that once a certain level of healthy lifespan has been achieved, what we gain by further increases is revalued, and these gains are discounted in our deliberations about public spending. Once this point has been crossed we cannot be said to need further increases in healthy lifespan in the way that we can be said to need further reductions in the burden of ill-health carried in that period that succeed the healthy lifespan. Without this appeal to the idea of need in justifying the expenditure of collective resources in health care, it seems impossible to avoid the conclusion that the issue turns on our assumptions about the marginal utility of additional healthy life years. If we doubt the coherence of such an appeal to the idea of need[8] – or indeed the coherence of the distinction between (i) interventions that would enable individuals to achieve the full potential of our species for a long and healthy life and (ii) interventions that would enhance this potential, is actually incoherent – then neither position can be sustained. Which would mean that the only reason for desisting from continuing to improve and apply the technologies which produce gains in HLE without expanding morbidity is that there are better things on which to spend our collective resources. Or perhaps we would have to say that there are other things which exert a stronger claim on our collective resources. And would this also require us to explain how the claim of gains in HLE (which we now think relatively strong) could start to weaken in relation to other claims?

Notes

1.   Although both Fukuyama (2002) and Callahan (2003) take their arguments beyond the pros and cons of public funding to consider the role of private capital in developing a new generation of age-retarding technologies, they also acknowledge that an outright "ban" on

private investment in research would be an extraordinary encroachment on well-established freedoms.

2. Like the War against Cancer launched by the U.S. Congress in 1971.

3. It should be remembered also that many of the countries which are most likely to be able to afford these technologies already have fertility rates well below replacement level – and there are some in which the populations are already in natural decline. It would be interesting to consider whether and how an assessment of the demographic risk associated with the widespread uptake of effective fertility-depressing technology would differ from an assessment of an effective longevity-extending technology. There is, after all, not much doubt that the widespread uptake of an effective and cheap fertility-depressing technology has played a major role in causing fertility rates to drop as low as they have in much of Europe and East Asia. A major change in the age structure of the population – a social experiment – is occurring at least partly as a result of lots of individual decisions to delay or refrain from childbirth. In the short to medium term, this means that there will be much less human capital available to provide for the needs of the baby-boom generation in old age; which is something that worries many policy-makers and analysts. The point is that we can see how a fall in fertility rates makes people better-off – and also how too large a fall in fertility rates might generate economic and social problems.

4. So, for example, we have to ensure that the ratio of people who are economically inactive to those who are active should be kept as low as possible.

5. Perhaps they stayed in work quite a bit longer than we do – and could pay for more years of retirement as a result – but still not enough to cover the full costs of their increased longevity.

6. That is, although HLE is increasing as well as life expectancy, the latter is increasing faster than the former.

7. Although the number of life years spent in poor health remains unchanged, there is a continuing *relative* compression of morbidity. The proportion of life spent in good health continues to increase.

8. Or think that what counts as a need may shift over time to reflect our increasing mastery over the world.

References

Callahan, D. (2003). *What Price Better Health? Hazards of the Research Imperative.* Berkeley: University of California Press.

Fries, J. (2004). Robine and Michel's "Looking forward to a general theory on population ageing." *Journals of Gerontology A,* **59**, M603–5.

Fukuyama, F. (2002). *Our Posthuman Future: Consequences of the Biotechnology Revolution.* New York: Picador.

Lutz, W., Sandersen, W. & Scherbov, S. (2004). *The End of World Population Growth in the 21st Century: New Challenges for Human Capital Formation and Sustainable Development.* London: Earthscan.

Oeppen, J. & Vaupel, J.W. (2002). Broken limits to life expectancy. *Science,* **296**, 1029–31.

Olshansky, J. *et al.* (2006). In pursuit of the longevity dividend: What should we be doing to prepare for the unprecedented aging of humanity? *The Scientist,* **20**(3), 28–36.

President's Council on Bioethics (2003). *Beyond Therapy: Biotechnology and the Pursuit of Happiness.* Washington, DC: President's Council on Bioethics.

Robine, J.-M. & Michel, J.-P. (2004). Looking forward to a general theory on population ageing. *Journals of Gerontology A,* **59**, M590–7.

Part VI
Moral Enhancement

34

Moral Enhancement[1]

Thomas Douglas

Biomedical technologies are routinely employed in attempts to maintain or restore health. But many can also be used to augment the capacities of already healthy persons. Without thereby attributing any value to these latter alterations, I will refer to them as *biomedical enhancements*.

Biomedical enhancement is perhaps most apparent in sport, where drugs have long been used to improve performance (Verroken, 2005), but it is also widespread in other spheres. Some musicians take beta-blockers to calm their nerves before performances (Tindall, 2004), a significant proportion of U.S. college students report taking methylphenidate (Ritalin) while studying in order to improve performance in examinations (Johnston *et al.*, 2003; Teter *et al.*, 2006), and then, of course, there is cosmetic surgery. Research on drugs that may enhance memory (Lynch, 2002; Scott *et al.*, 2002; Tully *et al.*, 2003), the retention of complex skills (Yesavage *et al.*, 2001), and alertness (Caldwell *et al.*, 2000; Turner *et al.*, 2003) suggests that the possibilities for biomedical enhancement are likely to grow rapidly in coming years. However, the *morality* of using biomedical technologies to enhance remains a matter of controversy. Some argue that it would be better if people were more intelligent, longer lived, and physically stronger, and that there is no objection to using biomedical technologies to achieve these goals. But others hold that biomedical enhancement ought to be avoided.

The Bioconservative Thesis

The opponents of enhancement do not all set out to defend a common and clearly specified thesis. However, several would either assent or be attracted to the following claim (henceforth, the bioconservative thesis): Even if it were technically possible and legally permissible for people to engage in biomedical enhancement, it would not be *morally permissible* for them to do so.[2] The scope of this thesis needs to be clarified. By "people," I mean here to include all currently existing people, as well as those people that may exist in the medium-term future – say, the next 100 years – but not people who may exist in the more distant future. Similarly, I mean to include under "biomedical enhancement" only those enhancement practices that may plausibly

Enhancing Human Capacities, edited by Julian Savulescu, Ruud ter Meulen and Guy Kahane.
© 2011 Blackwell Publishing Ltd

become technically feasible in the medium-term future. The opponents of enhancement may justifiably have little to say about enhancements that would take place in the distant future, or would require far-fetched technologies.

In what follows, I argue that the bioconservative thesis, thus qualified, is false.

A Possible Counter-Example to the Bioconservative Thesis

The bioconservative thesis may be defended in various ways. But many of the most prevalent arguments for it are based on social considerations: though enhancement might be good for the enhanced individuals, it could well be bad for others (Annas, 2002; Fukuyama, 2002; McKibben, 2003; Mehlman, 2005).

Thus, regarding intelligence enhancement it could be argued that if one person makes herself more intelligent she will disadvantage the unenhanced by, for example, outcompeting them for jobs, or by discriminating against them on the basis of their lower intelligence (Buchanan *et al.*, 2000; Farrah *et al.*, 2004; McKibben, 2003; Sandel, 2007, pp.8–12, 15).

These arguments may be persuasive when directed against the most commonly discussed biomedical enhancements – physical ability enhancements, intelligence and memory enhancements, and natural lifespan enhancements. But there are other types of biomedical enhancement against which they appear much less persuasive. In this chapter I will focus on one such possibility: that future people might use biomedical technology to *morally* enhance themselves.

There are various ways in which we could understand the suggestion that we morally enhance ourselves. To name a few, we could take it as a suggestion that we make ourselves more virtuous, more praiseworthy, more capable of moral responsibility, or more disposed to act or behave morally. But I will understand it in none of these ways. Rather, I will take it as a suggestion that we cause ourselves to have morally better motives (henceforth often omitting the "morally"). I understand motives to be the psychological – mental or neural – states or processes that will, given the absence of opposing motives, cause a person to act.[3]

Since I focus only on motives, I will not claim that the morally enhanced person *is* more moral, has a more moral character, or will necessarily act more morally than her earlier, unenhanced self. I will also try to avoid committing myself to any particular view about what determines the moral goodness of a motive. For example, I will, insofar as possible, remain neutral between the views that the moral goodness of a motive is determined by the sort of acts it motivates, the character traits it partially constitutes, the consequences of its existence, or its intrinsic properties.

With these qualifications in hand, I now set out my formula for moral enhancement: A person morally enhances herself if she alters herself in a way that may reasonably be expected to result in her having morally better future motives, taken in sum, than she would otherwise have had.

This formula strikes me as a natural way of capturing the idea of moral enhancement given our focus on the moral goodness of motives. However, it has three noteworthy features. First, it compares *sets* of motives, rather than individual motives. More specifically, it compares the full set of future motives that an agent would have following enhancement with the one he would have without it. Second, it focuses on whether an alteration may *reasonably be expected* to result in the agent having morally better motives (or, as I will henceforth say, whether it will *expectably* lead the agent to have better motives), not on whether it actually succeeds in bringing about those motives. Without this second condition it would be difficult to know in advance whether some alteration would constitute a moral enhancement. Third, my formula allows that a moral enhancement may be achieved through non-biomedical means. I will focus specifically on the case of *biomedical* moral enhancement later.

Unlike the most frequently mentioned varieties of enhancement, enhancements satisfying this formula for moral enhancement could not easily be criticized on the ground that their use by some would disadvantage others. On any plausible moral theory, acquiring morally better motives will tend to be to the advantage of others. Indeed, on some views, the fact that having some motive would tend to advantage others is what makes it a morally good motive. Admittedly, acquiring a better set of future motives may sometimes cause a person to inflict disadvantage on other persons, but it will do this only when (a) the better motives fail to have their typical effects (as where an appropriate desire to help others has, due to unforeseen circumstances, harmful effects); (b) the disadvantage serves some moral purpose (as where a concern for justice leads someone to inflict an appropriate punishment on a wrongdoer); or (c) having a morally better overall set of future motives involves having some worse individual motives. One could not object to moral enhancement on the ground that it would systematically impose morally gratuitous disadvantage on others.

Indeed, I will argue that, when performed under certain conditions, there would be no good objection to biomedical moral enhancement. I will suggest that it would, contrary to the bioconservative thesis, be morally permissible for people to undergo such enhancements. Before proceeding to my argument, however, it is necessary to say something more about how moral enhancement might work.

The Nature of Moral Enhancement

There is clearly scope for most people to morally enhance themselves. According to every plausible moral theory, people often have bad or suboptimally good motives. Moreover, according to many plausible theories, some of the world's most important problems – such as developing-world poverty, climate change, and war – can be attributed to these moral deficits.

However, it is not immediately clear what sorts of psychological changes would count as moral enhancements. There are at least three reasons for the lack of clarity.

First, what counts as a good motive will depend on a person's context. For a judge, a certain sort of legal reasoning, relatively detached from feelings of sympathy, might be the best motive, at least when she is at work. For a parent interacting with his children, a feeling of love might be more appropriate.

Second, what sorts of psychological changes should be expected to improve a person's motives will depend on what sort of moral psychology that person has to begin with. For a person who feels little sympathy for others, an increase in sympathy might count as a moral enhancement. But for someone who is already overwhelmed by feelings of sympathy, any such increase is unlikely to count as an improvement. Some people are violent, deceitful or morally apathetic, others less so. And these differences will have important implications for what counts as a moral enhancement.

Third, even if a person's context and starting psychology could be fully specified, there would, I think, often be significant and reasonable disagreement about whether some particular change to that person's psychology would qualify as a moral enhancement. There is substantial disagreement about what types of mental states or process can qualify as morally good motives. Whereas some would claim that it is good to be motivated by normative beliefs formed as a result of correct reasoning processes,[4] others would emphasize the importance of moral emotions such as sympathy (Mill, 1979). Others still would favor some mixture of the two (Aristotle, 1985). There would also be disagreement between the adherents of different normative theories about what particular motives are good. For example, we can imagine an act utilitarian and a deontologist agreeing that sentiments count as good motives whenever they motivate right action, but disagreeing on what particular sentiments tend to do this: the utilitarian might focus on benevolent feelings, whilst the deontologist might instead emphasize sentiments related to fairness or fidelity.

Despite these difficulties, I think it would be possible to identify several kinds of psychological change that would, for some people under some circumstances, uncontroversially qualify as moral enhancements. I will focus solely on one possibility here. My thought is that there are some emotions – henceforth, the counter-moral emotions – whose attenuation would sometimes count as a moral enhancement regardless of which plausible moral and psychological theories one accepted. I have in mind those emotions which may interfere with all of the putative good motives (moral emotions, reasoning processes, and combinations thereof) and/or which are themselves uncontroversially *bad* motives. Attenuating such emotions would plausibly leave a person with better future motives, taken in sum.

One emotion that might frequently qualify as a counter-moral emotion is a strong aversion to members of certain racial groups. Such an aversion could be a bad motive. It might also *interfere with* what would otherwise be good motives. It might, for example, lead to a kind of subconscious bias in a person who is attempting to weigh up the claims of competing individuals as part of some reasoning process. Alternatively, it might limit the extent to which a person is able to feel sympathy for a member of the racial group in question.

A second example would be the impulse towards violent aggression. This impulse may sometimes count as a good motive. If I am present when one person attacks another on the street, impulsive aggression may be exactly what is required of me. But, on many occasions, impulsive aggression seems to be a morally bad motive to have – for example, when one has just been mildly provoked. Moreover, as with racial aversion, it could also interfere with good motives. It might, for example, cloud a person's mind in such a way that reasoning becomes difficult and the moral emotions are unlikely to be experienced.

I suspect, then, that for some people in some contexts, the mitigation of an aversion to certain racial groups or a reduction in impulsive violent aggression would qualify as a moral enhancement – that is, it would lead those people to expectably have better motives, taken in sum, than they would otherwise have had. However, I do not want, or need, to commit myself to this claim here. Rather, I will stake myself to the following weaker claim: there are some emotions such that a reduction in the degree to which an agent experiences those emotions would, under some circumstances, constitute a moral enhancement.

Two broadly Kantian objections might be made to this claim. First, it might be objected that when a person brings about certain motives in herself, the moral goodness of those motives is wholly determined by the earlier motives for bringing them about. The locus of moral appraisal is shifted from the (later) motives that are brought about to the (earlier) motives for bringing them about. Thus, though it might normally be true that the attenuation of some emotion would improve one's motives, this will not necessarily be the case when the attenuation of the emotion is itself a motivated action. If, say, one is motivated to alter one's emotions by some bad motive, the badness of the earlier motive may infect the subsequent motives.

It is implausible, however, that the goodness of a person's motives at some time is determined wholly by the earlier motives that brought those later motives about. Suppose that a neo-Nazi attends an anti-Semitic rally in order to protest against an influx of Jews into his city. But suppose that he is, unexpectedly, sickened by the behavior of his co-protestors, and impressed by the conduct of the horrified Jewish onlookers. The upshot is that he is left with a greatly diminished aversion to Jewish people. Intuitively, this person has better motives after the rally than he had before. But it is difficult to see how this improvement in his motives could be explained by reference to the motives which brought it about. Those earlier motives were, after all, racist ones.

A second objection to my account of moral enhancement would maintain that nothing which alters only emotions could truly give an agent better motives. The only thing susceptible of moral appraisal is, it might be argued, the will. Thus, the only motives capable of being good or bad are those that consist in the exercise of the will. And whether one experiences certain emotions or not is simply irrelevant to the question whether one has such motives, for emotions lie outside of the boundaries of the will. Rather, the will is exercised through engagement in reasoning processes that are independent of emotional states: these reasoning processes are the only motives that can be good or bad (they will be good, on the Kantian view, when they are properly directed by the moral law – or, as I will henceforth say, when they are *correct*).[5]

The view that reasoning processes are the only motives susceptible of moral appraisal strikes me as implausible. Intuitively one can sometimes morally improve one's motives by, for example, cultivating feelings of sympathy. But this could not count as an improvement on the Kantian view just sketched, since being moved by sympathy surely does not count as engaging in reasoning. Moreover, even if we accept that reasoning processes are the only motives susceptible of moral appraisal, *attenuating* an emotion might still count as a moral enhancement. Though emotions may lie outside the will, they may interfere with its exercise by corrupting reasoning processes. Thus, attenuating the problematic emotions may allow an agent to engage in correct practical reasoning processes when that would not otherwise have been possible.

There is, it must be admitted, a stronger version of the Kantian position. It could be argued that one exercises one's will only when one engages in reasoning processes that are *insusceptible to emotional interference*. On this view, even though attenuating counter-moral emotions might enable an agent to engage in correct reasoning processes, those processes could not themselves count as good (or bad) motives, precisely because they were susceptible to emotional interference.

I cannot adequately respond to this objection here. However, since I doubt that many people will subscribe to the strong view about the nature of the will that it presupposes, I am not sure that any response is called for. I will simply record that, like the weaker Kantian view, this stronger view implies that cultivating certain emotions cannot in any way morally improve one's motives. Unlike the weaker view, it also implies (in my view counter-intuitively) that neither training oneself to suppress emotions such as racial aversion, nor avoiding circumstances known to provoke them, could affect the goodness of one's motives.

The Possibility of Biomedical Moral Enhancement

I will tentatively argue that it would sometimes be morally permissible for people to biomedically mitigate their counter-moral emotions. But first I want to briefly consider a prior question. Will this sort of biomedical moral enhancement be possible within the medium-term time span that we are considering?

There are two obvious reasons for doubting that biomedical moral enhancement will, in the medium term, become possible. The first is that there are, on some views about the relationship between mind and brain, some aspects of our moral psychology that cannot in principle be altered through biological intervention.[6] This is not the place to explore this claim. I hope it suffices merely to note that it is not a mainstream philosophical position. The second ground for doubt is that our moral psychology is presumably highly complex – arguably, so complex that we will not, within the medium-term future, gain sufficient understanding of its neuroscientific basis to allow the informed development of appropriate biomedical interventions.

There are surely some aspects of our moral psychology that are exceedingly complex. We probably will not, in the medium term, properly understand the neuroscientific basis of belief in Kant's categorical imperative. But there are other elements of our moral psychology that may be more amenable to understanding, and these would plausibly include at least some of the counter-moral emotions.

Consider the two emotions that I mentioned earlier – aversion to certain racial groups, and impulses towards violent aggression. Work in behavioral genetics and neuroscience has led to an early but growing understanding of the biological under-pinnings of both. There has long been evidence from adoption and twin studies of a genetic contribution to aggression (Cadoret, 1978; Crowe, 1974; Grove *et al.*, 1990), and there is now growing evidence implicating a polymorphism in the monoamine oxidase A gene (Brunner *et al.*, 1993a, 1993b; Caspi *et al.*, 2002), and, at the neurophysiological level, derangements in the serotonergic neurotransmitter system (Caspi *et al.*, 2002; de Almeida *et al.*, 2005).

Racial aversion has been less well studied. However, a series of recent functional magnetic resonance imaging studies suggest that the amygdala – part of the brain already implicated in the regulation of emotions – plays an important role (Cunningham *et al.*, 2004; Hart *et al.*, 2000; Phelps *et al.*, 2000). Further developments in these fields may, perhaps, enable the intentional development of moral enhancement technologies. But of course, even if they do not, such technologies may be discovered accidentally, perhaps through mainstream psychiatric research.

The Scenario

I am now in a position to set out the conditions under which it would, I will argue, be morally permissible for people to morally enhance themselves. These conditions are captured in a scenario consisting of five assumptions.[7]

The first assumption simply specifies that we are dealing with an enhancement that satisfies my formula for moral enhancement:

- **Assumption 1:** Through undergoing some biomedical intervention (for example, taking a pill) at time T, an agent Smith can bring it about that he will expectably have better post-T motives than he would otherwise have had.

In order to focus on the situation where the case for moral enhancement is, I think, strongest, I introduce a second assumption as follows:

- **Assumption 2:** If Smith does not undergo the intervention, he will expectably have at least some bad (rather than merely suboptimally good) motives.

A third assumption captures my earlier claim about how, as a matter of psychology, moral enhancement might work:

- **Assumption 3:** The biomedical intervention will work by attenuating some emotion(s) of Smith's.

And finally, the fourth and fifth assumptions rule out objections that are unlikely to apply to *all* moral enhancements: that it might have adverse side effects, and that it might be done coercively or for other unnecessarily bad reasons:

- **Assumption 4:** The *only* effects of Smith's intervention will be (a) to alter Smith's psychology in those (and only those) ways necessary to bring it about that he expectably has better post-T motives, and (b) consequences of these psychological changes.
- **Assumption 5:** Smith can, at T, freely choose whether or not to morally enhance himself, and if he chooses to do so, he will make this choice for the best possible reasons (whatever they might be).[8]

Would it be morally permissible for Smith to morally enhance himself in these circumstances? I will argue that, probably, it would.

Reasons to Enhance

Smith clearly has some moral reason to morally enhance himself: if he does, he will expectably have a better set of motives than he would otherwise have had, and I take it to be uncontroversial that he has some moral reason to bring this result about. (I henceforth omit the "moral" of "moral reason".)

Precisely why he has such reason is open to question. One explanation would run as follows. If Smith brings it about that he expectably has better motives, he expectably brings at least one good consequence about: namely, his having better motives.[9] And, plausibly, we all have at least some moral reason to expectably bring about any good consequence.

This explanation is weakly consequentialist in that it relies on the premise that we have good reasons to expectably bring about any good consequence. But thorough-going nonconsequentialists could offer an alternative explanation. They could, for example, maintain that Smith's *act* of moral enhancement has some intrinsic property – such as the property of being an act of self-improvement – that gives him reason to perform it. But regardless of *why* Smith has reason to morally enhance himself in our scenario, I take it to be intuitively clear that he has such reason.

This intuition can, moreover, be buttressed by intuitions about closely related cases. Suppose that some agent Jones is in precisely the same position as Smith, except that in her case, the moral enhancement can be attained not through biomedical means but through some form of self-education – for example, by reflecting on and striving to attenuate her counter-moral emotions. Intuitively, Jones has some reason to morally enhance herself – or so it seems to me. And if pressed on why she has such reason, it seems natural to point to features of her situation that are shared with Smith's – for example, that her morally enhancing herself would have expectably good conse-quences, or that it may express a concern for the interests of others.[10]

Reasons Not to Enhance

Smith may also, of course, have reasons not to morally enhance himself, and I now turn to consider what these reasons might be.[11]

Objectionable motives

One possibility is that Smith has reason not to enhance himself because he could only do so from some bad motive. I assumed, in setting up the Smith scenario, that if he enhances himself, he will do so from the best possible motive. But the best possible motive may not be good enough.

There are various motives that Smith *could* have for morally enhancing himself. And some of these seem quite unobjectionable: he may believe that he ought to morally enhance himself, he may have a desire to act morally in the future, or he may be moved simply by a concern for the public good. However, we should consider, at this point, an objection due to Michael Sandel. Sandel (2004, pp.50–65, 2007) argues that enhance-ment is invariably driven by an excessive desire to change oneself, or insufficient acceptance of "the given." And since we have reasons not to act on such motives, we have, he thinks, reasons to refrain from enhancing ourselves.

It would be difficult to deny that Smith's moral enhancement would, like any voluntary instance of enhancement, be driven to some extent by an unwillingness to accept the given (though this need not be his conscious motive). Here, we must agree with Sandel. But what is less clear is that this gives Smith any reason to refrain from enhancement. Leaving aside any general problems with Sandel's suggestion, it faces a specific problem when applied to the case of Smith. Applied to that case, Sandel's claim would be that Smith has reason to accept his bad motives, as well as that which interferes with his good motives. But this is implausible. Surely, if there are any features of himself that he should not accept, his bad motives and impediments to his good motives are among them. The appropriate attitude to take towards such properties is precisely one of *non-acceptance* and a *desire for self-change*.

Objectionable means

A second reason that Smith might have not to morally enhance himself is that the biomedical means by which he would do so are objectionable.

We can distinguish between a weak and a strong version of the view that Smith's proposed means are objectionable. On the weak version, his means are objectionable in the sense that it would be *better* if he morally enhanced himself via non-biomedical means. There is certainly some intuitive appeal to this view. It might seem preferable for Smith to enhance himself through some sort of moral training or self-education. When compared with self-education, taking a pill might seem "all too easy" or too disconnected from ordinary human understanding (Kass, 2003; President's Council on Bioethics, 2003). Arguably, given the choice between biomedical moral enhancement and moral enhancement via self-education, Smith would have strong reasons to opt for the latter.

Note, however, that Smith's choice is not between alternative means of enhancement, but simply between engaging in biomedical moral enhancement or not. Reasons that Smith has to engage in moral enhancement via other means will be relevant to Smith's choice only to the extent that whether he engages in biomedical moral enhancement will influence the extent to which he seeks moral enhancement through those other means. If Smith's morally enhancing himself through biomedical means would lead him to engage in *less* moral enhancement through some superior means (say, via self-education), then Smith may have some reason not to engage in biomedical moral enhancement. But it is difficult to see why Smith would regard biomedical enhancement and self-education as substitutes in this way. It seems at least as likely that he would regard them as complementary; having morally enhanced himself in one way, he may feel more inclined to morally enhance himself in the other (say, because he enjoys the experience of acting on good motives).

One might, at this point, turn to a stronger version of the "objectionable means" claim, arguing that to adopt biomedical means to moral enhancement is objectionable not just relative to alternative means, but in an *absolute* sense. Indeed, it is so absolutely objectionable that any moral benefits of Smith's morally enhancing himself would be outweighed or trumped by the moral costs of using biomedical intervention as a means.

Any claim that biomedical means to moral enhancement are absolutely objectionable is likely to be based on a claim that they are unnatural. Certainly, this is a common means-based criticism leveled at biomedical enhancement (Kass, 2003, pp.17, 20–4; President's Council on Bioethics, 2003, pp.290–3). But the problem is to come up with some account of naturalness (or unnaturalness) such that it is true both that:

1. using biomedical means to morally enhance oneself *is* unnatural; and that:
2. this unnaturalness gives a person reason not to engage in such enhancement.

Can any such account be found?

David Hume distinguished between three different concepts of nature; one which may be opposed to "miracles," one to "the rare and unusual," and one to "artifice" (Hume, 1888, pp.473–5). This taxonomy suggests a similar approach to the concept of unnaturalness. We might equate unnaturalness with miraculousness (or supernaturalness), with rarity or unusualness, or with artificiality. In what follows I will consider whether any of these concepts of naturalness succeeds in rendering both [1] and [2] above plausible.

Unnaturalness as supernaturalness

Consider first the concept of unnaturalness as supernaturalness. On one popular account of this concept, something like the following is true: something is unnatural if, or to the extent that, it lies outside the world that can be studied by the sciences (Moore, 1903, p.92). It seems clear, on this view, that biomedical interventions are not at all unnatural. For example, interventions are precisely the sort of thing that *could* be studied by the sciences. The concept of unnaturalness as supernaturalness renders [1] clearly false.

Unnaturalness as unusualness

The second concept of unnaturalness suggested by Hume's analysis is that which can be equated with unusualness or unfamiliarity. Leon Kass's idea of unnaturalness as disconnectedness from everyday human understanding may be a variant of this concept (Kass, 2003, pp.22–4).

Unusualness and unfamiliarity are relative concepts in the following way: something has to be unusual or unfamiliar *for* or *to* someone. Thus, whether Smith's biomedical intervention would qualify as unnatural may depend on whom we relativize unusualness and unfamiliarity to. For us, the use of biomedical technology for the purposes of moral enhancement certainly does qualify as unusual and unfamiliar, and thus, perhaps, as unnatural. But for some future persons, it might not. Absent any specification of how to relativize unusualness or unfamiliarity, it is indeterminate whether [1] is true.

We need not pursue these complications, however, since regardless of whether [1] comes out as true on the current concept of unnaturalness, [2] appears to come out false. It is doubtful whether we have any reason to avoid adopting means merely because they are unusual or unfamiliar, or, for that matter, disconnected from everyday human understanding. We may often prefer familiar means to unfamiliar ones on the grounds that predictions about their effects will generally be better informed by evidence, and therefore more certain. Thus, if I am offered the choice between two different drugs for some medical condition, where both are thought to be equally safe and effective, I may choose the more familiar one on the grounds that it will probably have been better studied and thus have more certain effects. But the concern here is not ultimately with the unnaturalness – or any other objectionable feature – of the means, but rather with the effects of adopting it. I will return to the possible adverse effects of Smith's enhancement below. The position I am interested in here is whether the unfamiliarity of some means gives us reasons not to use it *regardless* of its effects. To affirm that it does seems to me to involve taking a stance that is inexplicably averse to novelty.

Unnaturalness as artificiality

Consider finally the concept of unnaturalness as artificiality. This is arguably the most prevalent concept of naturalness to be found in modern philosophy (Heyd, 2003). It may be roughly characterized as follows: something is unnatural if it involves human action, or certain types of human action (such as intentional action).

Claim [1] is quite plausible on this concept of unnaturalness. Biomedical interventions clearly involve human action – and almost always intentional action. However, [2] now looks rather implausible. *Whenever* we intentionally adopt some means to some end, that means involves intentional human action. But it does not follow that we have reason not to adopt that means. If it did, we would have reason not to intentionally adopt any means to any end. And this surely cannot be right.

The implausibility of [2] on the current concept of unnaturalness can also be brought out by returning to the case where moral enhancement is achieved through self-education rather than biomedical intervention. Such enhancement seems unproblematic, yet it clearly involves unnatural means if unnaturalness is analyzed as involving or being the product of (intentional) human action.

We should consider, at this point, a more restrictive account of unnaturalness as artificiality: one which holds that, in order to qualify as unnatural, something must not only involve (intentional) human action, it must also involve *technology* – the products of highly complex and sophisticated social practices such as science and industry. Moving to this account perhaps avoids the need to classify practices such as training and education as unnatural. But it still renders unnatural many practices which, intuitively, we may have no means-based reasons to avoid. Consider, for example, the treatment of disease. This frequently involves biomedical technology, yet it is not clear that we have any means-based reasons not to engage in it. To avoid this problem, the concept of unnaturalness as artificiality would have to be limited still further, such that technology-involving means count as unnatural only if they are not aimed at the treatment of disease. On this view, Smith's means are not unnatural in themselves. Rather the unnaturalness arises from the combination of his means with certain intentions or aims. Perhaps by restricting the concept of unnaturalness in this way, we avoid classifying as unnatural practices (such as self-education, or the medical treatment of diseases) that seem clearly unobjectionable. However, it remains unclear *why*, on this account of the unnatural, we should have reasons to avoid unnatural practices. In attempting to show that Smith has reason not to engage in biomedical moral enhancement, it is not enough to simply stipulate some concept of unnaturalness according to which his engaging in moral enhancement comes out as unnatural while seemingly less problematic practices come out as natural. It must be shown that a practice's being unnatural *makes* it problematic, or at least provides evidence for its being problematic. Without such a demonstration, the allegation of unnaturalness does no philosophical work, but merely serves as a way of asserting that we have reasons to refrain from biomedical moral enhancement.

Objectionable means

I have argued that none of the three concepts of unnaturalness suggested by Hume's analysis renders both [1] and [2] plausible. If my conclusions are correct, it follows that none of these concepts of unnaturalness points to any means-based reason for Smith to refrain from moral enhancement. There may be some further concept of unnaturalness on the basis of which one could argue more convincingly for [1] and [2]. Or there may be some way of showing that biomedical moral enhancement involves means that are objectionable for reasons other than their unnaturalness. But I am not sure what the content of these concepts and arguments would be.

Objectionable consequences

Would the consequences of Smith's enhancement provide him with reasons to refrain from engaging in that enhancement? Two points about this possibility need to be noted up front. First, since we are assuming that Smith's moral enhancement will have no side effects (Assumption 4), the only consequences that his action will have are:

a. that he will expectably have better post-T motives than he would otherwise have had;
b. those, and only those, psychological changes necessary to bring about (a);
c. consequences that follow from (a) and (b).

Thus, if Smith has consequence-based reasons to avoid moral enhancement, those reasons must be grounded on the features – presumably the intrinsic badness – of (a), (b), or (c).

Second, there are some moral theories which constrain whether, or to what extent, consequences (a) and (c) could be bad. Consider theories according to which only hedonistic states (such as states of pleasure or pain) can be intrinsically good or bad. On these theories, (a) could not be intrinsically bad since motives are not hedonistic states. Consider, alternatively, a consequentialist moral theory according to which the moral goodness of a motive is determined by the goodness of the consequences of a person's having it. On this theory, if Smith indeed has better post-T motives, then the consequences of his having those motives – these fall under (c) – must be better than the corresponding consequences that would have come about had he had worse motives. Smith's having better motives is guaranteed to have better consequences than his having worse motives because having good consequences is what makes a motive good.

In what follows, I will assume, for the sake of argument, that moral theories which limit the possible badness of (a) and (c) in these ways are false.

Identity change

One bad effect of Smith's morally enhancing himself might be that he loses his identity. Worries about identity loss have been raised as general objections to enhancement, and there is no obvious reason why they should not apply to cases of moral enhancement (President's Council on Bioethics, 2003, p.294; Wolpe, 2002).

Clearly, moral enhancement of the sort we are considering need not be identity altering in the strong sense that Smith will, post-enhancement, be a different person than he was before. Our moral psychologies change all the time, and sometimes they change dramatically, for example, following particularly traumatic experiences. When these changes occur, we do not think that one person has literally been replaced by another. However, perhaps Smith's moral enhancement would be identity altering in the weaker sense that it would change some of his most fundamental psychological characteristics – characteristics that are, for example, central to how he views himself and his relationships with others, or that pervade his personality (Schectman, 1996, pp.74–6).

Suppose we concede that Smith's moral enhancement would be identity altering in this weaker sense. This may not give Smith any reason to refrain from undergoing the change. Plausibly, we have reasons to preserve our fundamental psychological characteristics only where those characteristics have some positive value. But though Smith's counter-moral emotions *may* have some value (Smith may, for example, find their experience pleasurable), they need not.

Restricted freedom

By morally enhancing himself Smith will bring it about that he has better post-*T* motives, taken in sum, than he would otherwise have had. However, it might be thought that this result will come at a cost to his freedom: namely, he will, after *T*, lack the freedom to have and to act upon certain bad motives. And even though having and acting upon bad motives may itself have little value, it might be thought that the *freedom* to hold and act upon them *is* valuable. Indeed, this freedom might seem to be a central element of human rational agency. Arguably, Smith has reasons not to place restrictions on this freedom.

The objection that I am considering here can be captured in the following two claims:

3. Smith's morally enhancing himself will result in his having less freedom to have and to act upon bad motives.
4. Smith has reason not to restrict his freedom to have and act upon bad motives.

Claim [4] is, I think, problematic. It is not obvious that the freedom referred to therein has any value. Moreover, even if this freedom does have value, there may be no problem with restricting it provided that the restriction is itself self-chosen, as in Smith's case it is. However, I will focus here on [3]. The proponent of [3] is committed to a certain understanding of freedom. She would have to maintain that freedom consists not merely in the absence of external constraints, but also in the absence of internal psychological constraints, for it is only Smith's internal characteristics that would be altered by his moral enhancement. This view could be sustained by regarding the self as being divided into two parts – the true or authentic self, and a brute self that is external to this true self. One could then regard any aspect of the brute self which constrains the true self as a constraint on freedom (Taylor, 1979, pp.175–93). And one could defend [3] on the ground that Smith's enhancement will alter his brute self in such a way that it will constrain his autonomous self.

There would be some justification for thinking that Smith's moral enhancement would alter his brute self rather than his true self. We are assuming that Smith's enhancement will attenuate certain emotions, so it will presumably work by altering the brain's emotion-generating mechanisms, and these mechanisms are arguably best thought of as part of the brute self. Certainly, it would be strange to think of the predominantly subconscious mechanisms which typically call forth racial aversion or impulsive aggression as part of the true autonomous self.

However, the view that moral enhancement would alter Smith's brute self in a way that would *interfere with* his autonomous self seems to be at odds with my assumption (Assumption 3) about the mechanism of that enhancement. Since Smith's enhancement is assumed to attenuate certain emotions, it presumably works by *suppressing* those brute mechanisms that generate the relevant emotions. The enhancement seems to work by *reducing* the influence of Smith's brute self and thus allowing his true self *greater* freedom. It would be more accurate to say that the enhancement increases Smith's freedom to have and to act upon good motives than to say that it diminishes his freedom to have and to act upon bad ones.

Inducing free-riding

The final possibility that I want to consider is that Smith might have reason to refrain from moral enhancement because his having better motives would induce others to free-ride.

Why this might occur can be illustrated through the following scenario. Suppose that Jack and Jim are the only fishermen who work in a certain bay. Fish stocks have become depleted in the bay, and both would prefer it if the stocks rose, but neither wants to limit his or her catch. Nevertheless, they formulate a plan: they will for the next month limit themselves to a quota of 20 fish each per day – significantly fewer than either would otherwise expect to take even with depleted stocks.

Each fisherman can either stick to the plan ("respect the quota") or not ("overfish"). There are, then, four possible action-pairs (Jack respects the quota, Jim overfishes; Jim respects the quota, Jack overfishes; etc.). The payoffs (i.e., values) for each fisherman from each of these action-pairs are depicted in Figure 34.1. They have been chosen to reflect the fact that each fisherman's payoff is negatively correlated with the extent to which future stocks are depleted, but positively correlated with the number of fish caught by himself in the present.[12]

Suppose that neither fisherman can observe the number of fish caught by the other, but each can observe the other's motives. Suppose further that Jim's motives are *Self-Interested*, meaning that he always does whatever maximizes his own payoff, whereas Jack's are either *Morally Good* – meaning that he always sticks to the plan,

	Respect Quota	Overfish
Respect Quota	(10,10)	(5,11)
Overfish	(11,5)	(1,1)

Figure 34.1   Jack and Jim

respecting the quota – or *Morally Bad* – meaning that he always reneges on the plan, overfishing.

If Jack's motives are *Morally Bad*, then Jim will know that Jack will overfish. He will thus face a choice between respecting the quota and getting a payoff of 5, or overfishing and getting a payoff of 1. Since his motives are *Self-Interested*, Jim will respect the quota.

But now suppose that Jack's motives are *Morally Good*. Jim will thus know that Jack will not overfish. Hence, he faces a choice between respecting the quota, and getting a payoff of 10, or overfishing, and getting a payoff of 11. Having *Self-Interested* motives, Jim will overfish. By having *Morally Good* motives, rather than *Morally Bad* ones, Jack induces Jim to overfish rather than respecting the quota. That is, he induces Jim to take advantage of his good motives in a way that harms him, reduces their combined payoff, and disrespects their earlier agreement.

This is a rather stylized scenario. Nevertheless, it illustrates one way in which one person's having better motives could, by altering the payoff structure faced by others, induce those others to free-ride in ways that might well be regarded as morally bad.

However, just as we can construct scenarios in which one person's having good motives induces another to act badly, so too we can construct scenarios in which it has the opposite effect. Consider a variant of the Jack and Jim scenario in which Sally and Sam face a similar problem but this time with the payoffs shown in Figure 34.2.

Sally's payoffs are the same as Jack's and Jim's, but Sam's payoffs have changed to reflect that he has a slightly different value function over future fish population.[13] Assume again that the fishermen cannot observe each other's catch, but can observe one another's motives. Assume also that Sam has *Self-Interested* motives. Then if Sally has *Morally Bad* motives, so that she always overfishes, Sam will face a choice between respecting the quota and getting a payoff of 1 or overfishing and getting a payoff of 5. Having *Self-Interested* motives, Sam will overfish. On the other hand, if Sally has *Morally Good* motives, so that she always respects the quota, Sam will have a choice between respecting the quota and getting a payoff of 10, or overfishing and getting a payoff of 9. He will respect the quota.

We thus have an interaction in which one person's having better motives induces the other *not* to free-ride. The effect is the opposite of that seen in the Jack and Jim scenario. There are also, of course, many collective action problems in which a change in one person's motives will simply have no effect on whether the other free-rides. (The standard Prisoner's Dilemma is an example. A self-interested agent will always free-ride in this scenario.)

Moral enhancement may sometimes induce free-riding via the mechanism illustrated by the Jack and Jim scenario. But I see no reason to suppose that it will do so any more frequently than it does the opposite, as in the Sally and Sam scenario. The payoff structure of the latter scenario is just as realistic as that in the former scenario. Merely

	Respect Quota	Overfish
Respect Quota	(10,12)	(5,9)
Overfish	(11,3)	(1,5)

Figure 34.2   Sally and Sam

pointing out the possibility of scenarios like Jack and Jill does not show that Smith's moral enhancement will certainly, or even probably, lead to a net increase in free-riding.

Implications

I have argued that Smith has some reason to morally enhance himself via biomedical means. I have also rejected several arguments for the existence of good countervailing reasons. Thus, I hope that I have offered some support for the claim that it would be morally permissible for Smith to engage in biomedical moral enhancement. But if it would be permissible for Smith to morally enhance himself, then the bioconservative thesis is almost certainly false. For as I claimed earlier, it is plausible that biomedical moral enhancement technologies will become technically feasible in the medium-term future. And it is almost certain that, if they do become feasible, some – probably many – actual future people will find themselves in scenarios sufficiently like Smith's that our conclusions about Smith will apply to them also: contrary to the bioconservative thesis, there will be people for whom it would be morally permissible to engage in biomedical enhancement.

I should end, however, by noting that the bioconservative thesis is not the only claim advanced by the opponents of enhancement. As well as claiming that it would not be morally permissible for people to enhance themselves, many bioconservatives would assert that it would not be permissible for us to *develop* technologies for enhancement purposes, nor for us to *permit* enhancement. For all that I have said, these claims may well be true. It would not follow straightforwardly from the fact that it would be permissible for some future people to morally enhance themselves – given the presence of the necessary technology and the absence of legal barriers – that they could permissibly be allowed to do so, or that we could permissibly develop the technologies whose availability we are taking as given. Other factors would need to be considered here. It may be, for example, that if we were to develop moral enhancement technologies, we would be unable to prevent their being used in undesirable ways – for example, to enhance self-interestedness or *im*morality. Whether we could permissibly develop or permit the use of moral enhancement technologies might thus depend on a weighing of the possible good uses of those technologies against the possible bad ones.

Acknowledgments

I would like to thank, for their comments on earlier versions of this paper, Julian Savulescu, David Wasserman, Matthew Liao, Ingmar Persson, Allen Buchanan, Rebecca Roache, Roger Crisp, two anonymous reviewers for the *Journal of Applied Philosophy*, and audiences at Otago, Oxford, and Hong Kong Baptist Universities.

Notes

1. This essay originally appeared as Douglas, T. (2009). Moral enhancement. *Journal of Applied Philosophy*, 25(3), 228–45.

2. Some critics of enhancement are opposed only to certain kinds of enhancement, but others appear to find *all* enhancement problematic, and perhaps impermissible, preferring that biomedical technology is used only maintain and restore health. See, for example, Fukuyama (2002), President's Council on Bioethics (2003), Sandel (2004, 2007).

3. I focus on the morality of motives because I take this to be common ground. Some Kantians might deny that acts or behavior are the proper objects of moral appraisal, and some of those who regard acts as the most basic units of moral appraisal might shy away from making judgments of moral character. But I think that all, or nearly all, would accept that motives come in varying degrees of morality, even if their morality derives ultimately from the behavior that they motivate or the virtues they derive from or constitute.

4. Immanuel Kant (1993) is of course the classic exponent of this of view, claiming as he did that the only thing "good in itself" is a good will, where the good will is understood as the capacity to engage in operations of practical reason that are governed in the right way by the moral law.

5. I assume, for argument's sake, that reasoning does not itself involve the emotions. For a denial of this view, see Damasio (2006).

6. Most obviously, this would be held by mind-body parallelists who believe that mind and brain are causally insulated from one another. The most famous exponent of this view is G.W. Leibniz (1973).

7. I also assume, as a background to the listed assumptions, that Smith is a normal person living in a world similar to our own – that is, a world governed by the scientific and social scientific principles that we take to govern our own world.

8. I take it that Assumption 5 entails at least that there is no physical or legal constraint on Smith's morally enhancing himself.

9. Smith might also bring many other expectably good consequences about – for example, those that follow from his expectably having good motives.

10. I do not claim that Smith's reason to engage in moral enhancement is as strong as Jones's.

11. The reasons considered in this section are based on a range of different substantive moral views. I do not claim that there is any one moral viewpoint which could accommodate all of the putative reasons discussed.

12. These payoffs are generated from the following assumptions. Assume that if each fisherman respects the quota, the fish population will be high by the end of the month, if only one respects the quota, the population will be low, and if neither respects the quota, the population will be very low. The value to each of having high population is 16, of having a low population is 11, and of having a very low population is 1. Suppose, moreover, that the short-term value to each of respecting the quota is -6 and the value of not doing so is 0. Thus, the value to one neighbor of respecting the quota when the other also respects the quota is $16 - 6 = 10$, of respecting the quota when the other overfishes is $11 - 6 = 5$, of overfishing when the other respects the quota is $11 - 0 = 11$, and of overfishing when the other also overfishs is $1 - 0 = 1$.

13. For Jack, Jim and Sally, the value of a low future fish population is much greater than that of a very low population, but there is little further gain from having a high rather than a low population. For Sam, having a high population has a much higher value than having a low population, whereas there is relatively little difference in value between a low and a very low population. The payoffs for Sam presented in Figure 34.2 reflect the following underlying values: value of a high fish population, 18; value of a low fish population, 9; value of a very low fish population, 5; short-term value of respecting the quota, -6; short-term value of overfishing, 0.

References

Annas, G.A. (2002). Cell division. *Boston Globe*, April 21.

Aristotle (1985). *Nicomachean Ethics*, Irwin, T. (trans.). Indianapolis: Hackett.

Brunner, H.G., Nelen, M.R., Breakefield, X.O. *et al.* (1993a). Abnormal behaviour associated with a point mutation in the structural gene for Monoamine Oxidase A. *Science*, **262**(5133), 578–80.

Brunner, H.G., Nelen, M.R., van Zandvoort, P. *et al.* (1993b). X-linked borderline mental retardation with prominent behavioural disturbance: Phenotype, genetic localization, and evidence for disturbed monoamine metabolism. *American Journal of Human Genetics*, **52**, 1032–9.

Buchanan, A., Brock, D., Daniels, N. & Wikler, D. (2000). *From Chance to Choice: Genetics and Justice*. Cambridge: Cambridge University Press.

Cadoret, R.J. (1978). Psychopathology in adopted-away offspring of biologic parents with antisocial behaviour. *Archives of General Psychiatry*, **35**, 176–84.

Caldwell, J.A., Caldwell, J.L. & Smythe, N.K. (2000). A double-blind, placebo-controlled investigation of the efficacy of Modafinil for sustaining the alertness and performance of aviators: A helicopter simulator study. *Psychopharmacology*, **150**, 272–82.

Caspi, A., McClay, J., Moffitt, T. *et al.* (2002). Evidence that the cycle of violence in maltreated children depends on genotype. *Science*, **297**, 851–4.

Crowe, R.R. (1974). An adoption study of antisocial personality. *Archives of General Psychiatry*, **31**, 785–91.

Cunningham, W.A., Johnson, M.K., Raye, C.L. *et al.* (2004). Separable neural components in the processing of black and white faces. *Psychological Science*, **15**, 806–13.

Damasio, A. (2006). *Descartes' Error: Emotion, Reason and the Human Brain*. London: Vintage.

de Almeida, R.M.M., Ferari, P.F., Parmigiani, S. *et al.* (2005). Escalated aggressive behavior: Dopamine, serotonin and GABA. *European Journal of Pharmacology*, **526**, 51–64.

Farah, M.J., Illes, J., Cook-Deegan, R. *et al.* (2004). Neurocognitive enhancement: What can we do and what should we do? *Nature Reviews Neuroscience*, **5**, 421–5.

Fukuyama, F. (2002). *Our Posthuman Future: Consequences of the Biotechnology Revolution*. New York: Farrar, Straus, and Giroux.

Grove, W.M., Eckert, E.D., Heston, L. *et al.* (1990). Heritability of substance abuse and antisocial behavior: A study of monozygotic twins reared apart. *Biological Psychiatry*, **27**, 1293–304.

Hart, A.J., Whalen, P.J., Shin, L.M. *et al.* (2000). Differential response in the human amygdala to racial outgroup vs. ingroup face stimuli. *Neuroreport: For Rapid Communication of Neuroscience Research*, **11**, 2351–5.

Phelps, E.A., O'Connor, K.J., Cunningham, W.A. *et al.* (2000). Performance on indirect measures of race evaluation predicts amygdala activation. *Journal of Cognitive Neuroscience*, **12**, 729–38.

Heyd, D. (2003). Human nature: an oxymoron? *Journal of Medicine and Philosophy*, **28**(2), 151–69.

Hume, D. (1888). *A Treatise of Human Nature*, Selby-Bigge, L. A. (ed.), Oxford: Clarendon Press.

Johnston, L.D., O'Malley, P.M. & Bachman, J.G. (2003). *Monitoring the Future National Survey Results on Drug Use, 1975–2002: II. College Students and Adults Ages 19–40*. Washington, DC: US Department of Health and Human Services.

Kant, E. (1993). *Critique of Practical Reason*, 3rd edition, Beck, L. W. (trans.), New York: Macmillan.

Kass, L.R. (2003). Ageless bodies, happy souls: biotechnology and the pursuit of perfection. *The New Atlantis*, **1**, 9–28.

Leibniz, G.W. (1973). New system, and explanation of the new system. In *Philosophical Writings*, Parkinson, G.H.R. (ed.), Morris, M. (trans.). London: Dent.

Lynch, G. (2002). Memory enhancement: The search for mechanism-based drugs. *Nature Neuroscience*, **5**, 1035–8.

McKibben, B. (2003). Designer genes. *Orion*, April 30.

Mehlman, M.J. (2005). Genetic enhancement: Plan now to act later. *Kennedy Institute of Ethics Journal*, **15**(1), 77–82.

Mill, J.S., (1979). *Utilitarianism*, Sher, G. (ed.) Indianapolis: Hackett.

Moore, G.E. (1903). *Principia Ethica*. Cambridge: Cambridge University Press.

President's Council on Bioethics (2003). *Beyond Therapy: Biotechnology and the Pursuit of Happiness*. Washington, DC: President's Council on Bioethics.

Sandel, M.J. (2004). The case against perfection. *The Atlantic Monthly*, **293**(3), 50–65.

Sandel, M.J. (2007). *The Case Against Perfection: Ethics in the Age of Genetic Engineering* (pp. 12, 47–9) Cambridge, MA: Harvard University Press.

Schectman, M. (1996). *The Constitution of Selves*. Ithaca, NY: Cornell University Press.

Scott, R., Bourtchouladze, R., Gossweiler, S. *et al.* (2002). CREB and the discovery of cognitive enhancers. *Journal of Molecular Neuroscience*, **19**, 171–7.

Taylor, C. (1979). What's wrong with negative liberty. In A. Ryan (ed.), *The Idea of Freedom* (pp. 175–93) Oxford: Oxford University Press.

Teter, C.J., McCabe, S.E., LaGrange, K. *et al.* (2006). Illicit use of specific stimulants among college students: Prevalence, motives, and routes of administration. *Pharmacotherapy*, **26**(10), 1501–10.

Tindall, B. (2004). Better playing through chemistry. *New York Times*, October 17.

Tully, T., Bourtchouladze, R., Scott, R. *et al.* (2003). Targeting the CREB pathway for memory enhancers. *Nature Reviews Drug Discovery*, **2**, 267–77.

Turner, D.C., Robbins, T.W., Clark, L., Aron, A.R., Dowson, J. & Sahakian, B.J. (2003). Cognitive enhancing effects of Modafinil in healthy volunteers. *Psychopharmacology*, **165**, 260–9.

Verroken, M. (2005). Drug use and abuse in sport. In D.R. Mottram (ed.), *Drugs in Sport* (pp. 29–63) London: Routledge.

Wolpe, P.R. (2002). Treatment, enhancement, and the ethics of neurotherapeutics. *Brain and Cognition*, **50**, 387–95.

Yesavage, J., Mumenthaler, M., Taylor, J. *et al.* (2001). Donezepil and flight simulator performance: Effects on retention of complex skills. *Neurology*, **59**, 123–5.

35

Unfit for the Future? Human Nature, Scientific Progress, and the Need for Moral Enhancement

Ingmar Persson and Julian Savulescu

Human Psychology and Commonsense Morality

Even if human beings were psychologically and morally fit for life in those natural conditions in which they have lived during most of human history, humans have now so radically affected their conditions of living that they might be less psychologically and morally fit for life in this new environment which they have created for themselves. These new conditions consist principally of enormously populous societies with advanced science and technology which enable their citizens to exercise an influence that extends all over the world and far into the future. A hypothesis which we will explore in this chapter is that if human beings do not better adapt psychologically and morally to these new conditions, human civilization is under threat. We will begin by a rough sketch of some of the relevant traits of human psychology and primordial commonsense morality, before we turn to the problems which threaten us. It is important to recognize that we are not here discussing what would constitute a correct or justified morality (like some version of Kantianism, other deontological theory, virtue ethics, or consequentialism). Rather we are concerned with moral dispositions as they occur in ordinary people, across cultures, in virtue of their evolutionary history. Of course, today, many more sophisticated moral beliefs, ideals, and ideologies form a "super-structure" upon these basic dispositions.

Since human beings compete with each other over the scarce resources of nature, they are prone to cause harm to one another. It is in general easier to cause harm than to do good, e.g. easier to kill than to save life, to wound individuals than to heal their wounds, and to rob individuals of their sustenance than to provide them with sustenance. This is to be expected in a world in which beings, when they have matured, are normally fit to survive by their own means, to find the food, shelter, and other things that they need. A world inhabited by beings which were constantly dependent upon aid

Enhancing Human Capacities, edited by Julian Savulescu, Ruud ter Meulen and Guy Kahane.
© 2011 Blackwell Publishing Ltd

from others to survive would not be functional; there would not be enough people around to supply all the aid needed.

Through nearly all of human history, humans have lived and cooperated within small units of around 150 people (Dunbar *et al.*, 2007). Rival groups often fought with each other over limited resources. Commonsense morality evolved because it enabled humans to live more fruitfully together in smaller groups. Owing to the relative ease of causing harm, commonsense morality places more stress on not causing harm than on doing good. This finds expression in the so-called *act-omission doctrine*. According to this doctrine, it is harder to justify morally causing harm than letting harm occur or, put another way, there are stronger moral reasons not to cause harm than to prevent harm from occurring. Such a principle also makes for a more practicable morality, which is not as demanding as a morality that requires us to relieve harm, or provide good, whenever we can (as some utilitarians now claim we should).

Historically, our sphere of influence as humans was very limited. The tools at our disposal in the long pre-scientific period of our history enabled us to affect only our immediate environment during the imminent future. The most urgent dangers which threatened our ability to survive and reproduce typically were (or appeared to be) in our immediate environment, in the near future. So we have a *bias towards the near (future)*.[1] It is this bias which manifests itself when we are relieved as something unpleasant due to happen to us in the immediate future is postponed, and disappointed or impatient as something pleasant in store for us is postponed.

Some discounting of the distant future is rational. It is true that when an event is in the more remote future, it is less certain to occur than one that is more imminent. This lower probability makes it rational to be proportionally less concerned about the future. But it would be a mistake to think that the bias towards the near consists in being less concerned about a future event only because it is estimated to be less probable. For we could be greatly relieved when an unpleasant event, such as a painful piece of surgery, is postponed for just a day, although this delay may make it only marginally less probable. To the extent that our lesser concern for what is more distant in the future is out of proportion to its being (rationally) estimated to be less probable, it is arguably irrational.

Many thinkers in the history of philosophy have believed that human beings are exclusively egoistic, i.e. concerned only about their own well-being for its own sake. However, this sits ill both with everyday experience and evolutionary theory. From an evolutionary point of view, the most uncontroversial kind of altruism is *kin altruism*, i.e. altruism as regards our children, parents, and siblings. Kin altruism is straightforwardly explicable in evolutionary terms, since each child shares 50% of each of its parent's and 50% of each sibling's genes. Consequently, caring about kin would be caring about somebody who carries similar genes to oneself. But, although this is the evolutionary explanation or reason why we are altruistically disposed to our kin, it is not *our* reason for being concerned about the welfare of our kin, for we hardly possess any sensor which tracks genetic relations (Joyce, 2006, pp.16–17). Instead, we seem to care about our kin for their own sakes, at least in part, because we have during a longer period met them on a daily basis and have grown accustomed to them. Such close encounters with individuals tend to breed sympathy with and liking for them.

This mechanism of habituation could generate altruism also for non-kin whom we regularly meet on a daily basis, e.g. the people who live in our neighborhood since, as remarked, we do not register the presence or absence of close genetic ties. Thus, we have an explanation of how our altruism could spill over to individuals who are not our kin especially those in our group with whom we cooperate and depend upon for support, as we shall now argue.

It might seem that such a wider range of altruism would be disadvantageous from an evolutionary point of view – such a broader altruistic disposition is likely to make altruists do favors to others, and this is liable to put these others who are favored in a better position to survive and reproduce if they are inclined to free-ride. But this will not happen if those who are benefited by altruists feel *gratitude* which impels them to return the favors that the altruists have done to them. If not only altruism, but also this disposition to feel gratitude is widespread in a group or population, this group or population is likely to do better than groups or populations in which these motivational traits are rare or non-existent. For instance, if someone who has been groomed gratefully returns the service, this mutually beneficial cooperation is more likely to continue, with the result that the probability of the cooperators being infested by parasites decreases. Thus, if we throw in something like a disposition to experience gratitude in the evolutionary mix, we have the beginnings of an explanation of why a more extensive altruism than kin altruism would not be wiped out in the course of evolution, even in the presence of a number of free-riders.

Still, free-riders who receive favors, but do not return them, are likely to do better than the grateful individuals who do return favors, unless there is also among benefactors and third parties a widespread disposition to react to ungrateful behavior with *anger* or *aggression*, i.e. an emotion that issues in tendencies to punish those who do not return favors. So, we should suppose that a disposition to feel a proportionate anger on proper occasions is equally widely spread and beneficial, from an evolutionary point of view. There are also other emotions that belong to this set of emotions which promote cooperation – a set which could be called *tit-for-tat*[2] – like the emotions to feel *guilt* and *remorse* when you yourself have acted wrongly, and *forgiveness* when someone else has acted wrongly and feels guilt and remorse.

It seems plausible to hypothesize that the emotions which make up the tit-for-tat bundle are bound up with the concepts of *desert* and *justice* or *fairness*. When we feel gratitude towards somebody, we take it that this individual deserves a good turn and, so, that it is just or fair that she have it. When we are angry at somebody, we see this individual as deserving to be punished or harmed in return and, so, that this treatment is just, etc. In other words, when we are in the grip of these emotions, we regard individuals as deserving and justice as requiring the kind of treatment that we are inclined to deal them in virtue of these emotions.

The strength of this sense of justice or fairness can be tested in so-called *ultimatum games*. In these games there are two players, a proposer and a responder. The proposer proposes a certain division of some benefits. If the responder rejects the offer, neither the proposer nor the responder gets anything of the benefits. When the players are human, responders normally reject offers which would give them significantly less than an equal share, apparently because their feeling of being offended by an unfair division then becomes stronger than their desire for the benefit (Persson & Savulescu, 2008).

Tit-for-tat and the cooperation it is conducive to is beneficial to populations in which they are widely distributed: these populations tend to grow faster in number than populations in which they are more sparsely distributed or non-existent. Even so, those who benefit most from the schemes of cooperation are inevitably the free-riders of these populations; therefore, the percentage of free-riders in cooperative populations will steadily increase. But, as Elliot Sober and David Sloan Wilson (1998) contend, this is not fatal to the number of altruistic and cooperative individuals if we assume that the faster growing cooperative populations have opportunities of regrouping and that altruistic and cooperative individuals will then tend seek each other out. If this happens, their total number could continue to increase. Thus, we have an evolutionary explanation of how, once they have a foothold, altruistic and cooperative dispositions will spread instead of being erased.

However, this explanation presupposes that altruism and invitations to cooperation do not extend indiscriminately to strangers, e.g., members of non-cooperative populations, for this would mean exposure to too great a risk of being exploited by free-riders. Suspicion against strangers, then, is called for, since human beings often try to get the better of each other. This is presumably the explanation of why *xenophobia* is a widespread characteristic of humanity. As we mentioned, work by Robin Dunbar *et al.* (2007) suggests that the group of people with whom we are personally acquainted, have to some extent collaborated with, and so on, is limited to about 150. These are the people we are inclined to put trust in as cooperative partners.

It should not be assumed, however, that this group is by necessity limited to people who live in one's neighborhood, as it presumably has been in the past. The globalization of the modern world, the fact that people nowadays travel and do business more internationally could make us include people of different races and cultures in the trusted circle. This is entirely in line with Sober and Wilson's explanation which presupposes that we could open ourselves to cooperation with people outside our original group. As a result, our inborn tendency to racism, i.e. to view racial features like skin color or facial appearance as reasons for suspicion or maltreatment, could weaken. This effect could be strengthened by reflection upon the superficiality and moral irrelevance of such features. But, although such "cognitive therapy" has been shown to have effects, it is probably not as effective as the cooperative mechanisms that are rooted in human nature based on tit-for-tat.

The Possibility of Intentional Misuse of Science

Armed with this rough sketch of some primordial psychological and moral dispositions of human nature, let us now look at how they play out in the modern world. As remarked, it is generally much easier to harm than to benefit. It is quite easy for virtually anyone to do serious harm, say, to shoot a number of people dead in a minute, but almost nobody is ever capable of saving as many in the same period of time. People can be killed at any point in their lives, but it is only in exceptional circumstances, such as when we can save them from death, that we can benefit them as much as we harm them when we kill them. The claim that we would now like to put forward is that this greater ease of causing harm rather than doing good is magnified as our powers of action increase through science and technology. This is because the expansion of scientific knowledge and technological prowess will put in the hands of an increasing number of people weapons of mass destruction. In so far as this is so, this growth of knowledge will be instrumentally bad for us on the whole, by seriously augmenting the risk that many people will die, or be seriously harmed, within the near future. For if an increasing percentage of us acquires the capacity to destroy an increasing number of us, it is enough if very few people are malevolent or deranged enough to use this power for all of us to run a significantly greater risk of death and suffering.

The present technological know-how makes it possible for small groups, or even single individuals, to kill millions of people. Nuclear weapons are one well-known example, which have been feared since the 1950s. To make a nuclear bomb out of fissile material, such as highly enriched uranium or plutonium, seems not beyond the capacity of a well-organized terrorist group (Ackerman & Potter, 2008). If set off in a mega-city, such a bomb could kill millions of people and create panic among billions, causing directly medical disaster and indirectly social catastrophe. Dozens of countries have poorly secured stockpiles of enriched uranium, and Richard Posner (2004) surmises that "there may be enough plutonium outside secure military installations to furnish the raw material for 20,000 atomic bombs." Some of this fissile material might fall into the lap of terrorist groups. A technological breakthrough might also enable non-state agents to enrich uranium. Another possibility is that terrorists succeed in stealing nuclear weapons from a state. Nor can we exclude the possibility of a nuclear state willingly supplying a terrorist group with nuclear weapons, e.g. Pakistan supplying al-Qaeda with such weapons.

Another, even scarier, threat is biological weapons. This threat is scarier for the reason that biological weapons are much easier to fabricate – indeed, a single individual could do so with a crude backyard laboratory. Infectious diseases could spread extensively before they are discovered, especially if their incubation time is relatively long, such as a week or more. This is true of smallpox which kills one out of three infected. Biological weapons are harder to control and outlaw than nuclear weapons because they are the downside of research which has the laudable aim of curing diseases; in other words, it is research whose products have a dual use, both a beneficial and a harmful use.

Some scientists have modified mousepox to make it lethal in 100% of mice. Mousepox is similar to human smallpox, which was eradicated from the globe in the 1970s by vaccination. The study of mousepox was published on the internet, making it indiscriminately available. Genetic engineering of smallpox could create a new strain with a mortality of 100% instead of 30%, and with a resistance against current vaccine. A small group of terrorists could fly around the world and deposit aerosolizes with fluids of this virus in airport terminals, shopping malls, indoor stadiums, etc. Within a few minutes these aerosolizes could infect thousands of people at each location, most of whom would in their turn infect others, and so on. Since the incubation period of smallpox is one to two weeks, the disease would have spread widely before it was even detected, and even after detection there would be no effective way of preventing further dissemination. Below we shall consider what means are available keep these kinds of threats in check.

The Omission of Aid to the Developing World

We turn now to some consequences of our intuitive endorsement of the act-omission doctrine. Despite belief in the act-omission doctrine, the more wide-ranging the powers of action which science and technology put in our hands, the greater our moral responsibility. This holds, of course, under the assumption that we are also aware of what these powers enable us to do, since this is a necessary condition for it to be true that we let or allow something to happen by not putting these powers to use. If we know that it is in our power to prevent some harm, and we refrain from so doing, we are arguably as responsible for its occurrence as we would be had we knowingly caused it (Singer, 1993; Unger, 1996). If this is right, people in developed, affluent countries would be responsible for a lot of misery in developing countries. They act morally wrongly by not abolishing it.

The developed nations have to a large extent shirked to shoulder their responsibilities with respect to the developing world. For instance, in 2008 only five countries (Sweden, Luxembourg, Norway, Denmark, and the Netherlands) had reached the modest goal that the United Nations set decades ago of aid amounting to 0.7% of a country's GDP. The average for OECD nations is 0.47%; the two biggest world economies, the United States and Japan, lie at the bottom, at around 0.2%. One factor behind the weakness of the inclination to aid is surely the hold the act-omission doctrine has on our minds. Another factor is our limited altruism or selfishness. For instance, Cass Sunstein (2007, p.46) refers to "a "revealed preference" study of American taxation and foreign aid which suggests that Americans value a non-American life in the poorer nations at 1/2000 of the value they put on an American life.

But there is also a further factor that we have not yet mentioned: the sheer *number* of subjects to whom we have to respond can also present an obstacle to a proper response. While many of us are capable of vividly imagining the suffering of a single subject before our eyes and, consequently, feel strong compassion, we are unable vividly to imagine the suffering of 100 subjects even if they be in sight, let alone 1,000 subjects, and so on. Nor could we feel a compassion which is 100 times (or more) as strong as the compassion we feel for a single sufferer. Rather, the degree of compassion which we experience is likely to remain more or less constant when we switch from reflecting upon the suffering of a single subject to the suffering of 100 subjects. This *insensitivity or numbness to numbers of sufferers* is prone to make us seriously underestimate the amount of suffering that we could (but fail to) alleviate in the developing world. Hence, we are unlikely to be willing to pay the costs required to alleviate this suffering.

Failures of Cooperation and the Environment

Environmental problems probably provide the most worrying example of the limitations of our cooperative dispositions in the contemporary world. Important environmental problems include: a global climate change to which our emissions of greenhouse gases, like carbon dioxide and methane, contribute substantially; loss of biodiversity due to our destruction of forests, wetlands, and coral reefs; wasteful use of non-renewable energy sources, in particular oil, and of vital resources like water. Some of the mechanisms in operation can be illustrated on a smaller scale by *the problem of the tragedy of the commons* (Hardin, 1968).

Imagine a group of herdsmen who share a common pasture upon which their cattle graze. And imagine that if the herdsmen let their cattle continue to graze the pastures that they share to the current extent, there will be overgrazing of the pastures in the near future. As a consequence, the herdsmen will be able to feed fewer cattle in the course of time. They and their families will eventually starve. Suppose further that if a few herdsmen reduce the grazing of their cattle, but most of the other herdsmen do not do so, there will still be overgrazing, though it will occur somewhat later. Almost all of them will have to effect a reduction if overgrazing is to be avoided.

Under these circumstances, it might not be rational for any individual herdsman to cut down on the grazing of his cattle. This will be rational only if he has good reason to believe that his signing up for reduction is necessary for there to be a sufficient number of herdsmen who do so in order for overgrazing to be prevented. That is, that his reduction in grazing will contribute to an actual preservation of the pasture. Thus, if concern for or trust in the fellow-herdsmen is faltering, there is a risk that each herdsman will let his cattle continue to graze as before, with the result that there will be overgrazing and starvation in the future. There is a self-interested reason to reduce grazing only if one's reduction is necessary to make up a number of reductions that together are sufficient to prevent overgrazing. This is also an altruistic or utilitarian reason, since the prevention of overgrazing is what is best for the collective. If this degree of cooperation appears unlikely, there is a strong self-interested reason to defect from the cooperative endeavor.

As long as the number of herdsmen involved is small (e.g. in the range of 150), the herdsmen are more likely to know each other personally and to have developed concern and trust for each other. Likewise, if their number is small, it will be easier for them to keep an eye on each other and detect free-riders. For these reasons, the tragedy of the commons on a smaller scale presents a cooperation problem that is more tractable than environmental problems in the modern world. Environmental problems are caused by huge states with millions of citizens who are largely anonymous to each other and, so, have little reason to trust each other. Moreover, the masses of people make it easy for free-riders and defectors to escape notice.

There are, however, further reasons why modern environmental problems are harder to solve. As long as the total number of the herdsmen is small enough, there *could* be some self-interested reason for the herdsmen to opt for a reduction of grazing. If there is a chance that one individual herdsman's reduction is necessary for there to be a sum of reductions which is minimally sufficient to prevent overgrazing, there is an altruistic or utilitarian reason for him to cut down his grazing, since this will yield an outcome that is best for all. And as each herdsman is a member of the collective that is benefited, there is also something to be gained in terms of self-interest by cutting down. Thus, as long as one herdsman's reduction makes a noticeable or measurable difference to the outcome, there might be a self-interested reason for him to cut down because it is then possible that his reduction is necessary to produce, in conjunction with the other reductions in fact made, a set that is sufficient for the most beneficial outcome for himself and his collective. All the same, the self-interested reason not to reduce grazing is normally greater for each and every herdsman, since the chance that his particular reduction will tip the scales is likely to be slim.

As the number of agents involved in a cooperation problem grows, a stage is eventually reached at which the contribution of each agent to the total outcome becomes *negligible* or *imperceptible*. Then an individual agent can have no altruistic and, *a fortiori*, no self-interested reason to contribute. This is because there is then no determinate threshold of contributions which makes them sufficient to produce the beneficial outcome for all. Now, with regard to the environment, the contribution to each of us to environmental degradation is imperceptible or negligible. Apart from the fact that there is then no altruistic reason that is also a self-interested reason to adopt environmental-friendly policies, this means that the prohibition of commonsense morality against causing harm does not kick in. Consequently, the problem of the tragedy of the commons becomes more acute, and more certain.

What *could* make us cooperate in these circumstances would be *a feeling of justice and fairness*, that it would be unfair to those who contribute by cutting down on their consumption of natural resources and their release of waste to free-ride upon their sacrifices. We found earlier that there is a ground for thinking that human beings are equipped with such a feeling of justice or fairness. If – but only if – one believes that a sufficient number of other parties might make sacrifices, it would then be unfair to them to be a free-rider, who takes advantage of their sacrifices without making any sacrifice oneself. But this feeling of unfairness will be weaker when many of the other parties are anonymous to the individual agent. Moreover, in these circumstances, it is also often harder to be confident that they will make the requisite sacrifices. Any sense of unfairness is further undermined by the fact that, to a large extent, one will not be in a position to take advantage of the sacrifices of others: those who will benefit most from contemporary environmental-friendly policies are likely to be future generations rather than those who are alive today. This is because environmental processes in most cases are slow-working and will take decades before they make themselves felt. Therefore, there might not be any gain upon which one "rides" unfairly.

This implies that the bias towards the near future comes into operation as well, making it even more difficult for us to impose upon ourselves the consumptive restraints necessary to save the environment. Moreover, there is the complication that the nations which per capita are the worst sinners as regards the emission of greenhouse gases – in particular the United States, which is responsible for one-fifth of the world's emission of carbon dioxide – will not be among those which will suffer most because of global warming. This will rather be coastal lowland, like Bangladesh and Oceania, which risks being inundated when the sea-level rises owing to the melting of the inland ice of Greenland and Antarctica, and Africa which is threatened by desertification. Thus, our lack of concern for strangers (or innate xenophobia) will also come into play.

A final hurdle to addressing these environmental problems is an enormous global economic inequality. For instance, the Kyoto Protocol of 1997 proposed no restrictions on the emission of carbon dioxide by populous nations like China and India. Indeed it is not easy to think of a regulation that would be acceptable to the United States, on the one hand, and China and India, on the other. A *sustainable* rate of emissions which is proportionate to the population of a nation would scarcely be acceptable to the United States, since it would mean a massive reduction in their current level of emissions. On the other hand, a more modest reduction of the emissions of the United States would put China and India in a position to claim rights to much larger emissions, in view of their much larger populations, and in view of the fact that they have hitherto contributed relatively little to the greenhouse effect. So, this proposal would lead to rights to emissions which are far too permissive from an environmental perspective.

Could Liberal Democracies Cope with These Problems?

This brief survey is enough to make it apparent that the advance of science and technology has brought in its wake some serious moral problems. Indeed, the eminent British scientist Martin Rees (2003, p.8) estimates that "the odds are no better than fifty-fifty that our present civilisation on the Earth will survive to the end of the present century." Such an estimate would have been wildly implausible in recent centuries prior to the development of nuclear weapons. But exponential technological advance has brought with it much greater threats of worldwide catastrophe, for reasons some of which we have detailed (and some further ones which Rees reviews).

Certainly, the progress of science has also had countervailing good effects: thanks to it, far more people lead longer and better lives than ever before. But this must be weighed against the fact that far more people than ever live in deep misery, as a result of vast global inequality. To illustrate: "the difference between the per capita incomes of the richest and the poorest countries was 3 to 1 in 1820, 11 to 1 in 1913, 35 to 1 in 1950, 44 to 1 in 1973, and 72 to 1 in 1992" (Seitz, 2008, p.3). At the beginning of the present millennium the wealthiest fifth of the world's population stood for 86% of the world's GNP, while the poorest fifth stood for only 1% of it, and the richest three individuals owned as much as 600 million people in the poorest countries.

So, it is certainly not obvious that the progress of science has led to a better world, all things considered. On the contrary, it is likely that if this progress were soon to lead us into a global catastrophe, the final judgment will have to be that this progress has been for the worse, all things considered. The question we would like to raise is, however, what means liberal democracies have of averting these catastrophes. We define liberal democracy ostensibly or "demonstratively" as the form of government found in the affluent nations of the European Union, the United States, and members of the British Commonwealth like Canada, Australia, and New Zealand. We prefer an ostensive definition because we want to present an argument which applies to these affluent nations or societies, not to the societies, if any, which fit some abstract conception. But if something were to be said by way of characterizing the ideal of liberal democracy (which these states might not fully realize), it would run along the following lines. A fully liberal state is a state in which every citizen has equal rights and liberties which are as extensive as they could be, consistently with all others having the same rights and liberties. The requisite rights and liberties comprise equal rights before the law, equal rights to acquire property – thus, a liberal state has a market economy – and freedom of speech, press, assembly, and religion. A liberal state is ideally a state in which the citizens can decide the course of their own lives, and the state interferes only when the citizens encroach upon the equal freedom of other citizens. It is natural to assume that the equal rights include an equal right to determine who shall have the political power. Accordingly, a liberal state is naturally, but not necessarily, a democracy in which, by definition, every citizen has a right to vote in general elections which by majority decision determine who should govern.

As regards terrorist threats discussed earlier, the advance of science has equipped societies with more effective means of surveillance. Their intelligence agencies may be able to monitor all electromagnetic transmissions – phone calls, e-mail communication, etc. – which involve their societies, unless they are unbreakably encrypted. They could survey public places by CCTV and record face-to-face conversations. Digitization and computerized data processing could make possible the storage of an overwhelming mass of recorded information about individual citizens. But if authorities were to employ these wide-ranging means of intelligence, they would seem to set aside a right to privacy, which has been considered one of the characteristics of a liberal state, and turn it into something uncomfortably like the totalitarian state depicted by George Orwell's novel *Nineteen Eighty-Four*.

However, it is doubtful whether there is any moral *right* to privacy, i.e. a right that outsiders do not gain such information about the right-holders that they would be embarrassed if anyone but themselves and a select few were to possess it. Even such a staunch defender of rights as Judith Thomson (1990, p.280) denies its existence. It should, however, be noticed that, even if there is no such right, other rights, like property rights, could provide some of the protection of privacy that a right to privacy would provide. For instance, if you own a house and, thereby have a right that others do not enter it without your permission, you could normally ensure the privacy of some of your activities by performing them in your home. But suppose that I could gain intimate information about your life, without violating your property rights, or physically affecting anything belonging to you, e.g. by simply by looking you in the eye, would you then have a right against me that I do not look you in the eye? This seems questionable because such a right would appear to restrict my freedom severely.

Even if we do not have any right to privacy, it cannot be denied that we have an interest in privacy, and this interest needs to be weighed against other interests we have, such as an interest in security. Terrorist threats jeopardize this security, and close surveillance of citizens may prove to be necessary to counteract them. The need for such surveillance may seem particularly acute in liberal democracies. This is because they are to an increasing degree *multicultural*. Historically speaking, human societies have tended to be culturally homogeneous. This appears to be so for two reasons. First, there is a strong tendency in human nature towards conformism. When children grow up, they do not merely acquire knowledge of the cultural traditions of their society, its language, religion, etc.; most of them readily adopt these traditions and regard them as superior to alternatives. Secondly, in the past there was comparatively little mobility between one society and another, as a rule people stayed put in the society into which they were born. But in the world of today there is an unprecedented mobility which has resulted in modern liberal democracies being mixes of people from innumerable cultures. Liberal democracies are as a matter of ideology tolerant of this cultural diversity. They allow minorities with different political and religious ideals to be cultivated in their midst. This brings along an inescapable risk that some of these minorities will contain subgroups that are prepared to resort to violence to promote their divergent ideals – and modern science and technology are liable to provide them with ever more powerful weapons.

One could imagine the majority in democracies voting in favor of extended surveillance in the interest of their security. But it is harder to imagine the majority voting in favor of the substantial cutbacks of welfare that seem necessary to tackle the problems of climate change and global inequality. In this case the majority will have to make much more tangible sacrifices to benefit, not themselves, but individuals remote in time and place. Since the majority has limited altruism, is biased towards the near, and does not experience itself as causing harm, it appears very unlikely that it will vote in favor of such sacrifices.

Are liberal democracies really in such trouble? The so-called *jury theorem* has led some to think that some very modest epistemic assumptions could justify high hopes about the righteousness of democracy. Suppose that, when voting about two alternatives, each voter is slightly more likely to be right than a random process, say, right 51% of the time. Then, the theorem declares that, if the number of voters is huge, it is virtually certain that the majority of them will come down in favor of the right alternative. This is as obvious as that, if we weight a huge number of coins such that there is a 51% probability that they will show heads if they are flipped, then, if we flip them all, it is virtually certain that a majority of them will show heads. This might sound reassuring for liberal democracy, but it should be borne in mind that there is downside of the coin: If each voter is slightly *less* likely than a random process to be right about some kind of issue, say, right 49% of the time, then the majority will almost certainly be wrong about an issue!

Indeed, it has been noted that, if there is in a democracy a minority which is hated by the majority, it may be more likely that the majority will not vote for a morally acceptable treatment of this minority. (The prevalent maltreatment of asylum-seekers might be one example.) Likewise, if human nature is as we have described it earlier, it seems more likely than not that the majority will be inclined to vote for policies that will disfavor or discriminate against individuals who are remote in time and place, owing to their biases. This is a problem of democracy which is amplified by the growth of the powers that science has given us to affect the whole globe far into the future. In the past, when we could not affect what was remote in time and place, it did not morally matter that we do not care much about it. But today, we can drastically affect events remote in time and place, though our moral dispositions have not much changed.

What would be needed to rectify this situation would seem to have to be a moral enhancement of human beings, which would make them less biased towards what is near in time and place and feel more responsible for what they collectively cause and let happen. We should not think that a moral development of human nature is impossible. As already noted, there is a strong tendency in human nature towards conformism. Societies have always taken advantage of this fact by imprinting upon their members moral norms conducive to their survival and prosperity. These norms include not only norms to refrain from certain kinds of behavior, such as killing innocent members of society against their will, or stealing their property, but also norms to contribute positively to the public good by paying taxes. Most citizens abide by these norms, without it being necessary to bring in the legal sanctions to enforce them.

These traditional means of moral education and training seem not to have been put to full use. Perhaps the ideological and evaluative neutrality espoused by liberal tradition bears some of the responsibility for this. As remarked, the ideal of classical liberalism was to abstain from interfering with the lives of citizens as long as they do not harm other citizens; this ideal is most famously expressed by J.S. Mill's principle of liberty in his *On Liberty* (1859). Despite this ideal, liberalism has developed into a social liberalism which acknowledges the need for state interference to neutralize glaring welfare inequalities within a society, by a welfare system funded by taxation. We now suggest that it is necessary for liberalism to take the further step of becoming a *global*(ly responsible) liberalism, which extends the welfare thinking globally and into the remote future. Liberalism is right in thinking that citizens should be permitted to live out their individualities, but citizens in affluent societies must learn to do this without wasting the resources of the planet. In the world of today, when scientific progress has vastly increased our powers of action, and connected societies all over the world by means of travel and commerce, intra-societal norms are not enough. Societies need to inculcate norms that are conducive to the good of the world community of which these societies are an integral part.

We might have witnessed the beginning of this process with the increased stress in politics upon international organizations like the United Nations, and upon the doctrine of the equality of all human beings. But in spite of these efforts, global inequality is growing rather than shrinking. It is one thing to endorse a moral principle intellectually, but quite another, and much more difficult thing to internalize it to the degree that one's life is regulated by it.[3] Overcoming our biases towards what is near us in time and place and our truncated sense of responsibility is a tall order.

The Further Future?

In this chapter, we have identified the problems created by the misfit between a limited human moral nature and globalized, highly advanced technology. The 21st century is the century in which humans will pose the greatest threats to themselves, in virtue of their nature.

We have sketched several ways of addressing the potential catastrophic consequences of this mismatch. We considered the development of a globally responsible liberalism, with the restriction of traditional liberal neutrality, inculcation of values and "moral education" to achieve restraint, promote cooperation, respect for equality, and other values now necessary for our survival as a global community. We also considered the possibility of greater infringements of privacy and heightened surveillance. But we should also consider the possibility that the very scientific progress that has created this mismatch could be employed to ameliorate it, by delivering methods of enhancing our capacity for moral behavior.

We have argued that concepts of justice and fairness are central to tit-for-tat behavior which characterizes primordial morality. There are reasons to believe that behavior relating to justice and fairness is partly biologically determined. When ultimatum games are performed with chimps, responders generally accepted 2/8 distributions without any sign of dissatisfaction even when there was an equal distribution of five raisins in each pot on the alternative tray. In contrast, under similar conditions adult human responders as a rule respond by rejecting the offer, thereby forgoing a smaller reward in order to punish the proposers for their blatant unfairness.

However, humans differ in terms of how much unfairness they will tolerate in the ultimatum game. Some will accept a 4/6 distribution; others only 5/5. What is remarkable is not that humans differ from each other, but that when human identical twins play the proposer and responder roles of the ultimatum game, there is a striking correlation between the average division with respect to both what they propose and what they are ready to accept as responders. There is no such correlation in the case of fraternal twins. Since identical twins share the same genes (and these twins have been separated at birth), this strongly suggests that the human sense of fairness has some genetic basis. In humans, the rejection of unfair offers is >40% genetically determined, with a very modest role for environmental influences.

Another example of the contribution of biology to moral behavior is violent aggressive behavior. Caspi and colleagues investigated the relationship between the presence of a change in the gene encoding for monoamine oxidase A (MAOA), a neurotransmitter metabolizing enzyme, and the tendency towards antisocial behavior in a large cohort of New Zealand males. They found that men who had been mistreated as children and were positive for the polymorphism conferring low levels of MAOA were significantly more likely to exhibit antisocial behavior than those who had been mistreated but lacked the change. Both groups were more likely to exhibit antisocial behavior than those who were not mistreated. This suggests a possible interaction between mistreatment and MAOA deficiency in causing antisocial behavior. (Needless to say, this does not imply that it would be morally acceptable to use knowledge of this interaction in order to prevent antisocial behavior simply by pharmacological manipulation of MAOA, without attempting to eliminate the social condition of mistreatment.)

The neurotransmitter serotonin has been linked to less aggressive behavior. There is an inverse relationship between levels of this transmitter and impulsive aggressive behavior (O'Keane et al., 1992). Serotonin appears to suppress aggressive behavior (Haller et al., 2005). For example, depleting serotonin leads to more aggressive behavior. And drugs such as selective serotonin reuptake inhibitors like Prozac increase cooperation and reduce aggression.

Oxytocin, a hormone released by the hypothalamus, facilitates birth and breastfeeding, and, in at least nonhuman mammals, it also appears to mediate pair bonding, maternal care, and other pro-social behaviou (Insel & Fernald, 2004). It has been shown to influence ability to infer another's mental state (Domes et al., 2007). It increases willingness to trust, but this does not extend to all risk taking, only social risks. For example, it prevents decrease of trust after betrayal and even after several betrayals. It also reduces fear of social betrayal (Baumgartner et al., 2008; Kosfeld et al., 2005). That is to say, oxytocin may mediate trustworthiness. Signals of trust are associated with increases in oxytocin in the person receiving the signal of trust (Zak et al., 2004). Tom Douglas (2008) reviews other potential ways of biologically enhancing moral behavior.

To be sure, such findings are a long way from yielding effective biomedical techniques of moral enhancement. But we think that the enormity of the moral problems that face us makes it reasonable to explore the possibility of such techniques, though their discovery may prove to lie too far into the future for such techniques to offer us any realistic hope of helping us with the urgent moral problems that we have reviewed. Biomedical moral enhancements, were they feasible, would be the most important biomedical enhancement. However, it must not be forgotten that they raise the same moral problems as all technological innovations: that of a proper application of them. In the case of techniques of moral enhancement this takes the form of a bootstrapping problem: it is human beings, who need to be morally enhanced, who have to make a morally wise use of these techniques.

Acknowledgments

We would like to thank Tom Douglas, Russell Powell, Guy Kahane and audiences at the Sydney Dangerous Ideas Festival, Brocher Conference on Human Enhancement and Princeton Center for Human Values in 2009 for valuable comments.

Notes

1. This is the name that Derek Parfit (1984) gives to this trait. But the trait has been discussed by many others, and has been experimentally studied in various ways.
2. This term sometimes designates a somewhat simpler pattern of reactions: when the response to a failure to return a favor does not include anger, but simply consists in the discontinuation of the doing of favors. However, this simpler pattern seems less useful, since it allows the ungrateful to get away too easily.
3. There is evidence, though, that general cognitive enhancement and higher average intelligence in a group may issue in more cooperative behavior, see Jones, 2008.

References

Ackerman, G. & Potter, W.C. (2008). Catastrophic nuclear terrorism: A preventable evil. In N. Bostrom & M.M. Cirkovic (eds.), *Global Catastrophic Risks* (pp. 412–14). Oxford: Oxford University Press.

Baumgartner, T., Heinrichs, M., Vonlanthen, A., Fischbacher, U. & Fehr, E. (2008). Oxytocin shapes the neural circuitry of trust and trust adaptation in humans. *Neuron*, **58**(4), 639–50.

Domes, G., Heinrichs, M., Michel, A., Berger, C. & Herpertz, S.C. (2007). Oxytocin improves "mind-reading" in humans. *Biological Psychiatry*, **61**(6), 731–3.

Douglas, T. (2008). Moral enhancement. *Journal of Applied Philosophy*, **25**(3), 228–45.

Dunbar, R., Barrett, L. & Lycett, J. (2007). *Evolutionary Psychology*. Oxford: One World.

Haller, J., Mikics, É., Halász, J. & Tóth, M. (2005). Mechanisms differentiating normal from abnormal aggression: Glucocorticoids and serotonin. *European Journal of Pharmacology*, **526**(1–3), 89–100.

Hardin, G. (1968). The Tragedy of the Commons. *Science*, **162**, 1243–8.

Insel, T.R. & Fernald, R.D. (2004). How the brain processes social information: Searching for the social brain. *Annual Review of Neuroscience*, **27**, 697–722.

Jones, G. (2008). Are smarter groups more cooperative? Evidence from prisoner's dilemma experiments, 1959–2003. *Journal of Economic Behavior and Organization*, **68**(3–4), 489–97.

Joyce, R. (2006). *The Evolution of Morality*. Cambridge, MA: MIT Press.

Kosfeld, M., Heinrichs, M., Zak, P., Fischbacher, U. & Fehr, E. (2005). Oxytocin increases trust in humans. *Nature*, **435**(2), 673–6.

O'Keane, V., Moloney, E., O'Neil, l.H., O'Connor, A., Smith, C. & Dinan, T. (1992). Blunted prolactin responses to d-fenfluramine in sociopathy. Evidence for subsensitivity of central serotonergic function. *British Journal of Psychiatry*, **160**(5), 643–6.

Parfit, D. (1984). *Reasons and Persons*. Oxford: Clarendon Press.

Persson, I. & Savulescu, J. (2008). The perils of cognitive enhancement and the urgent imperative to enhance the moral character of humanity. *Journal of Applied Philosophy*, **25**, 162–77.

Posner, R.A. (2004). *Catastrophe: Risk and Response*. Oxford: Oxford University Press.

Rees, M. (2003). *Our Final Century*. Oxford: Heinemann.

Seitz, J.L. (2008). *Global Issues*, 3rd edition. Oxford: Blackwell.

Singer, P. (1993). *Practical Ethics*. Cambridge: Cambridge University Press.

Sober, E. & Wilson, D.S. (1998). *Unto Others*. Cambridge, MA: Harvard University Press.

Sunstein, C. (2007). *Worst-Case Scenarios*. Cambridge, MA: Harvard University Press.

Thomson, J. (1990). *The Realm of Rights*. Cambridge, MA: Harvard University Press.

Unger, P. (1996). *Living High and Letting Die*. New York: Oxford University Press.

Zak, P., Kurzban, R. & Matzner, W. (2004). The neurobiology of trust. *Annals of the New York Academy of Sciences*, **1032**, 224–7.

Part VII
General Policy

36

Of Nails and Hammers: Human Biological Enhancement and U.S. Policy Tools

Henry T. Greely

"I suppose it is tempting, if the only tool you have is a hammer, to treat everything as if it were a nail" (Abraham Maslow, 1966)

Tools are humanity's greatest enhancers. We use them to make ourselves better at almost everything we do, from hunting and gathering to sending missions to other planets. And, confronted with any task, among the first questions asked are "What tools do I have available?" and "What tools do I need?" Less often asked, but sometimes more important, is the question, "Are the tools I have sufficient?"

Advances in biomedical sciences, driven by the search for solutions to human suffering, are increasingly creating opportunities for other kinds of enhancers, those that act by modifying our bodies, and our brains. These human biological enhancements, of one sort or another, are being used to improve our looks, our athletic abilities, our moods, our intellectual productivities, and perhaps our lifespans. The currently available enhancements are not terribly impressive, but enhancements are likely to become more powerful and less dangerous, and hence both more attractive and more common.

I have argued elsewhere that we should not categorically reject human biological enhancements (Greely, 2004a, 2004b, 2005/2006, 2008a, 2008b). The arguments made against the whole category of such enhancements are, I believe, seriously flawed. Yet I have also argued that human biological enhancements do raise three real issues, problems that our societies will need to manage, if not perfectly solve. These issues are safety, coercion, and fairness.

Like the humans who constitute them, human societies rely on tools, specifically, on policy tools. These allow us, collectively, to respond to problems. The tools can be government dictats, the policies of private organizations, educational campaigns, or other intentional efforts to affect society. They can be very general, like the legislative power of the U.S. Congress, or very specific, like the authority of the U.S. Food and Drug Administration (FDA) to regulate dietary supplements. They can be powerfully coercive, like criminal sanctions, or much more subtle, like advertising campaigns.

Enhancing Human Capacities, edited by Julian Savulescu, Ruud ter Meulen and Guy Kahane.
© 2011 Blackwell Publishing Ltd

This chapter explores the questions "What policy tools do we have to deal with human biological enhancements?" as well as "What policy tools do we *need*?" The chapter discusses the United States because that is the society I know best – and looking at the policy tools available to even one country is a substantial effort. After discussing, in general, the policy tools available in the United States, I will examine their adequacy in coping with human biological enhancements in two respects – how easy they would be to adopt and how easy they would be to enforce. In each category, I will look at the three major issues raised by human biological enhancement: safety, coercion, and fairness. I conclude that some of the policy tools we need to deal with enhancement already exist but need to be better focused. In other cases, appropriate tools do not yet exist. And in all situations, we need to pay more attention to human biological enhancements and how we want to manage them.

U.S. Policy Tools

Policy formation in the United States is complicated, perhaps more complicated than in most societies. U.S. governments are both numerous and simultaneously strong and weak. Non-governmental actors also have broad scope to make policy, but face some special limitations. This section describes both *de jure* and *de facto* aspects of first governmental and then non-governmental policy making in the United States. It provides an oversimplified analysis of a very complicated political system, but it should be useful in setting the scene for consideration of policy tools for managing enhancement.

The federal government

In theory, the United States federal government should be weak. It has only the powers delegated to it by the Constitution; all other powers, including the inherent powers of sovereignty, remain with the states. In reality, at least since the mid-1930s, the federal government has been dominant, although the states – and the counties, cities, special districts, and other governmental bodies created by the states – continue to play crucial roles in some policy fields.

New legislation is the most direct way for the federal government to implement policy, but it is rarely easy.[1] The U.S. Congress has long been made up almost exclusively of members of either the Democratic or Republican parties – the 100-member Senate currently has 98 Democrats or Republicans and two independents, both of whom vote mainly with the Democrats; the 435-member House of Representatives currently has no members who are not Democrats or Republicans. This two-party dominance, with its consequence that one party or another almost always has a majority, does not, however, make new legislation easy to pass because party control in Congress is quite weak. Nomination and election to seats is controlled locally, and not nationally. Senators and representatives care more about pleasing their voters and campaign contributors – many of whom are independents or voters who regularly cross party lines – than their party leadership. As a result, neither party can count on controlling its members' votes.

Congress presents other obstacles to effective policy implementation. Passage of a controversial measure in the Senate effectively requires 60 votes, not 51, as the side opposed can threaten to "filibuster" – to speak indefinitely – in order to block consideration of a bill. Under Senate rules, it takes 60 votes to close debate. Although no such effective super-majority requirement exists in the House of Representatives, both houses have complex committee systems. Legislation will usually have to be approved by one, two, or even three committees in each house before it can reach the floor. Committee or subcommittee chairs with particular policy or political interests can bottle up proposed legislation indefinitely.

The Congressional system makes it very easy to stop legislation and hard to pass it, particularly if politically significant interests are opposed. If all of the interest groups are aligned, legislation can go through quickly, but that rarely happens. Sometimes legislation passes as a result of a perceived crisis or scandal. Both the Pure Food and Drug Act of 1906 and the Federal Food, Drug, and Cosmetics Act of 1938, along with its crucial 1962 amendments, followed events that focused public attention on problems in food and drug regulation. Sometimes legislation passes as a result of years of negotiation, consensus building, and compromise, often pushed over the edge by a significant change in the party balance of power in Congress. The passage of Medicare and Medicaid in 1965 provides an example of this dynamic; an effort to provide health insurance for elderly Americans that began in the late 1950s finally was successful after the 1964 election proved a landslide for the Democrats. The 2010 major health care financing reform in the United States provides a contemporary example.

The passage of new statutes by Congress is difficult, but new regulations issued by federal agencies provide a much easier policy tool. The FDA, for example, can adopt new regulations without any new legislative action, as long as it acts within the powers given it by earlier legislation and follows certain procedural requirements. The procedures can be time-consuming, but, fundamentally, rule-making is something an agency can just *do*, and ultimately something a president can have done through officials whom he commands.

Federal agencies can take major action through methods other than rule-making, of course. For example, the FDA often avoids some of the procedural requirements of formal rule-making by posting "guidance" that, although not legally binding, is very likely to be followed (Noah, 1997). Agencies can also spend money in ways that have policy implications, through grant programs or through more direct expenditures. Similarly, a federal agency could provide grants to support research or education (or propaganda) about an issue, with policy implications. Or the agency could spend the money directly on a public relations campaign. These kinds of actions can be compelled by Congress or can be forbidden by Congress, but most fall into a vast middle ground of being authorized, but not required, by often-broad Congressional language about the agency's power.

Of course, a federal agency's power does have some legal and practical limits. Most directly, Congress can pass legislation halting or overturning such regulations. Less formally, important members of Congress, particularly those who sit on Congressional committees or subcommittees with policy oversight or budgetary authority over the agency, can express objections or concerns, which the agency will find it prudent to consider. Affected persons can sue to block an action, claiming that it exceeds the agency's power under its authorizing legislation, that it conflicts with other federal statutes, or that it violates the federal constitution. Such litigation, even if ultimately unsuccessful, could impose serious costs on the agency, particularly by delaying implementation of the regulation. The White House can pose barriers to actions by agencies that, in theory, it controls, if, for example, a new regulation that seems sensible to the agency offends the policy, or political, judgments of the highest levels of the Administration. (The Bush Administration was widely thought to have interfered with FDA decisions about contraceptives for political reasons.) And people, companies, or industries made unhappy by the regulation can go to Congress or the White House, seeking either to have the regulation overturned or to take other actions against the agency. Issuing or amending regulations is less politically constrained than passing or amending statutes, but it is not free from political pressure.

State and local governments

Under the U.S. system of federalism, the 50 state governments have governmental powers that are not delegated, through the Constitution, to the federal government. In practice, since the 1930s and President Franklin Roosevelt's "New Deal," the federal government has played the most important role in governing, but many governmental powers are still primarily exercised by the states, including the bulk of the criminal law, regulation of education, and control over the professions, including especially medicine. The states, in turn, created a myriad of lesser jurisdictions to serve broad or narrow governmental ends, from counties and cities to special districts for the control of mosquitoes or the provision of water supplies. States are constrained mainly by federal laws, including the federal constitution and its amendments, but also by their own constitutions.

The states have their own legislatures and their own regulatory agencies. State legislation and state regulation are often easier to achieve than their federal equivalents. Partially this is because states are "narrower." Legislation in favor of rural interests, for example, may be more easily passed in predominantly farming states, while in the federal Congress urban constituencies counterbalance rural desires. Similarly, some individual states will be more thoroughly dominated by one party or one ideological position than the overall nation.

At the same time, groups with major political interests will focus more closely on federal action, because it affects the whole country. An action by Wyoming, the state with the smallest population (less than 0.2% of the country's population), will be less important than a similar action by California, with the largest population, at more than 12% of the national total and an even larger portion of the national economy. Both will pale in importance compared to federal action.

Thus states often take more diverse positions than the federal government, serving as, in the famous idea of U.S. Supreme Court Justice Louis Brandeis, "laboratories of democracy" (*New State Ice Co. v. Liebmann* 1932). Sometimes those positions spread broadly through the rest of the states; sometimes they languish. State action can also importantly drive federal action. Often, groups with interests in many states, such as broad-based industries, will prefer federal regulation that, by "preempting" state action with an exclusively federal scheme, sets uniform policies throughout the country, to a patchwork of friendly and unfriendly state laws. This is particularly true for products that are to be sold throughout the country; having different sets of legal requirements for each state is difficult for manufacturers.

The federal constitution imposes some constraints on the ability of the federal government to preempt state law, based either on limits of federal power or on concern about federal interference with state sovereignty. These limits will not stop a determined Congress, as the federal government can "bribe" states to accede to its wishes by conditioning their receipt of various federal grant moneys on their adoption of particular policies. For example, every state sets the age for the legal purchase of alcoholic beverages at 21, not because federal law requires it but because federal law reduces federal highway aid by 10% to any state not complying with the law.

Non-governmental actors

Non-governmental actors also play a major role not only in influencing government policy-making, but also in setting policy directly. Professional organizations or accrediting bodies are particularly important. For example, assisted reproduction technologies are almost entirely unregulated in the United States, but the trade association representing reproductive clinics, the American Society for Reproductive Medicine, issues guidelines and ethical standards that seem to affect how these services are delivered.

For the most part, these professional standards do not have the direct force of law, although occasionally regulatory authority is formally delegated to them. For example, most states will license any hospital that is accredited by the Joint Commission (formerly known as the Joint Commission on Accreditation of Healthcare Organizations and still widely referred to as the JCAHO), although it is a private, non-profit body dominated by the hospital industry and the medical profession. Even when private standards are not expressly made legally binding, they may serve to set the standard of practice in the relevant area, with or without government intervention. Consider practice guidelines issued by a medical specialty society about how best to treat a particular medical problem. Those guidelines will likely be accepted by most practitioners in the field as an expert statement of appropriate care. In addition, a doctor's failure to follow a relevant practice guideline can be evidence in a civil suit that the doctor's actions were negligent or otherwise inappropriate. Such a guideline might also determine whether either a private insurer or a government program pays the doctor for the treatment.

The Role of the Courts in Reviewing Policy

The U.S. judicial system can become involved in almost any part of policy-making. All actions by governments in the United States must comply with the applicable portions of the federal constitution, including particularly its Bill of Rights and the Equal Protection Clause and Due Process Clause of its Fourteenth Amendment. State and local governments also must comply with federal statutes and regulations, as do federal agencies and officials. The federal government need not, however, generally comply with state or local laws. Private organizations or individuals are supposed to comply with all applicable constitutional provisions, statutes, or regulations, whether federal, state, or local.

Over the last century the courts, both federal and state, have become more active in striking down federal and state laws or actions that violate federal or state constitutions. Almost any major new governmental policy initiative will be tested in court. New statutes will be judged against the relevant constitutions, new regulations will be judged against the constitutions and the statutes, and other actions will be judged against constitutions, statutes, and regulations. Similar oversight may be brought to bear on private policy-making activities (although the federal constitution, which mainly binds governmental action, will rarely apply). One special source of statutory review of private policy-making will be the federal (and often state) antitrust laws, which broadly ban combinations or conspiracies "in restraint of trade." A professional or trade association's standards, if applied forcefully, are sometimes held to be illegal efforts to restrain the trade of covered parties who disagree with the standards.

Enforcing policy

It is one thing to make policy; it is another thing to implement it. Murder has been illegal for millennia, but it still happens. Policies are particularly difficult to implement when they seek to limit behavior that some people strongly desire, especially when and if the behavior is relatively easy to conceal. History – perhaps especially U.S. history – is littered with failed crusades against drugs, from alcohol to marijuana, and other disfavored activities, such as prostitution.

Illicit activities are easier to enforce if they require difficult manufacturing processes. Even so, people have run illegal stills for centuries; amateur chemists have synthesized illegal methamphetamine and LSD for decades. Similarly, it is easier to limit procedures that require skilled intermediaries, such as surgeons, but even if there are some professionals who may choose openly to violate the law, others will operate at or beyond the edge of the law, and some amateurs will learn to provide the services. The history of abortion in restrictive legal regimes provides examples of all three–doctors providing abortion as a matter of principle, doctors illegally performing abortions for financial gain, and midwives or other non-physicians acting as abortionists.

Few if any regulatory schemes will be perfectly implemented. Imperfection is not, in itself, a decisive argument against regulation. Laws against murder have never made it disappear, but they have, almost certainly, reduced its incidence. Still, the likely costs and efficacy of implementation need to be considered before adopting any new policy.

After this brief survey of policy-making in the United States, it is time to apply those lessons to the regulation of human biological enhancements. The remainder of this chapter looks first at the adoption of, then at the enforcement of, policy tools available in the United States to cope with three real problems raised by such enhancements: safety, coercion, and fairness. The discussion is necessarily fairly general. Any particular enhancement will generate its own set of issues. The analysis below seeks to provide both some general approaches and some examples of specific problems.

Adopting Policies on Human Biological Enhancement

Some kinds of policies about human biological enhancement will be easier or harder to adopt than others. In general, it will be easier (though not easy) to adopt policies regulating the safety of such enhancements and harder to adopt those dealing with coercion or fairness.

Safety

The safety of human biological enhancements should be a major concern. Although we need to be concerned about the safety of our external tools, from automobiles to cell phones, enhancements that take place within our complex and still-poorly understood biological organism seem, on the face of it at least, to raise more serious issues of safety. And, in general, products that are intended to affect how our bodies (including our brains) function are already regulated for safety and efficacy as drugs, medical devices, or dietary supplements. The existence of this kind of regulation makes it easier to extend regulation to human biological enhancements. This section will first describe the existing regulatory structure, before laying out the kinds of extensions that would need to be adopted to handle the safety of enhancements.

Existing safety regulation   The FDA has the main responsibility for regulating the safety of categories of activities that would make up most of the plausible forms of human biological enhancement: drugs, biologics, medical devices, and dietary supplements. The Food, Drug, and Cosmetics Act defines drugs primarily as "articles intended for use in the diagnosis, cure, mitigation, treatment, or prevention of disease in man or other animals" *or* as "articles (other than food) intended to affect the structure or any function of the body of man or other animals." Biologics have an odd definition, but by and large can also be regulated as "drugs." A regulated "device" is "an instrument, apparatus, implement, machine, contrivance, implant, in vitro reagent, or other similar or related article" intended for the same uses, as long as it does not achieve its goal primarily through chemical action. (In that case, it would be a drug.) The statute defines a dietary supplement as "a product . . . intended to supplement the diet that bears or contains . . . a vitamin, a mineral, an herb or other botanical, an amino acid . . . or a concentrate, metabolite, constituent, extract, or combination of [the above]."

Drugs and most biologics are heavily regulated. They may not legally be sold or used in the United States until the FDA has been convinced, generally by controlled clinical trials, that they are safe and effective. Particularly novel or dangerous medical devices are subject to similar regulation; simpler or less novel devices undergo much more cursory review before marketing. Dietary supplements are subject to almost no regulation as long as they make claims only to affect "the structure or any function" of the body and do not claim to treat a disease or medical condition. (Thus, dietary supplements may, and often do, claim to "strengthen the cardiovascular system," but may not claim to "treat heart disease.")

The FDA already regulates human biological enhancements, but generally as treatments for diseases or other medical conditions. Their enhancing uses are so-called "off-label" uses, generally permissible under existing law. Thus, recombinant eryth-ropoietin, a drug of choice for athletes seeking more endurance through greater blood oxygen capacity, has been approved by the FDA for the treatment of various forms of anemia, but once it was approved for one purpose, doctors can ordinarily prescribe it for any other purpose. Very few products have actually been approved and sold as human biological enhancements even though such enhancements would meet the statutory definition by affecting "the structure or any function" of the body. Almost all are approved as treatments for disease. One of the only FDA-regulated products approved as an enhancement is the cosmetic contact lens, which is regulated, with other contact lenses, as a medical device.

The federal government is not the only regulator of drug, device, and supplement safety. State governments, and to some extent local governments, could regulate such products, typically by imposing more stringent restrictions on them than the federal government does. Thus, states sometimes act earlier or more strongly than the federal government in regulating certain drugs of abuse. State governments also can act to hold professionals, manufacturers, or distributors liable for problems with these products through the tort system. Professionals are typically liable only if they acted negligently, but manufacturers are often held to strict liability for any harm they cause. States may also take disciplinary action, including license suspension or revocation, against health professionals misusing such products.

The private sector also has a role. Notably, professional organizations or other non-governmental actors can prescribe guidelines for the uses of such products. These guidelines may serve to limit the misuse of the products directly. They may also serve, indirectly, to set the "standard of care" in lawsuits for professional negligence.

Extensions needed to regulate the safety of enhancements   The laws of negligence, product liability, and professional discipline exist and can be applied to enhancements just as easily as to treatments. Private organizations can continue their existing activities to extend voluntary guidelines and standards to the use of enhancements. And even FDA regulation already covers enhancements. If a firm were to seek approval to sell a new drug for enhancement purposes, no new safety regulation would be needed in the United States. The company would have to conduct serious clinical trials and to demonstrate to the satisfaction of the FDA that the drug was safe and effective for the intended use. But the FDA process, which probably provides the greatest assurance of safety, will not necessarily function well with regard to enhancements.

Of course, the existence of a rigorous regulatory regime can drive firms to look for alternative, and easier, ways to bring their product to market. For example, genetic tests would be regulated as medical devices in the United States if sold as "kits" to consumers, physicians, hospitals, or other health care organizations. If, however, they are provided as services by clinical laboratories, using their own "home brew" materials to do the tests, they are not regulated. Of the hundreds of genetic tests currently marketed in the United States, fewer than five have had FDA approval conferred – or even sought (Javitt, 2007). For human biological enhancements, the regulatory schemes would need to be tightened in at least two ways to provide for better assurances of safety: regulation of off-label use for enhancement purposes and increased regulation of dietary supplements.

The FDA's regulation of drugs and similar products has long been said *not* to include any power to regulate "the practice of medicine." This exception, beloved by the American Medical Association, is, of course, not all it seems. If a drug cannot be used without FDA approval, the FDA's failure to approve it surely regulates at least one aspect of the practice of medicine. But this phrase has been held to allow physicians to prescribe drugs that were approved by the FDA for one use – to treat sleep disorders, for example – for any other legal purpose –such as to help academics stay up late to finish writing projects. The FDA has not substantially regulated such off-label prescriptions (although it has tried to regulate company promotion of regulated products for off-label uses) and has stated that its legislation limits its power to do so. To what extent this off-label use exception is required by the statute has never been clear.

Many, and probably the vast majority, of human biological enhancements will be off-label uses of drugs or other products approved to treat disease. To a large extent, that will be the result of the likely financial rewards of selling drugs for disease, where the customer's need for the product is great and the purchase is usually paid for by some kind of health care coverage.

It is also the case that, for any given level of safety risks, the FDA is more likely to approve a drug for use against a disease than for use to "enhance" an otherwise healthy or normal individual. Safety will always be assessed relative to the risks of the underlying condition. Consider a hypothetical drug for metastatic pancreatic cancer, a disease with a truly dismal prognosis – over 95% of those diagnosed with the condition are dead within a year. If such a drug cured half of those with the disease instantly but killed the other half equally instantly, it would be a wonderfully safe and effective drug for metastatic pancreatic cancer. Its off-label use, however, to treat common teenage acne, or to improve a normal person's memory by 50%, would not be safe.

Drugs can be approved as safe and effective for one use against one disease, based on clinical trial evidence, but then prescribed off-label for uses in people without that disease, or perhaps any disease, without *any* proof that the drug is either safe or effective for the prescribed uses. Because the burden of proving safety is likely to be especially high in enhancement products, where the user does not suffer from a disease that is to be treated by the product, off-label use provides a major loophole for the sale and use of drugs that are unsafe as human biological enhancements.

If the FDA had to get new legislation from Congress to regulate off-label enhancing uses, the prospects for effective regulation would be dim. Drug makers, physician groups, and eager possible users would likely combine to block any effective reforms. This barrier might be breached, however, if there were public scandals involving injury or death from such off-label uses, creating powerful political sentiment for regulation.

But it is not clear that the FDA would need new legislation to increase its regulations of off-label enhancement uses of drugs – and not just because of the lack of certainty about the scope of the off-label use doctrine. Rather than seeking to restrict doctors' prescription practices, the FDA might focus on drug companies by requiring (or even strongly requesting) them to submit clinical trial data of enhancement uses of regulated products when those uses were, or were expected to become, common. That kind of expanded control might not need new legislation; new regulations, or even "guidances," might suffice.

Similar kinds of constraints could even come about as part of the back and forth of the normal regulatory process. For example, the FDA has negotiated certain limits on what kinds of physicians can prescribe Accutane, a powerfully effective anti-acne drug that is also a powerful cause of birth defects if taken by women in the early stages of pregnancy. These limits have not been "imposed" by the FDA as an agency incursion into the practice of medicine, but "voluntarily" by the manufacturer, in an effort to influence the FDA's assessment of the safety of the product (Krause, 1991–2; Noah, 2007).

Many enhancements are likely to take the form of dietary supplements, in part because the regulation of such supplements is minimal. The manufacturer does not have to prove to the FDA that the supplements are safe and effective in order to market them; the FDA has to prove to a court that a supplement is unsafe in order to have it removed from the market. Already, supplements offer to boost energy, strength, concentration, memory, and many other "enhancement" traits.

My favorite example is "Think Gum," a chewing gum that has been sold at my institution's student snack bar. According to its website (2009, http://thinkgum.com/about.html):

> Think Gum is a sugar-free candy-coated chewing gum carefully designed to enhance mental performance. It contains potent herbs and herbal extracts that are scientifically demonstrated to improve concentration, increase alertness, reduce careless errors and enhance information recall.

As required by the Dietary Supplement Health and Education Act (DSHEA), which defined the FDA's power to regulate dietary supplements, the Think Gum website and the packaging of the product both state that "Think Gum has not been evaluated by the FDA and is not intended to diagnose, treat, cure or prevent any disease."

It is harder to see any feasible ways to extend regulation of dietary supplements to improve the safety of human biological enhancements. DSHEA intentionally gives the FDA only very limited power over supplements. The Act, passed in 1994, was the backlash of an FDA attempt to tighten the regulation of supplements after use of the supplement L-tryptophan caused over 1,500 cases of permanent disability and at least 37 deaths. The supplement industry had massive popular support from scores of millions of committed supplement users, as well as powerful political help from, among others, members of Congress from states with high levels of supplement production, such as Utah. The result was a law that, intentionally, served more to limit the FDA's authority over supplements than to enhance it. This strong backing for supplements makes it unlikely that the supplements' loophole for human enhancement can be closed short of a major scandal – and as the L-tryptophan experience indicates, it would probably have to be a very large scandal indeed. It will prove very hard to adopt serious safety regulation of human biological enhancements that are capable of being sold as dietary supplements.

With the existing laws of negligence, product liability, and professional discipline, and with the adoption of some non-statutory changes to the FDA regime, some – admittedly imperfect – safety regulation of human biological enhancements seems plausible. Other, more novel, regulatory methods can also be imagined. One might choose not to limit the right to sell or use enhancements (at least for or by adults), but instead only require that the enhancements be tested for safety and the resulting information be made publicly available. Whatever its attractions, such a regulatory scheme would require new legislation, which makes it, barring scandals, highly unlikely at the federal level and difficult, though less implausible, at the state or local level.

Coercion

The situation is much different with respect to coercion. There are few situations where existing law would allow someone to be frankly coerced into using enhancement. But, importantly, there are equally few mechanisms that prohibit what would be, in effect, coercion in the use of enhancements. Adopting new limits on *de facto* coercion may not prove easy.

To the extent enhancements require some intrusion into an individual's body – by a drug, supplement, medical device, or otherwise – underlying U.S. law protects people from such unwanted touchings. Competent adults can only rarely be subjected to those kinds of intrusions without their consent. Examples include mandatory treatment for those with certain infectious diseases. Mandatory treatment also exists for some of the mentally ill but they are typically not viewed as competent. Members of the military may be subjected to mandatory intrusions, such as vaccinations. And minor children are often frankly coerced, usually by their parents but sometimes by other authorities. (One could consider mandatory education as a coercive enhancement, but, for the purposes of this chapter, it does not count as a human *biological* enhancement, even though it acts on the brain, a biological entity.)

The main problem with coercive enhancements is when the coercion is not so direct. The coercer does not insist on the enhancement but conditions something else on the enhancement. An employer might offer an employee a choice between accepting an enhancement and losing a promotion or even being fired. Or a government might require a citizen to accept an enhancement in order to get a benefit, such as a license to drive or to practice a profession.

U.S. law provides only limited checks on the powers of employers to make demands on employees. Practices that discriminate based on race, color, sex, national origin, religion, disability, and genetic information are banned by federal law. States sometimes ban other kinds of discrimination, such as discrimination based on marital status or sexual orientation. Particular practices may be banned – working too many hours, paying too low wages, and occupational health hazards, for example. But employment in the United States is predominately "employment at will," allowing the employer to hire or fire, promote or demote, for any reason or no reason at all – as long as it is not an expressly forbidden reason. If an employer were to say, "take this enhancement or you are fired," it is difficult to see what existing law that would violate (apart from a possible religious discrimination claim where the employee could show that using the enhancement somehow violated his or her religious beliefs).

Not all employees are quite so unprotected. Employees covered by union-negotiated collective bargaining agreements usually have broader contractual rights against the employer, but they make up fewer than 8% of the private work force in the United States. Government workers also have broader rights, in part because of union contracts (more than a third of government workers are unionized), but in part because of regulatory, statutory, and even constitutional protections. These workers might be able to argue that the forced enhancement violated the existing contract or legal regime, or, for union workers, might be able to force the negotiation of protective terms in the next contract.

Of course, employers coerce employees regularly in ways that might be seen as related to enhancements, such as forcing them to have or maintain licenses or to attend training courses. Some employers coerce actions even more closely related to enhancements. Health care workers in some contexts are required by their employers to get prophylactic vaccinations (medical interventions to enhance the immune system, not to treat disease) both to protect patients and to ensure a sufficient supply of health care workers to cope with an epidemic. One might argue from those precedents that employers should be allowed to require human biological enhancements. In many cases, though, these enhancements will be much more intrusive than training seminars or even vaccinations, which might be seen as a valid distinction.

The key point for our purposes is that if one thought that such coercion to enhance should not be allowed, new legislation, at either a state or federal level, would generally be required. Unionized employees would be a partial exception in that they might be able, if they chose, to avoid the coercion through collective bargaining, up to and including strikes. Apart from unions, however, no other private organizations seem likely to play a protective role, though it is conceivable that employer groups could draw up some voluntary guidelines that might be helpful.

New legislation is often difficult to pass, especially legislation limiting the powers of employers over employees (or, to put it another way, giving employees rights, and possible lawsuits, against employers). The Genetic Information Nondiscrimination Act was first introduced in the U.S. Congress in 1995. It had broad popular support as well as the (at least nominal) support of most members of Congress, as well as the support of the Clinton Administration and, eventually, the Bush Administration. It still did not become law for 13 years, largely as a result of the opposition of employer groups working through sympathetic committee chairs in Congress.

Legislation protecting employees from coercive enhancements is likely to have substantial popular support – far more Americans, and even American voters, are employees than are employers – but that support is unlikely to be intense, focused, or expert at influencing Congress. The opposition from employers would be all of those things. Without a scandal – some example of deeply offensive, risky, or harmful enhancements forced upon employees – new legislation will face difficult barriers. Those barriers, again, are likely to be higher in Congress than in state legislatures.

Apart from employers, three other examples of possible coercive enhancement deserve attention. Schools might require students to undergo enhancements. Schools already make requirements of students, from academic (no admission without various prerequisites) to mechanical (requiring calculators or computers) to physical (requiring proof of certain vaccinations). The compulsory governmental primary and secondary schools would perhaps be limited in what they could require, but, without new legislation, it is hard to see what would limit private elementary or secondary schools or private or public colleges or universities.

The military is a special case. The military and naval forces do not technically "employ" uniformed service personnel and their powers are extremely broad. For example, the U.S. forces in the Persian Gulf region after the first Gulf War were required to accept anthrax vaccinations, for fear of possible biological warfare by the Hussein government in Iraq. Military personnel who refused were subject to court-martial (Katz, 2001). It is perhaps not surprising that, in a context where a soldier can be ordered to make a suicidal attack or defense, his superiors have enormous power. It is interesting that the U.S. military uses enhancements, in the form of stimulant drugs, in some circumstances, particularly for pilots on long flights. It is also interesting that the Defense Department is thought to have funded substantial research on enhancements. If we conclude that service members should be protected from coercive enhancements, new legislation may well be required.

The final example is the most difficult. Children, particularly young children, are *always* coerced, typically by their parents. Even when a five year old does something happily, she is not making an informed, competent decision. Parents coerce their children into pre-school, into violin lessons, into language classes, and into sports, among other things. It is not just the parents' right, but, at some level, their duty to enhance their children from infancy to (at least) adolescence. The United States gives parents great latitude in deciding how to raise their children; some decisions of the U.S. Supreme Court find constitutional protection for such decisions (*Meyer v. Nebraska* 1923; *Pierce v. Society of Sisters* 1925; *Stanley v. Illinois* 1972; *Troxel v. Granville* 2000).

Yet one can easily imagine parents going too far in seeking to enhance their children, giving them unreasonably dangerous drugs or implants to improve their athletic or cognitive function. At the extreme, when parental decisions become the equivalent of abuse, U.S. law will step in. But should the use of enhancements by minor children, at the instance of or with the permission of their parents, be further regulated? Any such legal restriction of enhancements to adults would run afoul of the general spirit of parental discretion in childrearing. It would require new legislation and might face constitutional challenges. Barring a compelling scandal, the difficulties of regulating how parents provide their children with, or coerce their children into, such enhancements seem to make such legislation unlikely.

Fairness

The concern about fairness is primarily a concern about competition. It stems from a fear that enhancements would give one person, or group, an unfair advantage over another – in school, in the employment market, in sports, or elsewhere. This fairness concern can have a micro-focus, looking at two individuals in competition, but it also has macro implications. If enhancements are both powerful and expensive, one could justly worry that only the rich would be able to use them, further cementing their positional advantages.

Like coercion, "fairness" in the use of enhancements is scarcely subject to any current regulation. There is no general legal structure requiring fairness in human affairs, however that may be defined.[2]

Sports are the only area where enhancements are regulated for reasons that seem importantly to include fairness. This regulation is a combination of government-based prohibitions and private regulation through the Olympic Movement and other sports bodies, focused through the World Anti-Doping Agency (WADA). Of course, regulation of performance-enhancing drugs in sports is not solely about fairness, or it would seek to ensure only that competitors had equal enhancements or equal opportunities for enhancement. And WADA defines fairness quite narrowly, as no one using *any* performance-enhancing drug. As we will see, that is not the only plausible definition.

One might look at various employment-related laws as examples of fairness regulation. Bans of various kinds of discrimination in employment (and other contexts) are at least in part born of a concern with fairness. But that potential unfairness, that uneven metaphorical playing field, does not result from the actions of the employees but from the decisions of the employer. With enhancements, the unfairness would come from the differential use, or access to, an enhancement by some, but not all, of the "competitors."

It is also important to consider the many different ways one might intervene to avoid this unfairness. One might, with WADA, try to level the playing field by prohibiting all enhancements. One might, as with childhood education, level the playing field by *requiring* that everyone be enhanced. One might make the enhancement equally available to all without requiring anyone to use it. One might require disclosure by "competitors" of their use of enhancements and adjust their "score" as a result.

Except in sports, there are no structures for this kind of fairness regulation. They would have to be created and, if done by the government, that would require new legislation. Even apart from the difficulties of adopting legislation, there are other reasons to question the value of government solutions here.

Both the problems of unfairness and the best solutions for those problems may vary quite substantially. One school, dealing with the use of memory-enhancing pills by students, may reasonably come to a different decision than another school. A recreational basketball program for young women may reach a different decision than the National Basketball Association. One acting company might want to ban actors who had had cosmetic surgery, while another might seek them out. Fairness, at least at the micro-level, seems so nuanced and variable that local solutions should be encouraged.

And the policy tools already exist for local solutions through the decisional autonomy created by the absence of governmental mandates. And if different people have different views of fairness, they may be able to "vote with their feet," by moving from one school or job or sports league to another.

There is an exception to this "small is beautiful" response to fairness issues. If an enhancement has powerful general effects and if its availability is likely to be narrowly limited (most likely through high costs), the entire society may have an strong interest in ensuring fair access to, or perhaps use of, that enhancement across lines of income, class, or ethnicity. At this point, it is hard to conceive of a plausible enhancement technology that meets those criteria – perhaps if gene therapy for, say, intelligence were both possible and expensive it might qualify. But there is a possibly useful example from an older and enormously powerful "non-biological" enhancement technology – education.

It is hard to imagine any human biological enhancement changing the cognitive powers of a normal individual as much as education can. The differences in potential between the literate and the illiterate in modern societies are vast. Five hundred years ago, only the wealthy (or the very lucky) were literate. But today that enhancing skill is so important that we have responded, not by making literacy available to everyone, but by making it mandatory for every child who has the ability to learn. And, as higher education has become increasingly important, most rich societies have, one way or another, made it available to everyone who can master it, though not (yet) mandatory. Similarly, many countries have encouraged the widespread availability of internet access to their citizens.

Should a broadly powerful but expensive enhancing technology appear, overall governmental action may be required, but that action may be more likely to lead to social fairness by an expansion of the enhancement as to social fairness by an effort (most likely futile) to ban it.

Enforcement

Adopting policies with regard to human biological enhancement is not the same as enforcing them. Of course, for some purposes, enforcement may be unnecessary. In some cases the proponents of regulation may seek only a symbolic rejection of enhancements, without concern about their actual use. In others, it may be thought that the mere statement of regulation will be self-enforcing. Still, for the most part, if we want to regulate enhancements, we presumably will want that regulation to be at least somewhat effective. The likely effectiveness of enhancement regulation is likely to vary, based in part on the goal of the regulation.

Safety

Note first that safety regulation would presumably involve a user willing to take the safety risks. Otherwise, an informational campaign about those risks should be sufficient. If the user is willing to take the risks, the situation appears to be a classic "victimless crime." Neither the provider of the enhancement nor its user is unhappy about the transaction. No witness has an incentive to report the transaction. So technical methods of detection will be needed, like drug tests.

These are cumbersome, expensive, and invade the privacy of both enhancement users and non-users. We also know, from experience with regulation of performance-enhancing drugs in sports, that they are not perfect. They can lead to a dance where, for example, as soon as the testers start looking for a compound, the producers subtly change the compound in ways that continue to produce the desired effect but without being detectable by the existing test. From prostitution to prohibition of alcohol to contemporary efforts to control drugs of abuse, the record of enforcing victimless crimes, though not completely futile, is not encouraging.

On the other hand, some kinds of regulation might be very effective, at least in some cases. If FDA-type safety regulation prevented any production of an enhancing substance or device, anyone seeking to use it illicitly, in spite of the safety risks, would need to create it.

For some types of enhancement, that might be fairly simple. For example, an athlete can enhance the oxygen-carrying capacity of her blood not just with erythropoietin but also by sleeping under a tent that keeps the percentage of oxygen in the breathed air below normal levels. These tents are available for purchase, but even if entirely banned, would not be hard for someone to manufacture, either for her own use or for resale.

Other kinds of enhancers would be more difficult to manufacture illicitly. Small molecule drugs, like Adderall or Ritalin, might require complex chemical labs. These might be available to criminal organizations, like those that make methamphetamine, or gifted quasi-amateurs, who apparently provided much of the supply of LSD in recent decades, but the complexity of the work would restrict the supply and make detection somewhat easier. Still other kinds of drugs, such as recombinant proteins like erythropoietin, seem likely to remain basically impossible for anyone except a skilled biotechnology company to create.

The harder problem for safety regulation will be dual-use products, those that have a legitimate, non-enhancing use and a prohibited, or heavily regulated, enhancing use. Keeping track of the uses to which such products are put will be very difficult. It is here that the all the problems of victimless crimes re-emerge. Neither the physician prescribing the drug, the pharmacist dispensing it, nor the consumer is necessarily unhappy with the transaction. Probably the best method of control is through professionals controlling the supply of the product, such as physicians who control access to prescription drugs and devices. A combination of their sense of professionalism and their fear of disciplinary sanctions might serve to limit the leakage of products into prohibited enhancement uses.

On the other hand, we know from the experience of "pill mills" where doctors over-prescribe stimulants or painkillers that these incentives are not perfectly effective. It is worth noting, though, that the degree of effectiveness may vary with the breadth of legitimate use. Opiates for pain relief, amphetamines, and cocaine all have legitimate medical uses. Opiates have very broad legitimate medical uses and amphetamines have substantial medical uses, but the legitimate medical uses of cocaine are very narrow, primarily as a local anesthetic in some nasal procedures. Diversion from medical use has been a major source of supply for the first two drug types, but not for cocaine.

Similarly, the degree of medical intervention needed will affect how easy it is to prevent unauthorized leakage. Deep brain stimulation, for example, might well become a method of cognitive enhancement, but it requires delicate neurosurgery and substantial "tuning" and care after placement. It is much less likely that such a procedure, involving many skilled health care personnel over a long period of time, would generate a large illicit market.

Coercion

Rules against coercion should, in general, be the easiest to enforce. These do not involve a willing user and hence a "victimless crime." Like those protected by employment rules against racial discrimination or from bad working conditions, those who feel victimized by the violation have strong incentives to report it (particularly if they could receive damages or other compensation for the coercive action).

The aggrieved workers would, of course, need to feel confident that they would be protected against retaliation from the employer. Although such protection can never be guaranteed, U.S. law has substantial experience with anti-retaliation provisions, as well as "whistleblower" provisions to protect and reward informants. Coercion in employment or secondary or higher education should be relatively easy to detect and prevent, though never, of course, to eliminate completely.

Parental coercion is the great exception here. With parental coercion of minor children, we return to the situation of a victimless crime. Even if the child is actually a victim, she does not realize it or have much ability to act on it. This could also be true of coercion in primary education, although in that case the child's parents may be an effective proxy for enforcement purposes.

Fairness

Regulation based on fairness seems much like regulation based on safety. Again, the supplier and the user will be happy with the transactions. Without either physical control or control through the gatekeeper of a trusted professional (and one with too much at stake to risk sanctions lightly), enforcement seems difficult. It should be even more difficult to keep these kinds of enhancements under control because they will be more attractive to users, who do not necessarily have any good reason to fear that the enhancement may injure them.

The very intrusive, but imperfectly effective, schemes for regulating performance-enhancing drugs in sports may be a preview of a broad scheme for regulating enhancements based on fairness. Sports regulation, though, seeks to control a relatively narrow part of the population, and, at its most intensive levels, elite athletes who are easy to identify and track. Extending that kind of regulation to any sizable part of the population seems fraught with difficulties.

Conclusion

Not all tools are hammers, not all subjects of tools are nails. When considering the real-world regulation of human biological enhancements, it is crucial to consider what policy tools are available and just *how* available they, in fact, are. It is also vital to assess how well the policies can be enforced. Good policies that cannot be adopted have little value; good policies that are adopted but cannot be enforced may bring substantial harms. As our societies' contacts with human biological enhancements move increasingly from the hypothetical and academic to the real and practical, we will have to face these possibly less intellectually engaging, but ultimately essential, questions.

Acknowledgments

The author would like to thank his indomitable research assistant, Mark Hernandez.

Notes

1. The discussion of policy options is, I fear, very amateur political science. It derives largely from my own observations and not substantially from my now long-distant undergraduate

degree in political science or from more recent reading of scholarly sources. I do want to acknowledge the strong influence of David Mayhew's (2004) work on my views about Congress.

2. The Fifth and Fourteenth Amendments to the U.S. Constitution state that neither the states nor the federal government may deprive a person of "life, liberty, or property" without "due process of law." These due process clauses have been held to require some kinds of fair procedures, in some circumstances – but only with respect to government actions.

References

Greely, H.T. (2004a). Disabilities, enhancements, and the meanings of sport. *Stanford Law and Policy Review*, **15**, 99–132.

Greely, H.T. (2004b). Seeking more goodly creatures. *Cerebrum*, **6**(4), 49–58.

Greely, H.T. (2005/2006). Regulating Human biological enhancements: Questionable justifications and international complications, the mind, the body, and the law. *University of Technology, Sydney, Law Review*, 7, 87–110 and *Santa Clara Journal of International Law*, **4**, 87–110 (joint issue).

Greely, H.T. (2008a). Remarks on human biological enhancement. *University of Kansas Law Review*, **56**, 1139–57.

Greely, H.T. *et al.* (2008b). Towards responsible use of cognitive-enhancing drugs by the healthy. *Nature*, **456**, 702–5.

Javitt, G. (2007). In search of a coherent framework: Options for FDA oversight of genetic tests. *Food and Drug Law Journal*, **62**, 617–52.

Katz, R.D. (2001). Friendly fire: The mandatory military anthrax vaccination program. *Duke Law Journal*, **50**, 1835–65.

Krause, J.H. (1991–2). Accutane: Has drug regulation in the United States reached its limits? *Journal of Law and Health*, **6**, 1–29.

Maslow, A. (1966). *The Psychology of Science: A Reconnaissance*. New York: Harper & Row.

Mayhew, D. (2004). *Congress: The Electoral Connection*. New Haven: Yale University Press.

Meyer v. Nebraska, 262 U.S. 390 (1923) (invalidating a state law banning the education of children in private or public schools, before the eighth grade, in modern foreign languages).

New State Ice Co. v. Liebmann, 285 U.S. 262, 311 (1932) (Brandeis, J., dissenting). Interestingly, this opinion, the always-cited source of the Brandeis view, never uses the term "laboratories of democracy."

Noah, L. (1997). The FDA's new policy on guidelines: Having your cake and eating it too. *Catholic Law Review*, **47**, 113–42.

Noah, L., (2007). Too high a price for some drugs? The FDA burdens reproductive choice. *San Diego Law Review*, **44**, 231–58.

Pierce v. Society of Sisters, 268 U.S. 510 (1925) (invalidating a state law requiring all children between the ages of 8 and 16 to attend public schools).

Stanley v. Illinois, 405 U.S. 645 (1972) (invalidating a state law that automatically made the children of single women wards of the state upon the mother's death without regard to the claims of the biological father).

Troxel v. Granville, 530 U.S. 57 (2000) (invalidating an order that gave visitation rights to grandparents over the mother's objection).

37

The Politics of Human Enhancement and the European Union

Christopher Coenen, Mirjam Schuijff, and Martijntje Smits[1]

Though still rarely discussed outside expert circles, human enhancement issues are not merely academic: the technologies and trends involved give rise to new needs and social demands, provide opportunities for individuals and society, and present new risks. They also challenge crucial cultural notions, social concepts and views of the human condition, and may cause new forms of social pressure and social exclusion. These developments not only require public debate and the articulation of normative positions, but also some action by policy-makers. As tensions are likely to be caused in the future as a result of member states of the European Union adopting different stances on these issues, a European approach to the issue of human enhancement is needed.

This chapter reports on a systematic attempt by the European Technology Assessment Group, conducted on behalf of the Science and Technology Options Assessment panel of the European Parliament, to suggest policy options on this issue. The authors argue for a notion of enhancement which includes "therapeutic enhancements" and excludes traditional means of improving performance such as physical exercise and education. They sketch the current politics of human enhancement by discussing various tendencies which appear to be veering towards an "enhancement society." The chapter then outlines and discusses a number of strategies for dealing with the issue in a European policy context, identifying a reasoned pro-enhancement approach, a reasoned restrictive approach, and a systematic case-by-case approach as viable options. It is argued that a temporary European body should be established by EU policy-makers. This body should be charged with developing a normative framework to guide EU policies in this area. Moreover, it could initiate and promote broad public deliberation on human enhancement issues.

Enhancing Human Capacities, edited by Julian Savulescu, Ruud ter Meulen and Guy Kahane.
© 2011 Blackwell Publishing Ltd

Introduction

How should European policy-makers respond to the political challenges raised by the phenomenon of human enhancement? New human enhancement technologies (HET) promising to improve bodily functions have unleashed vehement and polarized reactions among international experts and, to a lesser extent, among a broader public, in Europe and elsewhere. Obviously, human enhancement and its supposed effects on individuals and society are highly normative subjects, involving a broad range of social and ethical issues.

These technologies signal the blurring of boundaries between restorative therapy and improvements extending beyond such therapy. As most of them stem from the medical realm, they can boost societal tendencies of medicalization when increasingly used to treat non-pathological conditions. They will affect various policy fields and raise challenges to normative concepts such as "health," "normalcy," or "(dis)ability." At the same time, the discourse on HET touches on several contested issues in European history and culture.

For the purposes of a project of the Science and Technology Options Assessment (STOA) panel of the European Parliament and conducted by the European Technology Assessment Group (ETAG), we analyzed several trends which can be regarded as tendencies towards an "enhancement society," and examined their political consequences. The main goal of the project was to make a policy proposal specifically for the European Union (EU) level. We developed our proposal after consulting experts in the field, and subsequently deliberated it in a workshop with members of parliament.

In order to develop sound policy recommendations, we had to tackle three major challenges: First, we needed to find or develop a concept of human enhancement that would be suitable for a policy context, against the backdrop of an ideologically heated debate characterized by considerable conceptual unclearness. Second, we were confronted with a complex "politics of human enhancement" in which several interrelated tendencies currently appear to be converging towards an enhancement society, embraced by some and fiercely rejected by others. To establish a sound basis for the development of policy proposals, we therefore needed to obtain as encompassing and differentiated a picture of the issue of human enhancement as possible. This needed to include the state of the art in selected HET and a rather wide range of social, ethical, political, and cultural aspects which have an impact on the development and public acceptance of these technologies. Finally, our task was to draft a policy proposal, specifically suited to the EU and reflecting the complexity of the issue. For this purpose, an approach was needed that would take into account the diverse normative aspects of the issue of enhancement, while being sufficiently concrete to allow for at least some form of political action.

In this chapter we will present and discuss the main findings of our study (Coenen *et al.*, 2009). First, we argue for a definition of enhancement which includes "therapeutic enhancements" and excludes such traditional means of improving performance as physical exercise and education. Next, we sketch the politics of human enhancement, pointing out that several societal tendencies are veering towards an enhancement society. Finally, we outline strategic options for a policy on human enhancement in Europe, and explain and discuss our specific policy proposal concerning the EU level.

A Policy Oriented Concept of Human Enhancement

Human enhancement debates were still in their early stages when it was argued that conceptual clarity and knowledge about the various uses of the term "enhancement" are needed in a policy-making context (Parens, 1998). The older discourse on enhancement had revolved mainly around doping, the off-label use of drugs, and certain biomedical technologies, and had its antecedents in the decades-old debates on genetic engineering and eugenics. The new discourse on enhancement also encompasses emerging "second-stage" enhancement technologies (Khushf, 2005), such as new brain–machine interfaces, and has been propelled forward by the often highly speculative debates on nanotechnology (Coenen, 2009; Nordmann, 2007). However, the core conceptual challenge, at least as regards policy issues, remains the same, namely to clarify how the notion of enhancement relates to the notion of therapy.

Two widely used approaches find radical solutions to this challenge (for an overview, see for example Lin & Allhoff, 2008). The first approach, often taken by promoters of HET, regards therapy as a special case of enhancement. Any intervention to improve the body is regarded as enhancement. Its exponents see new HET as the logical successor to physical exercise, the consumption of coffee etc. They present HET as the expression of an innate human striving for self-improvement and as being related to fundamental tenets of civilization, such as religion, education, medicine, and the creation of tools. While usually conceding that differentiation is sometimes difficult, the exponents of the second approach oppose enhancement to therapy and define the former *ex negativo* as any improvement-oriented intervention not aimed at healing or sustaining good health. From this viewpoint, enhancement is outside the medical realm, and tendencies such as the rise of "cosmetic" plastic surgery are considered aberrations. Some exponents of this approach use strong normative assumptions or give historical reasons (such as eugenicist crimes) to denounce enhancement. Others argue that we should adhere to a rather strict therapy–enhancement distinction for pragmatic reasons.

In the first approach, qualitative differences are ignored and the term "enhancement" becomes useless, because it is taken as a synonym for "progress" or similar terms. In the second approach, the dichotomy of therapy and enhancement is often based on questionable notions of health, disability, or normalcy – without enabling us to make clear distinctions either. Proponents of such viewpoints often simply ignore the blurring of boundaries between therapeutic and other improvement-oriented interventions which takes place under the influence of new HET. The distinction between therapeutic and non-therapeutic interventions, however, should not be abandoned – if only for the pragmatic reason that one needs to decide which interventions should be paid for by health insurance companies and which should not.

We therefore chose a third approach: it acknowledges that notions of "health," "normalcy," and "disability" are highly normative notions and change their meaning over time. Moreover, it does not define away the qualitative difference between science-based interventions into the human body and such activities as physical exercise. Our approach also distinguishes between therapeutic and non-therapeutic enhancements without regarding therapy as a special case of enhancement and without classifying all enhancements as non-medical. This approach agrees that "restoring a previous condition after disease or injury" (*restitutio ad integrum*) can serve as a concise definition of a therapy which is clearly not an enhancement (Wiesing, 2008). Moreover, we took into account that some therapies can have effects that go beyond merely restoring good health and may enable better-than-average and even species-untypical functioning (e.g. in the case of emerging prosthetic technologies).

In our definition, the term "human enhancement" refers to any modification aimed at improving individual human performance and brought about by science-based or technology-based interventions in the human body. This definition includes "strong," second-stage forms of human enhancement with long-term, permanent or not easily reversible results (e.g. genetic modifications and any enhancement requiring major surgery) as well as "temporary" science-based enhancements (e.g. the use of new drugs). We distinguish between three categories of intervention in the human body:

- restorative or preventive, non-enhancing interventions;
- therapeutic enhancements;
- non-therapeutic enhancements.

The first type aims at *restitutio ad integrum* or the prevention of diseases. Since there is no intended or accidental enhancement effect, we will not discuss this category in the present chapter. Therapeutic enhancements are interventions whose effects, intentionally or not, allow the patient to perform better than before his disease or accident, or provide the patient with entirely new abilities. If for example progress in the field of artificial limbs continues, people who have lost a natural limb in an accident may experience therapeutic enhancements of this kind. The aim of non-therapeutic enhancements may be to improve natural human abilities (even to a degree not previously seen in any human being, like the ability to run faster than a cheetah), or to create characteristics or abilities that no human has ever possessed before (e.g. extra senses).

HET include a wide range of existing, emerging and envisioned technologies or pharmaceutical products, such as neuroimplants that provide artificial senses, drugs for "brain doping," human germline engineering, existing reproductive technologies, nutritional supplements, new brain stimulation technologies, gene doping in sports, cosmetic surgery, growth hormones for children of short stature, anti-aging medication, and highly sophisticated limb prostheses.

The Politics of Human Enhancement

The politics of human enhancement shape the way the technologies in question are envisioned, developed, marketed, used, and governed. Due to the manifold nature of HET and the significant differences between them, common features of these technologies are hard to identify. Moreover, the politics of enhancement encompass a wide variety of individual decisions and lifestyle choices. These in turn have to be seen against the background of socioeconomic, cultural, ethical, and other frameworks within which individual decisions are taken. These frameworks constantly change over time, a process which is often driven by broader societal tendencies. Longstanding cultural and ideological traditions permeate these ever-changing frameworks, and are themselves continuously transformed. In new governance structures, policy action is influenced by increasingly complex interaction between institutions and diverse networks. Popular culture (e.g. science fiction) and the public communication of science by research policy actors and journalists influence the public's image of HET and its views on their future prospects. All of these factors interact and together determine which and how technologies are imagined, developed, and publicly accepted.

Accordingly, our goal was to obtain as encompassing and differentiated a picture of the issue of human enhancement as possible, as a basis for a sound policy proposal. In order to reach this goal, we distinguished between three main groups of tendencies shaping the current politics of human enhancement:

- new demands, desires, and lifestyle choices of individuals ("bottom-up tendencies");
- changes to socioeconomic, ethical, and other frameworks ("broader societal tendencies");
- the promotion of HET and human enhancement as a public issue ("top-down tendencies").

All these tendencies have to be seen against an internally diverse, and in some respects even incoherent European value system. It is in turn based on longstanding traditions, including the forerunners of those ideologies and sociocultural practices that characterize the current discourse on human enhancement.

Non-therapeutic enhancements: from visions to applications?

A basic requirement for an analysis of the factors shaping the politics of enhancement is to identify the state of the art in the relevant fields of research, development, and technology application. So what actual evidence is there that effective and, in particular, non-therapeutic HET exist?

One can distinguish here between direct and indirect means of enhancing an individual's performance. The latter encompass, for example, cosmetic surgery and the use of drugs to enhance mood, both of which are well-established practices. They may indirectly help to improve cognitive or physical performance by changing the mood of the treated persons. However, evidence of performance enhancement in healthy, non-depressive people is still scarce.

As regards the direct enhancement of cognition, perception, motor skills and strength, the majority of HET are still therapeutic and do not offer their users significant advantages over "non-enhanced" humans; indeed, the level of improvement often remains well below the level of normal function. However, there are some cases of highly remarkable progress in therapeutic and in particular prosthetic technologies. Moreover, there are several instances of moderate success of non-therapeutic enhancements. Drugs that are used to treat sleep deprivation, stress or extreme nervousness, for example, can evidently enhance performance in some healthy individuals to a modest

526   *Christopher Coenen, Mirjam Schuijff, and Martijntje Smits*

extent. However, these decreased conditions are more similar to a disease than to a state of well-being.

On the other hand, there are also strong indications that more and more effective means of non-therapeutic enhancement will be developed in the near future, and that some existing lines of research and development already have the potential to significantly alter human corporeality and cognition. If, for example, the development of medication to improve performance in healthy people were allowed, more targeted research may lead to effective and safe drugs with significant market potentials. Many experts also agree that man–machine interrelations may be fundamentally changed in the foreseeable future, leading also to prosthetic applications that will provide specialized sensory input or mechanical output. They might thus begin to put competitive pressure on traditional human corporeality, at least in a military context.

While we often still have to deal with mere potentialities in the discussions about non-therapeutic enhancements, there are realistic prospects of near-term progress in several fields of research and application. These developments may be significantly accelerated by regulatory and funding measures and may turn out to be economically attractive, for example in the field of cognitive enhancement. Nevertheless, the efficacy of HET still often pales in comparison with the efficacy of technologies that do not modify the human body and even of traditional means of enhancing performance, such as the consumption of tea or coffee.

The promotion of human enhancement

While non-therapeutic HET are still rare and their effects moderate, visions of significant improvements of human performance are already shaping the politics of enhancement. By staging debates on far-reaching visions – which relate to the very distant future of (post)humanity and even extend to eschatological questions such as those concerning immortality and the end of the universe (e.g., Kurzweil, 2005) – promoters and some critics of human enhancement have managed to raise attention for their goals and their ideologies at large.

This is true, for example, of the debate on "converging technologies" which focuses on HET on the basis of nanotechnology, brain–machine interfaces, artificial intelligence, and other cutting-edge research fields. This debate and similar discussions in recent years have been driven forward by a number of influential networks in research policy and society. They include, for example, important representatives of the IT industry, the organizations of the transhumanists – a technofuturist movement which has lately risen to some prominence – and a political initiative on "converging technologies" in the United States (Roco & Bainbridge, 2002). Moreover, ethicists, high-level policy advisors and leaders of Western Christianity animatedly discuss the topic of enhancement, often in a way that can be deemed purely "speculative ethics" (Nordmann, 2007) and even including its most visionary aspects, such as the hope of overcoming death. These discussions on enhancement are at the heart of a broader controversial discourse on an "ideology of extreme progress," on eugenics and on dystopias of the *Brave New World* kind. This discourse is rooted in the early twentieth-century European, and in particular British, history of ideas (cf. for example Coenen, 2009; Hughes, 2008).

The far-reaching visions are combined with short-term-oriented promotion of specific HET. Calls to legalize the non-therapeutic use of certain drugs (Greely *et al.*, 2008), for example, radicalize older pro-enhancement positions by initiating a discussion on "mandatory" enhancements. The U.S. initiative on "converging technologies," albeit highly visionary, also placed emphasis on short-term applications, for example in the field of military applications.

The (often deliberate) mixing of facts and visions, of realistic projections and ideological fantasies constitutes a specific challenge for political decision making – in research policy in particular, and for the public discourse on science and technology as a whole. The handling of visions is not a merely academic, literary or marketing-related activity, but has political relevance. There is, for example, the danger of a vicious circle in research policy in which all the players involved compete to promote the most spectacular visions of the future. A better understanding of the ideological background and driving forces behind such highly visionary and irrational modes of communicating and marketing science and technology is needed – also in EU-funded accompanying research on emerging technologies. Moreover, the ideology of extreme progress presents itself, and is seen by some of its critics, such as the Vatican, as the culmination of the strivings of Enlightenment thinkers and the progressives of modernity. If such an understanding of European history were to gain further ground, Europe would run the risk of experiencing conflicts about HET that may even result in a culture conflict similar to those in the United States on Darwinism and certain reproductive technologies.

Bottom-up tendencies in the politics of enhancement

On the demand side we see a widespread public willingness to adopt or at least consider interventions that may enhance performance and (often irreversibly) change the body (Van Est *et al.*, 2008). Examples are the rise of cosmetic surgery, the growing demand for pre-implantation genetic diagnosis (PGD), and the use of drugs such as Ritalin and Prozac. This trend further blurs the distinctions between therapeutic and non-therapeutic enhancements. Moreover, certain areas of application, such as military research, prosthetics or doping in sports, obviously serve as testbeds for emerging HET.

Certain HET, as well as technologies which may pave the way for more effective HET, appear to be growing increasingly attractive within the population – and some have significant market potential. If these bottom-up tendencies in the politics of human enhancement continue, there will also be a host of policy implications and challenges.

Medical tourism, for example, which already exists (e.g. in the case of PGD) between EU Member States and elsewhere, will increasingly encompass "enhancement tourism." This could aggravate problems of distributive justice in and between health systems. It could also lead to medical risks for patients, since the medical expertise to provide follow-up treatment in the home country might be insufficient.

In research, technology, health and education policies, controversies may arise on whether invasive means of enhancing individual performance should be prioritized over infrastructural improvements in the broadest sense. In such controversies, undesired consequences of new HET, such as the physical or psychological side effects of (long-term) use or negative impacts on social cohesion would probably play an important role.

A spread of effective HET could even influence the competitiveness of European economies: directly by creating relevant international markets for such technologies and indirectly by affecting the productivity of employees.

The bottom-up tendencies in the politics of enhancement constitute challenges to existing regulations (e.g. in the case of doping in sports, drug use, and certain reproductive technologies) and may create new regulatory wastelands. Moreover, they raise questions concerning broader normative frameworks. This relates, for example, to such concepts as "health," "normalcy," and "(dis)ability" as well as to questions of distributive justice. A rise in effective HET could affect the degree and quality of solidarity with the weak and poor who cannot gain access to these HET, and with the conscientious objectors who simply choose not to use it.

Broader societal tendencies

The bottom-up tendencies in the politics of enhancement are shaped by individual "consumers" rather than by state intervention. They contribute to a new kind of "biopolitics." New in this context is also the focus on improving the individual body by technological interventions, as opposed to traditional biopolitical interventions that enhance the external conditions of the body of a population, for example hygiene policy or education and training (Van Est *et al.*, 2008). However, the bottom-up tendencies are in turn fostered by wider socioeconomic and cultural trends, and individual decisions are taken in light of social and economic pressures. This relates, for example, to the medicalization of society, to the commercialization of medicine, to new ways of seeing one's body and abilities, and to new working life challenges in a globalised economy.

Medicalization occurs when previously nonmedical social problems are treated as medical problems. In the domain of HET, too, what was formerly regarded as being "unfavorable," a "weakness," or a "bad habit" is increasingly being redefined as a disease or disability when an effective (or allegedly effective) treatment is at hand (Conrad, 2007). Disabled people are often highlighted as potential beneficiaries of advanced HET. However, within a "transhumanized model of health" (Wolbring, 2008), all human bodies are seen as limited, defective, and as being in need of constant improvements by technoscientific means. In any case, the rise of HET and the promotion of human enhancement threaten to marginalize those concepts of disability that focus on the social and normative aspects of disability rather than on medical categories or technological fixes.

In a policy context, these tendencies raise the general question of whether invasive HET or an infrastructure supported by high technology should be prioritized. In the case of "disabilities," one can either invest more heavily in an intelligent, barrier-free public infrastructure and new assistive technologies, for example, or focus on how to change the bodies of disabled persons. There is also a need to critically reflect on the roles of the targets or "poster boys" often assigned to disabled people in the science system and in technology policy, and to ascertain their demands and wishes by empirical means.

In light of these tendencies, the promotion of human enhancement by influential networks in research and technology policy appears to indicate that the new biopolitics also integrate significant top-down components. The far-reaching visions of a future society based on new forms of brain–computer interaction, for example, build on problematic elements of the existing normative framework, such as the ideology of ableism (Wolbring, 2008). By emphasizing and sharpening these elements, individual options are further reduced, at least for some social groups.

In the politics of human enhancement, bottom-up, top-down, and broader societal tendencies interact in a way that can be said to amount to a trend towards a new kind of society: There is growing evidence of a transition from a performance-oriented society, in which the fulfillment of predefined tasks is rewarded, to an *enhancement society*. In such a society, individuals would feel under strong pressure to constantly improve their bodily preconditions for successful performance by all means. Recently it has been argued that the tendencies towards an enhancement society necessitate a reframing of the debate on enhancement (Grunwald, 2008): The focus should shift from rather conventional short- or mid-term ethical questions to a more comprehensive discussion of our social systems and the implications of HET for human corporeality. This would also raise questions regarding guiding visions in research and other policies.

Towards a European Policy on Human Enhancement

Tendencies towards an enhancement society increasingly have an impact on a number of policy fields and European normative frameworks. Until now, however, virtually no hard governance measures or other actions on the part of key political institutions have explicitly targeted the topic of "human enhancement." Moreover, the pertinent activities at EU level are only loosely interconnected. The discussions and activities display a remarkable degree of diversity as regards topics and normative stances, as will be briefly shown in the following.

In 2003, the EU reacted to the new debate on enhancement in the context of activities on nanotechnology and "converging technologies" (Coenen, 2009). In its final report (EU HLEG FNTW 2004), an EU High-Level Expert Group on "converging technologies" openly criticized visions of nanoconvergence which center on HET. According to the expert group, these visions advocate an "engineering of the mind" and "of the body." The group also warned against misallocating public funds. Its work ushered in a whole series of EU-funded research activities and discussions on the topic of enhancement. The topic of enhancement has also attracted considerable attention from the staff of the Directorate-General for Research of the European Commission.

The European Group on Ethics in Science and New Technologies (EGE) has tackled the issue of enhancement in its Opinion No. 20 on information and communication technology (ICT) implants and in its Opinion No. 21 on nanomedicine. The EGE argued that maintaining the distinction between medical and nonmedical uses is important with respect to European research funding policies. The group proposed that therapeutic applications should be given priority. In its Opinion on ICT implants (EGE, 2005) the group identified a number of ICT implants for which special caution and regulation would be necessary, such as implants that change psychic functions, or implants that could be misused for social surveillance and manipulation. Certain uses of ICT implants should be banned (e.g. implants used to change identity, memory, self-perception, and perception of others). Moreover, the EGE made the general point that nonmedical applications of ICT implants pose a potential threat to human dignity and democratic society. At the same time, the EGE argued that access to HET should be allowed in certain cases (always on the basis of a precautionary approach), for example to bring children or adults into the "normal" range for the population. In its view, broad public debate is needed on what kind of applications for ICT implants should be legally approved, particularly concerning surveillance and enhancement.

Given the rather numerous policy-related advisory and research activities, how does "human enhancement" figure at the highest level of EU policy? Official political statements on the topic are still rare: the subject has only been explicitly raised within the discourse on nanotechnology. Documents that mention the term "enhancement" do not contrast it with "therapy," but speak of "non-therapeutic enhancement" if they wish to draw attention to ethical concerns. In 2008, for example, following a public consultation which even included a proposal to ban a wide range of HET, the European Commission proposed a "code of conduct" for responsible nanosciences and nano-technologies research. Under the heading "Prohibition, restrictions or limitations," it states that "nanosciences and nanotechnologies research organisations should not undertake research aiming for non-therapeutic enhancement of human beings leading to addiction or solely for the illicit enhancement of the performance of the human body" (European Commission, 2008, p.9).

Challenges and strategic options for a European policy on human enhancement

The brief overview above shows that discussions and activities at the EU level are diverse and have been loosely interconnected until now. It indicates a lack of any coherent and comprehensive approach to the issues of human enhancement in Europe. Against this background we developed a proposal concerning the governance of human enhance-ment at EU level, building on inputs from two expert meetings in 2008 and a workshop in the European Parliament in February 2009. During the meetings, several elements for such a proposal were assembled.

A number of specific issues for regulation were identified, such as practical require-ments when it comes to the professional self-regulation of new HET and the regis-tration of certain interventions, access to orphan technologies, and the use of HET in military and nonmedical domains. Moreover, a number of overarching challenges for regulation were identified, such as the cultural and institutional diversity of the EU Member States, and the fact that new HET may potentially be stumbled upon in the course of standard therapeutic treatments. There was broad consensus among the experts that an attempt should be made for the sake of consumer protection to regulate all practitioners, including those outside the public medical system. Furthermore, it became obvious that a first step towards possible governance of human enhancement is to make proposals for initiating and politically organizing deliberation on the issue. The participants agreed that the European Parliament should play an important role as the interface between policy-makers and the public.

As regards legal and regulatory aspects of human enhancement, only a small number of possible starting points exist as yet: Legal stipulations which already exist in the medical sector do not cover central problems connected with HET, such as the distinction between therapeutic and non-therapeutic applications. What is more, the case of sports doping, where this distinction is already relevant in a regulatory context, reveals the existence of practical problems (such as the difficulty to keep pace with technological advances) and of doubts concerning the logic of the existing legal framework. As regards the possible interference of HET with human rights and human dignity, the notions of personal autonomy and human freedom are crucial. Although regulatory restrictions of the freedom of individual choice could be legitimized if the use of HET conflicted with the principle of fairness of competition and the equal distribution of chances, autonomy and fairness can be regarded as providing guiding principles for regulatory intervention.

In principle, five approaches to a European policy of human enhancement are conceivable (for a similar analysis, see: CSPO, ACG, 2006):

- a total ban on any technology that alters "human nature";
- a laissez-faire approach;
- a reasoned pro-enhancement approach;
- a reasoned restrictive approach; and
- a systematic case-by-case approach.

However, we deem the first two approaches to be neither desirable nor realistic in the European context (cf. Coenen *et al.*, 2009, section 4.2) which leaves us with three viable options.

In a *reasoned pro-enhancement approach*, the creation of a competitive, dynamic European knowledge society would form a starting point for discussion. EU policy would explicitly fund the development of non-therapeutic HET, while preserving all applicable elements of existing ethical frameworks and, as a matter of course, respecting fundamental European values. In such a strategy the EU would stimulate a societal dialogue about innovations which might run counter to traditional value systems. This strategy could include initiatives to discuss deregulation in areas as drug and doping policies or reproductive technologies.

However, it is far from clear, ethical concerns aside, whether non-therapeutic HET really would facilitate the achievement of competitive goals. Accordingly, a *reasoned restrictive approach* would always have to consider whether proposed HET solutions to social and individual problems really do have added value when compared with non-technological or other technological solutions. Moreover, the precautionary principle would have to be applied as systematically and comprehensively as possible, since – from this viewpoint – individual enhancements should never be allowed to threaten the social fabric and fundamental cultural values. The social prejudices and the ideologies underlying the recent trend towards human enhancement would have to be subjected to further scrutiny and critical examination, with particular attention given to the ideology of extreme progress and its roots in European history. Some kinds of research into HET, such as research for military purposes, might be banned altogether.

Finally, in a *systematic case-by-case approach*, action would always be taken whenever an intervention with non-therapeutic enhancement potential is proposed. Any decision on whether to allow such an intervention or to fund relevant research and development would be based on a process involving consultation of all groups directly affected by such interventions as well as on expertise from all relevant fields and disciplines (selected to reflect the cultural diversity of Europe). This approach does not demand a single large regulatory system: instead, specific regulations tailored to fit within an overall framework would be drawn up as new technologies appeared on the scene. This overall framework would also include some fundamental norms, while allowing existing human enhancement trends to be systematically taken into account and deliberated on in due course, with input from those most closely affected.

Our proposal

Potential human enhancement technologies need to be evaluated on the basis of *shared* European values and beliefs. Accordingly, the normative framework should be based on fundamental and uncontroversial values such as autonomy, fairness, and the right to physical integrity. Moreover, any approach will need some kind of participation by European citizens.[2]

Staman *et al.* (2008, p.153ff.) emphasized that it is doubtful whether the two main levels of public and private decision making, namely the state and the individual, suffice to collectively deal with emerging HET. However, on their view, the emergence and foreseeable future development of such technologies pose questions that demand a wider, collective approach. They argue that such an approach must take into account the "terrifying examples" of state-driven collective endeavors like the old eugenics programs and the fact that, "despite apparent individualism and its inherent freedom of choice," many people tend to make the same technological and lifestyle choices. Accordingly, neither an individualistic ethics nor a state-driven top-down approach will be appropriate when it comes to the social shaping of emerging potential HET. What is needed are new venues for public deliberation and new forums for societal deliberations on scientific, medical and cultural norms, identities and practices.

Bearing these considerations in mind, the essence of our proposal is to set up a temporary European body to develop a normative framework for human enhancement in order to guide EU policy-making in this field. We believe there are two institutional options for such a body: the European Parliament could decide to set up a temporary committee; or the Commission could decide to put together a working group also comprising members of parliament. The remit of such a body would be to further explore the topic and pave the way for possible further regulation of HET.

The temporary body would help to

- organize a comprehensive impact assessment of HET;
- identify further research needs;
- define the limits within which each country can regulate HET;
- prevent undesirable effects and serious inner-European inequalities; and, finally,
- prepare the ground for a funding policy on HET and a broader societal dialogue about the topic as a whole.

To achieve these objectives, the body's work must not be overloaded by the highly visionary or ideological aspirations currently triggered by the term "enhancement." It should, however, monitor relevant activities, in Europe or elsewhere, in which more radical visions of enhancement are promoted.

The mandate of the body could be supported by a range of specific activities (for a full list, see Coenen *et al.*, 2009, section 4.3), such as a thorough analysis of risks to individuals (e.g. addiction and the adverse health effects of surgical interventions) and the use of state-of-the-art public participation tools and surveys to learn more about European public opinion on the various facets of the issue. As regards the composition of the proposed body, it is important for it to reflect European cultural diversity and the interdisciplinary character of the issue. This body would thus not only function as an intermediary between science and technology and EU policy, but would also be a forum for broad, normative discussion of the technologies in question and the related public issues.

Some recent developments after the STOA study

Whatever the prospects may be of these matters becoming institutionalized within the European Parliament and within a broader European dialogue, the topic of enhancement is obviously here to stay – as is also shown by some recent EU activities in this context.

Answering a written question about human enhancement by Bart Staes (Member of the European Parliament), EU Health Commissioner Androulla Vassiliou stated that adjustments to existing European policies or legislation will depend on the specific issues concerned (European Parliament, 2009). In addition, the Commissioner recalled that the Member States are responsible for the regulation and delivery of health services in their countries, which includes taking measures against the illicit trading of cognitive enhancers. The final question put by Staes, namely what the Commission is doing to inform the general public about human enhancement, was not answered at all. In August 2009, a new STOA project entitled "Making *Perfect* Life" started. Conducted by ETAG and managed by the Rathenau Instituut, it analyzes tendencies in converging fields of research and development, including HET, which may lead to more and more aspects of life being fundamentally altered. The project will focus on four such developments and their ethical, legal, and social implications. The provisional edition of the European Parliament Resolution of April 24 2009 on Regulatory Aspects of Nanomaterials states that stringent ethical guidelines need to be developed in good time, particularly for nanomedicine, and must include limits imposed on non-therapeutic human enhancement. The parliament also asked the EGE to draw up another opinion on these ethical aspects of nanotechnology.

These and other examples show that existing ethical advisory institutions and publicly funded research projects are increasingly addressing the issue of human enhancement. There is a tendency towards further politicization of the topic of human enhancement.

Conclusion

Human enhancement technologies and the public's interest in them may have both beneficial and adverse effects on several policy domains at EU level. Differences between EU Member States and the lack of a coherent normative framework for dealing with enhancement issues will likely lead to significant tensions in the future. These issues not only require public debate and the articulation of normative positions, but also some policy measures and a strategic and comprehensive approach in Europe. Current activities do not yet meet these requirements.

The EU should therefore seek new ways to address the complex and cross-border challenges triggered by the trend towards an enhancement society. This needs to be done on the basis of conceptual clarity and a nuanced and balanced account of the politics of human enhancement. A temporary European body could help to develop a normative framework for dealing with human enhancement issues and promote a broad public deliberation on them.

Notes

1. This chapter is based on our STOA report *Human Enhancement* (Coenen *et al.*, 2009), which was co-authored by Leonhard Hennen, Michael Rader, Gregor Wolbring, and Pim Klaassen. We could not have written the chapter without the invaluable contributions to this project of our co-authors and of our colleagues Rinie van Est, Huub Dijstelbloem, and Frans Brom.
2. One problem in this context is the fact that only few survey results are available which reveal anything about the views of the public on human enhancement, prenatal genetic engineering being a major exception.

References

Coenen, C. (2009). Deliberating visions: The case of human enhancement in the discourse on nanotechnology and convergence. In M. Kaiser, M. Kurath, S. Maasen & C. Rehmann-Sutter (eds.), *Governing Future Technologies* (Sociology of the Sciences Yearbook, Vol. 27) (pp. 73–87). Dordrecht: Springer.

Coenen, C., Schuijff, M., Smits, M., Klaassen, P., Hennen, L., Rader, M. & Wolbring, G. (2009). Human enhancement, Brussels (European Parliament; IPOL/A/STOA/2007-13; PE 417.483); www.europarl.europa.eu/stoa/publications/studies/stoa2007-13_en.pdf.

Conrad, P. (2007). *The Medicalization of Society: On the Transformation of Human Conditions into Treatable Disorders.* Baltimore: The Johns Hopkins University Press.

CSPO, ACG, (Consortium for Science, Policy & Outcomes at Arizona State University, Advanced Concepts Group, Sandia National Laboratories) (2006). Policy Implications of Technologies for Cognitive Enhancement, www.cspo.org/documents/FinalEnhanced-CognitionReport.pdf.

EGE (European Group on Ethics in Science and New Technologies), (2005). Ethical aspects of ICT implants in the human body. Opinion No. 20. Brussels.

EU, HLEG, FNTW, (EU, High Level Expert Group "Foresighting the New Technology Wave") (2004), Converging Technologies (Rapporteur: Nordmann, A.). Brussels, http://ec.europa.eu/research/conferences/2004/ntw/pdf/final_report_en.pdf

European Commission (2008). Commission Recommendation of 07/02/2008 on a code of conduct for responsible nanosciences and nanotechnologies research, C(2008) 424 final. Brussels.

European Parliament (2009). Answer given by Ms. Vassiliou on behalf of the Commission (Parliamentary Question E-2200/2009, May 15, 2009).

Greely, H., Sahakian, B., Harris, J., Kessler, R.C., Gazzaniga, M., Campbell, P. & Farah, M.J. (2008). Towards responsible use of cognitive enhancing drugs by the healthy. *Nature*, **456**, 702–5.

Grunwald, A. (2008). *Auf dem Weg in eine nanotechnologische Zukunft.* Philosophisch-ethische, Fragen. Freiburg, München: Verlag Karl Alber.

Hughes, J. (2008). Back to the future. Contemporary biopolitics in 1920s' British futurism. *EMBO Reports* **9** (special issue), 59–63.

Khushf, G. (2005). The use of emergent technologies for enhancing human performance: Are we prepared to address the ethical and political issues? *Public Policy & Practice (E-Journal)*, **4/2**, www.ipspr.sc.edu/ejournal/Archives0805.asp.

Kurzweil, R. (2005). *The Singularity is Near. When Humans Transcend Biology.* New York: Viking.

Lin, P. & Allhoff, F. (2008). Untangling the debate: The ethics of human enhancement. *Nanoethics*, **2**(3), 251–64.

Nordmann, A. (2007). If and then: A critique of speculative nanoethics. *Nanoethics*, **1**(1), 31–46.

Parens, E. (1998). Special Supplement: "Is better always good? The Enhancement Project." *The Hastings Center Report*, **28**(1), 1–17.

Roco, M. & Bainbridge, W. (eds.) (2002). Converging Technologies for Improving Human Performance, http://wtec.org/CT/Report/NBIC_report.pdf.

Staman, J., Dijstelbloem, H. & Smits, M. (2008). Afterword. In L. Zonneveld, H. Dijstelbloem & D. Ringoir (eds.), *Reshaping the Human Condition: Exploring Human Enhancement.* Amsterdam: Elsevier.

Van Est, R. Klaasen, P., Schuijff, M. & Smits, M. (2008). *Future Man – No Future Man. Connecting the Technological, Cultural and Political Dots of Human Enhancement.* Den Haag: Rathenau Instituut.

Wiesing, U. (2008). The history of medical enhancement: From restitutio ad integrum to transformatio ad optimum? In B. Gordijn & R. Chadwick (eds.), *Medical Enhancement and Posthumanity* (pp. 9–24). The International Library of Ethics, Law, and Technology, Vol. **2** (pp. 9–24). Dordrecht: Springer.

Wolbring, G. (2008). Why NBIC? Why human performance enhancement? *Innovation. European Journal of Social Science Research*, **21**(1), 25–40.

Index

Locators to figures/tables are denoted in *italics*

Enhancing Human Capacities, edited by Julian Savulescu, Ruud ter Meulen and Guy Kahane.
© 2011 Blackwell Publishing Ltd

540 *Index*